69 —
39. —
¢

Neurobiological Approaches
to Human Disease

Neuronal Control of Bodily Function: Basic and Clinical Aspects

Volume 2

Neurobiological Approaches to Human Disease

Edited by

Dirk Hellhammer
University of Trier
Irmela Florin
University of Marburg
Herbert Weiner
University of California, Los Angeles

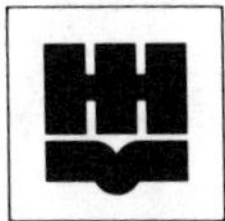

Hans Huber Publishers
Toronto · Lewiston, NY · Bern · Stuttgart

Library of Congress Cataloging-in-Publication Data

Neurobiological approaches to human disease

(Neuronal control of bodily function)
The proceedings of a symposium held in Bielefeld, FRG in Oct. 1985.
Includes bibliographies and index.

1. Medicine, Psychosomatic – Congresses. 2. Psychobiology – Congresses. 3. Neurotransmitters – Physiological effect – Congresses. 4. Central nervous system – Congresses. I. Hellhammer, Dirk. II. Florin, Irmela. III. Weiner, Herbert. IV. Series. [DNLM: 1. Central Nervous System – physiology – congresses. 2. Disease – psychology – congresses. 3. Peripheral Nerves – physiology – congresses. 4. Psychophysiology – congresses. 5. Psychosomatic Medicine – congresses. WL 103 N4932 1985]

RC49.N47 1987 616'.08 87-16813
ISBN 0-920887-27-9

Canadian Cataloguing in Publication Data

Main entry under title:

Neurobiological approaches to human disease

(Neuronal control of bodily function. Basic and clinical aspects)
Proceedings of a symposium held in Bielefeld, Federal Republic of Germany, in October 1985.

Bibliography: p.
Includes index.
ISBN 0-920887-27-9

1. Nervous system – Congresses. 2. Neurobiology – Congresses. 3. Psychobiology – Congresses. I. Hellhammer, Dirk, 1947– . II. Florin, Irmela, 1938– . III. Weiner, Herbert, 1921– . IV. Series.

RC327.N48 1987 616.8 C87-094331-6

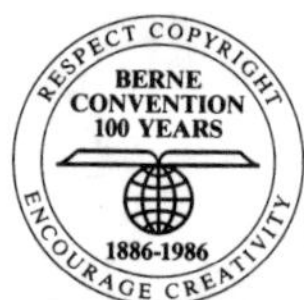

14 Bruce Park Ave.
Toronto, Ontario M4P 2S3

P. O. Box 51
Lewiston, NY 14092

Printed in Germany

ISBN 0-920887-27-9
Hans Huber Publishers · Toronto · Lewiston, NY · Bern · Stuttgart

ISBN 3-456-81638-3
Hans Huber Publishers · Bern · Stuttgart · Toronto · Lewiston, NY

Acknowledgement

The editors gratefully acknowledge the support and encouragement of the Volkswagen Foundation (Hannover), the Center for Interdisciplinary Research (Bielefeld), the Dresdner Bank AG (Frankfurt), the Janssen GmbH (Düsseldorf), Wyeth Pharma GmbH (Münster), and Philipps University (Marburg), without which this conference and proceedings would not have been possible.

Contents

Introduction

1. Brain Systems as Mediators Between Behavior and Bodily Disease

2. Central Control of the Gastrointestinal System

3. Central Control of the Cardiovascular System

4. Recent Approaches in Psychobiological Research

5. Central Control of the Pituitary-Adrenal Axis I

6. Central Control of the Pituitary-Adrenal Axis II

7. Brief Communications

Introduction

Hugh C. Hendrie

"This (nervous) system is the least understood of any in the body. Indeed if we understood it perfectly, we should know the nature of the union between soul and body."
(William Hunter, circa 1770)[1]

The need for a comprehensive biopsychosocial approach to health and illness has long been recognized. A vast body of data exists correlating psychological and social events with alterations in physical function. However, in order to construct scientifically valid hypotheses to incorporate all these data into models for disease pathogeneses, it is necessary to provide a plausible biological system which could connect psychosocial factors and physiological systems. The vast accumulation of knowledge of the central nervous system and of its widespread connections make the brain the current focus of interest in most psychosomatic speculations.

In Indianapolis, in October of 1984, a symposium was held, the first of an intended annual series, where invited guests, both basic scientists and clinical researchers, gathered together for three days of intensive meetings. The[a] shared their knowledge and perspectives regarding the function of the nervous system (central and peripheral) and the way in which it controls, and is in turn controlled by the internal milieu of the body, and speculated on how perturbations in these interacting systems could produce illness. It was, to the knowledge of the organizers, the first major occasion when neurobiologists, neuropharmacologists, neurochemists, immunologists, internists, cardiologists, neurologists, psychiatrists, psychologists and others could meet in this way to exchange views and to discuss possible research strategies.

The program of the first symposium was constructed to present a broad overview of our current understanding of body-brain interactions. It included information on central neurotransmitter systems, including the monoaminergic system, the putative amino acid neurotransmitters and neuropeptides. The autonomic system, endocrine system and the immune system were discussed in subsequent sessions focussing on their interactions with the brain. Finally an attempt was made to integrate the new knowledge of brain mechanisms in order to construct models of disease. A book based on this symposium was published and constitutes the first volume in the current series.

1. Lectures Anatomical and Chirurgical Vol. 1. Glasgow University Library. Hunterian Museum, Special Collection.

It was the intention of the organizers that the contents of the first program would provide the framework for future meetings alternating in Europe and North America, each of which would discuss in more depth one aspect of the general topic, neuronal control of bodily function. In the present volume, based on the second symposium held in Bielefeld, Federal Republic of Germany, Drs. Florin and Hellhammer have chosen to focus on psychological and biological approaches to the understanding of human disease. Future symposia already planned include the titles "Neurobiology of Amino Acids, Peptides and Trophic Factors" and "The Consequences of the Aging Process" amongst others.

As a member of the original planning committee it is exciting to see the series develop and the list of participants grow. Neuronal control of bodily function represents one of the most exciting frontier areas in the medical sciences. The development of research in this area requires the interaction and exchange of knowledge between basic scientists and clinicians from many disciplines. We hope that the planned symposia and the subsequent publications provide a vehicle for this informational exchange.

1.

Brain Systems as Mediators Between Behavior and Bodily Disease

Brain Monoamine Systems and Personality

Marvin Zuckerman

The idea that basic human temperaments are based on "humors" of the body is not new, originating in the fifth century B.C. Hippocrates and other Greek physicians felt there was a link between the sanguine disposition and blood, the phlegmatic and phlegm, the choleric and yellow bile, and the melancholic and black bile. A normal person had an optimal balance of all of the humors, but an imbalance with excess or deficit of one of them led to a personality disorder related to that humor. Today, psychologists can recognize and even measure the personality dispositions described by Hippocrates, although they now conceive of them as continuous trait dimensions rather than pure types. The "humors" are neurotransmitters, enzymes and hormones, and our reductionist goals are much more empirical, even if equally fantastic and impossible. How could the complex behavior patterns which define personality traits be related to the equally complex biochemical systems? Even if these parameters are related, how can one measure or assess either the mysterious hypothetical construct of "personality" or the more tangible biochemistry of the brain in living humans in any meaningful fashion?

There is a particular personality trait that my research has become identified with over the years. Some years ago I was involved in experimental research on the phenomenon of "sensory deprivation." Noticing that there was a wide range of individual variation in response to confinement in a stimulus-invariant environment, an attempt was made to predict the individual susceptibilities to the stress of uncertainty or boredom. Since the personality psychologist cannot follow persons around, observing and rating their everyday behaviors, they usually end up devising a questionnaire in which they are asked to describe their usual behaviors, moods, and attitudes. Such scales are not like those you see in popular magazines since each is subject to scientific standards of reliability and validity before being accepted as valid measures.

A test was developed called a "Sensation Seeking Scale" (1) which consisted of items asking whether one does or would like to engage in certain kinds of sometimes risky activities which provide novel or intense sensations and experiences. It was hypothesized that there was such a broad trait that would predict preferences and behavior in natural settings and in experiments. The finding of a general factor was encouraging. Hundreds of studies have been done relating the questionnaire-measured trait to behaviors like reactions to sensory deprivation or confinement, volunteering for unusual activities, engaging in risky sports, choice of vocation, preferences in art, music, and films, sensory and cognitive styles, sexual experience, use of drugs and alcohol, and many other phenomena (2, 3, 4). Such studies have confirmed the basic validity of the scale. Since research has demonstrated the reliability and concurrent and predictive validity of the instrument, the scale could then be used to explore the sources of the trait in biological or social variables. The research has thus far focused largely on biological correlates of sensation seeking (5), although the model (2, 4) is certainly a psychobiological or a biosocial one. It has generated interest in biological bases of other personality traits like extraversion, impulsivity, and anxiety (6), with the ultimate goal of developing a more comprehensive psychobiological model of personality.

There are four subscales contained in our more recent versions of the Sensation Seeking Scale (SSS). The four basic scales were developed from factor analyses (7, 8) of items beyond the factor analysis (1) that established the *General* scale. The factor structure has been generally replicated in studies done in America, England, Australia, Israel and other countries. In form V of the SSS, a *Total* score is used which is the sum of scores on the four subscales. The subscales may be described as follows:

Thrill and Adventure Seeking (TAS):
The desire to engage in sports which provide unusual sensations produced by speed or the defiance of gravity, and the willingness to take physical risks.

Experience Seeking (ES):
The desire to try new ways of stimulating the mind and senses through travel, music, art, drugs, living in an unconventional style, and associating with unusual people.

Disinhibition (DIS):
The desire to seek excitement through other persons, parties, and a hedonistic, disinhibited life style.

Boredom Susceptibility (BS):
A tendency to become easily bored and restless when things, situations or persons are constant or unvarying.

Biochemical Correlates of Sensation Seeking

The research for biological bases of the sensation seeking trait was first based on a theory that the trait-reflected individual differences in optimal levels of stimulation and cortical arousal and arousability. This led to psychophysiological studies of cortical (EEG) evoked potentials, electrodermal, and cardiovascular responses to simple stimuli varying only on the dimensions of intensity and novelty (5). These studies are not described here; instead this paper will concentrate on the biochemistry of sensation-seeking and related traits.

Gonadal Hormones

The fact that sensation seeking was higher in males than in females in many different countries, and showed a peak in the late teens and a decline thereafter, suggested that the trait might have something to do with testosterone which shows similar sex and age differences. Studies by Daitzman et al. (9) and Daitzman and Zuckerman (10) did show positive relationships between one type of sensation seeking, *Disinhibition* (DIS), and androgens in males, but these data also showed relationships with estrogens as well. Both forms of gonadal hormones were positively related to *Disinhibition*, and heterosexual experience, and negatively related to socialization (conformity) and self-control (10). Testosterone alone correlated positively with extraverted traits like sociability, social presence, dominance, activity, and self acceptance, and negatively with neurotic traits like depression and psychasthenia scales on the Minnesota Multiphasic Personality Inventory (MMPI). Estradiol in males correlated with permissive attitudes toward sex, homosexual experience, psychological feminity and psychopathological scales on the MMPI, including *Psychopathic Deviation, Schizophrenia, Hypomania*, and *F* (general response deviancy) scales.

Broverman et al. (11) suggest that gonadal hormones activate the central nervous system through depression of monoamine oxidase (MAO), an enzyme that regulates the monoamine system in the brain.

Monoamine Oxidase (MAO)

Six studies involving nine groups of male, female, or mixed subjects, have reported correlations between the General or Total SS scales, contained in forms IV and V respectively, and platelet MAO.

Table 1: Correlations: Platelet MAO vs. Sensation-Seeking Scales.

Authors	Subjects	n	r Total Gen. scales[1]	Significantly correlated subscales[2]
Murphy	F students	65	0.17	none
et al. (15)	M students	30	-0.45**	DIS
Schooler	F students	47	-0.43**	TAS,ES
et al. (16)	M students	46	-0.52**	TAS,ES,BS
Ballenger et al. (17)	M & F adult	36	-0.17	none (TAS -0.30)
Schalling et al. (12)	M students	40	-0.25	DIS (-0.26)*
Von Knorring et al. (13)	M soldiers	1129	-0.06*	BS
Arqué	M & F adult	13	-0.66**	TAS, ES, DIS
et al. (14)	M & F pts.	44	-0.25*	ES, DIS

1. Gen. = General Scale from form IV, Total = sum of 4 subscales, form V
2. TAS = Thrill and Adventure Seeking, ES = Experience Seeking, DIS = Disinhibition, BS = Boredom Susceptibility; see above for specific descriptions of subscales.

* $p<0.05$, ** $p<0.01$

In all but one of these studies, the correlation was negative, and in 6 of the 9 samples the correlation was significant. There is a large range in the values of the correlations, and the median correlation is only -0.25.

However, there is no question that there is a relationship between the sensation-seeking trait and the biological marker MAO in platelets. The first three studies in Table 1 were done at the National Institute of Mental Health in the USA, whereas the studies by Schalling et al. (12) and von Knorring et al.

(13) were done in Sweden; the study by Arqué et al. (14) was completed in Spain, all using translated SS scales. In Sweden the researchers also developed their own form of a sensation seeking scale which was called *Monotony Avoidance* (MoAv). The data in Table 2 show the platelet MAO-MoAv correlations in 3 normal and 3 patient samples. All of the correlations are negative, and 3 of the 6 are significant. The median correlation is -0.22, close to the median value of -0.25 obtained with the sensation seeking scales (Table 1).

Although the MAO Sensation-Seeking relationship cannot be attributed to chance, it is clearly not a strong one. But why would one expect it to be higher? Although MAO activity is highly correlated between different parts of human brain (21), one does not know if platelet MAO is a good index of brain MAO. Since the influence of MAO in personality must be a function of brain MAO rather than MAO in the peripheral blood, the correlation with platelet MAO must be an attenuated one. Secondly, the personality trait is likely to be related to characteristics of the monoamine systems themselves as well as to other neurotransmitter systems and enzymes. The interactions between and within systems suggest that MAO is just one piece in a very complex puzzle. What the low but significant MAO-SSS correlation does is point to the involvement of the monoamine systems in the personality trait.

Table 2. Correlations: Platelet MAO vs. monotony avoidance[1].

Authors	Subjects	n	r
Schalling et al. (12)	M students	40	-0.30*
	M adults	58	-0.16
Fowler et al. (18)	M & F adults	59	-0.17
Perris et al. (19)	M & F dep. pts.	24	-0.55**
Perris et al. (20)	M & F dep. pts.	143	-0.18**
	M dep. pts.	60	-0.05
	F dep. pts.	83	-0.26**

1. A sensation-seeking-type scale developed by Schalling et al. (12)
* $p<0.05$, ** $p<0.01$

Before leaving the topic of MAO, it should be pointed out that the platelet measure shows relationships with behavior and demographic characteristics that are consistent with its relationships with the personality measure (5). Low platelet MAO levels are found in males as opposed to females, and in younger persons as opposed to elder ones. Low MAO levels are found in neonates who are more active in the first 72 hours of life (22). The relationship with the personality trait of sociability is confirmed in two species: Humans with low platelet MAO report more time spent in social activities than those with high MAO levels (23); low MAO monkeys are observed to spend more time in social and play activity than highs (24). Low MAO human males smoke more, use more drugs, and alcohol (13, 24, 25) and are more likley to get in trouble with the law (23). All of these habits and vulnerabilities are characteristics of high sensation seekers as well. Sensation seekers as are attracted to risky sports such as mountain climbing, hang-gliding, parachuting, etc. (26). Fowler et al. (18) found that mountain climbers, or those just interested in the sport, have low platelet MAO levels relative to those who are not interested. In the realm of psychopathology, both high sensation seeking scores and low MAO levels in platelets have been found in manic-depressives, even when they are not in the manic state (27).

Monoamines, Their Metabolites, and Enzymes

The enzyme dopamine-ß-hydroxylase (DBH) in noradrenergic neurons in the brain converts dopamine to noradrenaline (NA) and therefore is important in keeping NA from being depleted by activity of the system. Three studies (17, 28, 29) have reported negative correlations between serum of plasma DBH and sensation seeking; however, one study (15) failed to find a significant relationship. If DBH in blood is a reliable index of DBH in brain neurons, then low levels of DBH could be related to low levels of NA in the brains of high sensation seekers. Ballenger et al. (17) did find that NA in cerebrospinal fluid (CSF) was significantly and negatively correlated with sensation seeking in normal males and females. The direction of this relationship was a surprise, since the earlier model (2) had predicted that high sensation seekers would have high levels of catecholamines (NA and dopamine) in brain. In CSF, dopamine and serotonin metabolites, HVA and 5-HIAA respectively, did not correlate with sensation seeking in this study.

Schalling et al. (30) reported the results of studies of CSF metabolites of the monoamines in normal and patient groups, using the KSP scale to assess personality traits. One of the most consistent findings in this study were negative correlations between CSF 5-HIAA and Eysenck and Eysenck's (31) P scale in normal and patient samples. While this scale is labelled *Psychoticism*, it actually seems to measure a broad factor consisting of socialization, aggression, impulsivity and sensation seeking (32). A better diagnostic label for the scale would be *Psychopathy*, the term used to describe the sociopathic and antisocial personality. The low levels of 5-HIAA in high *P* scores are consistent with the clinical data showing low levels of 5-HIAA in brain or CSF of persons attempting or committing violent suicide or homicide (33). *KSP Impulsivity* and *Monotony Avoidance* scales are also correlated negatively with CSF 5-HIAA in most of the patient groups, but the correlations with these traits in the normal group were not significant.

The dopamine and noradrenaline metabolites, HVA and MHPG, produced few consistent correlations with personality measures. HVA, like 5-HIAA, correlated negatively with the *P* scale and tended to correlate negatively with the *Monotony Avoidance* scale in normals. The parallel results of HVA and 5-HIAA are not suprising since these two measures derived from CSF correlated high and positively, as they also did in the Ballenger et al. study (17). There is no reported association between dopamine and serotonin in the brain and their behavioral effects tend to be antagonistic, so the high positive correlation in their CSF metabolites raises questions about the adequacy of the CSF measures as indices of brain activity.

Other Biochemical Systems

Sensation seeking was found to be negatively correlated with endorphin levels in the CSF in a group of chronic pain patients (34), but this finding was not replicated in normals (17). Arqué et al. (14) found negative correlations between thyroid stimulating hormone (TSH) and sensation seeking, and between peripheral acetylcholinesterase (AChE) and sensation seeking in both normal and patient groups. AChE is a catabolic enzyme which destroys ACh by its action usually at the postsynaptic membrane. These recent findings underscore the growing conviction that one must look beyond the monoamine systems for a full understanding of the biological substrate of sensation seeking and related traits.

Comparative Theories and Research on the Monoamine Systems

So far, this work has only dealt with correlational studies of humans. Ethical limitations prevent investigators from doing drastic experiments that might alter the biochemistry of the brain in healthy, living humans. Patients are given psychotropic drugs to alleviate their disorders, and much of our knowledge comes from these "natural" manipulations. Since the pre-illness biological or behavioral baselines are not generally known, the changes observed during drug treatment are problematical. For these reasons, many investigators have turned to comparative studies of other species where the brain can be directly manipulated and specific systems can be lesioned or stimulated in order to understand their behavioral functions. This literature has been reviewed in an attempt to understand the significance of the correlational data relating sensation seeking to the monoamine systems (4, 35).

Serotonin

Low levels of the peripheral serotonin metabolite in humans are related to unsocialized and impulsive behaviors and traits. Experiments with rats have led to theories that serotonin serves to inhibit behavior in conflict situations (36). Panksepp (37) has emphasized the inhibition of all emotional systems. Crow (38), Gray (39) and Stein (40) have all implicated serotonergic systems in trait or state anxiety. Gray has suggested that serotonin mediates a "Behavioral Inhibition System" triggered by either novel stimuli or stimuli associated with punishment. While acknowledging the behavioral inhibitory effects of serotonin, Soubrié says that the animals with lesions of the serotonin systems are impulsive in spite of anxiety rather than because of its absence. Panksepp sees lowered serotonin levels as disinhibiting fear and other emotional reactions rather than eliminating them. The depletion of serotonin in forebrain and brain stem also produces an animal that is aroused, active, aggressive, and sexually responsive in a familiar colony environment (41). These descriptions are compatible with the idea that serotonin may be low in some high sensation seekers. However, the fact that the same animals may behave in a fearful fashion in an unfamiliar, non-social environment suggests that low serotonin levels may be more characteristic of the DIS rather than the TAS type of sensation seeking.

Dopamine

The dopaminergic system has been suggested as one that energizes or activates behavior directed toward primary biological rewards (37, 38, 40, 42). The Crow and Stein theories had been largely based on the studies of intracranial self-stimulation (ICSS) in rats. Such stimulation seems to be effective in primary reward centers in the brain. While earlier studies seemed to identify these reward systems with both catecholamines (dopamine and NA), recent summaries (42, 43) rather convincingly suggest that only dopamine is involved in the intrinsic reward systems. The drugs, like amphetamine and cocaine, that promote dopamine release are sought after by high sensation seekers. Rats and primates can also be addicted to these drugs and learn to self-administer them. As Stellar and Stellar comment: "It is difficult to imagine why these organisms would perform these behaviors unless the action of dopamine in the brain were rewarding" (p. 158). In addition to mediation of primary reward or "pleasure," dopamine seems to be necessary for motivation or the initiation of activity leading to primary rewards. The motor system needs little dopamine for actual execution of actions but requires it to stimulate the initiation of action. Animals or humans (e.g., Parkinson's disease patients) who are dopamine depleted have difficulty in executing voluntary movements, tend to be inactive and unreactive to their environments. However, when influenced by strong stimuli or situations, they are capable of vigorous movements.

All of these findings from animal models suggest that dopamine activity should be high in sensation seekers. However, the recent Zuckerman (4) model, which does not distinguish between effects of dopamine and NA, suggests that low levels of tonic catecholamine activity with high levels of reactivity to novel stimuli might provide the basis for the need to seek stimuli or use drugs that increase catecholamine system activity to an optimal level. The present methods of assessing central dopaminergic activity in living humans (e.g., CSF HVA) do not seem adequate for the testing of this theory.

Noradrenaline

The behavioral significance of the noradrenergic system, particularly the dorsal ascending noradrenergic bundle that originates in the locus coeruleus has been the source of considerable speculation and controversy. Both Gray (39, 44) and Redmond (45, 46) suggest that this system is an alarm mechanism that is triggered specifically by stimuli identified as noxious, threatening or merely novel. The central arousal stimulated by activity in the system is the basis of the emotion of fear or anxiety, according to these models. It is interesting that Gray includes reactions to novel stimuli as unconditioned stimuli for anxiety. For a rat, or a very low human sensation seeker, novelty may be intrinsically linked to anxiety. However, for high sensation seekers or even average ones, novelty dissociated from threat is positive or neutral rather than anxiety provoking. Novelty commands attention, regardless of its emotional valence, and that is what accounts for its link to a behavioral inhibition mechanism. You have to stop in order to look and listen. In contrast to the anxiety theories of NA function, Crow (38) and Stein (40) claimed that NA mediates reward. This claim rested largely on the ICSS studies and, as noted in the previous section, the consensus of recent investigators is that dopamine, not NA, is involved in the reward of ICSS behavior. Panksepp (37) maintained that NA mediates a general arousal function for all emotional systems, including those related to appetite and sex, as well as fear and rage ones. Experimental evidence, based on recording electrodes planted in the locus coeruleus (47), has shown that activity in these largely noradrenergic neurons reflect the tonic level of general arousal (sleep to waking and alertness), and phasic reactions to novel stimuli, whether noxious or non-noxious. Mason and Fibiger (48) suggest that the system not only sensitizes the reactions to novel stimuli, but facilitates subsequent approach to such stimuli. Zuckerman (4) has proposed that at optimal levels of activity of NA or dopamine, social behavior, activity, and positive emotions are common, while dysphoric reactions (fear, anger, depression), social withdrawal or aggressiveness, are characteristic of extreme low *or* high levels of NA or dopamine activity. Studies of human drug abusers, and rats subjected to increasing dosages of stimulant drugs, suggest that curvilinear relations between catecholaminergic activity and behavioral and emotional reactions are possible.

Future Research

The major limitations of the current research relating personality dispositions to the biochemistry of the brain cannot be overstressed. Uncertain relationships between peripherally obtained measures and the activity of neurotransmitters and enzymes in the brain are a major barrier to an understanding of how the brain neurons affect behavior. The correlational nature of most of the research is another problem, since one cannot disentangle cause and effect. As one example of this, it is not certain as to whether the levels of neurotransmitters, metabolites, and enzymes in the CSF are correlated with personality traits because they affect behavioral reactions, or because people differ in their reactivity to a lumbar puncture. Although experimental methods would be difficult to apply to measures relying in CSF samples, there are some new methodologies that offer the possibility of directly imaging and recording activity in specific neurotransmitter systems, i.e., Position Emission Tomography (PET), and the neurochemically selective techniques being developed for the major monoamine and opiate systems. Using such methods, it would be possible to observe the activity of the dopamine system at specific brain sites before and after the administration of some experimental treatment.

References

1. Zuckerman, M., Kolin, E.A., Price, L. & Zoob, I. (1964). Development of a sensation seeking scale. J. Consult. Psychol., 28: 477-482.

2. Zuckerman, M. (1979). Sensation seeking: Beyond the optimal level of arousal. Erlbaum, Hillsdale, N.J.
3. Zuckerman, M. (1983). A biological theory of sensation seeking. In M. Zuckerman (Ed.), Biological bases of sensation seeking, impulsivity and anxiety. Erlbaum, Hillsdale, N.J., p. 37-76.
4. Zuckerman, M. (1984). Sensation seeking: A comparative approach to a human trait. Behav. Brain Sci., 7: 413-471.
5. Zuckerman, M., Buchsbaum, M.S. & Murphy, D.L. (1980). Sensation seeking and its biological correlates. Psychol. Bull., 88: 187-214.
6. Zuckerman, M. (1983). Sensation seeking and sports. Pers. Individ. Differ., 4: 285-292.
7. Zuckerman, M. (1971). Dimensions of sensation seeking. J. Consult. Clin. Psychol, 36: 45-52.
8. Zuckerman, M., Eysenck, S.B.G. & Eysenck, H.J. (1978). Sensation seeking in England and America: Cross-cultural, age and sex comparisons. J. Consult. Clin. Psychol., 46: 139-149.
9. Daitzman, R.J., Zuckerman, M., Sammelwitz, P.H. & Ganjam, V. (1978). Sensation seeking and gonodal hormones. J. Biosoc. Sci., 10: 401-408.
10. Daitzman, R.J. & Zuckerman, M. (1980). Disinhibitory sensation seeking, personality, and gonadal hormones. Pers. Individ. Differ., 1: 103-110.
11. Broverman, D.M., Klaiber, E.L., Kobayashi, Y. & Vogel, W. (1968). Roles of activation and inhibition in sex differences in cognitive abilities. Psychol. Rev., 75: 23-50.
12. Schalling, D., Edman, G. & Åsberg, M. (1983). Impulsive cognitive style and inability to tolerate boredom. In M. Zuckerman (Ed.), Biological bases of sensation seeking, impulsivity, and anxiety. Erlbaum, Hillsdale, N.J., p. 125-147.
13. Von Knorring, L. & Oreland, L. (1985). Personality traits and platelet monoamine oxidase in tobacco smokers. Psychol. Med., 15: 327-334.
14. Arqué, J., Segurn, R. & Torrubia, R. (1985). Biochemical correlates of sensation seeking and susceptibility to punishment scales: A study in individuals with somatoform disorders and normals. Paper presented at the second meeting of the International Society for the Study of Individual Differences, San Feliu, Spain, June 20-24, 1985.
15. Murphy, D.L., Belmaker, R.H., Buchsbaum, M.S., Martin, N.F., Ciaranello, K. & Wyatt, R.J. (1977). Biogenic amine related enzymes and personality variations in normals. Psychol. Med., 7: 149-157.
16. Schooler, C., Zahn, T.P., Murphy, D.L. & Buchsbaum, M.S. (1978). Psychological correlates of monoamine oxidase in normals. J. Nerv. Ment. Dis., 166: 177-186.
17. Ballenger, J.C., Post, R.M., Jimerson, D.C., Lake, C.R., Murphy, D.L., Zuckerman, M. & Cronin, C. (1983). Biochemical correlates of personality traits in normals: An exploratory study. Pers. Individ. Differ., 4: 615-625.
18. Fowler, C.J., von Knorring, L. & Oreland, L. (1980). Platelet monoamine oxidase activity in sensation seekers. Psychiatry Res., 3: 273-279.
19. Perris, C., Jacobsson, L., von Knorring, L., Oreland, L., Perris, H. & Ross, S.B. (1980). Enzymes related to biogenic amine metabolism and personality characteristics in depressed patients. Acta Psychiat. Scand., 61: 477-484.
20. Perris, C., Eisemann, M., von Knorring, L. & Perris, H. (1984). Personality traits and monoamine oxidase activity in platelets in depressed patients. Neuropsychobiology, 12: 201-205.
21. Adolfsson, R., Gottfries, C.G., Oreland, L., Roos, R.E. & Winblad, B. (1978). Monoamine oxidase activity and serotonergic turnover in human brain. Prog. Neuropsychopharmacol., 2: 225-230.
22. Sostek, A.J., Sostek, A.M., Murphy, D.L., Martin, E.B. & Born, W.S. (1981). Cord blood amine oxidase activities relate to arousal and motor functioning in human newborns. Life. Sci., 28: 2561-2568.
23. Coursey, R.D., Buchsbaum, M.S. & Murphy, D.L. (1979). Platelet MAO activity and evoked potentials in the identification of subjects biologically at risk for psychiatric disorders. Br. J. Psychiat., 134: 372-381.
24. Redmond, D.E.Jr., Murphy, D.L. & Baulu, J. (1979). Platelet monoamine oxidase activity correlates with social affiliative and agonistic behaviors in normal rhesus monkeys. Psychosom. Med., 41: 87-100.
25. Von Knorring, L., Oreland, L. & Winblad, B. (1984). Personality traits related to monoamine oxidase activity in platelets. Psychiatry Res., 12: 11-26.
26. Zuckerman, M. (1983). A summing up with special sensitivity to signals of reward in future research. In M. Zuckerman (Ed), Biological bases of sensation seeking , impulsivity, and anxiety. Erlbaum, Hillsdale, N.J., p. 24.
27. Zuckerman, M. (1985). Sensation seeking, mania, and monoamines. Neuropsychobiology, 13: 121-128.

28. Kulcsár, Z., Kutor, L. & Arató, M. (1984). Sensation seeking, its biochemical correlates, and its relation to vestibulo-ocular functions. In H. Bonarius, G. van Heck & N. Smid (Eds.), Personality psychology in Europe: Theoretical and empirical developments. The Netherlands: Swets and Zeitlinger, Lisse, p. 327-346.
29. Umberkoman-Wiita, B., Vogel, W.H. & Wiita, P.J. (1981). Some biochemical and behavioral (sensation seeking) correlates in healthy adults. Res. Commun. Psychol. Psychiat. Behav., 6: 303-316.
30. Schalling, D., Åsberg, M. & Edman, G. (1984). Personality and CSF monoamine metabolites. Preliminary manuscript. Dept. of Psychiatry and Psychology, Karolinska Hospital, University of Stockholm, Sweden.
31. Eysenck, H.J. & Eysenck, S.B.G. (1975). Manual of the Eysenck Personality Questionnaire. Hodder & Stoughton, London.
32. Zuckerman, M., Kuhlman, D.M. & Camac, C. (in press). What lies beyond E and N? Factor analyses of scales believed to measure basic dimensions of personality. J. Pers. Soc. Psychol.
33. Lidberg, L., Tuck, J.R., Åsberg, M., Scalia-Tombia, G.P. & Bertilsson, L. (1985). Homicide, suicide, and CSF 5-HIAA. Acta Psychiat. Scand., 71: 230-236.
34. Johansson, F., Almay, B.G.L., von Knorring, L., Te enius, L. & Åstrom, M. (1979). Personality traits in chronic pain patients related to endorphin levels in cerebrospinal fluid. Psychiatry Res., 1: 231-239.
35. Zuckerman, M., Ballenger, J.C. & Post, R.M. (1984). The neurobiology of some dimensions of personality. In J.R. Smythies & R.J. Bradley (Eds.), International review of neurobiology, Vol. 25., Academic Press, N.Y., p. 391-436.
36. Soubrié, P. (1986). Reconciling the role of central serotonin neurons in human and animal behavior. Behav. Brain Sci., 9: 319-364.
37. Panksepp, J. (1982). Toward a general psychobiological theory of emotions. Behav. Brain Sci., 5: 407-422.
38. Crow, T.J. (1977). Neurotransmitter-related pathways: The structure and function of central monoaminergic neurons. In A.N. Davidson (Ed.), Biochemical correlates of brain structure and function. Academic Press, N.Y., p. 137-174.
39. Gray, J.A. (1982). The neuropsychology of anxiety: An enquiry into the functions of the septo-hippocampal system. Oxford University Press, N.Y.
40. Stein, L. (1978). Reward transmitters: Catecholamines and opioid peptides. In M.A. Lipton, A. di Mascio & K.F. Killam (Eds.), Psychopharmacology: A generation of progress. Raven Press, N.Y., p. 569-581.
41. Ellison, G.D. (1977). Animal models of psychopathology: The low-norepinephrine and low-serotonin rat. Am. Psychol., 32: 1036-1045.
42. Mason, S.T. (1984). Catecholamines and behavior. Cambridge University Press, N.Y.
43. Stellar, J.R. & Stellar, E. (1985). The neurobiology of motivation and reward. Springer-Verlag, N.Y.
44. Gray, J.A. (1985). Issues in the neuropsychology of anxiety. In A.H. Tuma & J.D. Maser (Eds.), Anxiety and the anxiety disorders. Erlbaum, Hillsdale, N.J., p. 5-25.
45. Redmond, D.E.Jr. (1977). Alterations in the function of the nucleus locus coeruleus: A possible model for studies of anxiety. In I. Hanin & E. Usdin (Eds.), Animal models in psychiatry and neurology. Pergamon Press, N.Y., p. 293-305.
46. Redmond, D.E.Jr. (1985). Neurochemical basis for anxiety and anxiety disorders: Evidence from drugs which decrease human fear or anxiety. In A.H. Tuma & J.D. Maser (Eds.), Anxiety and the anxiety disorders. Erlbaum, Hillsdale, N.J., p. 533-555.
47. Aston-Jones, G. & Bloom, M.E. (1981). Norepinephrine-containing locus coeruleus neurons in behaving rats exhibit pronounced responses to non-noxious environmental stimuli. J. Neurosci., 8: 887-900.
48. Mason, S.T. & Fibiger, H.C. (1979). Current concepts. I Anxiety: The locus coeruleus disconnection. Life Sci., 25: 2141-2147.

Transformation of Emotion into Motion: Role of Mesolimbic Noradrenaline and Neostriatal Dopamine

Alexander R. Cools

Whenever an organism faces a threat, various physiological, endocrinological and behavioral changes occur. It is the overall outcome of these concertedly working changes that determine the organism's response to threat. It is widely accepted to refer to these changes as phenomena inherent in emotion. Although there is little agreement about the term emotion, the following changes occur together in many instances: Changes in inner feelings (man), changes in the objective state of bodily arousal, and changes in the display of ongoing behavior. The fact that a healthy organism always acts as an integrated whole gives rise to the notion that the bodily substrates involved in each of these changes require a very close and intense "cross-talk."

Today, the vast majority of research in this field attempts to lay the foundation for understanding how physiological and endocrinological processes are mutually tuned in order to produce certain changes in the objective state of bodily arousal. The latter research mainly focuses the attention upon the cross-talk between limbic structures such as hippocampus, amygdala, septum, preoptic area, hypothalamus and the pituitary adrenal-cortical axis (Bohus, this volume).

The present-day research about the mutual tuning of processes underlying changes in inner feelings to processes underlying changes in the objective state of bodily arousal is limited. Anyhow, it is not unlikely that the cross-talk between cortical structures such as the prepiriform and entorhinal cortex and limbic structures such as the hippocampus and amygdala plays an important role.

Research that focuses the attention upon the tuning of processes underlying changes in the display of ongoing behavior to processes underlying changes in the objective state of bodily arousal is just started (1, 2). Again, it seems that the limbic-hypothalamo-pituitary-adrenal circuitry plays an essential part.

Until now, very little attention is paid to the "tuning" of processes underlying changes in the objective state of bodily arousal to processes underlying changes in the display of ongoing behavior. This is probably because the brain structures involved in the manifestation of each of these changes are regarded as independent mechanisms localized in separate parts of the brain. Thus, changes in the objective state of bodily arousal are regarded as due to alterations in the above-mentioned limbic structures including the pituitary-adrenal axis, whereas changes in the display of ongoing behavior are regarded as due to alterations in pyramidal and/or extrapyramidal structures.

Recently, however, it has been found that the nucleus accumbens forms a crucial link between limbic and extrapyramidal structures (3-11). This finding arises the question whether limbic information actually serves two purposes: (1) directing changes in the objective state of bodily arousal via the limbic-hypothalamo-pituitary-adrenal circuitry, and (2) directing changes in the display of ongoing behavior via the limbic-mesolimbic-neostriatal circuitry. This article deals with the second part of this question. The role of the nucleus accumbens in the transformation of limbic information into neostriatal information occupies a central part (Figure 1).

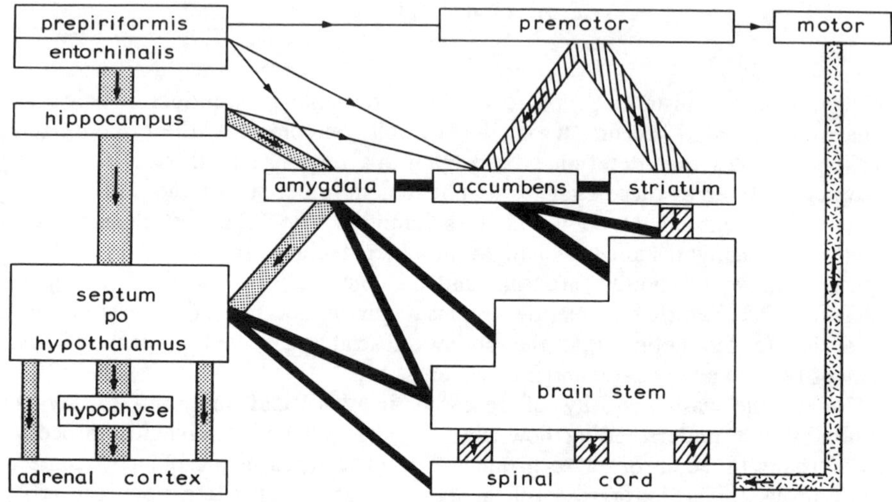

Figure 1. Schematic diagram of the main connections between the limbic-hypothalamo-pituitary-adrenal axis, i.e., the circuitry that mediates changes in the objective state of bodily arousal, and the limbic-mesolimbic-neostriatal axis, i.e., the circuitry that mediates changes in the display of emotional behavior. The nucleus accumbens occupies a central position in the transformation of limbic information into neostriatal information, i.e., the transformation of Emotion into Motion.

This article consists of three parts. The first part deals with the causal relationship between the functional activity within the nucleus accumbens of rats and the display of certain emotional behaviors in a so-called defeat-test. It is shown that the neurochemical state of the mesolimbic, noradrenergic activity directs the display of behavior in the defeat-test. The data imply that limbic information that directs changes in the display of certain emotional behavior indeed arrives at the level of the nucleus accumbens. The second part deals with the relation between the display of behavior in the defeat-test and the functional activity within the neostriatum. It is shown that the behavior in the defeat-test nicely correlates with the susceptibility of dopaminergic mechanisms within the neostriatum to the dopaminergic agonist apomorphine. The data imply that the functional activity within the nucleus accumbens controls the functional activity within the neostriatum and its output-stations. The third part deals with the impact of the above-mentioned findings for the insight into the role of the nucleus accumbens in the transformation of limbic information into neostriatal information, i.e. the transformation of Emotion into Motion.

Nucleus Accumbens and the Display of Emotional Behavior

When limbic information that directs changes in the display of emotional behavior indeed arrives at the level of the nucleus accumbens, changes in the

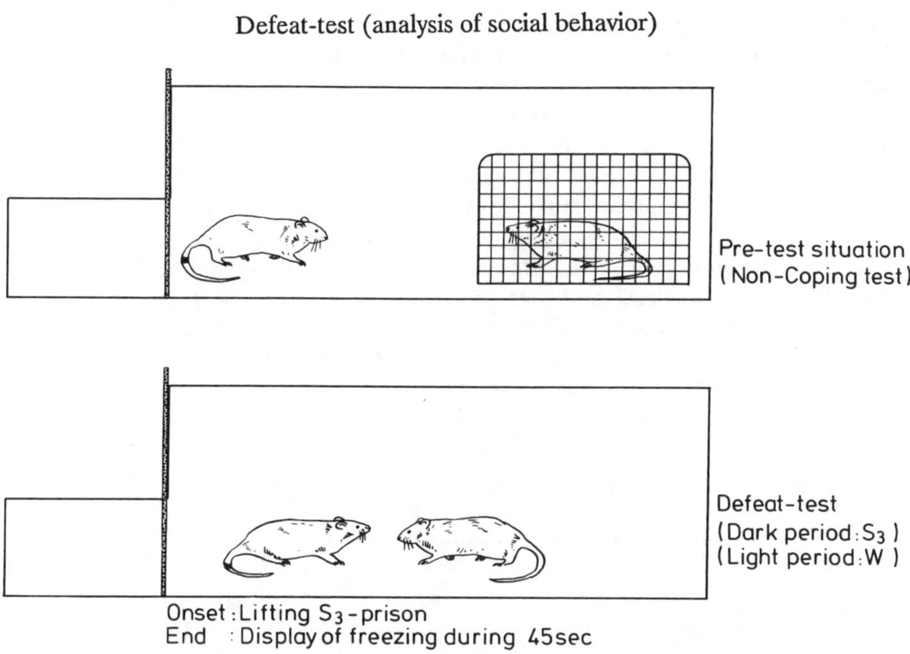

Figure 2. Defeat-test. *Pre-test situation*: The female Wistar partner of the Tryon-maze-Dull S3 male rat is removed, and the S3 rat itself is put into a small enclosure. Then, the experimental male Wistar rat (± 200 g) is gently placed into the start box (20 x 15 x 15 cm) depicted at the left side of the S3 home cage (80 x 40 x 75 cm). The Wistar rat is allowed to enter the territory of the S3 rat. As soon as the Wistar rat has entered the arena, the door of the start-box is closed. It is allowed to explore the territory for a period of 5 min. *Test-situation*: Lifting the S3-enclosure implies the onset of the defeat-test. The number of fleeing and freezing spells shown by the Wistar rat is counted. As soon as the Wistar rat freezes for a continuous period of 45 sec, the test is terminated. Note that the S3 rat is tested during the dark period of its day/night cycle in contrast to the Wistar rat, which is tested during the light period of its day/night cycle; the test itself is performed under infrared light.

functional activity of the nucleus accumbens should have direct consequences for changes in the display of emotional behavior. Below it is illustrated that this is indeed the case. When rats differ in their emotional behavior, they also differ in their functional activity within the nucleus accumbens. It is also shown that changing the functional activity of the nucleus accumbens has direct consequences for the display of emotional behavior.

Wistar rats belonging to an inbred strain show individual differences in the display of defensive behavior when confronted with a Tryon Maze Dull S3 rat on the territory of the latter (12). Since the S3 rat always becomes the winner and may ultimately kill the wistar rat, this so-called defeat-test (Figure 2) is terminated as soon as the wistar rat displays freezing for a continuous period of 45 sec. In practice, it is possible to classify individual rats according to the number of freezing spells, fleeing spells, or the ratio of both. Thus, the defeat-test allows one to classify rats according to their individual display of certain emotional behaviors (13).

Table 1. Percentage of rats showing explosive motor behavior (EMB) after intra-accumbens (ACC)-injections of l-phenylephrine (500 ng/0.5 μl per side) given 5 min prior to the subthreshold dose of intra-collicular injections of picrotoxin (<100 ng/0.5 μl per side) during two successive trials with an interval of 24 h. Two categories of rats were discerned: Rats that displayed EMB on the first test-day, i.e. responders; and rats that did not display EMB on that day, i.e. non-responders. As discussed elsewhere (15), the latter feature was intrinsic of the animal: When the test-interval was greater than 48 hours, all responders remained responders, and all non-responders remained non-responders.

		% Rats showing EMB				
ACC-treatment	(n)	Responders		(n)	Non-responders	
		day 1	day 2		day 1	day 2
Phenylephrine	(22)	100	0	(22)	0	100

In order to investigate whether individual differences in defensive behavior are anyhow related to individual differences in the functional activity within the nucleus accumbens, it is necessary to use an *in vivo* measure of the latter activity. For that purpose, the susceptibility to intra-accumbens injections of the α-noradrenergic agonist phenylephrine (PE: 500 ng/ 0.5 μl per side) was measured in rats treated with bilateral injections of a subthreshold dose of picrotoxin into the deeper layers of the superior colliculus, i.e., a dose that is 10 ng smaller than the dose required for eliciting explosive motor behavior (EMB, 14, 15): Administering 500 ng PE together with a subthreshold dose of collicular picrotoxin also results in the display of EMB under certain circumstances. This PE-test allows one to separate rats into responders and non-responders. Responders show EMB during the first trial of the PE-test, but become insensitive to this treatment during the second trial given 24 h later, whereas non-responders are insensitive to the PE-treatment during the first trial, but become susceptible to this treatment during the second trial given 24 h later (15; Table 1).

Percentage of responders (•) and non-responders (o) showing a phenylephrine-induced shift in responsivness to phenylephrine on the second day

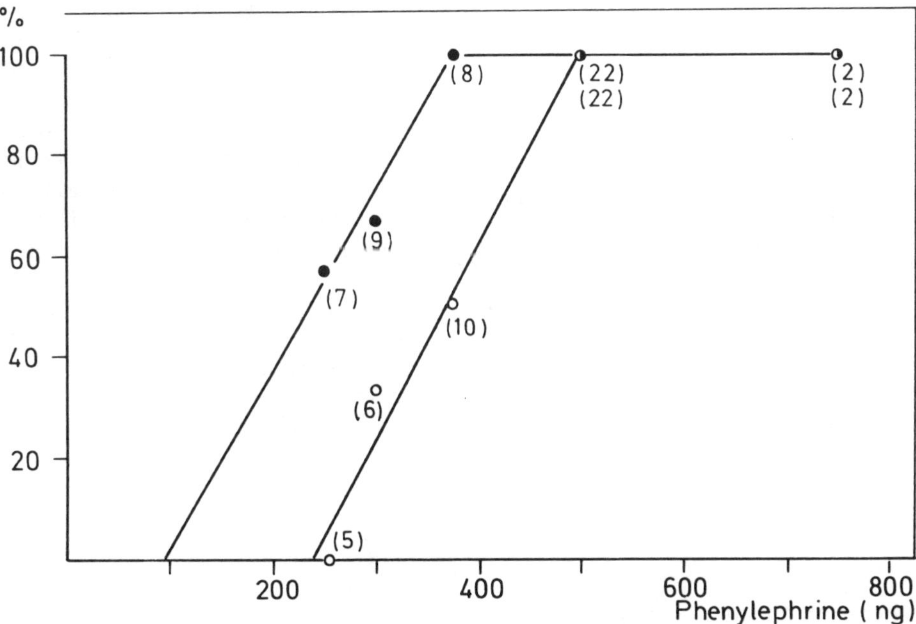

Figure 3. Dose-dependency of the phenylephrine-induced shift in responders, i.e., rats that display EMB on the first test-day, but become temporarily insensitive to phenylephrine on the second test-day, and non-responders, i.e., rats that do not display EMB on the first test-day, but become temporarily sensitive to phenylephrine on the second test-day. The intercept of the regression line for responders (correlation coefficient, 0.981 for the effects of 250, 350 and 375 ng phenylephrine) differed significantly from that of the regression line of non-responders (correlation coefficient, 0.989 for the effects of 250, 350, 375 and 500 ng phenylephrine): $p < 0.001$ (two tailed t-test).

This together with the fact that the dose dependency of the drug-induced shift in responders significantly differs from that in non-responders (Figure 3) has led to the conclusion that the neurochemical state of the mesolimbic, noradrenergic activity anyhow differs between responders and non-responders; below, additional support in favor of this conclusion is given.

This rather complex paradigm allows one to analyze the causal relation between the functional activity of the nucleus accumbens and the display of emotional behavior in the defeat-test.

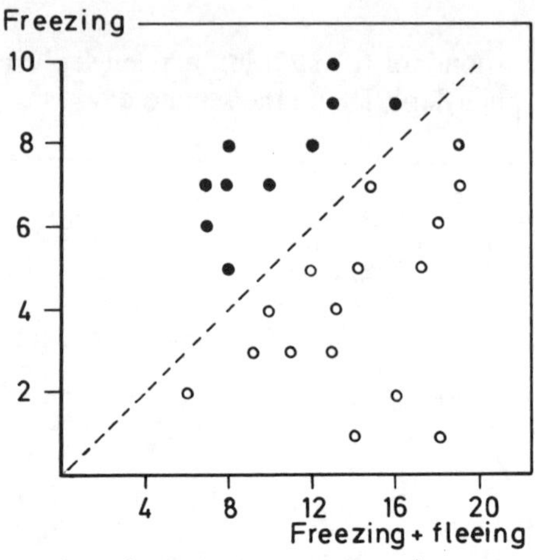

Figure 4. The correlation between behavior shown in the defeat-test and that shown in the phenylephrine-test; the latter was performed 24 h after the former. All rats that primarily freeze (ratio of freezing vs. freezing *plus* fleeing >0.5) turn out to be responders, i.e., rats that display EMB in the phenylephrine-test, whereas all rats that primarily flee (ratio of freezing vs. freezing *plus* fleeing <0.5) turn out to be non-responders, i.e., rats that do not display EMB in the phenyl-ephrine-test: $p<0.01$ (point-biserial correlation between the amount of fleeing in responders and non-responders).

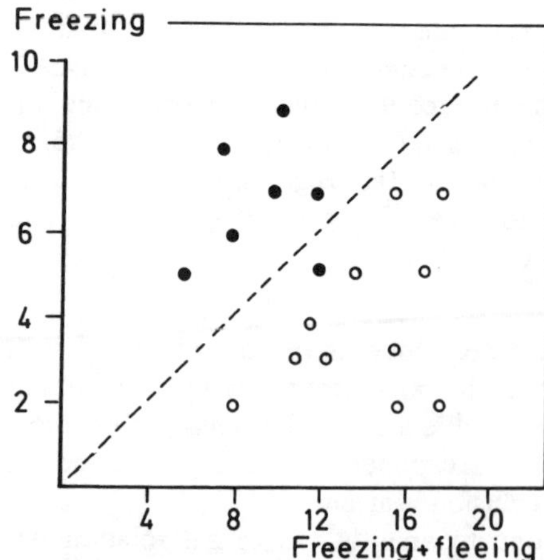

Figure 5. The correlation between behavior shown in the phenylephrine-test and that shown in the defeat-test. Since the latter was performed 24 h after the former, responders were changed into non-responders, and vice versa: Phenylephrine temporarily reverses the sensitivity to phenylephrine (see also Table 1). Resonders that have been changed into non-responders do not freeze anymore, but flee: $p<0.01$ (point-biserial correlation between the amount of fleeing in responders and non-responders).

Combining the defeat-test with the PE-test, for instance, results in the finding that the behavior in the defeat-test significantly correlates with the susceptibility to PE (Figure 4). Thus, non-responders primarily freeze in the defeat-test, whereas responders primarily flee in the defeat-test. Since the first trial of the PE-test alters non-responders in responders, and vice versa, it becomes possible to analyse thc consequences of such a shift in the susceptibility to PE for the behavior in the defeat-test. As shown in Figure 5, responders that have been changed into non-responders do not flee anymore, but freeze; and non-responders that have been changed into responders do not freeze anymore, but flee.

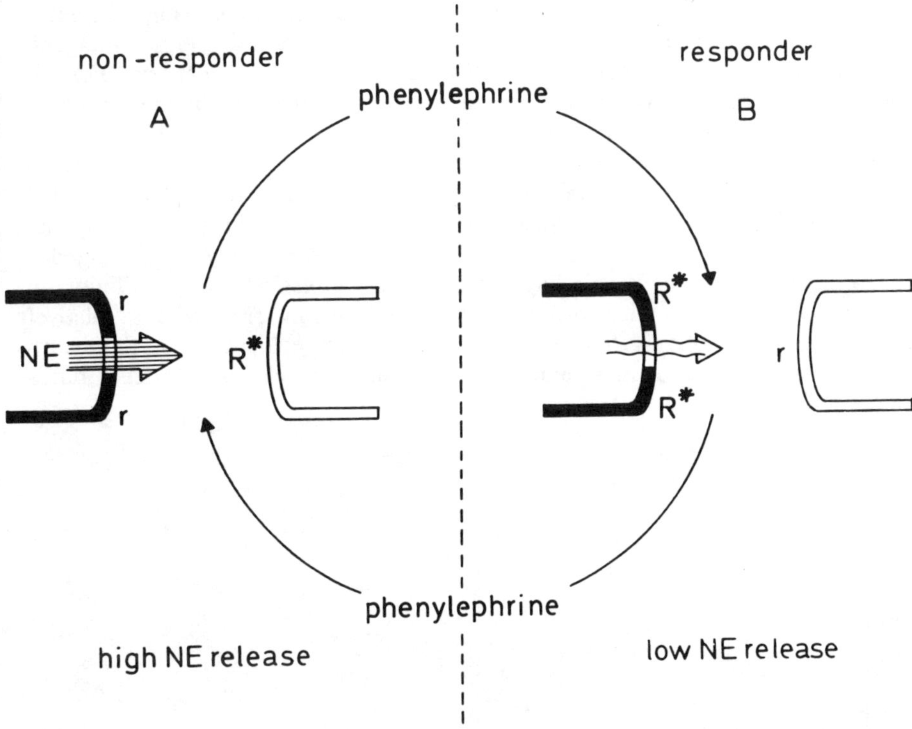

Figure 6. Schematic diagram of the relation between the amount of noradrenaline (NE) released in the synaptic cleft and the functional state of post- and presynaptic noradrenergic receptors in non-responders (left side) and responders (right side). Synapses with a high NE release (left side) have postsynaptic NE receptors in the "antagonist" state, i.e., receptors that are sensitive to NE antagonists and insensitive to NE agonists (R*), and presynaptic NE receptors in the "agonist" state, i.e., receptors that are sensitive to agonists and insensitive to NE antagonists (r). The mirror image holds true for synapses with a low NR release (right side). The circular arrows reflect the phenylephrine-induced, short-term shift in sensitivity to phenylephrine in non-responders (upper part) and responders (lower part).

Thus, it is the degree of susceptibility to PE that determines the behavior in the defeat-test, indicating a causal relation between the neurochemical state of the mesolimbic, noradrenergic activity and the display of emotional behavior. Since limbic structures such as the medial amygdala directs the emotional behavior under discussion (16), the present data imply that limbic information that directs changes in the display of emotional behavior does indeed arrive at the level of the nucleus accumbens.

Elsewhere we have provided evidence in favor of the hypothesis (1) that non-responders are marked by a predominance of postsynaptic noradrenergic receptors in the antagonist state, and (2) that responders are marked by a predominance of postsynaptic noradrenergic receptors in the agonist state (15; Figure 6). In view of this hypothesis, it was of interest to investigate whether the affinity of mesolimbic binding sites for the α-noradrenergic antagonist prazosin shows any correlation with the behavior in the defeat-test. For, the hypothesis predicts that mesolimbic, noradrenergic receptors in the antagonist state, i.e., receptors that have a high affinity for the antagonist, are characteristic for non-responders, i.e., rats that primarily freeze, but not for responders, i.e., rats that primarily flee. As shown in Figure 7, the amount of fleeing significantly correlates with the affinity of prazosin for binding sites within the nucleus accumbens. Thus, rats that display nearly no fleeing and, accordingly, freeze have binding sites with a relatively high affinity for prazosin, whereas rats that primarily flee have binding sites with a relatively low affinity for prazosin. These data provide direct evidence that the neurochemical state of the mesolimbic, noradrenergic mechanism indeed differs between rats that freeze and rats that flee.

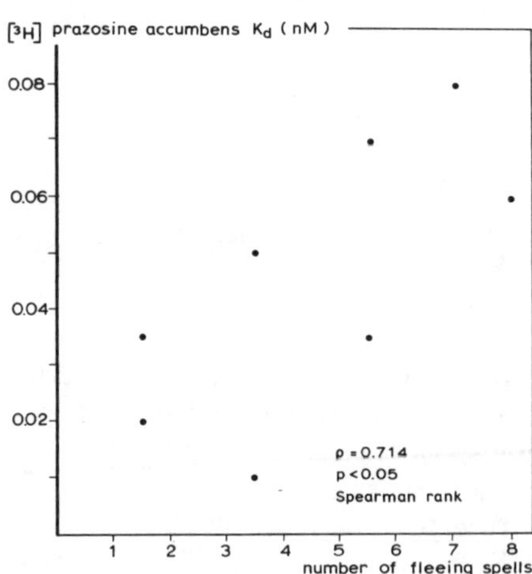

Figure 7. Correlation between the K_d or the α_1-noradrenergic antagonist (^3H) prazosine for binding sites within the nucleus accumbens and the behavior shown in the defeat-test.

Concerning the nature of the neurochemical state of the noradrenergic mechanism within the nucleus accumbens, it is relevant to consider the following. Non-responders, i.e., rats that are insensitive to the α-noradrenergic agonist PE during the first PE-trial, apparently lack mesolimbic, noradrenergic receptors in the agonist state: No response is elicited. This together with the fact that such rats are marked by binding sites with a high affinity for the α-noradrenergic antagonist prazosin has led to the hypothesis that non-responders are marked by a relatively high noradrenaline turnover (15; Figure 6). On the other hand, responders must have mesolimbic, noradrenergic receptors in the agonist state, since they immediately respond to the α-noradrenergic agonist PE. This together with the fact that responders have binding sites with a low affinity for the α-noradrenergic antagonist prazosin has led to the hypothesis that responders are marked by a relatively low noradrenaline turnover (15; Figure 6).

The above-mentioned data provide evidence that individual differences in the display of certain emotional behavior are *inter alia* directed by the neurochemical state of the noradrenergic mechanism within the nucleus accumbens.

Neostriatum and the Display of Emotional Behavior

Since the nucleus accumbens sends fibers to the substantia nigra, pars compacta, i.e., the origin of dopaminergic, nigro-striatal fibers (4), the question arises whether individual differences in the functional activity of the nucleus accumbens are anyhow reflected by individual differences in the neostriatal, dopaminergic activity. When such a relation indeed exists, it becomes evident that limbic information that arrives in the nucleus accumbens may indirectly control the functional activity of brain structures that direct changes in on-going behavior.

Given the causal relation between the behavior in the defeat-test and the neurochemical state of the mesolimbic, noradrenergic mechanism (see above), the behavior shown in the defeat-test was correlated with the animal's susceptibility to the dopaminergic agonist apomorphine. The latter compound is known to activate dopaminergic receptors within the neostriatum and to elicit a number of behavioral changes, of which the gnawing response can be quantitatively measured with the help of the so-called gnawing-box (17). When apomorphine (1.5 mg/kg) is subcutaneously given 24 h after the defeat-test, a significant correlation between the amount of fleeing in the defeat-test and the amount of gnawing in the apomorphine-test is found (Figure 8). Thus, rats that primarily flee have a relatively high gnawing score, and rats that nearly do not flee, and accordingly primarily freeze, have a relatively low gnawing score. In order to investigate whether the individual differences in the gnawing score are anyhow related to individual differences in the functional activity of the dopaminergic mechanism within the neostriatum, use was made of the fact that animals with a low neostriatal, dopaminergic activity have a low GABA-ergic activity at the level of the substantia nigra, pars reticulata, i.e., a structure that is innervated by striato-nigral, GABA-ergic fibers (18). Since a decreased GABA-ergic activity within the substantia nigra, pars reticulata worsens the ability to use static, proprioceptive stimuli for adjusting the position of the organism (for review, 19), the latter ability was measured in rats showing individual differences in their response to apomorphine. These experiments, which are described elsewhere in detail (15), have shown that there exists a significant, negative correlation between the strength of the apomorphine-response and the ability to adjust the position with the help of static, proprioceptive stimuli. Thus, rats with a weak response to apomorphine correctly adjust their position, whereas rats with a strong response to apomorphine have difficulties in that respect. On basis of these data, it is justified to state (1) that rats with a weak response to apomorphine have a relatively high dopaminergic activity within the neostriatum, and (2) that rats with a strong response to apomorphine have a relatively low dopaminergic activity within the neostriatum.

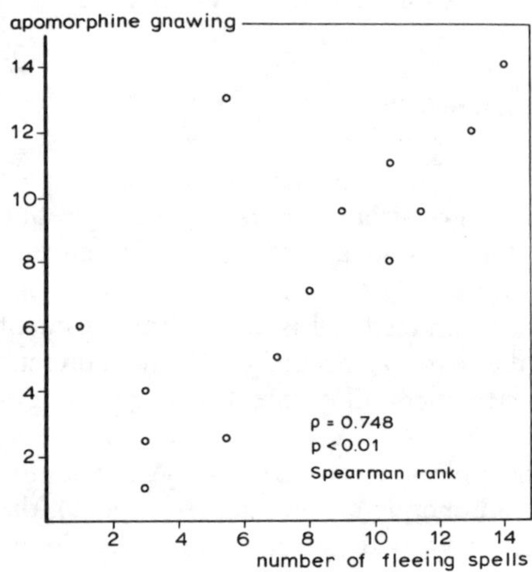

Figure 8. Correlation between behavior shown in the apomorphine gnawing-test and that shown in the defeat-test ($p < 0.01$).

Summarizing the data collected in the various tests, the following picture emerges:

1) There is a significant, negative correlation between the strength of the response to amorphine and the degree of the functional, dopaminergic activity within the neostriatum: Rats with a strong apomorphine response have a relatively low functional, dopaminergic activity within the neostriatum, whereas rats with a weak apomorphine response have a relatively high functional, dopaminergic activity within the neostriatum.
2) There is a significant, positive correlation between the strength of the response to apomorphine and the amount of fleeing shown in the defeat test: Rats with a weak apomorphine-response show a small amount of fleeing, whereas rats with a strong apomorphine-response show a high amount.
3) There is a significant, negative correlation between the amount of fleeing shown in the defeat-test and the degree of the mesolimbic, noradrenergic activity within the nucleus accumbens: Rats with a small amount of fleeing have a relatively high functional, noradrenergic activity, whereas rats with a

high amount of fleeing have a relatively low functional, noradrenergic activity.

4) Changing the neurochemical state of the noradrenergic mechanism within the nucleus accumbens alters rats that primarily freeze in rats that primarily flee, and vice versa.

All these data together imply that rats having a high noradrenergic activity within the nucleus accumbens are marked by a high dopaminergic activity within the neostriatum, and vice versa. Since the nucleus acccumbens sends information towards the neostriatum, and not vice versa (4), it seems justified to state that the neurochemical state of the noradrenergic mechanism within the nucleus accumbens directs the neurochemical state of the dopaminergic mechanism within the neostriatum. The impact of the latter will be discussed below.

Transformation of Emotion into Motion

Before considering the impact of the above-mentioned data, it is relevant to recall the following about the neostriatum, c.q. caudate nucleus in higher mammals (for review, 19). First, the neostriatal, dopaminergic activity stimulates the GABA-ergic activity at the level of the substantia nigra pars reticulata via the striato-nigral, GABA-ergic fibers; the nigral, GABA-ergic activity, in turn, inhibits the GABA-ergic activity at the level of the deeper layers of the superior colliculus *via* the nigro-collicular, GABA-ergic fibers (for review, 18). Thus, animals with a high neostriatal, dopaminergic activity have a high nigral, GABA-ergic activity together with a low collicular, GABA-ergic activity, whereas animals with a low neostriatal, dopaminergic activity have a low nigral, GABA-ergic activity together with a high collicular, GABA-ergic activity.

Today, there is hard evidence that a high neostriatal, dopaminergic activity allows the organisms to shift arbitrarily behavioral programs in rats, cats, monkeys, and man; a low dopaminergic activity, however, just allows the organism to shift behavioral programs with the help of conditioned, proprioceptive and/or exteroceptive stimuli (for review, 19, 20). Furthermore, evidence is available that a high nigral, GABA-ergic activity allows the organism to shift behavioral programs with the help of static, proprioceptive stimuli; a low nigral, GABA-ergic activity, however, just allows the organism to shift behavioral programs with the help of dynamic proprioceptive stimuli, conditioned and/or exteroceptive stimuli (for review, 19). Finally, there is evidence that a low collicular, GABA-ergic activity allows the organism to shift behavioral programs with the help of static exteroceptive stimuli; a high collicular, GABA-ergic activity, however, just allows the animal to shift behavioral programs with the help of dynamic exteroceptive stimuli, conditioned and/or dynamic proprioceptive stimuli (for review, 19, 21). Thus, animals with a high neostriatal, dopaminergic activity and, consequently, a high nigral, GABA-ergic activity as well as a low collicular, GABA-ergic activity have the highest degree of freedom in shifting arbitrarily their ongoing behavior; such animals are labeled "non-stimulus bound" (22-24). In contrast, animals with a low neostriatal, dopaminergic activity and, consequently, a low nigral, GABA-ergic activity together with a high collicular, GABA-ergic activity can only shift their ongoing behavior with the help of conditioned, dynamic proprioceptive and/or dynamic exteroceptive stimuli; accordingly, they are labeled "stimulus bound" (22-24).

Recalling the present findings about the functional relation between mesolimbic, noradrenergic activity and neostriatal, dopaminergic activity, it becomes now possible to understand the individual behavior displayed in the defeat-test. Rats with a high mesolimbic, noradrenergic activity and, consequently, a high neostriatal, dopaminergic activity are non-stimulus bound. It is this feature that allows them to shift arbitrarily their ongoing behavior and, accordingly, to select the best strategy in order to be sacred from the attack: They freeze. On the other hand, rats with a low mesolimbic, noradrenergic activity are stimulus-bound, so that they only shift their ongoing behavior on the condition that the attacker changes its behavior: They flee as soon as the attacker moves.

The insight that the individual differences in the defeat-test may be considered as the consequences of a particular neurochemical state within the brain lays the foundation for the hypothesis that rats with a neurochemical state characterized by a relatively high mesolimbic, noradrenergic activity and, accordingly, a relatively high neostriatal, dopaminergic activity are always superior to rats with a neurochemical state characterized by a relatively low mesolimbic, noradrenergic activity and, accordingly, a relatively low neostriatal, dopaminergic activity. The former rats have a higher degree of freedom in changing and/or maintaining their ongoing behavior. Against this background, it is relevant to recall the data of Koolhaas and his colleagues (1, 2, 13). Starting from a global classification of rats into: (1) a class of socially active and/or competitive rats that rapidly change their display of emotional behavior and (2) a class of socially inactive and/or non-competitive rats, it has become possible to show that the former animals have a relatively high (a) catecholaminergic output, (b) sympathetic tone and (c) reactivity, and that the latter animals have not only a relatively low (a) catecholaminergic output, (b) sympathetic tone and (c) reactivity, but also a relatively high parasympathetic tone (1). These and related data clearly show that rats changing rapidly their display of emotional behavior are marked by a relatively active limbic-hypothalamo-pituitary-adrenal axis, and that rats being less active in that respect are marked by a relatively inactive limbic-hypothalamo-pituitary-adrenal axis. Thus, processes that give rise to particular changes in emotional behavior are tuned to processes that give rise to changes in the objective state of bodily arousal. Since (a) rats changing rapidly their emotional behavior also have a high mesolimbic noradrenergic activity, and rats being less active in that respect have a low mesolimbic, noradrenergic activity (present study), it appears that rats having an active limbic-hypothalamo-pituitary-adrenal axis also have an active limbic-mesolimbic-neostriatal axis, and vice versa. This insight shows that li»bic structures indeed serve two purposes: Directing changes in the objective state of bodily arousal via the limbic-hypothalamo-pituitary-adrenal circuitry, and directing changes in the display of emotional behavior via the limbic-mesolimbic-neostriatal circuitry. Viewed in this light, it appears justified to state that the nucleus accumbens allows the organism to transform emotion into motion (8, 11).

References

1. Fokkema, D.S. (1985). Social behavior and blood pressure. A Study of rats. Thesis, State University of Groningen, The Netherlands.
2. Koolhaas, J.M. & Fokkema, D.S. (1984). Changes in blood pressure of individual male rats during and after defeat. In R. Bandler & R. Alan (Eds.), Modulation of sensimotor activity during alterations in behavioral states. Liss Inc., N.Y., p. 456-467.
3. De France, J.E. & Yoshihara, H. (1975). Fimbria input to the nucleus accumbens septi. Brain Res., 90: 159-173.
4. Domesick, V.B. (1981). Further observations on the anatomy of nucleus accumbens and caudatoputamen in the rat: Similarities and contracts. In R.B. Chronister and J.F. de France (Eds.), The neurobiology of the nucleus accumbens. Haer Inst., New Brunswick, p. 7-39.
5. Groenewegen, H.J., Becker, N.E.H.M. & Lohman, A.H.M. (1980). Subcortical afferents of the nucleus accumbens septi in the cat, studied with retrograde axonal transport of horseradish peroxidase and bisbenzimid. Neuroscience, 5: 1903-1916.
6. Groenewegen, H.J., Boom, P., Witter, M.P. & Lohman, A.H.M. (1982). Cortical afferents of the nucleus accumbens in the cat, studied with anterograde and retrograde transport techniques. Neuroscience, 7: 977-995.
7. Kelley, A.E., Domesick, V.B. & Nauta, W.J.H. (1982). The amygdalostriatal projection in the rat - An anatomical study by anterograde and retrograde tracing methods. Neuroscience, 7: 615-630.
8. Mogenson, G.J. & Yim, C.Y. (1981). Electrophysiological and neuropharmacological-behavioral studies of the nucleus accumbens: Implications for its role as a limbic-motor interface. In R.B. Chronister & J.F. de France (Eds.), The neurobiology of the nucleus accumbens. Haer Inst., New Brunswick, p. 210-229.
9. Siegel, A. & Tassoni, J.P. (1971). Different efferent projections from the ventral and dorsal hippocampus of the cat. Brain Behav. Evol., 4: 185-200.
10. Swanson, L.W. & Cowan, W.M. (1975). A note on the connections and development of the nucleus accumbens. Brain Res., 92: 324-330.
11. Taghzouti, K., Simon, H., Loilot, A., Herman, J.V. & le Moal, M. (1985). Behavioral study after local injection of 6-hydroxydopamine into the nucleus accumbens of the rat. Brain Res., 344: 9-20.
12. Schuurman, T. (1981). Endocrine processes underlying victory and defeat in the male rat. Thesis, State University of Groningen, The Netherlands.
13. Koolhaas, J.M., Fokkema, D.S. & Kalsbeek, A. (in press). Individual differentiation in behavior and hormonal response to psychosocial stress in male rats. Psychoneuroendocrinology.
14. Cools, A.R., Ellenbroek, B.A. & Van den Heuvel, C.M. (1983). Picrotoxin microinjections into the brain: A model of abrupt withdrawal "jumping" behavior in rats not exposed to any opiate? Eur. J. Pharmacol., 90: 237-243.
15. Cools, A.R., Ellenbroek, B., Van den Bos, R. & Gelissen, M. (in press). Mesolimbic noradrenaline: Specificity, stability and dose-dependency of individual-specific responses to mesolimbic injections of α-noradrenergic agonists. Behav. Brain Res.
16. Luiten, P.G.M., Koolhaas, J.M., de Boer, S. & Koopmans, S.J. (1985). The cortico-medial amygdala in the central nervous system: Organization of agonistic behavior. Brain Res., 332: 283-297.
17. Ljunberg, T. & Ungerstedt, U. (1978). A new method for simultaneous registration of 8 behavioral parameters related to monoaminergic neurotransmission. Pharmacol. Biochem. Behav., 8: 483-489.
18. Scheel-Krüger, J. (1983). The GABA receptor and animal behavior. In S.J. Enna (Ed.), GABA receptor. Hermana Press, Clifton, N.J., p. 215-265.
19. Cools, A.R., Jaspers, R., Schwarz, M., Sontag, K.-H., Vrijmoed-de Vries, M. & Van den Bercken, J. (1984). Basal ganglia and switching motor programs. In J.S. McKenzie, R.E. Kemm & L.N. Wilcock (Eds.), The basal ganglia. Plenum Publishing Corporation, p. 513-544.
20. Jaspers, R., Schwarz, M., Sontag, K.-H. & Cools, A.R. (1984). Caudate nucleus and programming behavior in cats: Role of dopamine in switching motor patterns. Behav. Brain Res., 14: 17-28.
21. Gelissen, M. & Cools, A.R. (1986). The interrelationship between superior colliculus and substantia nigra pars reticulata in programming movements of cats. Behav. Brain Res., 21: 85-93.

22. Cools, A.R. (1985). Brain and behavior: Hierarchy of feedback systems and control of input. In P.P.G. Bateson & P.H. Klopfer (Eds.), Perspectives in Ethology 6 (Mechanisms). Plenum Press, N.Y. and London, p. 109-168.
23. Vrijmoed-de Vries, M.C. (1985). Programming motor and non-motor behavior: Role of striatum in animals. Thesis, University of Nijmegen, The Netherlands.
24. Vrijmoed-de Vries, M.C. & Cools, A.R. (1986). Differential effects of striatal injections of dopaminergic, cholinergic and GABAergic drugs upon swimming behavior of rats. Brain Res., 364: 77-90.

The Role of Serotonin in Affective Disorders, Schizophrenia and Anxiety Disorders

Hugh C. Hendrie, Joseph N. Hingtgen and Morris H. Aprison

Serotonin, undoubtedly because of its ubiquitous presence in bodily fluid and tissues, has been implicated as a possible etiological factor in a multitude of behavioral disorders, either through direct action on the central nervous system or indirectly by influencing other neurotransmitters or neuromodulators. These disorders include the affective disorders and suicidal behavior, the schizophrenic disorders and hallucinatory states, anxiety states, personality disorders, particulary aggressive and antisocial, including homicidal behavior, the perception of pain, eating disorders and other illnesses of the GI tract, mental retardation, sleep disorders, various forms of sexual dysfunction, alcoholism and other drug addictions, migraine headaches and hyperactivity in children.

In this paper we will focus primarily on the evidence for the possible role of serotonin in the genesis of affective disorders, schizophrenic disorders and anxiety states; but first we review briefly the neurobiology of serotonin and discuss some of the types of studies, both human and animal, which have been conducted by basic and clinical researchers in this area.

Serotonin (5-HT) is synthesized from the essential amino acid L-tryptophan (TRY) by hydroxylation at the 5 position on the indole group to form 5-HTP, which is then quickly decarboxylated. The 5-HT is stored in intraneuronal vesicles from which it can be released on demand of the nervous system (nerve impulse) into the synaptic cleft. In the cleft, 5-HT may reversibly combine with receptors in the postsynaptic membrane and/or with presynaptic receptors. The latter are autoreceptors which function by modulating the synthesis and release of 5-HT by serotonergic neurons. The action of 5-HT on receptors is terminated by an uptake mechanism into the presynaptic serotonergic neuron, or into glia. When taken back into the neuron, 5-HT can either be stored in vesicles, or it can be oxidatively deaminated by monoamine oxidase (MAO) and then converted to 5-hydroxyindoleactic acid (5-HIAA), a major metabolite, by an aldehyde dehydrogenase.

Observations of the behavioral and biochemical actions of drugs in both humans and animals which have been found to alter the serotonergic physiological processes have provided one way of studying the role of serotonin in health and illness. A drug which acts directly on synaptic receptors mimicking 5-HT is a serotonergic agonist (e.g., quipazine, MK 212). A drug can block the action of 5-HT at the receptor site, functioning as an antagonist (e.g., methysergide, trazadone, cyproheptidine). Other drugs are available which can decrease or increase the level of serotonin reaching the receptor (e.g., synaptic serotonin can be reduced by the action of a synthesis inhibitor such as PCPA, and depletors like reserpine, p-chloroamphetamine, 5,7-dihydroxytryptamine; or synaptic serotonin can be increased by the action of precursors like tryptophan and 5-HTP, uptake inhibitors like fluoxetine, or degradation inhibitors like MAO inhibitors).

In addition to studies of drug interaction, four types of data derived from the basic and clinical literature have been used to implicate serotonin in disease states:

1) biochemical and pharmacological measurements on CSF, blood, serum, platelets or urine from patients;
2) biochemical and pharmacological measurements on autopsy tissues from patients;
3) biochemical and pharmacological measurements on brain and peripheral tissues from animals which may provide animal models for the functional illnesses;
4) a serotonergic neuroendocrine challenge method predicated on the observation that central serotonergic stimulation affects pituitary hormones such as prolactin and growth hormone or target gland secretion such as cortisol.

In affective disorders and anxiety states both human and animal studies have been conducted. In schizophrenia, since good behavioral animal models still elude us, most work has been on peripheral measurements in humans.

Affective Disorders

There have been many attempts to develop a biological theory explaining depressive disorders involving the monoaminergic neurotransmitter systems. While these explorations have led to the development of important new knowledge, no one theory has yet emerged which satisfactorily explains all the clinical manifestations of depression. Perhaps this is an impossible goal. It is probable that depressive disorders represent a heterogeneous etiological grouping.

Nevertheless, a hypothesis is presented for the etiology of depressive disorders involving the development of a postsynaptic hypersensitive serotonin receptor theory which has been constructed over the years by Aprison and colleagues (1, 2). We believe this hypothesis, which is being continually developed and tested, provides a framework for understanding at least some of the manifestations of depression (3-8).

A biological theory of depression should try to answer the following five questions:

1) What biological trait renders some individuals vulnerable to developing depression?
2) What biological event triggers the episode?
3) What biological state sustains the episode?
4) What biological event terminates the episode?
5) What is the biological mechanism of action in our current treatment methods?

Over the past 15 years, Aprison and Hingtgen (2, 7) have developed an animal model of behavioral supression which possesses characteristics which resemble some aspects of depressive disorders. Defense of this animal model in 1984 was summarized by Aprison and Hingtgen at the 15th Annual Meeting of the American Society for Neurochemistry (9) as follows:

In 1978 we reconciled our animal data with conflicting clinical data (i.e., the suppression of animal behavior is caused by an increase in 5-HT in the synaptic cleft in specific cerebral areas; human depression is associated with lowered cerebral 5-HT), by formulating a new theory of depression. This theory predicts the formation of hypersensitive postsynaptic serotonergic receptors in the brain of some individuals during their accomodation to chronic decreased release of 5-HT. Stress, occurring at a later date, causes a "subjective" increased release of 5-HT, which now interacts with these supersensitive postsynaptic receptors, resulting in depression. Providing conclusive proof for such receptors in man is very difficult. However, much new animal data fits predictions from this theory. Thus, (1) chronic administration of PCPA, a depletor of 5-HT, produced hypersensitive 5-HT receptors in 5-HT injected rats; (2) trazodone, mianserin, amitriptyline, imipramine and iprindole, currently used antidepressants, blocked 5-HTP induced depression postsynaptically; (3) the selective 5-HT_2 receptor antagonist, LY53857, an experimental drug used in blood vessel research, blocked the behavioral effect of large doses of 5-HTP, and hence is a potential antidepressive drug; (4) behavioral stress alone enhances sensitivity to 5-HTP induced depression in our model. Additional supporting clinical evidence shows (1) reduction of (^{3}H)-imipramine binding, a presynaptic event, in cortical tissues from depressed patients; (2) increase in number of 5-HT_2 receptors, a postsynaptic event, in the frontal cortex of a number of suicide patients; and (3) cyproheptadine appears to improve depression in some patients with associated pituitary-adrenal disinhibition.

We wish to briefly review some of these data. Animals were trained to work for a food reward (food reinforced operant schedule), and under certain conditions were injected with D,L-5-HTP, L-5-HTP, L-tryptophan, various drugs, etc., and their behaviors were quantitatively measured. Under certain biochemical conditions this behavior was suppressed even though the animals remained hungry and were capable of movement (10-13). This behavioral suppression could be considered analogous to the psychomotor retardation that may occur in depression. Figure 1 is a diagrammatic representation of a series of such early experiments using intraperitonal injections of D,L-5 HTP, showing the time course of the behavioral suppression and comparing it to elevations of cerebral 5-HT. In these experiments only total serotonin levels, not other measured neurotransmitters such as norepinephrine and dopamine, correlated with the time course of behavioral suppression and this only in the telencephalon and diencephalon, not in other parts of brain or peripheral tissues.

Then in a series of elegant experiments using drugs which affect various parameters of serotonin metabolism including p-chlorophenylalanine (PCPA) which inhibits tryptophan hydroxylase, as well as α-methyl-*m*-tyxrosine and tetrabenazine, both of which inhibit storage of bound forms of 5-HT, Aprison, Hingtgen, and their colleagues, together with Takahashi and his group in Japan, obtained sufficient data to conclude that this behavioral suppression was related to levels of free 5-HT in the synaptic cleft (1, 2, 7).

The conclusion from these studies that depression may be related to an increase in free synaptic serotonin conflicted, however, with at least one theory which proposed that depression results from serotonin *deficiency* not excess. This conflict and the examination of some pertinent clinical and experimental data led in 1978 to the first formulation of the present theory which we are currently testing (1).

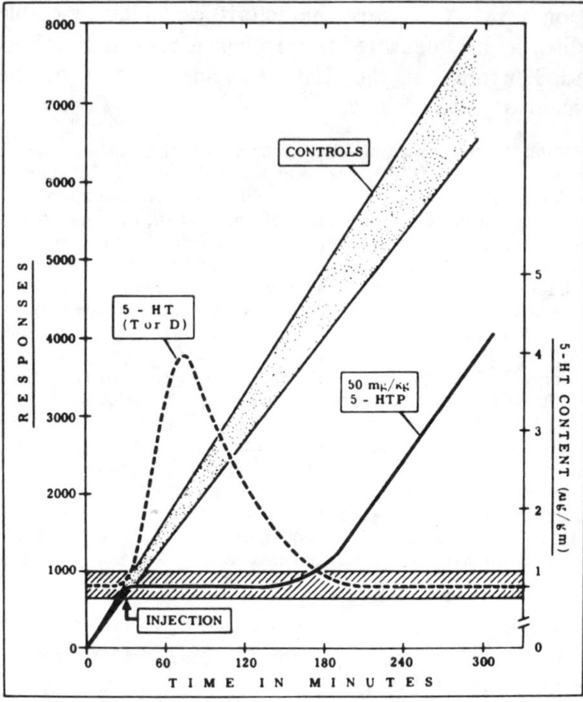

Figure 1. Diagrammatic presentation of the effect of an intramuscular (i.m.) injection of 50 mg/kg D,L-5-HTP on the approach response rate and 5-HT content in the telencephalon (T) or diencephalon plus optic lobes (D) of the pigeon. After the injection of 5-HTP, the 5-HT level increases, passes through a maximum and then decreases to normal; the behavior of the experimental animal was disrupted for a period of time (mean: 154 min) and then returned to normal at approximately the same time as the 5-HT levels return to normal. The speckled band indicates the extreme range of response rates during control sessions (with or without saline injections). The band at the bottom represents the range of the 5-HT concentration in the telencephalon from control pigeons. The broken line shows the chenge in 5-HT concentration in this brain part at different times after the 5-HTP injection. The data from the diencephalon were similar. From Aprison and Hingtgen (13), with permission. Copyright 1965 by Pergamon Press, New York.

For selective review of the relevant findings supporting both theories see references (1) and (2). In support of the serotonin deficiency theory are (1) the neuropharmacological data that reserpine and tetrabenazine, both serotonin depletors, produce depression, (2) the clinical data that low levels of serotonin are found in the brains of patients who have killed themselves, and (3) that low levels of 5-HIAA are found in the CSF of at least some patients who are depressed. In support of the new theory are (1) the experimental data already discussed suggesting that increases in free synaptic serotonin leads to behavioral suppression in animals, and (2) several interesting clinical studies suggesting that the levels of probencid enhanced CSF 5-HIAA in depressed patients were significantly decreased after one to three weeks of successful treatment with imipramine and amitriptylline (1, 2). The newer theory suggests the following: Individuals vulnerable to depression have chronically low levels of released serotonin. This prolonged reduction in serotonin release is compensated for by the development of hypersensitive receptors. The individual shows no evidence for depression at this stage as the hypersensitive receptor handles information as though a normal amount of serotonin were being released. However, any exogenous or endogenous factor, which led to more serotonin than normal to be released, would produce depression in individuals with hypersensitive postsynaptic receptors (1, 2).

Table 1. Percent blockade of 5-HTP induced depression in rats following acute pretreatment with a postsynaptic serotonergic receptor blocker or one of five clinically used antidepressive drugs.

Drug	Dose (mg)	% Blockade
Methysergide	1.0	70
Trazodone	2.0	62
Mianserin	1.0	53
Amitriptyline	2.5	49
Imipramine	2.5	40
Iprindole	1.5	22

The antidepressants were administered in doses based on the human clinical dose. Pretreatment was given 60 min prior to injection of D,L-5-HTP (50 mg/kg), which was given 15 min following the start of VI session. N= 6-10 per group. Adapted from Aprison, Hingtgen and co-workers (2, 4, 5, 6, 16).

One way of testing the new theory was to explore the mode of action of anti-depressant medication (3, 4), a traditional serotonin deficiency theory would predict that the drugs would act primarily presynaptically on uptake systems, thus increasing the levels of free synaptic serotonin, whereas the hypersensitive receptor theory would suggest that the drugs would act primarily post-synaptically rather than presynaptically, and the therapeutic action would be postsynaptic. To establish a behavioral paradigm for distinguishing presynaptic from postsynaptic effects, fluoxetine, a known serotonin uptake blocker, and methysergide, a known postsynaptic serotonin blocker were studied in the animal model (3). It was shown that fluoxetine (5 mg/kg) injected one hour previously potentiated the behavioral effects of a low dose of D,L-5-HTP (12.5 mg/kg) by 200% whereas methysergide again injected one hour previously almost completely blocked (93%) the effects of a much higher dose of D,L-5-HTP (50 mg/kg). Amitriptyline acted in a manner similar to methysergide, i.e., as a post-synaptic blocker (3, 4).

The data in Table 1 show the effects of acute injections of the anti-depressants trazodone, mianserin, amitriptyline, imipramine and iprindole in clinically relevant doses on the behavioral system. As can be seen, all act in a manner similar to methysergide as postsynaptic blockers with varying degrees of potency. PCPA acts as a potentiator only if given three times at two day intervals over the course of a week, not in one injection, and is associated with the development of receptor hypersensitivity (14).

These data do not suggest that the drugs are only acting postsynaptically or on one neurotransmitter system. However, if presynaptic and postsynaptic effects are occurring simultaneously it appears likely that at least with the more potent of these drugs, postsynaptic effects predominate.

Other data in the literature support this theory of action for at least some anti-depressants. Ogren et al. (15) in Sweden studied the effects of anti-depressants on (^{3}H)-d-LSD and (^{3}H)-5-HT binding *in vitro* to membrane sites in the rat neo-cortex, and concluded that many block postsynaptic serotonin in receptor sites as well as affect serotonin and NE uptake systems.

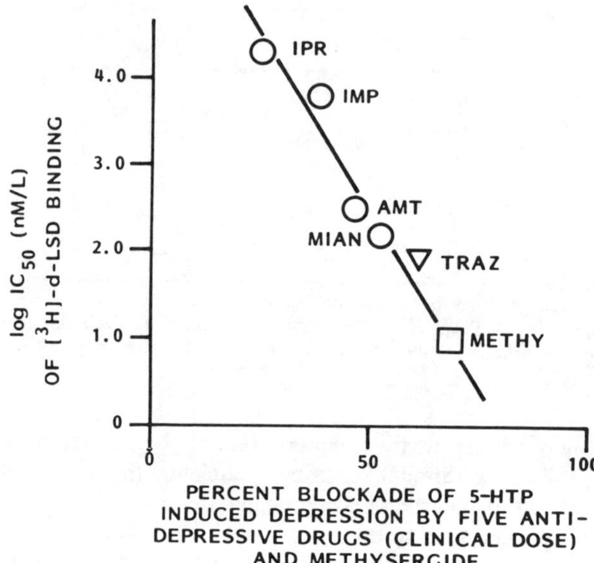

Figure 2. Relationship between the percent blockade of 5-HTP induced depression by the following five antidepressive drugs, 2 mg/kg trazodone (TRAZ), 1.0 mg/kg mianserin (MIAN), 2.5 mg/kg amitriptyline (AMT), 2.5 mg/kg imipramine (IMP), and 1.5 mg/kg iprindole (IPR), and 5 mg/kg methysergide (METHY), and their IC_{50} (nM/L) values obtained in (^{3}H)-LSD binding studies using rat brain (Fuller, personal communication). See (5) for similar data where the K_i values also were used for four of these drugs. The antidepressants were administered in a single dose within the range comparable to a daily clinical dose. From Hingtgen et al. (6) with permission. Copyright 1984 by Anklho International, Inc.

When the binding data, from the Ogren et al. study, expressed as log K_i (nM) of (^{3}H)-d-LSD binding (where K_i is the inhibitory dissociation constant), are compared to the behavioral data referred to above, an inverse linear relationship is found (5, 16, 17). A similar relationship (see Figure 2) was found using entirely independent but comparable IC_{50} data of (^{3}H)-d-LSD binding in the presence of five antidepressant drugs as well as for methysergide (6).

In clinical usage, however, anti-depressant drugs are administered chronically, not acutely. It is possible that while the predominant acute effects are postsynaptic, the chronic effects are presynaptic. Accordingly, first trazodone and then other anti-depressants were administered to the animals over a prolonged period of time. Data from such experiments show that after eight days pre-treatment with 2 mg/kg trazodone, the 5-HTP-induced depression was effectively blocked at the 75% level. Chronic treatment of up to 28 days with amitriptyline and mianserin also produced similar results (6). Mianserin maintained, but did not increase, its effectiveness in blockade with time whereas amitryptyline did. Thus, the chronic action of the three drugs tested appears to remain predominantly postsynaptic.

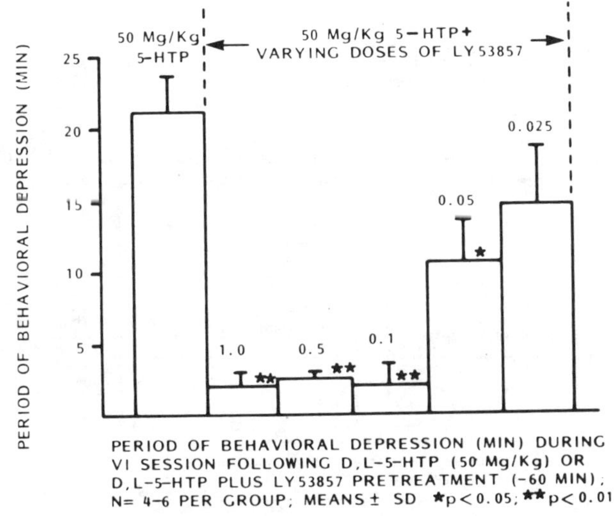

Figure 3. Period of behavioral depression (min) during VI session following D,L-5-HTP (50 mg/kg) or D,L-5-HTP plus LY53875 (mg/kg) pretreatment (-60 min); N=4-6 rats per group; means ± SD; $*p<0.05$, $**p<0.01$ (Student's t-test). Period of behavioral depression or "depth of depresssion" was determined by the amount of time required to make the same number of responses following the 5-HTP injection as made during the baseline period prior to the 5-HTP injection. From Hingtgen et al. (7) with permission. Copyright 1985, Elsevier Science Publishing Co., Inc.

At this point in the development of the Aprison-Hingtgen hypothesis it was suggested that an effective treatment of certain types of human depression would be to use a clinically potent postsynaptic serotonin blocker. The development of a new selective 5-HT_2 receptor antagonist, LY53857 (4-isopropyl-7-methyl-9 (2-hydroxy-1-methylpropoxycarbonyl) 4,6,6A,7,8,9,10,10A octahydroindolo (4,3-FG) quinoline maleate) (18, 19) made this suggestion feasible. To test the potential blockade effects of LY53857 on our model of depression, Aprison and co-workers studied the pretreatment effects of this drug given to rats 60 min prior to the administration of 5-HTP during a VI 1 schedule of reinforcement. As predicted, and shown in Figure 3, LY53857 pretreatment significantly blocked 5-HTP depression (90%) in doses as low as 0.1 mg/kg i.p. (7). When the dose of LY53857 was further reduced to 0.025 mg/kg, blockade of 5-HTP-induced depression was still greater than 30%. In doses as high as 5.0 mg/kg, LY53857 alone had no effect on the baseline performance of rats working a VI 1 schedule. Pretreatment with desipramine (2.5 mg/kg), an antidepressant characterized as having major noradrenergic effects, did not significantly block the 5-HTP-induced depression. These data suggest that the 5-HTP-induced depression is mediated by serotonergic mechanisms involving 5-HT_2 receptors, as LY53857 is a selective antagonist of these receptors (7).

The present state of this hypothesis is summarized in Figure 4. The depression-prone individual develops hypersensitive postsynaptic serotonin receptors as a result of chronically reduced serotonin release. This could be due to genetic or environmental factors.

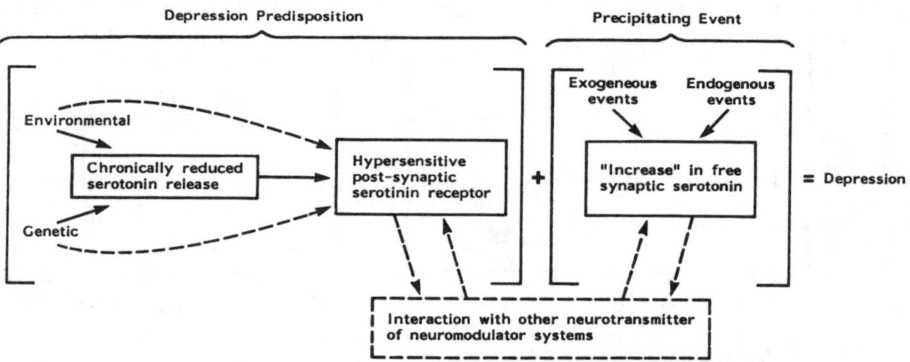

Figure 4. A diagrammatic representation describing the hypersensitive postsynaptic serotonergic receptor theory of depression based on the research studies of Aprison et al. (1) and Aprison and Hingtgen (2).

In our laboratories, chronic stress produced in rats by the Pare method (20), has been shown to reduce 5-HT levels in a number of brain areas including the cortex, hippocampus and midbrain (21). This may be due to an autoregulatory mechanism. The rats have been found to get ulcers in this procedure, and their body weight is greatly reduced. However, since we believe that depression does not develop until the hypersensitive receptor has to cope with increased release of serotonin into the key serotonergic synapses, this stress model may not be ideal to study depression but only to show the effect of stress on cerebral 5-HT levels.

Unfortunately, sufficient data are not available to determine why rapid down regulation does not occur in the case of the serotonergic hypersensitive receptor following injections of L-tryptophan or L-5-HTP. Perhaps the diffusional forces existing within the synapse are of such magnitude to prevent the maintenance of high synaptic concentrations of free serotonin for sufficiently long periods of time to permit the rapid down regulation of the hypersensitive receptor. Therefore, the latter process appears to take much longer.

Effective treatment for depression theoretically could be accomplished by one of the following four methods (see reference (2) for additional comments):

(1) reduction in free synaptic serotonin
(2) postsynaptic serotonin blockade
(3) down regulation of hypersensitive postsynaptic serotonin receptors
(4) some indirect effect through other interacting neurotransmitter systems.

If the first synaptic hypersensitive serotonergic receptor hypothesis is correct, one would expect to see in depression-prone individuals evidence of (1) persistently reduced serotonin metabolism and (2) hypersensitive postsynaptic receptors. The evidence for the former in the form of decreased measures of 5-HIAA in CSF of depressed patients has been well summarized by Van Praag (22). For the latter, the evidence is more scanty.

The data from a recent study of serotonin receptor properties in the frontal cortex from 11 suicide victims and controls (23), indicated a significantly higher (44%) number of 5-HT receptors in the suicide group using tritiated spiroperidol. This study incidentally also showed a significant drop in the number of imipramine binding sites in the frontal cortex of the same patients. The latter, evidence for reduced presynaptic uptake sites, fits with what we expect if less 5-HT is released during the development of hypersensitive receptors. A brief report by Perry (24), involving data from brains of either depressed, normal or demented patients, confirmed the latter finding on (^{3}H)-imipramine binding but did not detect any increase in post synaptic receptors using LSD binding.

In a review of seven separate studies of whole blood or platelet 5-HT levels in major depressive disorders by Stahl et al. (25), there were discrepancies not only in diagnostic criteria and use of medication, but also in levels of 5-HT in the various groups. Normal levels have beeen reported as well as high and low 5-HT concentrations in blood of depressed patients. Much additional work is required to clarify the relationship of blood 5-HT to depression.

The results of a study by DeMyer et al. (26) measuring circulating levels of tryptophan and five competing amino acids (5aa) are of considerable interest. They found reduced Try/5aa levels in depressed patients as compared to controls, indirectly suggesting the possibility of reduced central serotonin metabolism in depression (26).

However, it does appear that there is more consistency in studies reporting platelet 5-HT uptake, with the great majority finding *decreased* platelet 5-HT uptake in depressed patients (25). Subsequent work has revealed that it is the platelet site itself (as measured by imipramine binding) that is somehow deficient in this patient population. This finding of decreased platelet uptake may fit with our depression theory since it is possible that less 5-HT is released both centrally and peripherally.

Incidentally, although most studies report decreased platelet uptake in patients with depression as compared to controls there is usually considerable overlap in the results. Recently Lewis and McChesney (27) have suggested one possible reason for this overlap. In their study of tritiated imipramine binding sites, they found that these were significantly lower than controls only in depressed patients who had bipolar or familial pure depressive diseases and not in those depressed patients who fell into the depressive spectrum or sporadic depressive disease category. They suggested therefore an etiological heterogeneity among patients with depressive disorders.

Perhaps the most direct evidence in favor of the hypersensitive postsynaptic serotonergic theory comes from the work of Meltzer et al. (28). They found that serum cortisol concentration following administration of 200 mg of 5-HTP orally was significantly greater in unmedicated depressed and manic patients than in normal controls, indicating hypersensitivity as there is considerable evidence that serotonin secretion in man is under serotonergic control. While these data are encouraging, it must be pointed out that Heninger et al. (29) found exactly the opposite result when they measured serum prolactin levels in healthy subjects and depressed patients and following IV tryptophan. In depressed patients there was a marked blunting of maximal prolactin response, supporting the idea that the serotonergic function is impaired, but suggesting instead either subsensitive postsynaptic receptors in these patients or some other reason. These differences in the clinical studies are presently difficult to explain. Perhaps the high 7 g dose of tryptophan altered the catecholamine function in these patients. More research is indicated.

Meltzer and his co-workers (30) recently replicated their results showing an enhanced cortisol and an enhanced prolactin secretion but not growth hormone secretion in depressed patients using the direct acting serotonin agonist MK-212.

Schizophrenia

Most current interest in the biochemistry of schizophrenia concentrates on the dopaminergic system mainly because of the action of the antipsychotic drugs. However, interest in the serotonergic system's potential involvement has waxed and waned throughout the years. The previous interest in putative hallucinogens derived from methylated pathways of serotonin, e.g., dimethyltryptamine, has declined in the last decade. Post mortem examinations of brain tissue from schizophrenic patients looking at parameters of serotonin metabolism have yielded confusing and contradictory results (25).

One major research effort involving studies of the biochemical and pharmacological mechanisms utilizing human blood platelets has renewed interest in serotonergic involvement. Numerous investigators have noted that several biochemical analogies exist between blood platelets and CNS neurons, especially with serotonergic neurons. For instance, both platelets and serotonergic neurons appear to possess similar (1) storage properties, (2) active high affinity uptake mechanisms, (3) release properties involving a Ca^{++}-dependent, energy-dependent process, (4) (^{3}H)-imipramine binding sites, (5) mitochondria and (6) limiting membranes. The mitochondria differ somewhat in that human platelets contain only the B form of MAO whereas the brain contains A and B forms of MAO. However, there are a number of reports by investigators (25, 31, 32) who feel that human platelets are *not* an appropriate model for the norepinephrine or dopamine uptake sites of CNS neurons.

In studies of schizophrenic populations whole blood or platelets 5-HT concentrations appear to be generally elevated in the psychotic group. Although it has not been firmly established that changes in platelet 5-HT content reflect changes in cerebral 5-HT content, the finding of elevated platelet 5-HT in schizophrenic populations is not only replicable, but also very interesting. Stahl et al. (25) compiled these data from nine separate reports of whole blood or platelet 5-HT measurements in schizophrenic patients. They note that from the more than 200 chronic schizophrenic patients studied, seven reports indicate elevated whole blood or platelet mean 5-HT levels, whereas two reports found normal levels in the chronic schizophrenic patients as a group. There are a number of reasons why some of the data varied, i.e., various diagnostic critera used, whole blood was used in some studies and platelets in others, control for age, sex and medication status was generally lacking, etc. In order to make more meaningful generalizations, consistently better controlled experiments need to be carried out! But even with these limitations, there is an interesting new correlation with serotonin functioning.

Some evidence indicates that this serotonin increase or abnormality may be related to morphological differences as revealed by computer tomography (CT). Schizophrenic patients with abnormal CT brain scans had higher blood serotonin concentrations than patients with normal CT scans or control subjects. When the patients are subcategorized into a group with abnormal CT scan and a group with normal CT scans, only the patients with abnormal CT scans had significantly higher 5-HT levels when compared either to schizophrenics with normal CT scans or with controls (33). It was found that cerebral ventricular size was positively correlated with blood serotonin concentration.

A preliminary analysis of the data from a multiple brain imaging study of schizophrenic patients also indicates a significant correlation between the ventricular brain ratio measured from CT scan and whole blood serotonin levels in 16 schizophrenic patients (DeMyer et al., personal communication). It should be noted, however, that all of these patients were on some type of antipsychotic medication.

Anxiety

Although literature reviews on the psychobiology of anxiety, which include animal stress studies as well as human and animal anxiolytic drug studies, conclude that the serotonergic neurotransmitter systems as well as other systems are implicated in anxiety, the precise functions have not been delineated. Reports have been published indicating both increases and decreases in total serotonin levels and turnover in brain tissue of animal. The variability of design used in these studies (brain area studied, type of stress used, acute or chronic treatment used, etc.) no doubt can account for some of the apparent conflict in the reported data.

In a study by Hellhammer et al. in our laboratories in 1983 (21), it was suggested that the serotonin response to stress may be an initial increase in certain brain areas of rats followed by a decrease in serotonin metabolism and release. An important methodological problem to be addressed is the separate consideration of specific psychological responses and specific situational stresses. As applied to people, the range of situations included under conditions of "stress" is varied, heterogeneous, and not necessarily analogous to the intensive stressors to which animals are exposed. Direct measures of psychological responses to the stressors have been infrequently used.

A recent study from our research group was designed by Davis et al. to evaluate the relationship between the noradrenergic and serotonergic transmitter systems and anxiety as a subjective, psychological response among normal humans undergoing stress (34). Normal individuals undergoing the commonly encountered stress of academic exams were chosen as the focus of this investigation, which incorporated the methodological advantages of improved assay techniques for MHPG and whole blood serotonin. An assay for platelet imipramine binding was included as an indirect measure of platelet serotonin uptake. It was hypothesized that individuals who characteristically tended toward subjective anxiety (high trait anxiety) would have higher baseline levels of MHPG and serotonin. The second hypothesis suggested was that biological indices would vary across baseline, stressful, and poststress conditions, so that the stress condition would produce an increase in MHPG and serotonin.

Table 2. Psychological responses to stress conditions.

	State Anxiety	By Condition		
	Baseline	Pre-exam		Post-exam
Group	mean ± SD	mean ± SD	Paired t	mean ± SD
Low anxious (n = 18)	28.4 ± 4.4	32.3 ± 7.3	2.37*	28.9 ± 7.1
High anxious (n = 21)	40.3 ± 9.8	44.0 ± 13.4	1.08	40.2 ± 8.7
t	4.99**	3.45**		4.39**

* $p<0.05$, ** $p<0.001$. Adapted from Davis et al. (34).

A total of 192 students enrolled in three different sections of an undergraduate psychology course were administered the *Trait Anxiety Inventory* (A Trait). From the distribution of A Trait scores, the lowest and highest 20% were selected as low and high anxiety groups. Eighteen low anxious (LA) and 21 high anxious (HA) individuals participated in, and completed, the study.

A middle-term academic examination in psychology was designed as the situational stressor, and students were assessed under baseline (3 days pre-exam), pre-exam stress (morning of exam), and poststress (immediately postexam) conditions. Blood was analyzed for whole blood serotonin content, plasma MHPG, and platelet imipramine binding.

Preselection of subjects produced high and low anxious groups that significantly differed on trait anxiety. In responding to each of the three assessment conditions, high anxious subjects experienced significantly greater state anxiety than did anxious subjects. Table 2 summarizes these group mean scores for state anxiety across stress conditions. Thus, students differed consistently in the degree of their anxiety, but the subjective impact of the stress condition was most apparent among the generally calm students (34).

Among the biological variables, only serotonin was significantly higher at baseline for high anxious subjects compared with low anxious subjects.Baseline levels of platelet imipramine binding and MHPG did not significantly differ on the trait anxiety (34). Mean values for serotonin levels (pmol/ml whole blood) by anxiety group are summarized in Table 3. From these data, it is apparent that serotonin levels increased from baseline to pre-exam conditions. Highly anxious students had consistently higher serotonin levels, but between-group differences were significant only at baseline. Within high and low anxious groups, sertonin levels were not significantly correlated with any of the psychological measures (34).

Table 3. Changes in blood serotonin levels to stress conditions.

Group	Baseline mean ± SD	Pre-exam mean ± SD	Paired t	Postexam mean ± SD
Serotonin (pmol/ml whole blood)				
Low anxious (n = 18)	745.06 ± 402.7	865.72 ± 350.8	2.87**	855.11 ± 346.05
high anxious (n = 21)	945.76 ± 310.3	1004.86 ± 303.7	2.33*	1029.38 ± 319.36
t	1.72*	1.31		1.62

* $p < 0.05$, ** $p < 0.001$. Adapted from Davis et al (34).

The findings of the increase in whole blood serotonin concentrations by Davis et al. (34) posssibly could be used both as a biological marker for trait anxiety as well as a state response to stress. This conclusion is at least partly supported by other studies. For example, in studies of normal subjects, including our own, blood serotonin concentrations are remarkably stable over time, suggesting blood serotonin levels could be used as a trait marker. Other investigators have also found evidence of serotonin increases in periods of stress during the pregynaecological or presurgical period, suggesting serotonin levels are also state-dependent.

In an interesting animal study involving adult male vervet monkeys (35), it was demonstrated that spontaneous and induced changes in socio-environmental variables altered serotonin levels in monkeys. In particular elevated blood serotonin concentrations were a state-dependent consequence of active occupation of the dominant male social position. Central serotonergic reactions to stress in humans have yet to be delineated, as the whole blood measures assessed in this study only provide information about peripheral activity.

Other recent evidence has linked anxiety states to the serotonergic system. It has been proposed that the anxiolytic actions of benzodiazepines may be mediated by their effects on serotonergic neurotransmission (36). For example, dorsal raphe neurons have been shown to have both "autoreceptors" for 5-HT and independent receptors for GABA (37, 38). Consistent with this finding is the fact that benzodiazepines significantly reduce 5-HT turnover in the central nervous system (39). In addition, iontophoretic or systemic administration of benzodiazepines inhibits raphe cell firing (40-42). This physiological effect is identical to the effect of the new antianxiety drug buspirone on raphe cell activity (43).

Behavioral effects of systemic benzodiazepines can also be reproduced by microinjections of the drugs into dorsal raphe nuclei (44). However, the benzodiazephines have no effect in the same system if 5-HT neurons are first destroyed by 5,7-dihydroxytryptamine. Furthermore, studies of *in vivo* (^{3}H)-5-HT release suggest that benzodiazepines act directly on 5-HT cell bodies to inhibit release of 5-HT, but have no effect on 5-HT cell terminals in the basal ganglia (45).

As reported by Peroutka (46), the antianxiety action of novel drugs such as buspirone and TVX Q 7821 may be related directly or indirectly to their effect on central 5-HT receptors. The possible mediation of the anxiolytic effects of buspirone and TVX Q 7821 by 5-HT$_{1A}$ receptors may elucidate the pathophysiology of anxiety. The 5-HT$_{1A}$ site has a distinct regional localization, with highest densities found in the hippocampus, portions of the frontal cortex, and on the dorsal raphe nuclei (47). Importantly, these receptors are minimally present in the basal ganglia, a finding that may account for their lack of significant extrapyramidal effects. These anxiolytic effects of buspirone and TVX Q 7821 may therefore relate to their selective effects on a localized sub-population of 5-HT receptors. Thus, more and more evidence is accumulated which suggests an important role for serotonin in anxiety-related disorders.

With regard to the overall approach to studying serotonin involvement in psychiatric disorders, we would like to introduce one word of caution. We have been discussing both central and peripheral serotonergic biochemistry. However, it is not clear what relationship (if any) exists betwen the central and peripheral compartments of the serotonin system in the body. The bulk of serotonin in the periphery is generated and stored in the enterochromafin cells of the GI tract as well as some in the smooth muscles of the lung, heart, kidney as well as the GI system. Blood serotonin levels and urinary 5-HIAA are primarily related to the secretion of the serotonin by the enterochromafin cells (and of course the uptake system of the platelet) which are under complicated control mechanisms involving local factors (like acid secretion) as well as neuronal control from the vagal and splanchnic nerves. We are now conducting research on animal models to try to understand better the relationship between these central and peripheral events.

References

1. Aprison, M.H., Takahashi, R. & Tachiki, K. (1978). Hypersensitive serotonergic receptors involved in clinical depression - A theory. In B. Haber & M.H. Aprison (Eds.), Neuropharmacology and behavior. Plenum Press, N.Y., p. 23-53.
2. Aprison, M.H. & Hingtgen, J.N. (1981). Hypersensitive serotonergic receptors: A new hypothesis for one subgroup of unipolar depression derived from an animal model. In B. Haber, S. Gabay, M.R. Issidorides & S.G.A. Alivisatos (Eds.), Serotonin: Current aspects of neurochemistry and function. Plenum, N.Y, p. 627-656.
3. Nagayama, H., Hingtgen, J.N. & Aprison, M.H. (1980). Pre- and postsynaptic serotonergic manipulations in an animal model of depression. Pharmacol. Biochem. Behav., 13: 575-579.
4. Nagayama, H., Hingtgen, J.N. & Aprison, M.H. (1981). Postsynaptic action by four antidepressive drugs in an animal model of depression. Pharmacol. Biochem. Behav., 15: 125-130.
5. Hingtgen, J.N., Hendrie, H.C. & Aprison, M.H. (1984). Postsynaptic serotonergic blockade following chronic antidepressive treatment with trazodone in an animal model of depression. Pharmacol. Biochem. Behav., 20: 425-428.
6. Hingtgen, J.N., Fuller, R.W., Mason, N.R. & Aprison, M.H. (1985). Blockade of a 5-hydroxytryptphan induced animal model of depression with a potent and selective 5-HT_2 receptor antagonist (LY53857). Biol. Psychiat., 20: 592-597.
7. Aprison, M.H. & Hingtgen, J.N. (1970). Neurochemical correlates of behavior. Inter. Rev. Neurobiol., 13: 325-341.
8. Hingtgen, J.N., Gerometta, J.S. & Aprison, M.H. (1984). Behavioral stress enhances sensitivity to 5-hydroxytryptophan administration in animal model of depression. Fed. Proc., 43: 572.
9. Aprison, M.H. & Hingtgen, J.N. (1984). Is depression related to postsynaptic serotonergic hypersensitivity? Proc. Am. Soc. Neurochem., 3: 11-12.
10. Aprison, M.H. & Ferster, C.B. (1961). Neurochemical correlates of behavior. I. Quantitative measurement of the behavioral effects of serotonin precursor, 5-hydroxytryptophan. J. Pharmacol. Exp. Ther., 131: 100-107.
11. Aprison, M.H. & Ferster, C.B. (1961). Neurochemical corrrelates of behavior. II. Correlation of brain monoamine oxidase activity with behavioral changes after iproniazid and 5-hydroxytryptophan administration. J. Neurochem., 6: 350-357.
12. Aprison, M.H., Wolf, M.A., Poulus, G.L. & Folkerth, T.L. (1962). Neurochemical correlates of behavior. III. Variation of serotonin content in several brain areas and peripheral tissues of the pigeon following 5-hydroxytryptophan administration. J. Neurochem, 9: 575-584.
13. Aprison, M.H. & Hingtgen, J.N. (1965). Neurochemical corelates of behavior. IV. Norepinephrine and dopamine in four brain parts of the pigeon during period of atypical behavior following the injection of 5-hydroxytryptophan. J. Neurochem., 12: 959-968.
14. Fleisher, L.N., Simon, J.R. & Aprison, M.H. (1979). A biochemical-behavioral model for studying serotonergic supersensitivity in brain. J. Neurochem., 32: 1613-1620.
15. Ogren, S.O., Fuxe, K., Agnati, L.F., Gustafsson, J.A., Jonsson, G. & Holm, A.C. (1979). Reevaluation of the indoleamine hypothesis of depression. Evidence for a reduction of functional activity of central 5-HT systems for antidepressant drugs. J. Neurol. Trans., 46: 85-103.
16. Aprison, M.H., Hingtgen, J.N. & Nagayama, H. (1982). Testing a new theory of depression with an animal model: Neurochemical-behavioral evidence for postsynaptic serotonergic receptor involvement. In S. Langer, R. Takahashi, T. Segawa & M. Briley (Eds.), New vistas in depression. Pergamon Press, N.Y., p. 171-178.
17. Aprison, M.H. & Hingtgen, J.N. (1983). Postsynaptic serotonergic action of antidepressive drugs. Behav. Brain Sci., 4: 549-551.
18. Fuller, R.W. & Snoddy, H.D. (1979). The effects of metergoline and other serotonin receptor antagonists on serum corticosterone in rats. Endocrinology, 105: 923-928.
19. Cohen, M.L., Fuller, R.W. & Kurz, K.D. (1983). LY53857, a selective and potent serotonergic (5-HT_2) receptor antagonist, does not lower blood pressure in the spontaneously hypertensive rat. Pharmacol. Exp. Ther., 227: 327-332.
20. Pare, W.P., Vincent, G.P., Ison, K.E. & Reeves, J.M. (1978). Restricted feeding and incidences of activity-stress ulcers in the rat. Bull. Psychoneurol. Sci., 12: 143-146.
21. Hellhammer, D.H., Hingtgen, J.N., Wade, S.E., Shea, P.A. & Aprison, M.H. (1983). Serotonergic changes in specific areas of rat brain associated with activity-stress gastric lesions. Psychosom. Med., 45: 115-122.
22. Van Praag, H.M. (1982). Depression. The Lancet, 2: 1259-1264.
23. Stanley, M. & Mann, J.J. (1983). Increased serotonin-2 binding sites in frontal cortex of suicide victims. The Lancet, 1: 214-216.

24. Perry, E.K., Marshall, E.F., Blessed, G., Tomlinson, B.E. & Perry, R.H. (1983). Decreased imipramine binding in the brains of patients with depressive illness. Brit. J. Psychiat., 142: 188-192.
25. Stahl, S.M., Ciaranello, R.D. & Berger, P.A. (1982). Platelet serotonin in schizophrenia and depression. In B.T. Ho, J.C. Schooler & E. Ursin (Eds.), Serotonin in Biological Psychiatry. Raven Press, N.Y., p. 183-198.
26. DeMyer, M.K., Shea, P.A., Hendrie, H.C. & Yoshimura, N.N. (1981). Plasma tryptophan and five other amino acids in depressed and normal subjects. Arch. Gen. Psychiat., 38: 642-646.
27. Lewis, D.A. & McChesney, C. (1985). Tritiated imipramine binding distinguishes among subtypes of depression. Arch. Gen. Psychiat., 42: 485-488.
28. Meltzer, H.Y., Umberkoman-Wiita, B., Robertson, A., Tricou, B.J., Lowy, M. & Perline, R. (1984). Effect of 5-hydroxytryptophan on serum cortisol levels in major affective disorders. I. Enhanced response in depression and mania. Arch. Gen. Psychiat., 41: 366-374.
29. Heninger, G.R., Charney, D.S. & Sternberg, D.E. (1984). Serotonergic function in depression. Prolactin response to intravenous tryptophan in depressed patients and healthy subjects. Arch. Gen. Psychiat., 41: 398-402.
30. Meltzer, H.Y., Koenig, J.T., Lowy, M., Koyama, T. & Robertson, A.G. (1985). Serotonergic neuroendocrine challenges in affective disorders. Proc. World Congr. Biol. Psychiat., 4: 355.
31. Solomon, H.M., Ashley, C., Spirt, N.M. & Abrams, W.B. (1969). The human platelet as model for dopaminergic neurons. Clin. Pharmacol. Ther., 10: 229-238.
32. Stahl, S.M. & Meltzer, H.Y. (1978). The human platelet as a model for the dopaminergic neurone: Kinetic and pharmacologic properties and the role of amine storage granules. Exp. Neurol., 59: 1-15.
33. DeLisi, L.E., Neckers, L.M., Weinberger, D.R. & Wyatt, R.J. (1981). Increased whole blood serotonin concentrations in chronic schizophrenic patients. Arch. Gen. Psychiat., 38: 647-650.
34. Davis, D.D., Dunlop, S.R., Shea, P., Brittain, H. & Hendrie, H.C. (1985). Biological stress responses in high and low trait anxious students. Biol. Psychiat., 20: 843-851.
35. Raleigh, M.J., McGuire, M.T., Brammer, G.L. & Yuwiler, A. (1984). Social and environmental influences on blood serotonin concentrations in monkeys. Arch. Gen. Psychiat., 41:405-410.
36. Stein, L., Belluzzi, J.D. & Wise, C.D. (1977). Benzodiazeptines: Behavioral and neurochemical mechanisms. Am. J. Psychiat., 134: 665-669.
37. Gallager, D.W. & Aghajanian, G.K. (1976). Effect of antipsychiotic drugs on the firing of dorsal raphe cells. II. Reversal by picrotoxin. Eur. J. Pharmacol., 39: 357-364.
38. Wang, R.Y. & Aghajanian, G.K. (1977). Physiological evidence for habenula as major link between forebrain and midbrainÞ+8Xraphe. Science, 197: 89-91.
39. Wise, C.D., Berger, B.D. & Stein, L. (1972). Benzodiazepines: Anxiety reducing activity by reduction of serotonin turnover in the brain. Science, 177: 180-183.
40. Gallager, D.W. (1978). Benzodiazepines: Potentiation of a GABA inhibitory response in the dorsal raphe nucleus. Eur. J. Pharmacol., 49: 133-143.
41. Hunkeler, W., Mohler, H., Pieri, L., Pole, P., Bonnestti, E.F., Cumin, R., Schaffner, R. & Haefely, W. (1981). Selective antagonists of benzodiazepines. Nature, 290: 514-516.
42. Trulson, M.E., Preussler, D.W., Howell, G.A. & Frederickson, C.J. (1982). Raphe unit activity in freely moving cats: Effects of benzodiazepines. Neuropharmacology, 21: 1045-1050.
43. Van der Maelen, C.P. & Wilderman, R.C. (1984). Iontophoretic and systemic administration of the nonbenzodiazepine anxiolytic drug buspirone causes inhibition of serotonergic dorsal raphe neurons in rats. Fed. Proc., 43: 947.
44. Thiebot, M.H., Hamon, M. & Soubrié, P. (1982). Attenuation of induced anxiety in rats by chlordiazepoxide: Role of raphe dorsalis benzodiazepine binding sites and serotonergic neurons. Neuroscience, 7: 2287-2294.
45. Soubrié, P., Blas, C., Ferron, A. & Glowinski, J. (1983). Chlordiazepoxide reduces in vivo serotonin release in the basal ganglia of encephale isole but not anesthetized cats: Evidence for a dorsal raphe site of action. J. Pharmacol. Exp. Ther., 226: 526-532.
46. Peroutka, S.J. (1985). Selective interaction of novel anxiolytics with 5-hydroxytryptamine$_{1A}$ receptors. Biol. Psychiat., 20: 971-979.
47. Marcinkiewicz, M., Verge, D., Gozlan, H., Pichat, L. & Hamon, M. (1984). Autoradiographic evidence for the heterogeneity of 5-HT$_1$ sites in the rat brain. Brain Res., 291: 159-163.

Discussion of Brain Systems as Mediators Between Behavior and Bodily Disease: Implications from a Psychological Viewpoint

Petra Netter

The present discussion will focus (1) on some general aspects inherent in studies designed to elucidate relationships between transmitter functions and behavior; (2) on the special aspect of biochemical identification of subgroups and (3) on future questions of research raised by the three papers. Since psychological aspects will dominate this part of the discussion, there will be more emphasis on individual differences and the catecholaminergic system as presented in Zuckerman's paper and less reference to the clinical and experimental data presented by Hendrie et al. and Cools. But this deficit will be compensated by Wesemann's discussion from the neurobiological viewpoint.

General Aspects

The papers discussed within the broad section of "brain systems as mediators between behavior and bodily disease" cover very different areas of neuropsychological research (clinical symptomatology in patients, Hendrie et al.; molecular behavior in animals, Cools; and personality dimensions in healthy subjects, Zuckerman). Moreover, they represent different scientific approaches ranging from strictly experimental manipulations of brain transmitter systems by chemical or surgical techniques to clinical observations and correlational analyses between psychiatric symptomatology, response to treatment or questionnaire scores on the one hand and biochemical data on the other. Finally they focus on different transmitter systems (serotonin, Hendrie et al.; dopamine (DA), Cools; and the noradrenergic (NE) system represented by platelet monoamine oxidase (MAO) and cerebral dopamine-betahydroxylase (DBH), Zuckerman).

Yet the three papers and the studies they report have some common problems: All three papers more or less explicitly demonstrated that three major difficulties are inherent in establishing cause/effect relationships between neurotransmitter processes and behavior:

1) Multidimensional relationships between stimuli and neurotransmitters as well as between neurotransmitters and behavior obscure straightforward inference as indicated in Figure 1.
(a) On the one hand different chemical compounds, sleep deprivation or electrical stimulation may be equally potent in eliciting the same

neurotransmitter increase or decrease and on the other hand one stimulus may effect several neurotransmitter changes at the same time.
(b) The same neurotransmitter increase or decrease may be related to different behavioral effects and one type of behavioral response, like increase in motor activity or decrease in depressive mood may be related to a variety of neurotransmitter and neuropeptide changes.

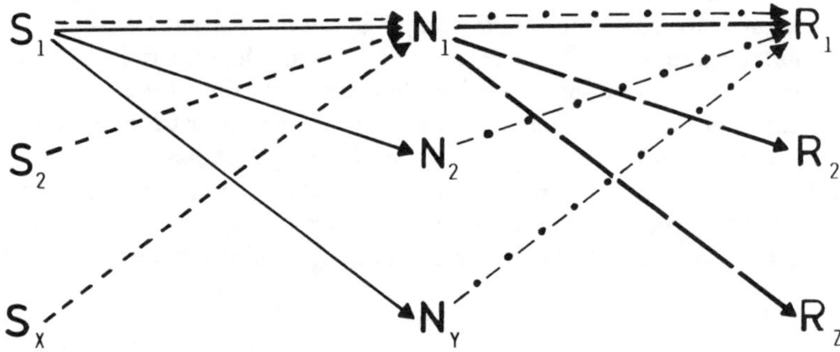

Figure 1. Graphic representation of possible relationships between stimuli ($S_1 ... S_x$), neurotransmitters ($N_1 ... N_y$) and behavioral responses ($R_1 ... R_z$).

2) Different behavioral effects are elicited by the same neurotransmitter released in different areas of the brain. This has particularly been demonstrated by Cools' paper on DA related behavior which differs according to whether neostriatal or limbic DA is manipulated.

3) Feedback loops between different systems compensate for deficits or surplus of neurotransmitter release or electrophysiological arousal. This kind of homeostatic counterbalance may not only be observed in different levels of the limbic-hypothalamic pituitary-adrenal (LHPA) axis (as discussed later in this volume) but also in α_2 receptor mediated inhibition of NE release upon increase of NE supply at the pre- and postsynaptic membranes. It also can effect receptor up- or down-regulation depending upon the amount of NE or 5-hydroxytryptamine (5-HT) at the postsynaptic receptor.

In response to these difficulties two general messages may be derived from all three papers:

1) The question to be asked about the role of transmitters in modulating behavior is no longer "Which transmitter is responsible for which kind of behavior?", but "Under which conditions and to what extent does a certain

transmitter or peptide contribute to a certain behavior?", which is linked to the question "Under which conditions may the transmitter act as a transmitter, a modulator or a hormone?", as pointed out by Cools.

2) Defining subgroups of individuals according to experimental conditions as well as to dispositional variables seems a promising approach to explain conflicting results in psychobiology because environmental as well as organismic variables to a large extent determine the quality and quantity of behavioral change elicited by changes in neurotransmitter output.

With regard to the *first message*, the following points should be considered: One of the conditions modifying behavioral effects of transmitter activity is, of course, location of neuronal nuclei and pathways. Thus, for example, dopaminergic functions, such as neurosecretory, motor and emotion-related functions have been demonstrated to be governed by tuberoinfundibular, nigrostriatal and mesolimbic pathways respectively (cf. 1). The concept contributed by *Cools'* experiments, however, demonstrates that the organismic response is determined by principles beyond a mere correspondence between localization and behavioral function. One of these was Cools' observation that chemically induced depletion of DA in the striatum did not result in simple blockade of behavior but in a change of behavior quality. Aspects like flexibility or capacity to change behavioral strategies proved to be promising interpretations of his results obtained by application of DA agonists or antagonists like apomorphine or haloperidol to the striatum. Furthermore, he could demonstrate that external factors were additionally relevant for determining whether the animal after inhibition of DA receptors was deprived of the capacity to switch his behavior by selecting the best behavior strategy for survival, since it was only in the absence of external cues that this ability was disrupted.

Another external condition relevant for DA modulated behavior is time of day which has been investigated with respect to its modification of DA induced hyperlocomotion after 6-hydroxydomamine (6-OHDA) induced ventral tegmental lesions (2, 3). Its dependence on type of stimulus (novel vs. habituated) could be demonstrated by Oades et al. (4).

An additional internal condition required for maintaining adaptive behavior could be shown to be intactness of corticostriatal glutaminergic input, as demonstrated by experimental evidence in Cools' presentation.

In *Hendrie, Aprison and Hingtgen's* contribution this question of modulating conditions for the causal relationship between neurotransmitter discharge and metabolism on the one hand and behavior on the other is put forward by asking which environmental events and biological states may be responsible for onset, maintenance and termination of affective illness episodes.Their theory on the role of serotonin in depression is an example of the way in which conflicting results can be explained by a common theory, if the course of regulatory processes within transmitter systems are taken into account. Thus the authors' interpretation of dispositionally low serotonin causing 5-HT-receptor supersensitivity with subsequent development of hyperreactions to any surplus of stress or 5-HTP induced serotonin release leading to depression could explain why in some individuals, 5-HT-precursors or reuptake inhibitors as well as postsynaptic-5-HT blockers may be effective in ameliorating depressive symptoms. Reduction of postsynaptic 5-HT levels as well as substrate induced postsynaptic 5-HT receptor down-regulation leads to the same desired effect.

Their contribution also revealed that these types of feedback loops not only operate in one transmitter system but represent mechanisms of functional linkage between the serotonergic and adrenergic systems.

Finally, the findings discussed by *Zuckerman* on correlations between plasma transmitter enzyme levels or cerebrospinal fluid (CSF) transmitter metabolite levels and sensation-seeking or psychopathy seem to raise puzzling questions on seemingly contradicting results similar to the ones observed with mutually antagonistic drugs in patient therapy reported by Hendrie et al. The findings of low homovanillic acid (HVA) in CSF and low plasma DBH suggest low DA brain levels if plasma DBH values may be taken (1) as indicators of brain levels, and (2) these again as indicators of low substrate supply. Low serotonin supply of the brain, on the other hand, is suggested by low 5-hydroxy-indoleaminoacid (5-H-IAA) levels in CSF and by low MAO B in platelets, if platelet MAO may be taken as an indicator of MAO B activity in the brain which is relevant for 5-HT-degradation. Thus, since both DA and 5-HT brain levels are negatively correlated to sensation-seeking or psychopathy, the puzzling question is raised why these two transmitter systems, generally associated with rather contrasting types of behavior, are correlated with the same personality dimension. So also these findings demonstrate that it would be wrong to associate certain transmitters linearly with certain types of behavior. Rather it seems that the (genetic?) transmitter deficit has probably produced compensatory behavior strategies, sensation-seeking possibly representing a coping behavior of the organism to counteract transmitter deficiency induced susceptibility to depression.

The *second message* emerging as a common idea in the three papers, which may help to explain contradicting results was the idea of identifying subtypes.

This idea was demonstrated by *Cools'* findings on different DA-NE-mechanisms characterizing animals of the submissive and the fleeing type of behavior, and by his observation that animals divided into responders and nonresponders according to reactions to NE receptor agonist injections into the nucleus accumbens could be changed with respect to their biochemical response as well as their behavior after having been exposed to a noncoping situation (being confronted with an aggression-provoking animal without the possibility of fighting).

These results nicely demonstrate that (1) dispositional differences of behavior may be reflected by different responsivity of noradrenergic receptors, and (2) environmental exposure to defined stimuli like the noncoping situation may change biochemical reactivity via homeostatic processes exerted on noradrenergic receptors by the nucleus accumbens.

Similarly, the need for analyzing subtypes of the population was demonstrated by *Hendrie et al.'s* discussion of the bimodal distribution of 5-HIAA in CSF of depressed patients, suggesting that deficient serotonergic functioning and resulting hypersensitivity of 5-HT receptors in a subgroup of depressed patients may serve as a predictor of differential antidepressant drug response to

5-HT-reuptake inhibitors as indicated by results reported by Van Praag (5). Thus, identification of subgroups was demonstrated to be a useful tool in explaining differences in patients' drug responses.

Finally, *Zuckerman's* data demonstrating correlational relationships between sensation-seeking and impulsivity on the one hand and several biological markers like low platelet MAO, low plasma DBH, low 5-HIAA in CSF and high testosterone levels on the other gave rise to the hypothesis that different sensation-seeking subscales, depending on their loading with antisocial and aggressive behavior, may be differently related to the serotonergic and dopaminergic system.

Since serotonin deficiency reported in clinical CSF studies has been more clearly related to the aggressive component of impulsivity, it should be worthwhile to investigate which subscales or behavioral characteristics are particularly related to low DBH levels.

Furthermore, the role of the noradrenergic system in sensation-seeking is rather unclear. On the one hand low NE levels should result from low DBH levels, but, as Zuckerman reported, MHPG levels in CSF were not clearly related to the clinical and behavioral symptoms typical for high impulsivity. Therefore in the following section an experiment will be reported which correlates epinephrine/norepinephrine levels and responses to the impulsivity dimension.

Identifying Impulsivity Subtypes by Biochemical Parameters

Since identification of subtypes as described in the previous section is a promising approach for elucidating the biological basis of individual differences, an example is demonstrated by which the broad concept of sensation-seeking and impulsivity may be subdivided according to biochemical parameters.

Impulsivity in the literature on personality dimensions is on the one hand conceived as an axis between the two orthogonal dimensions of neuroticism and extraversion which, according to Gray's concept (6) is related to susceptibility to reward as opposed to anxiety, which is located between neuroticism and the introversion pole of the extra-introversion dimension and being characterized by susceptibility to punishment. On the other hand, factor-analytic studies based on Eysenck's impulsivity scales (7) revealed their additional relation to the third dimension in the Eysenck personality system, namely psychoticism which is mainly characterized by antisocial behavior. Furthermore, four subfactors emerged which in a large correlational study on 430 pairs of twins by Martin et al. (8) were correlated with Zuckerman's four subscales of sensation-seeking and with the main personality dimensions extraversion-introversion (E), neuroticism (N), and psychoticism (P) of Eysenck's personality system. Similarities between two of the Eysenck impulsivity subfactors and two of the sensation-seeking scale factors could be established by their similarities in correlation patterns with E, N, P, and the lie scale L as represented by their sign patterns obtained in the male sample in Table 1.

Table 1. Correlation patterns of impulsivity subscales with P, E, N, L.

	Impulsivity Eysenck and Eysenck (1977/78)		Subscales		According Zuckerman (1976)			To
	Impuls "Narrow"	Risk Taking	Non-Planning	Live-liness	TAS	ES	DIS	BS
P	+	+	+	0	0	+	+	+
E	0	+	0	+	(+)	0	+	0
N	+	0	(-)	-	-	0	0	0
L	(-)	0	0	0	0	0	-	0

+ = positive, - = negative, 0 = no correlation, ( ) not observed in male sample of Martin, Eaves and Fulker (8).

TAS = Thrill and Adventure Seeking
ES = Experience Seeking
DIS = Disinhibition
BS = Boredom Susceptibility

P = Psychoticism
E = Extraversion
N = Neuroticism
L = Lie Scale

Table 2. Frequencies of cases classified according to their norepinephrine (NE) and epinephrine (E) response to pain and mental stress.

Reaction to Pain (NE E)	Reaction To Arithmetic Stress I: NE + (+) / E + +	NE + (+) + / E - - 0	NE - 0 (-) / E + + +	NE - (-) (-) 0 / E - - 0 -	Total	Type
+ + (+) +	7	4	1	6	18	1
+ - (+) - + 0	3	3	0	2	8	2
- + 0 + (-) +	1	3	3	6	13	3
- - (-) - (-) 0 0 -	1	2	0	2	5	4
Total	12	12	4	16	44	

+ = increase > 10%   - = decrease > 10%   0 = no change
(+) = increase < 10%   (-) = decrease < 10%

Another approach to subfactors is the definition of subgroups according to biochemical response patterns in a given experimental situation and relating these types to personality dimensions derived from questionnaire scores. This approach was applied to a set of data obtained in an experiment devoted to the study of plasma catecholamine response to stress and alcohol. Subjects were divided according to their plasma epinephrine (E) and norepinephrine (NE) responses to the pain of venipuncture as compared to a baseline obtained after one hour of rest. They were then classified according to patterns of increase (+), as compared to resting levels, or no increase (-) of each of the two hormones. The same procedure was performed for the subjects' response to mental arithmetic stress, resulting in the combined frequencies given in Table 2.

While comparisons of the four groups represented by the marginal sums of rows (=response types to mental stress) did not show substantial relations to impulsivity subscales, the pain response types displayed some interesting impulsivity related personality differences: Response types E+NE+ vs. E-NE- and types E+NE- vs. E-NE+ were compared with respect to their performance scores on a mental arithmetic test, their anxiety and aggression self ratings in the experiment, their trait scores on the Eysenck E, N, and impulsivity scales as well as on the Zuckerman sensation-seeking scales. Variables yielding significant differences between the two types within each pair of catecholamine types are listed in Table 3.

The table reveals that personality differences represent correlates of E, N, and P which closely resemble two of the impulsivity types listed in Table 2. The NE+E+ pain responder type 1, as compared to the NE-E- type 4 displays a behavior pattern similar to the Eysenck impulsivity type "in the narrow sense," a subtype showing neurotic anxiety as well as psychoticism related behavior. The NE-E+ type 3 as opposed to the NE+E- type 2 pain responder may be identified as a combination of Zuckerman's adventure seeker and disinhibitor or Eysenck's risk taking type and liveliness type characterized by a stable (non-neurotic) extraverted personality, however also high in psychoticism.

Although plasma catecholamines may not be related to MAO and DBH levels in the brain, and although the present subtypes in this investigation could not be characterized by their serotonergic activities (which would elucidate its relevance for the P component) or by their dopaminergic response (which might represent the dimension of susceptibility to reward as indicated by intracranial self stimulation experiments in rats; (9)), the response patterns of the two catecholamines to the painful injection of the catheter seem to reflect the controlled behavior of the neurotic type in the case of the NE+E+ response and loss of control in the case of the NE-E+ pattern, as reflected by the happy-go-lucky type with high adventure seeking and disinhibition scores.

The evaluation suggests that intraindividual relationships of monoamines rather than single parameters or linear combinations of scores should be analyzed when defining subtypes. Furthermore, the approach of starting from the biochemical response instead of from the personality dimension could be demonstrated to provide additional information on the possible behavioral concomitants of monoamine constellations.

Table 3: Variables yielding significant differences between two pairs of contrasting catecholamine response types to painful venipuncture (p values obtained by Student's t-Tests).

	Reaction	To Pain	
Psychological variable	NE E + + (n = 18) Type: 1	NE E - - (n = 5) Type: 4	significance p
Impulsivity (EPI)	high	low	0.001
Performance (no. of items)			
Test I: easy items	high	low	0.054
diff. items	high	low	0.029
Test II: easy items	high	low	0.019
State anxiety at test II	increase	decrease	0.002
Aggressiveness during 2nd half of experiment	constant	decrease	0.061

	Reaction	To Pain	
Psychological variable	NE E - + (n = 13) Type: 3	NE E + - (n = 8) Type: 2	significance p
Extraversion	high	low	0.043
Sensation-seeking total	high	low	0.056
Sensation-seeking TAS	high	low	0.038
Sensation-seeking DIS	high	low	0.025
Habitual alc. consump.	high	low	0.003
Performance test I (% errors) diff. items	bad	good	0.072
State anxiety test I	little incr.	large incr.	0.004
State anxiety test II	little incr.	large incr.	0.016
Mean elation score	high	low	0.007
Elation with test II	increase	decrease	0.024

Questions Relevant for Psychological Research Arising from the Presentations on Transmitters and Behavior

1) Cools' findings suggest
   (a) the elaboration of a possible correspondence between the neostriatal function described as the capacity "to shift ongoing behavior until the actual

situation matches the desired situation" and the septo-hippocampal comparator system as described by Gray (10). One might speculate that the neostriatal system is the effector analogue to the septo-hippocampal system which matches sensory input with internal expectations.
(b) A second point of interest arising from Cools' contribution is whether different types of experimentally induced coping behavior or noncoping situations would elicit different changes in noradrenergic response, since it seems worthwhile to relate the nucleus accumbens' adaptive capacity to Henry and Stephens' concept of the septum-hippocampus-related submissive and amygdala-related dominant behavior (11).

2) Questions emerging from Hendrie et al's presentation would concern further elucidation of the relationship between depression, anxiety, and aggression, since they all seem to be affected by the serotonergic system. If - as has also been suggested by Zuckerman's paper - low 5-HT activity and resulting hypersensitivity of 5-HT receptors is indicative of high vulnerability, the question should be raised as to the biochemical and psychological state and trait conditions which determine whether depression, antisocial behavior or panic attacks will be triggered by low 5-HT activity and resulting hypersensitivity of 5-HT receptors.

3) Zuckerman's data, being most closely related to personality research, raise many interesting issues to be taken up by future research on individual differences:
(a) A major question is whether the psychological relationships reported for the trait aspect would also hold for state variables. This question suggests experiments in which MAO inhibitors or NE reuptake inhibitors on the one hand and dopamine agonists on the other would be applied in order to test whether low DBH reflects accumulation of DA or low supply of DA as the NE precursor, and hence whether increase of DA or of NE could change sensation-seeking behavior. Similarly, 5-HT agonists and antagonists could be tested with respect to their effects on MAO levels and on reducing or increasing the subject's motivation for sensation-seeking activities. Results of this kind would help to answer the question whether the biochemical correlates of sensation-seeking are to be considered as genetic markers or as indicators of functional transmitter deficiencies.
(b) Analyses of the type illustrated by our own data could try to identify patterns of MAO-, DBH-, NE-, and 5-HT deficiencies and to relate these to different sensation-seeking and impulsivity subscales as has been tried by Kulczar et al. (12).
(c) Since low MAO in platelets is also observed in bipolar depression the relationship between depressive and impulsive reactions should be investigated with respect to further biochemical parameters suitable to predict the type of pathological behavior to be expected.
(d) Finally, the biochemical concommitants of the sensation seekers' reward should be identified in appropriate experimental conditions.

References

1. Taylor, D.P., Riblet, L.A., Stanton, H.C., Eison, A.S., Eison, M.S. & Temple, D.L.Jr. (1982). Dopamine and antianxiety activity. Dopamine receptors and their behavioral correlates. Pharmacol. Biochem. Behav., Suppl.1, 17: 25-35.
2. Joyce, E.M. (1980). On the nature and the function of the mesotelencephalic dopamine neurone system. Unpubl. Ph. D. Thesis, Cambridge Univ.
3. Brundin, P., Gage, F.H., Dunnet, S.B. & Bjoklund, A. (1985). Longterm locomotor and cognitive deficits in rats with 6-OHDA lesions of the ventral tegmental area: A model for transplantation studies. In C. Woodruff (Ed.), Dopaminergic systems and their regulation. McMillan Press, London.
4. Oades, R.D., Taghzouti, K., Rivet, J.M., Simon, H. & Le Moal, M. (1986). Locomotor activity in relation to dopamine and noradrenaline in the nucleus accumbens septal and frontal areas: A 6-hydroxydopamine study. Neuropsychobiology, 16: 37-42.
5. Van Praag, H.M. (1981). Central monoamines and the pathogenesis of depression. In M. van Praag, M. Lader, O.J. Raffaelson & E.J. Sachar, Handbook of biological psychiatry IV: Brain mechanisms and abnormal behavior. Marcel Dekker, N.Y., p. 159-205.
6. Gray, J.A. (1972). The psychophysiological nature of introversion-extraversion. A modification of Eysenck's theory. In V.D. Neblitsyn & J.A. Gray (Eds.), Biological basis of individual behavior. Academic Press, London.
7. Eysenck, S.B.G. & Eysenck, H.J. (1978). Impulsiveness and venture-someness: Their position in a dimensional system of personality description. Psychol. Rep., 43: 1247-1255.
8. Martin, N.G., Eaves, L.J. & Fulker, D.V. (1979). The genetical relationship of impulsiveness and sensation-seeking to Eysenck's personality dimensions. Acta Genet. Med. Gemellol., 28: 197-210.
9. Mason, S.T. (1984). Catecholamines and behavior. Cambridge Univ. Press, Cambridge.
10. Gray, J.A. (1982). The neurophysiology of anxiety: An inquiry into the functions of the septo-hippocampal system. Clarendon Press, Oxford.
11. Henry, J.P. & Stephens, P.M. (1977). Stress, health, and the social environment, a sociobiologic approach to medicine. Springer-Verlag, Berlin.
12. Kulcsár, Z., Fogarassy, E. & Arató, M. (1986). Sensation-seeking, paired associate learning and brain catecholamines. Neuropsychobiology, 15: 43-48.

Brain Systems as Mediators Between Behavior and Bodily Disease

Wolfgang Wesemann

The discovery and characterization of Otto Loewi's vagus and acceleration substances were followed by a period of intense activity in neurobiology. Meanwhile the concept of chemical transmission of nerve impulses was consolidated. The neuronal systems were mapped according to the transmitter substance. Experiments were performed to elucidate the mechanisms of neurotransmission on the molecular level including the transmitter substances, their transport, and metabolism as well as the receptors and the signal transducing systems like ion channels, cyclic AMP or protein kinase C. This type of research was performed in many laboratories and was assumed to be the most straightforward approach for the understanding of brain function. Though our knowledge about the transmitter systems is still insufficient, it soon turned out that this strategy would provide only an incomplete picture as long as the effects of endogenous and exogenous factors on the neuronal systems were neglected. Apparently the brain does not consist simply of neuronal systems each well-defined by a specific neurotransmitter.

I would like to mention briefly only a few factors which influence the function of the neuronal systems. Intensified studies of these factors will be a promising trend in neurobiology.

1) It was realized that different neurotransmitter systems interact with each other. If the activity of one transmitter system is changed, other systems will also affected. Moreover, as Cools pointed out in his lecture, we cannot define a neuronal system only in terms of its transmitter. There is accumulating evidence that there exists, e.g., more than one serotonergic or dopaminergic system. Strictly speaking, in addition to its neurotransmitter each neuronal system has to be characterized by other parameters like morphology, physiology or behavioral response.
2) Already several decades ago the coexistence of more than one neural active substance in one neuron was discovered by histochemical techniques. This finding implicates that the same neuron may release different neurotransmitters at different synapses. The action of coexisting neuroactive substances simultaneously released from a neuron may modify the information content of the neuron.
3) Besides acting as a transmitter, the same substance may have different other functions acting for instance as a neuromodulator or a hormone.

These are only three endogenous parameters which suggest that some basic programms must be given to regulate the interaction of different neuronal systems and to coordinate the function of different neurotransmitters. Moreover, the neuronal systems are affected by other factors, e.g., by hormones. Despite the tremendous development of neuroendocrinology our knowledge about the basic programs maintaining the interior milieu are rather scarce.

4) In addition to the endogenous factors mentioned above, the actions of the neuronal systems are changed by external stimuli. The mutual interaction between behavior and neuronal systems is well known. The observation that different individuals react differently to the same stimulus is in accordance with the concept that either the individuals differ in their basic programs or that the basic programs are differently affected. Another explanation for the various reactions of different individuals to the same stimulus could be given by a modification of the concept of Cannon and Hess: The basic programs are given; however, individual subprograms can be developed according to the demands of the environment. The organism develops new programs according to new inputs coming from a changing environment which leads to a behavioral response. But also manipulation of the neuronal program causes variations in the behavioral pattern. The interdependence of internal program and external stimuli was illustrated in Zuckerman's paper. The same manipulation, depletion of serotonin, produces either aggressive or fearful responses depending on the environment - familiar colony and unfamiliar, non-social environment, respectively.

I mentioned only a few parameters - interaction of neuronal systems, storage of different neuroactive substances in one neuron, regulation by hormones, and mutual interaction of internal programs and external stimuli. All these parameters complicate our brain model. But I think that the presentations of Zuckerman and Cools did show that the assessment of behavior and personality traits can help to understand the basic neuronal mechanisms and the underlying programs. Speaking about the catecholaminergic systems, Cools described how information, which is sent by the caudate nucleus downstream in the hierarchy of the central nervous system, is successively transformed at each level. At each level more details are added about the behavior to be executed.

Behavior is, according to Powers's definition, a process by which the organization i±side the organism controls its input. I think it is an interesting problem to study at which level incoming signals are discriminated and separated into signals which are suppressed, i.e., not followed by an internal reaction or a behavioral response, and those signals which trigger behavioral reactions.

Research work performed to elucidate the neurobiological basis of behavior follows two divergent but closely related lines. At one end of the spectrum neurotransmitters, receptors, and subcellular fractions are studied and at the other, studies of behavior in health and disease. The new theories of depression developed at the Medical School of Indiana University try to bridge the gap between studies on the molecular level and behavioral disturbances as we learned in the lecture of Hendrie. The studies performed in Indiana can help to understand the biochemical basis as well as the treatment of endogenous depression.

I would like to give just one example from our laboratory to illustrate how the concept, that supersensitve 5-HT[1] receptors are involved in depressive episodes, triggers work in this field.

It is well known that in some patients with depression the depressive episode can be overcome by sleep deprivation. In order to elucidate the mode of action of sleep deprivation, rats were sleep deprived for 12-72 hours. Since brain 5-HT and 5-hydroxyindoleacetic acid levels were only moderately affected, high affinity binding of 5-HT to crude brain membrane fractions was assayed (1). As compared with the controls, high affinity 5-HT binding was decreased by about 50% after sleep deprivation (Figure 1).

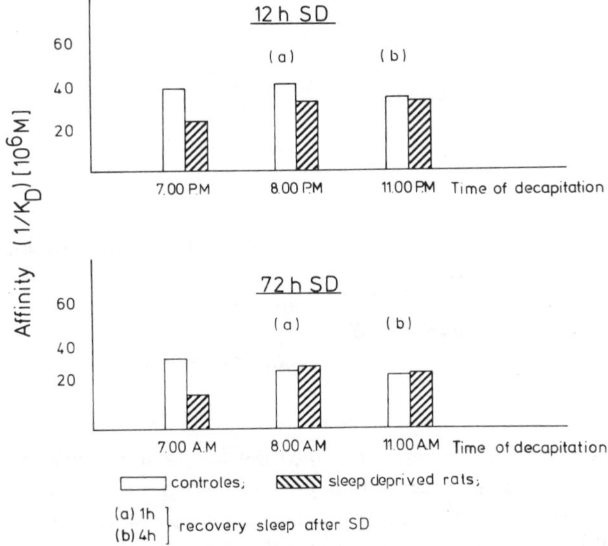

Figure 1. Effect of sleep deprivation (SD) on high affinity 5-HT binding to crude membrane fractions isolated from rat brain.

According to Fleisher, Simon and Aprison (2), supersensitive 5-HT receptors are involved in one subtype of endogenous depression. In the light of this theory, the result obtained with sleep-deprived rats could mean that in depressed patients supersensitive 5-HT receptors are down regulated towards normal sensitivity by sleep deprivation. The effect of sleep deprivation on 5-HT binding to rat brain membranes is reversible. If sleep deprivation is followed by recovery sleep, control values are obtained already after one hour. A parallel effect is observed in some patients: If sleep deprivation is interrupted by only a short sleeping period, the ameliorating effect of sleep deprivation is destroyed.

5-HT binding to rat brain membranes exhibits a circadian rhythm with a peak value at midnight and a through at noon (3). This rhythm is inverse to the circadian fluctuations of 5-HT concentrations, which show a maximum between

1. 5-HT = serotonin

10 and 12 a.m. and a minimum at 12 p.m. The circadian rhythms of 5-HT binding and concentration can be demonstrated as two sine functions with a phase shift of 180° (Figure 2).

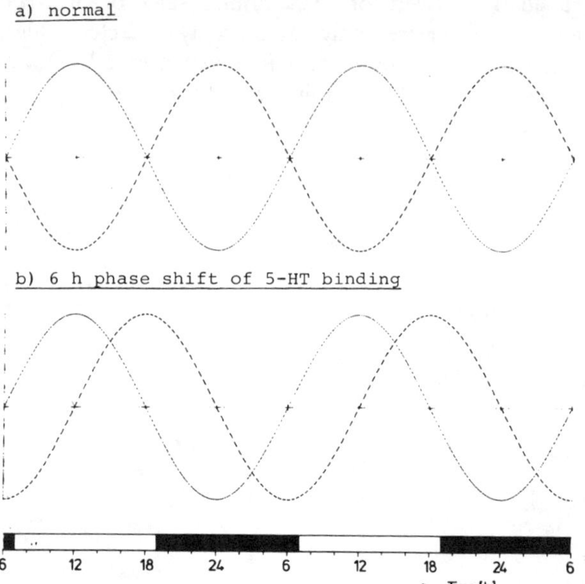

Figure 2. Circadian rhythm of 5-HT concentration (---) and binding (- - -) in rat brain. - Model 1: *Phase shift of 5-HT binding.*

On the basis of the findings that in depression some physiological parameters are phaseadvanced (e.g., temperature, REM sleep episodes) two models were developed to explain this depression. In contrast to the physiological conditions of inverse rhythms of 5-HT binding and concentration, desynchronization of the two rhythms could result in the coincidence of highly sensitive receptors with high 5-HT levels. The reason for desynchronization could be either a phase shift (Figure 2) or a deviation of the period length from 24 h (Figure 3).

The theory of the importance of supersensitive 5-HT receptors in depression has a couple of consequences: (1) This theory initiates further studies on the biochemical and physiological mechanisms involved in this disorder. (2) The mechanisms of current treatment applied in depression has to be reevaluated according to the theory of supersensitive 5-HT receptors and with regard to the hypothesis of the dissociation of the time structures of 5-HT binding and concentration. An antidepressant effect should be observed if a decrease in 5-HT receptor sensitivity and/or a phase shift of either 5-HT binding or concentration is induced by the treatment. The finding that the antidepressant imipramine decreases 5-HT binding by 50% and delays the circadian rhythm of 5-HT binding by 2 hours is in favor of the model, though it does not prove it (Figure 4). (3) Consequently, the theory of supersensitive 5-HT receptors can promote the development of drug design and of new strategies for the treatment of depressed patients.

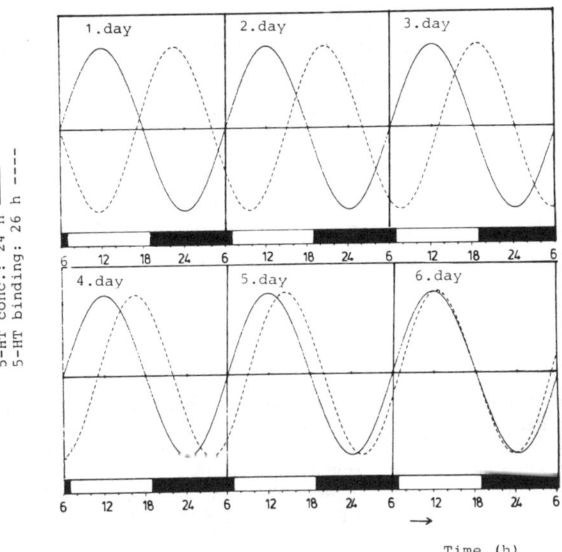

Figure 3. Circadian rhythm of 5-HT concentration (---) and binding (- - -) in rat brain. Model 2: *Frequency shift of 5-HT binding.*

(4) As a biochemist and speaking in more general terms, the theory of supersensitive 5-HT receptors is stimulating in the sense that besides substance concentration, enzyme activity, hormones, and neurotransmitters, receptor modulation plays an important regulatory function.

I think the presentation of this morning point in the direction of future research in behavioral neurobiology. We have got already some new insights by research work performed to explain personality traits and behavior on the molecular level.

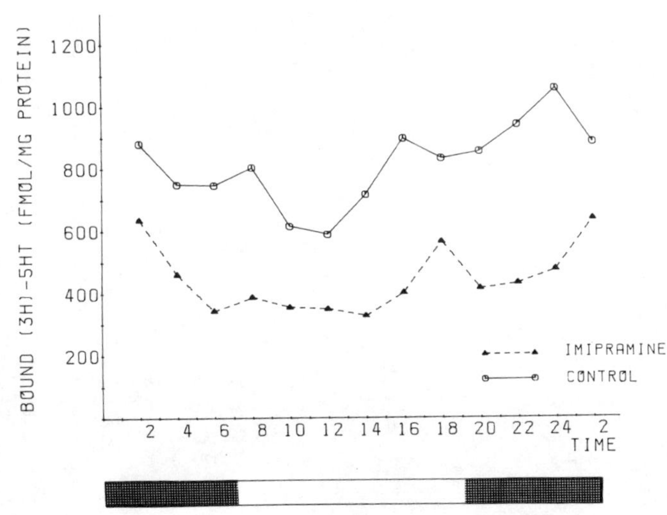

Figure 4. Influence of imipramine on circadian rhythm of 5-HT binding in rat brain.

New techniques like the Positron Emission Tomography (PET) will help to coordinate behavior and neurochemical changes in the living animal and man. However, the strategy should not be a one-way-street. In addition we should use behavior, manipulated behavioral changes, and diseases of the central nervous system as a tool to get a deeper insight into the basic programs of the neuronal systems. In my presentation only a few promising approaches could be mentioned. Other very interesting trends in neurobiology will be discussed in the forthcoming sessions, e.g., the interesting problems and parallels of memory in brain and the immune system.

References

1. Wesemann, W. & Weiner, N. (1982). Regulation of cerebral serotonin binding and metabolism in sleep deprived rats. Behav. Brain Res., 6: 79-84.
2. Fleisher, L.N., Simon, J.R. & Aprison, M.H. (1979). A biochemical-behavioural model for studying serotonergic supersensitivity in brain. J. Neurochemistry, 32: 1613-1619.
3. Wesemann, W., Weiner, N., Rotsch, M. & Schulz, E. (1983). Serotonin binding in rat brain: Circadian rhythm and effect of sleep deprivation. J. Neural Transm. Suppl., 18: 287-294.

2.

Central Control of the Gastrointestinal System

Innervation of the Gut:
Implications for Interaction Between the Nervous and Immune Systems

Paul F. Aravich, Barbara J. Davis, Celia D. Sladek, Suzanne Y. Felten and David L. Felten

The gastrointestinal tract is the largest and most diversified endocrine gland in the body. Some of the putative hormones it may secrete include serotonin, gastrin, secretin, cholecystokinin, gastric inhibitory polypeptide, somatostatin, motilin, enteroglucagon, neurotensin and corticotropin-releasing factor (1, 2). The gut also is an impressive neural organ, since it contains more intrinsic neurons than the spinal cord, and since most of these neurons are not connected directly to other parts of the nervous system (3). Finally, the gut has a remarkable immune system, which has an important and established role in overall immunocompetence (4, 5). In fact, the intestinal tract and mesenteric lymph nodes may contain twice as many lymphocytes as the spleen and other peripheral lymph nodes (6).

The purpose of this review is to describe the extrinsic and intrinsic neural innervation of the gastrointestinal (GI) tract; to review the organization of gut immune systems; and to consider the possibility that gut immune function is regulated by various neural systems, including the sympathetic nervous system.

Overview of the Neural Innervation of the Gut

Enteric neurons are contained essentially in two separate but interacting plexuses located within the outer layers of the GI tract. These thin plexuses, which extend continuously from the esophagus through the rectum (7), are the myenteric plexus (Auerbach's plexus) and the submucosal plexus (Meissner's plexus). The myenteric plexus is outermost and lies between the longitudinal and circular muscles; the submucosal plexus is closer to the lumen and lies within the submucosal layer. The number of neurons within each plexus varies fro» region to region, with more myenteric neurons in sphincter regions and fewer submucosal neurons in the stomach (7). In addition to intrinsic enteric systems, the neural innervation of the gut also consists of various extrinsic systems derived from sympathetic, parasympathetic, and sensory sources.

During development, neurons migrate from the neural crest to the enteric plexuses around gestational days 12-14 in the mouse (8). Migration is directed initially toward the developing myenteric plexus, and then subsequently to the submucosal plexus (9). The phenotypic maturation of enteric neurons progresses in an oral-anal direction, with cholinergic and serotonergic phenotypes expressed prior to peptidergic phenotypes (8). It is well documented that various aspects of gut function continue to develop into the early postnatal period in several species, with further marked changes occurring at weaning (10-12). It is therefore probable that significant enteric neural development occurs postnatally in most species. Furthermore, since a variety of microenvironmental, nutritional, hormonal and surgical alterations can affect the trophic regulation of the gut (8, 13-15), the phenotypic expression of enteric neurons may be subject to substantial modification throughout the lifespan of the animal.

In addition to developmental factors, the activity of the enteric nervous system can be modulated by the autonomic nervous system, by nutrient absorption, and by exocrine and endocrine secretions derived from the gut and other tissues (16). Conversely, the enteric nervous system may influence directly the autonomic nervous system and virtually all gut function, including motility, blood flow, absorption, secretion and immunoregulation. In addition to secretomotor fiber systems, the neural innervation of the gut also consists of an extensive sensory system, the importance and complexity of which is only now becoming appreciated. Finally, because of its similarities to the brain, the enteric nervous system has been proposed to serve as a particularly useful model for the exploration of a number of basic neurobiological (3) and immunological (8) questions.

Sympathetic Innervation of the Gut

Generally speaking, the majority of preganglionic sympathetic fibers originate in cell bodies in the intermediolateral cell column of the thoracolumbar spinal cord, through the nucleus intercalatus and the dorsal commissural nucleus (i.e., so-called central autonomic area) of the thoracolumbar spinal cord also contain preganglionic neurons (17, 18). Cells projecting to gut-related sympathetic ganglia extend primarily from mid-thoracic to upper-lumbar levels of the cord (19). These preganglionic cells receive diverse inputs from a variety of chemically identified transmitter substances. These inputs can originate from other preganglionic neurons, from dorsal horn neurons, and from supraspinal neurons in areas such as the paraventricular hypothalamic nucleus, the zona incerta, portions of the raphe complex, and certain brainstem catecholamine cell groups (20, 21). In the cat, the chemically identified neural input to preganglionic sympathetic neurons is derived more from enkephalin-, neurotensin-, and serotonin-containing fibers than it is from substance P-, vasopressin-, oxytocin- or somatostatin-containing fibers (22).

The axons of preganglionic sympathetic neurons contain acetylcholine and numerous peptides such as the enkephalins (23), neurotensin, somatostatin, substance P (20) and, at least in the frog, luteinizing hormone-releasing hormone (24). The sympathetic outflow of fibers from the spinal cord to the GI tract traverses the paravertebral ganglia in the sympathetic trunk and is directed primarily to the prevertebral (i.e., collateral) sympathetic ganglia in the abdomen, the most important of which include the celiac, superior mesenteric and inferior mesenteric ganglia, as well as ganglia scattered in the pelvic plexus. These various ganglia are interconnected by the intermesenteric and hypogastric nerves (25-27). Preganglionic sympathetic input to the prevertebral ganglia travels mainly via the splanchnic nerves, and is characterized by marked convergence onto individual ganglion neurons (27). While prevertebral neurons are responsible for most of the sympathetic innervation of the GI tract, neurons contained in paravertebral ganglia, such as the superior cervical, medial cervical, stellate, and selected lumbar ganglia also may provide sympathetic fibers to the GI tract (25, 28).

Postganglionic sympathetic fibers to the GI tract travel over the mesenteric, pelvic, hypogastric and colonic (i.e., inferior mesenteric) nerves. These fibers are distributed to the enteric plexuses and to intramural blood vessels (3, 10, 25, 29); relatively few fibers are directed to the muscularis externa. Sympathetic fibers also innervate the lamina propria, where most of the gut immune system is located (see below), but do not innervate directly the endocrine cells of the epithelium (i.e., enteroendocrine cells).

The majority of the postganglionic sympathetic projections originating from the prevertebral ganglia are noradrenergic and also may contain somatostatin (23, 24, 27). By contrast, noradrenergic neurons in paravertebral ganglia such as the superior cervical ganglion exhibit far less somatostatin immunoreactivity (24). Neuropeptide Y also has been co-localized in noradrenergic prevertebral ganglion cells, but in different neurons from those co-localizing somatostatin; another subset of noradrenergic prevertebral neurons have neither somatostatin nor neuropeptide Y (30, 31). These subsets of prevertebral noradrenergic neurons may subserve different functions: Noradrenergic neurons containing neuropeptide Y project to blood vessels; somatostatin-containing noradrenergic neurons project to the submucosa; and noradrenergic neurons containing neither neuropeptide Y nor somatostatin project to the myenteric plexus (32).

The sympathetic innervation of the gut influences a wide variety of functions. These include inhibition of non-sphincter motility, reductions in blood flow and oxygen extraction, and alterations in absorptive and secretory processes (16, 26, 33-35). The sympathetic nervous system also participates in the maintenance and replacement of mucosal epithelial cells, which is an impressive trophic function when it is recognized that the human replaces 300 g of these cells daily (36). Finally, as discussed below, the sympathetic nervous system also may participate in gut immune function.

The inhibitory effect of the sympathetic nervous system on gut motility is well established. Since sympathetic fibers do not innervate the muscularis externa to any considerable extent (10, 24, 29), sympathetic inhibition of gut smooth musculature may be mediated indirectly by projections to the enteric plexuses (but see Gershon, 3). This emphasis on an indirect action of the sympathetic nervous system on gut motility represents a major revision in the classical view of the neural innervation of the GI tract (29). However, noradrenergic varicosities projecting to the myenteric plexus tend to congregate around, rather than within, the plexus (3). This observation, coupled with other data (3), suggests that the sympathetic input to the enteric plexuses may terminate presynaptically upon incoming terminals, rather than postsynaptically upon enteric soma or dendrites.

Parasympathetic Innervation

The parasympathetic innervation of the GI tract derives from a craniosacral outflow of preganglionic fibers, and terminates upon postganglionic neurons contained within the enteric plexuses. The sacral contribution to this outflow is much less extensive than the cranial contribution. It originates primarily in the parasympathetic nucleus of the sacral cord (i.e., the sacral intermediolateral cell column), travels by way of the pelvic nerve through the pelvic plexus, and then branches into the colonic and rectal nerves to innervate primarily the descending colon and rectum (10). The enkephalins are included among the peptides in this outflow of fibers (37).

The cranial contribution to the parasympathetic outflow is derived from efferent vagal fibers, which are distributed throughout most of the GI tract, except for the distal colon. One way to appreciate the close association between the vagus nerve and the enteric nervous system is to recognize that most enteric neurons are embryological derivatives of the vagal portion of the neural crest; portions of the neural crest giving rise to the sympathetic ganglia, sensory ganglia, and the adrenal medulla appear not to contribute cells to the developing enteric nervous system, though some cells in the hindgut are derivatives of sacral portions of the neural crest (10, 13). Despite conflicting data (38), gut vagal fibers may originate in a topographic "columnar" fashion from the dorsal motor nucleus of the vagus (DMV) (39, 40): The cells of origin for efferent fibers to the stomach are located in the medial portion of the DMV, while efferent fibers destined for the intestines originate in more lateral portions of the nucleus. Some authors claim that a small number of cells within the rostral part of the nucleus ambiguus also contribute vagal efferents to portions of the stomach (38, 41, 42). Since neurons in the DMV have a broad dendritic plexus that extends into specific portions of the nucleus of the solitary tract, the fourth ventricle, and area postrema, they can be influenced by a wide variety of stimuli (42). Among the many factors affecting efferent vagal activity are the taste and smell of food, which induce the "cephalic" phases of digestion that are important to appetitive learning and, perhaps, to the etiology of obesity and the efficiency of food utilization (43, 44). Vagal efferents to the stomach and intestines travel largely via the gastric and celiac branches of the vagus nerve. The celiac branch ultimately traverses the celiac plexus and travels in the company of sympathetic mesenteric fibers to the intestine.

Vagal fibers to the gut subsume both secretory and motor actions. For example, vagal efferents induce epithelial cells to secrete gastric acid and a variety of peptides including gastrin, vasoactive intestinal polypeptide (VIP), substance P and somatostatin (45). The action of the vagus on gut smooth musculature, on the other hand, is generally regarded as excitatory. However, inhibitory as well as excitatory actions have been documented in the cat (46). It has been argued that excitatory gut motor function is mediated by low-threshold cholinergic fibers that terminate upon cholinergic ganglion cells. Contrarily, the inhibitory motor effects of vagal nerve stimulation have been attributed to high-threshold vagal efferents that terminate upon serotonergic neurons (46).

Vagal efferents are not only cholinergic in nature, but also contain met-enkephalin (47). Other efferent fibers travelling in the abdominal vagus nerve and distributed to the gut are noradrenergic and are derived from upper paravertebral sympathetic ganglia (e.g., the superior cervical ganglion) (48). This sympathetic system may participate in the release of serotonin from entero-endocrine cells (10, 48). Finally, preganglionic vagal efferent fibers, following the classical definition of the autonomic nervous system, putatively terminate upon cholinergic ganglion cells in the myenteric and submucosal plexuses. However, noncholinergic enteric ganglion cells containing peptides such as bombesin and gastrin/cholecystokinin, also may mediate the secretomotor effects of vagal nerve stimulation (45).

Sensory Reception

While the various nerves of the sympathetic and parasympathetic systems (e.g., splanchnic, vagus, pelvic and hypogastric nerves) transmit information from the central nervous system to the gut, these systems also carry numerous fibers relaying primary sensory information back to the central nervous system. Within the splanchnic nerves, substance P, somatostatin, VIP, cholecystokinin, vaso-pressin, oxytocin and calcitonin gene-related peptide fibers originating in dorsal root ganglion cells may participate in this function (23, 49, 50, 51). In the cat, primary afferents containing VIP are distributed predominantly to sacral levels of the cord, while substance P afferents are distributed more uniformly across all levels of the cord (52). Regardless of the transmitter type, sensory fibers outnumber secretomotor fibers in the splanchnic nerves by a ratio of 3:1 (53).

Sensory fibers in the vagus nerve, on the other hand, contain substance P, gastrin/cholecystokinin, somatostatin and VIP (54, 55). The sensory function of the vagus nerve seems especially important, since sensory fibers have been reported to outnumber secretomotor fibers in the abdominal vagus by a ratio of 9:1 (53) or 60:1 (48). These fibers represent the peripheral process of neurons contained within the nodose ganglia; some vagal sensory fibers also may be derived from neurons in the jugular (i.e., superior) ganglion (48). The central processes of vagal sensory neurons innervating the gut are directed to the nucleus of the solitary tract, directly upon the DMV cells, and possibly, in the case of some gastric sensory fibers, to the area postrema (41, 42, 56). Within the nucleus of the solitary tract, the medial subnucleus may be the primary receptive area for gut sensory information, although the dorsal, commissural, intermediate and gelantinosus portions of the nucleus also participate in this function (41, 42). The medial subnucleus of the solitary tract is innervated by a substantial number of substance P and neurotensin terminals that originate in various areas, but by relatively few enkephalin-, somatostatin- or vasopressin-like terminals (57, 58). From the nucleus of the solitary tract, second order vagal afferent information is distributed over a remarkably wide extent of the neuroaxis utilizing a variety of transmitter systems (56). Neural input to the nucleus of the solitary tract is likewise anatomically and biochemically diverse (56, 58, 59).

Gut sensory information is derived from receptors predominating in the upper portions of the GI tract (through the proximal jejunum) (60). Vagal sensory fibers outnumber splanchnic sensory fibers throughout the GI tract, with this disparity especially evident in the proximal small intestine (60). Several gut receptor types, many of which tend to be free nerve endings, have been identified or postulated (53, 60, 61, 62). In particular, specific mechano-, thermo-, osmo-, and chemoreceptors have been described for the vagal sensory system. Mechanoreceptors tend to be distributed throughout most layers of the gut, while the other receptors congregate in submucosal and mucosal areas. Vagal chemoreceptors may be specific for alkaline solutions, acid solutions, amino acids or glucose. Splanchnic sensory receptors predominate in submucosal areas and act as glucoreceptors or thermoreceptors. Glucoreceptors related to the vagus occur primarily in the duodenum and secondarily in the jejunum; splanchnic glucoreceptors are much less numerous and occur only in the jejunum (62).

Afferent sensory information from the gut may function in various aspects of feeding behavior (63, 64, 65), the affective response to taste (i.e., alliesthesia) (66), drinking behavior (67), gastric emptying (68), pancreatic polypeptide release (69), and the modulation of the neural activity of the lateral hypothalamus (70), which has been implicated in feeding behavior. From a basic neurobiological perspective, vagal sensory fibers show remarkable plasticity and, like vagal efferents (71), can be manipulated experimentally to innervate striated musculature and/or sympathetic ganglia (72).

One interesting aspect of gut sensory function concerns the prevertebral ganglia: In addition to sending efferent information to the gut, these ganglia are innervated in a reciprocal fashion by fibers originating from enteric neurons. These fibers may contain VIP, gastrin/cholecystokinin, or bombesin (10, 23, 24, 27). The VIP input to the prevertebral ganglia is primarily to neurons that contain norepinephrine alone, and to neurons containing both norepinephrine and somatostatin; noradrenergic neurons containing neuropeptide Y do not receive a prominent VIP innervation (30, 31). On the basis of the projections of these noradrenergic neurons noted previously (see above), fibers originating in the gut appear to innervate prevertebral neurons that project back to the enteric plexuses. Enteric efferent fibers directed to the prevertebral ganglia may therefore complete a putative peripheral reflex arc modulating motor (or secretory) responses (27, 30).

Enteric Nervous System

As noted above, the nervous system intrinsic to the gut is quite extensive, with the vast majority of its neurons not connected directly with the classically defined autonomic nervous system. In fact, when disconnected from the central nervous system (3, 10, 24), substantial gut motor function can be maintained (but see below). Many authors, starting with Langely, have viewed th enteric nervous system as a third component to the autonomic nervous system (3, 73). Unlike other peripheral ganglia, the organization of the enteric ganglia is quite similar to that of the central nervous system: There is tight packing of a large number of neurons; there are supporting cells that resemble astrocytes rather than Schwann cells; there is no internal collagen; the characteristic endoneurial and perineurial sheaths of the peripheral nervous system are lacking; and there is a blood-plexus barrier resembling the blood-brain barrier (3, 8, 10). For these reasons, the enteric nervous system has been called the "little brain" (74) and, as noted earlier, may be an excellent model system for the examination of a variety of basic neurobiological questions.

The enteric nervous system utilizes a large number of peptides, some of which also are contained within endocrine components of the gut. Enteroendocrine cells are confined generally to the mucosa, where they are distributed along with nonendocrine cells (primarily enterocytes, goblet cells and lymphocytes) in the epithelial lining of the lumen. In some instances, however, endocrine cells have been found in the lamina propria (15). Among the most widely distributed enteroendocrine cells are those that produce serotonin and somatostatin. Serotonin-producing cells also may produce substance P (15). Virtually all enteroendocrine cells are capable of monoamine precursor uptake; they are then capable of decarboxylating these precursors into specific biogenic amines. While a neural origin for gut amine precursor uptake and decarboxylation (APUD) endocrine cells has been debated (75), these endocrine cells contain a putative marker for neural tissue (i.e., neuron-specific enolase) and, along with cells distributed in other organs, have been considered to form part of the "diffuse neuroendocrine system" (76).

In contrast to enteroendocrine cells, enteric neurons are located primarily in the gut plexuses, though scattered neurons such as apparent sensory cells (77), may exist in the lamina propria. In general, the distribution of gut neuropeptides is quite broad within and across levels, whereas specific enteroendocrine peptides are more restricted to specific levels of the stomach and intestines (1). Also, neuropeptide projections to mucosal areas may originate primarily from cell bodies contained within the submucosal plexus (78), while projections to the circular muscle may originate in the myenteric plexus (32). Peptides such as cholecystokinin/gastrin, somatostatin, VIP, substance P, and serotonin may exist in both endocrine and neural components of the gut, while the enkephalins and calcitonin gene-related peptide are primarily or exclusively contained within neural components (1, 15, 24, 78, 79).

Enteric ganglion cells contain monoamines as well as peptides. The existence and distribution of various monoamines in the enteric nervous system have been the subject of intensive investigation for several years (3, 80). It is generally agreed that there are few, if any, intrinsic catecholamine (dopamine, noradrenaline, adrenaline) neurons. However, there is good pharmacological evidence for the existence of intrinsic serotonin and acetylcholine neurons (3, 80). Unfortunately, unequivocal anatomical confirmation for these two monoamines has not yet been provided. Immunoreactive serotonin-like cell bodies can be demonstrated in the myenteric plexus, and immunocytochemically identified fibers are localized in both enteric plexuses (81). However, neural serotonin systems in the gut cannot be demonstrated using the classic formaldehyde-induced histofluorescence technique (3, 80). An overwhelming amount of electrophysiological and pharmacological data indicate that the enteric nervous system also contains large numbers of cholinergic neurons, and that these neurons project to most areas of the gut. Nonetheless, anatomical confirmation for these systems has been hampered by the lack of a highly specific staining method for acetylcholine. The current methods involve markers for the cholinergic deactivating enzyme acetylcholinesterase (AChE), or for the cholinergic synthesizing enzyme, choline acetyltransferase (CAT). Unfortunately, each marker has its limitations, though the CAT technique appears superior to the AChE technique when the antibody staining works. A recent experiment utilizing a highly specific AChE staining procedure in the rat duodenum demonstrated cholinergic-like cell bodies in the myenteric plexus, but could not demonstrate unequivocally cholinergic neurons in the submucosal plexus (82). However, CAT staining of the guinea-pig small intestine indicates that the submucosal plexus has a large number of putative cholinergic soma (32).

Peptide systems within the enteric nervous system have diverse phenotypes and locations. It is not the purpose of this review to summarize all of these systems. Only some of the most prominent neural systems, which have been summarized by various authors (24, 78, 83, 84), will be noted here:

The most widespread peptides in the enteric nervous system are VIP and substance P. These neuropeptides are distributed extensively to nearly all components of the GI tract (muscularis externa, enteric ganglia cells, muscularis mucosa, blood vessels, lamina propria), except that they never penetrate the epithelium, and there are more fibers in the intestine than in the stomach. There are more enteric neurons containing VIP than any other peptide. VIP neurons are considerably more numerous in the submucosal plexus than in the myenteric plexus of the intestine. VIP cell bodies also have been described within the lamina propria (84); some of these cells may be neural (78). Although less numerous, substance P fibers exhibit a similar enteric distribution. In contrast to VIP, however, substance P soma tend to be in the myenteric plexus rather than in the submucosal plexus.

The enkephalins (met- and leu-) account for fewer enteric fibers and neurons than VIP and substance P. In the intestine, they are distributed primarily to the myenteric plexus and muscularis externa. In the stomach, however, enkephalin fibers are more numerous and can be observed in mucosal layers. Throughout the GI tract, cell bodies for the enkephalins are located in the myenteric plexus. Somatostatin-containing neural systems, on the other hand, are far less numerous than the previously noted peptide systems, and are distributed to both plexuses and to mucosal regions of the intestine, but not very extensively to the external muscle layers, nor to the stomach. Soma containing this peptide tend to be localized in the submucosal plexus. Cholecystokinin/gastrin neural systems are relatively restricted to the muscularis externa and enteric plexuses. Their cell bodies are found mainly in the submucosal plexus of the large intestine. Various other peptides such as bombesin, neurotensin, thyrotropin-releasing hormone, pancreatic polypeptide-neuropeptide Y and angiotensin II are present in varying amounts, and may be derived partly or totally from extrinsic sources. In this regard, however, it is worth noting recent data on submucosal neural phenotypes (32): Approximately half of the submucosal neurons in the guinea-pig small intestine contain VIP, while the other half contain the acetylcholine marker CAT. Three types of CAT cell bodies can be described: Those that contain three neuropeptides, viz., somatostatin, neuropeptide Y and cholecystokinin; those that contain one neuropeptide, viz., substance P; and those that contain CAT, but none of the other peptides.

Peptide and monoamine enteric neurons may directly affect virtually all functions of the gut. However, the activity of the enteric nervous system also is modulated by endocrine-paracrine factors, and by extrinsic neural sources. The regulation of gut motility, as reviewed by Costa and Furness (16) and Wingate (85), provides a good example of the interaction of these various systems:

It is quite clear that gut motility can be maintained when the enteric nervous system is disconnected from extrinsic neural influences. However, certain aspects of gut motility require the participation of extrinsic input. For example, during fasting (e.g., between meals), the gut exhibits a characteristic burst of motor activity every 80-170 minutes in some species. This burst of activity is often referred to as the migrating motor complex, since it propagates slowly from the proximal gut through the small intestine. Periodic migrating complexes persists until feeding is initiated and nutrients reach the duodenum. These migrating motor complexes are then abolished quickly and supplanted with another form of muscular activity that is prolonged but irregular. The purpose of this new form of activity ("postprandial" or "fed" activity) may be to alter mucosal blood flow for the promotion of nutrient absorption, and to aid digestion by mixing ingested nutrients and propelling them forward. The control of both migrating and postprandial motor activity is influenced by various endocrine factors. For instance, migrating motor complexes may be promoted by motilin, while postprandial motor activity, particularly in the proximal gut, is affected by cholecystokinin and several other gut peptides. When disconnected from external sources, the enteric nervous system is capable of initiating migrating motor activity, though there may be some abnormalities in the propagation of the motoric wave. Various phases of postprandial motor activity, on the other hand, are affected substantially by extrinsic denervation (16). For example, the first phase of "fed" activity has been called the "cephalic" phase. It occurs prior to the entry of nutrients into the gut, and is due to the taste of food. Vagotomy results in considerable disruption of this response. The second phase of the postprandial motor response is the "gastric" phase, which is due to the entry of nutrients into the stomach. Evidence has been provided for the participation of a reflex arc involving vagal sensory and motor fibers (i.e., a vago-vagal reflex), as well as the involvement of certain gut hormones in this response. The final phase of postprandial motor activity is the "intestinal" phase. In contradistinction to the other phases, this phase does not depend upon extrinsic neural factors. Thus, neuro-endocrine mechanisms intrinsic to the gut are sufficient for the intestinal phase of activity. It is evident, then, that the proper execution of gut motility requires not only the enteric nervous system, but also the integrated actions of various extrinsic sensory and motor systems, as well as a variety of endocrine-paracrine secretions.

Vasopressin in the Gut

As new brain peptides are characterized, there is great interest in determing their presence within the gut (2, 79, 86, 87). Vasopressin was one of the first brain peptides to be characterized, and is best known for its antidiuretic and pressor effects. However, perhaps for this reason, and because it has not been generally related to overall enteric function, systematic exploration of the GI tract for the presence of vasopressin has not, to our knowledge, been reported.

We have obtained preliminary data suggesting the existence of two independent vasopressin-like systems in the duodenum of the rat (88). The first system can be visualized immunocytochemically, and appears to be a neural system with fibers located mainly in the circular layer of the muscularis externa. Thus far, this system has been recognized by several different vaso-pressin-related antisera (Figure 1), and does not appear to be present in rats congentially deficient in brain vasopressin, i.e., Brattleboro rats. No immuno-reactive fibers have been observed in the mucosa, and immunoreactive cell bodies have not yet been located in the enteric plexuses. In some, but not in all experiments, the immunoreactivity of this system has been enhanced greatly by adrenalectomy, which caused an apparent increase in fiber size (Figure 2).

Another vasopressin-like system may be present in the lamina propria of both the normal rat and the Brattleboro rat. Radioimmunoassays with two different vasopressin antisera have detected vasopressin-like immunoreactivity in mucosal extracts obtained from adult rats. This reactivity diluted appropriately when compared to a vasopressin standard dilution curve, indicating a further similarity of the substance to vasopressin. Immunocytochemical examination of the mucosa utilizing various antisera has failed to demonstrate specific neural or enteroendocrine cell staining. The only observed immunoreactivity has been confined to non-neural cells in the lamina propria. These immunoreactive cells resemble plasma cells, though definitive identification is not possible at the light level (Figure 3).We have observed that these putative plasma cells generally react in a nonspecific fashion to immunocytochemical techniques. However, a slight diminution in putative plasma cell vasopressin staining was observed following vasopressin-blocking experiments. We therefore suggest tentatively that a subset of plasma cells may contain vasopressin. Further research is needed to confirm this speculation. In addition, elution studies and high performance liquid chromatography have not yet been performed on the circular muscle system nor the putative plasma cell system to establish with certainty the presence of vasopressin.

Figure 1. Vasopressin-like immunofluorescence in the circular muscle of the duodenum of Long-Evans rats. Fibers (arrows) were recognized by antibodies directed against vasopressin (A), against the neurophysin specific to vasopressin (B) and against the neurophysins common to both vasopressin and oxytocin (C). Abbreviations: VP (vasopressin), NPII (vasopressin-specific neurophysin), RNP (general rat neurophysin), L (longitudinal muscle), C (circular muscle). 375 x.

See opposite

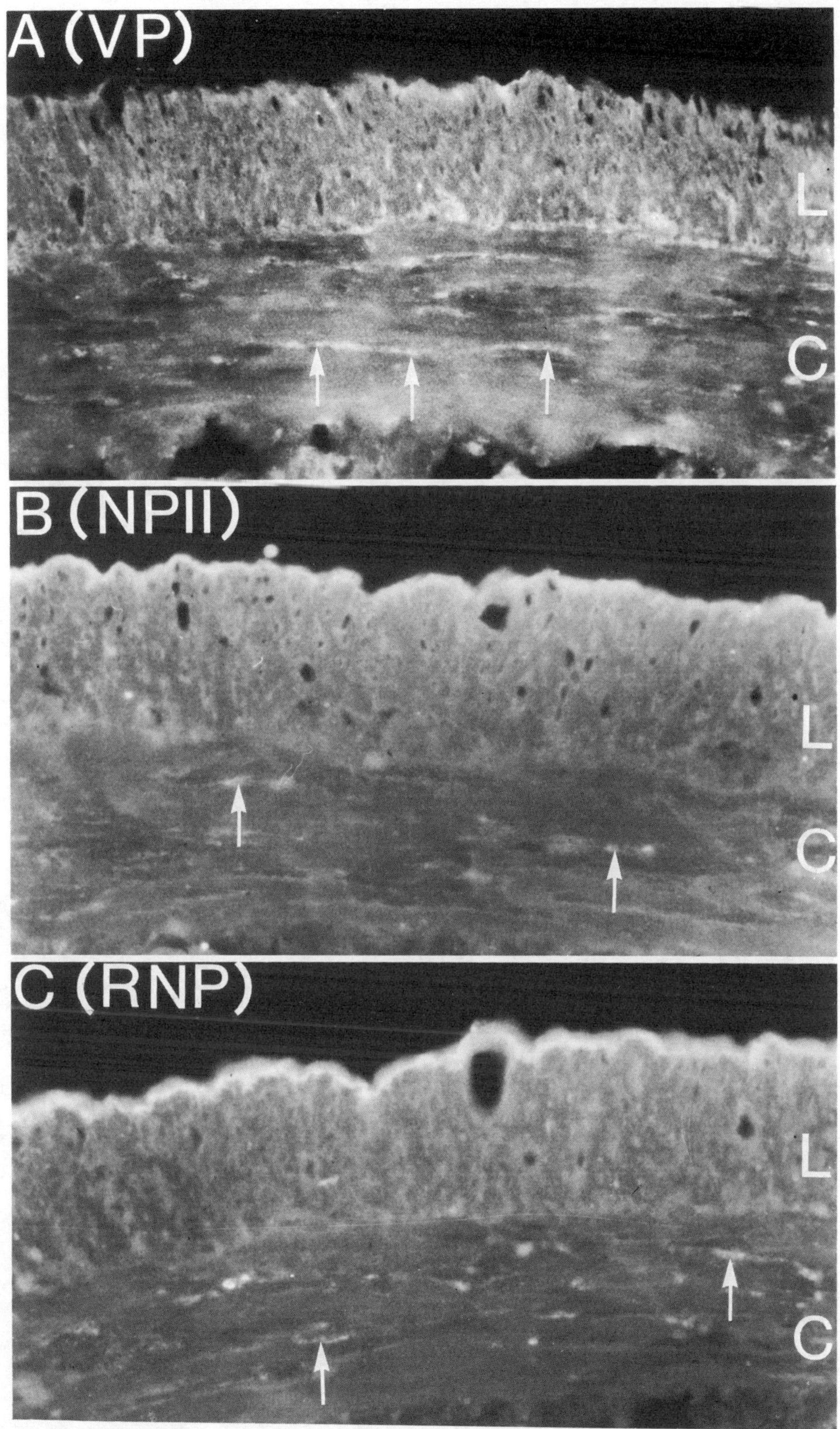

A (VP)
L
C
B (NPII)
L
C
C (RNP)
L
C

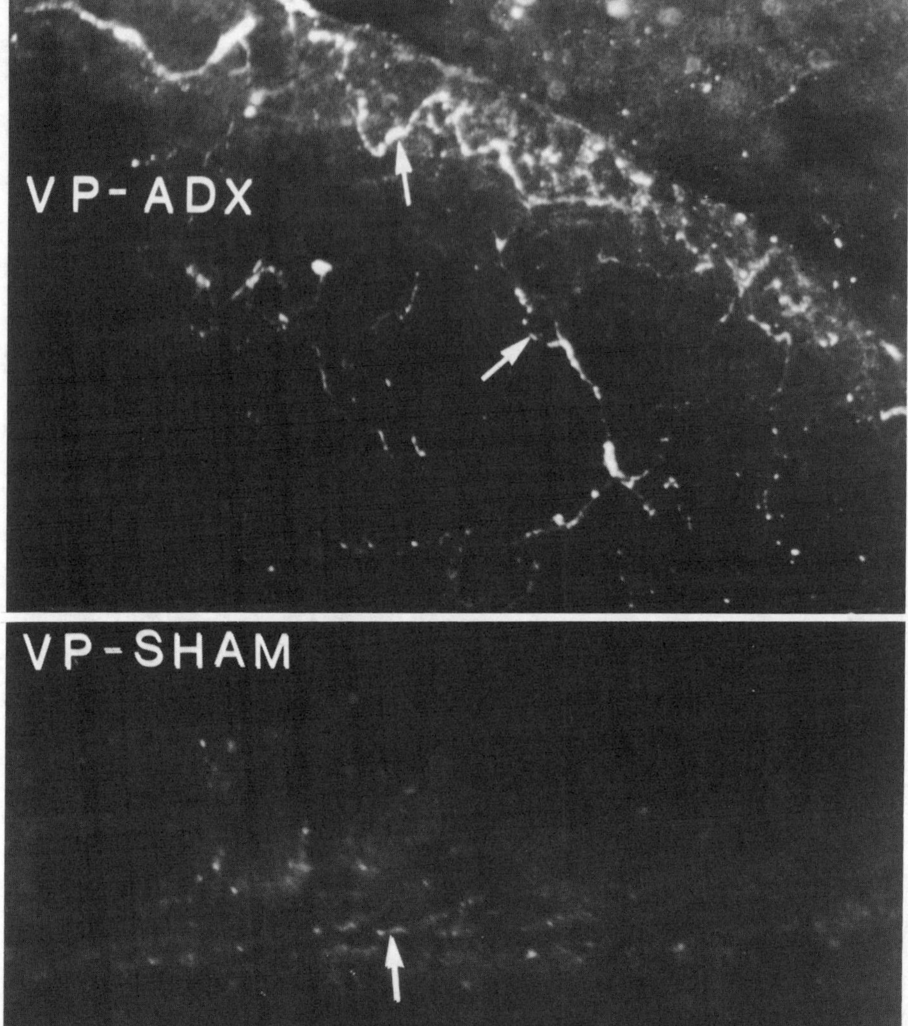

Figure 2. Anti-vasopressin immunofluorescence (arrows) in Long-Evans rats adrenalectomized (upper panel) or sham adrenalectomized (lower panel). In some, but not all experiments, adrenalectomy enhanced the immunoreactivity of neural vasopressin system. Abbreviations: VP (anti-vasopressin immunoreactivity), ADX (adrenalectomy), SHAM (sham adrenalectomy). 250 x.

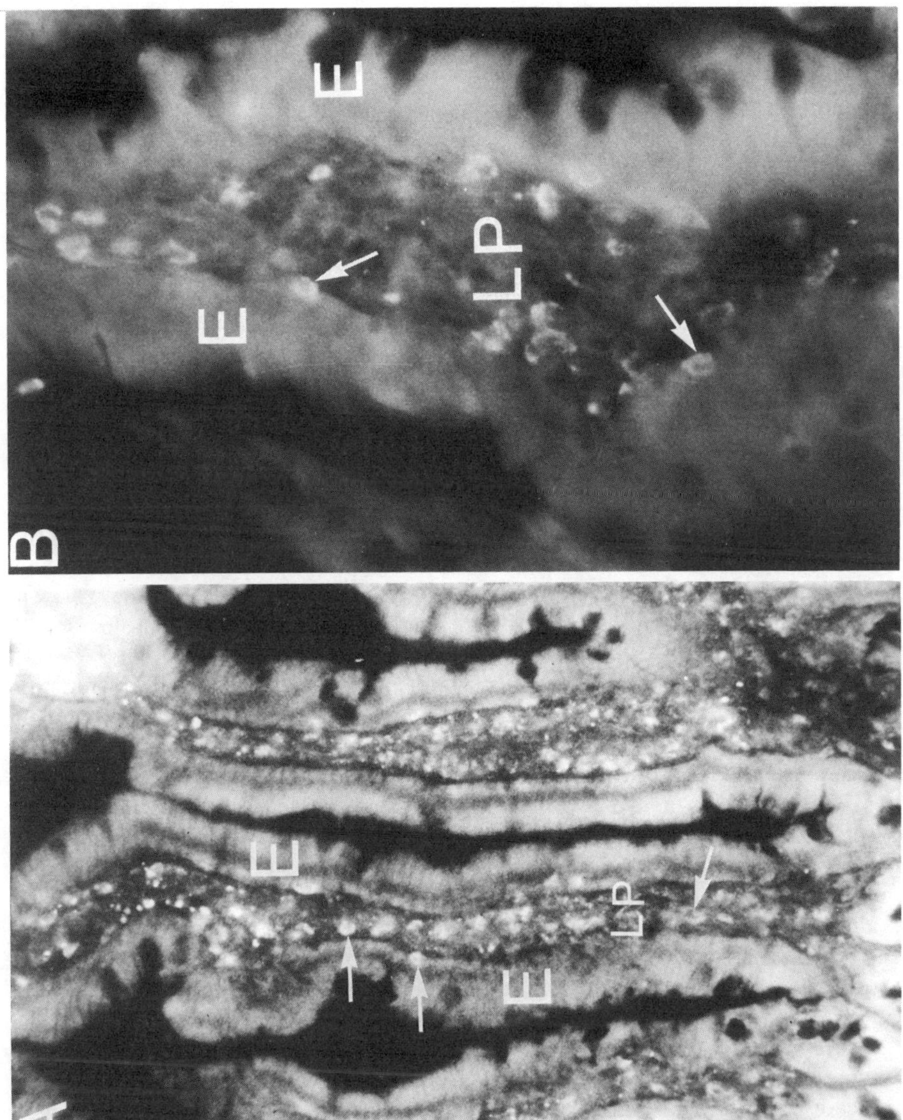

Figure 3. Immunofluorescence of putative plasma cells (arrows) in the lamina propria of the rat duodenum reacted with anti-vasopressin serum. A: Low magnification (375 x). B: Higher magnification (725 x). Abbreviations: E (epithelial lining of the lumen), LP (lamina propria).

Regardless of these reservations, our preliminary observations and other data suggest that vasopressin may influence gut function by several routes of action. One route may be related to the classic neurohypophysial vasopressin system

(89), which produces most of the vasopressin found in the circulation. Circulating vasopressin binds more avidly with the small intestine than with the kidney and liver (90), and may be able to affect gut blood flow and water absorption (34, 91-93). Recent data suggest that vasopressin release from the neural lobe of the pituitary participates specifically in stress-induced feeding and carbohydrate appetite, but not in other aspects of feeding behavior (94). It also has been shown that high-fat, high-sucrose diets induce changes in regional neurohypophysial vasopressin content, and that exercise protects against these changes (95, 96). Finally, vasopressin has been shown to have a lymphokine-like activity in the spleen (97) and to stimulate mitosis in bone marrow cells (98). On the basis of these various considerations, it is hypothesized that circulating vasopressin may influence gut function during times of acute stress; that stress-induced vasopressin release from the neural lobe may affect gut immunocompetence; and that at least some of the effects of nutrition on immune function (see below) may be mediated by vasopressin.

A second route by which vasopressin may influence gut function is via the putative neural system in the circular muscle. It is possible that this system participates in the control of gut motility. Vasopressin has been observed previously to enhance gut motility, but at fairly high doses (91). Relatively high doses of vasopressin may be needed to alter motility because the relevant receptor sites are within the wall of the gut, and are relatively inaccessible to circulating vasopressin.

Alternatively, the neural vasopressin system may subsume a sensory function related to gut motility. Since vasopressin-like enteric neurons have not yet been found, this system may derive from extrinsic sources. Among the sources to consider are the dorsal root ganglia and the nodose ganglia. As noted earlier, dorsal root ganglion neurons contain vasopressin (50), and may transmit primary sensory afferent information from the gut to the central nervous system. Since vasopressin also has been found in other sensory ganglia (50), vasopressin may exist in nodose ganglion cells. Consequently, vasopressin may be contained within vagal sensory fibers innervating the gut. While these various motor and sensory alternatives remain viable possibilities, the distribution of the putative vasopressin system in the circular muscle suggests that it is not a derivative of the sympathetic nervous system.

A final route by which vasopressin may influence gut function is via its possible existence within putative plasma cells in the lamina propria. This would implicate vasopressin directly in gut function (see below). It has been argued that lymphocytes produce various neuroendocrine peptides, such as oxytocin, adrenocorticotropin hormone and endorphin (99). Thus, the presence of a neuroendocrine peptide within important components of the immune system is not unprecedented. However, the complicated biochemical composition of plasma cells, coupled with the demonstration of vasopressin-like plasma cells in the Brattleboro rat, suggests that caution should be exercised in interpreting the specificity of the immunoreactivity.

Overview of the Gut Immunological System

The immune function of the gut is controlled by intrinsic lymphoid tissue located primarily in the mucosa, as well as by extrinsic tissue responsible for the collection of intestinal lymph (viz., the mesenteric lymph nodes). The intrinsic gut-associated lymphoid tissue (GALT) accounts for up to 25% of the entire tissue mass of the mucosa (100). Included among the important cell components of GALT are B and T lymphocytes, plasma cells, macrophages, eosinophils and mast cells. Lymphocytes are distributed to four major mucosal areas: Between the epithelial cells (intraepithelial lymphocytes); scattered throughout the lamina propria; aggregated into groups within the lamina propria (nodules or follicles); and aggregated into groups of nodules (e.g., Peyer's patches). Peyer's patches are found mainly in the distal ileum, while isolated follicles are found mainly in various portions of the small intestine and appendix. The follicles within a Peyer's patch are divided into a cell-poor subepithelial *dome* region, a *mantle* region characterized by tightly packed lymphocytes, and in an inner *germ center* (101). Within Peyer's patches, lymphocytes between follicles (i.e., in the interfollicular area) and within domal areas are thymus (T) dependent (101).

The immune system of the gut is inundated continually by antigens related to nutrients, chemicals, and microorganisms (102). For instance, it has been estimated that the gut is exposed to between 100 and 200 tons of food throughout the course of a lifetime in the human (103). Since many of the antigens exposed to the gut are needed for normal homeostatic functioning, gut immune responses are generally suppressed. This phenomenon has been attributed to "oral tolerance," and may be due to T-suppressor lymphocytes, certain classes of antibodies, and macrophage-prostaglandin synthesis (104). Inappropriate and excessive activation of the GALT system can have to wide spread consequences, resulting in food allergies (4), damage to gut epithelial cells (105), and the morbidity of Crohn's disease (5).

Many of the factors common to the secondary immune systems in other organs are common to the GALT system, though there are differences. As in other tissues, the precursor cells for gut lymphocytes originate in the bone marrow. Maturation of B lymphocytes takes place in the spleen, while T cell maturation first takes place in the thymus and then in the spleen. Following maturation, B and T Lymphocytes gain access to the gut mucosa through the blood and lymphatic circulations. The GALT system also participates in the two types of immune response characteristic of other tissues, viz. humoral (secretory) immunity and cellular immunity. Humoral immunity, which is conferred quickly and diffusely, is controlled by plasma cells scattered throughout the mucosa. These cells are formed from specific antigen-sensitive B lymphocytes. As in other tissues, antigen presentation to B cells is promoted by macrophages and T-helper lymphocytes. In addition to promoting the differentiation of B cells into plasma cells, T-helper cells also facilitate the replication of antigen-specific B cells, which contributes to immunological "memory" for subsequent exposure to the antigen. Some GALT T lymphocytes are combined helper/suppressor cells: They promote plasma cell antibodies of one class (immunoglobulin A antibodies) at the same time they inhibit plasma antibody formation from other types of immunoglobulins (4). These mixed action cells occur in Peyer's patches, and are peculiar to the gut and mesenteric lymphoid tissue (104).

Following differentiation from B cells, plasma cells begin specific antibody secretion. Unlike plasma cells in other tissues, most GALT plasma cell antibodies are class A immunoglobulins (IgA), though other classes of immunoglobulins also are produced (viz., IgD, IgE, IgG, IgM; 104). Upon leaving the plasma cell, antibodies are transported through epithelial cells, where they are modified and then released into the lumen. They then bind with specific antigens, rendering the antigen more susceptible to degradation by digestive enzymes; antibody secretion also causes epithelial goblet cells to secrete more protective mucus (104).

As in other secondary lymphoid organs, GALT cellular-mediated immunity is conferred by T lymphocytes. When a specific antigen is presented, T cells attack the antigen directly (t-killer cells) - forming the basis of cellular-mediated immunity - or secrete lymphokines. The lymphokines have varying effects, which can include the attraction of macrophages to degrade the antigen, the attraction of other lymphocytes to the antigenic area, and the induction of plasma cell antibody production. Because of various factors, Peyer's patches are especially amenable to antigenic activation. Antigenically activated T and B lymphocytes from this area gain access to the general circulation, and can be distributed to various tissues, such as the lungs and mammary glands. However, circulating lymphocytes derived from Peyer's patches have a propensity to migrate back into the lamina propria (4).

Since GALT is located in the mucosa, factors that alter mucosal function, might alter GAlt activity. Though this is an emerging area of interest, and few data are available, changes in blood flow, absorption, endocrine secretion, exocrine secretion and motility should affect mucosal cellular processing in general, and the mucosal immune system specifically. For example, during early infancy, the barrier function of the gut is not established fully and macromolecular absorption is much greater than in later life (102). Not surprisingly, it is at this time that the production of specific food antibodies is greatest (106). Other factors affecting nutrient absorption such as alterations in mucus secretion, malnutrition, local IgA deficiency and changes in motility also can affect antigen exposure to the GALT (102).

Increasing attention is being focused upon the modulation of GALT activity by nutritional factors. One example of such modulation is food intolerance due to food allergy. Food allergies are only one of many potential causes for specific food intolerances. Other mechanisms include specific toxic responses and enzyme deficiencies, as well as various psychological factors (107-110). Most food allergies are associated with antigens contained in milk, wheat, eggs, nuts and fish (106, 109). Much of the interest in food allergies has focused on humorally mediated mechanisms, particularly those involving IgA deficiencies and IgE excesses, though cellular-mediated components also have been implicated (111). Although various delayed responses are possible, allergic reactions to foods occur generally within a few hours of ingestion. These reactions are associated typically with IgE antibody production, and can involve several different target organs (107, 110, 111). Many otherwise normal infants and adults have circulating IgE, IgG and IgA antibodies to specific foods (4, 106). However, specific food allergies are less common than popularly believed, and tend to predominate in children (111). While the prognosis for childhood food allergies is quite good, such allergies may reflect an allergic predisposition during later life (106).

Aside from its relationship with food allergies, nutrient intake can have other effects on general immunocompetence. For example, malnutrition, overconsumption of high-fat diets and obesity can all reduce immune function (112-115). Thus factors that influence appetite may directly or indirectly affect immune function. Data relating gut factors to the control of appetite (64, 65, 116-118) may therefore be relevant to gut immunocompetence. Conversely, just as alterations in nonlymphoid gut tissue may affect immunocompetence, altered GALT immunoreactivity may affect various gut functions (100).

Neural Relationships with Gut-Associated Lymphoid Tissue

As documented previously, the gut contains an extensive nervous system as well as an extensive immune system. The possibility of interactions between these two systems has arisen from consideration of anatomical relationships in the gut (119, 120), and from evidence of functional interactions between the nervous and immune systems in otherþ1Xsecondary lymphoid organs (121-123).

The most prominent neural systems in the lamina propria of the gut, where immune cells are found, contain norepinephrine, acetylcholine, VIP, and substance P. The relationships of noradrenergic fibers and putative cholinergic (AChE-positive) fibers have been examined in rabbit GALT. The appendix, sacculus rotundus, and Peyer's patches all showed similar relationships between noradrenergic fibers and cells of the immune system. The noradrenergic fibers from the sympathetic nervous system entered the serosal surface of the gut in association with blood vessels; the cells of origin were found in adjacent prevertebral sympathetic ganglia. These fibers first traveled longitudinally inside the muscularis interna, and then abruptly turned radially to form long, linear varicose plexuses that ran inward towards the lumen. In the appendix, where nodules are located in orderly arrays, this plexus passed between adjacent nodules without sending collaterals into the nodules. As these fibers approached the interdomal regions of lamina propria, they passed directly through the thymus (T) dependent cell zones, and arborized extensively in the lamina propria. The arborizing fibers ran through the parenchyma of the GALT, and were located adjacent to lymphocytes, plasma cells and associated lymphoid cells such as eosinophils and mast cells. An extensive plexus of fibers arborized in the subepithelial region adjacent to the immunoglobulin-secreting plasma cells. In the appendix, noradrenergic fibers surrounded yellow fluorescent cells, tentatively identified as enteroendocrine cells; this relationship was less prominent in sacculus rotundus, and was infrequent in Peyer's patches, where fluorescent cells were less abundant. AChE-positive fibers also were present in the lamina propria, and arborized extensively among the lymphocytes and other cells of the immune system. These findings suggest that cells of the immune system, shown by previous studies to possess catecholamine and acetylcholine receptors, lie adjacent to nerve fibers and varicosities that utilize these neurotransmitters. We suggest that these relationships may provide the anatomical basis for neural influences over gut immunity, and may be important in immune-related disorders of the gut such as Crohn's disease.

Previous studies from the Felten's laboratories (121, 122) and Livnat's laboratory (123) have revealed a functional role for the noradrenergic innervation of secondary lymphoid tissue. In the spleen and lymph nodes, as in the GALT, the noradrenergic fibers end within the parenchyma adjacent mainly to T lymphocytes, macrophages, and associated cells such as eosinophils and mast cells. Chemical studies have revealed release of norepinephrine into these organs. Functional studies have revealed that chemical sympathectomy of spleen and lymph nodes in adults is followed by diminished primary and secondary antibody responses, diminished delayed-type hypersensitivity responses, and diminished mitogenic responses in lymph nodes. Since this collective body of evidence points towards the presence of noradrenergic nerves, the release of norepinephrine, and the functional "postsynaptic" interaction of norepinephrine with cells of the immune system, we suggest that norepinephrine serves the role of a neurotransmitter in the parenchyma of secondary lymphoid tissue. This opens up the possibility that various neurotransmitters may play an important role as immunomodulators, and may provide a direct link, perhaps supplementing classical neuroendocrine circuits, through which the brain can regulate immune responses, and through which psychosocial, stressful, and environmental factors may exert an influence over health and illness.

References

1. Grossman, M.I. (1981). General concepts. In S.R. Bloom & J.M. Polak (Eds.), Gut hormones. Churchill Livingstone, N.Y., p.17-22.
2. Petrusz, P., Merchenthaler, I., Ordronneau, P., Maderdrut, J.L., Vigh, S. & Schally, A.V. (1984). Corticotropin-releasing factor (CRF)-like immunoreactivity in the gastro-entero-pancreatic endocrine system. Peptides, 5, suppl. 1: 71-78.
3. Gershon, M.D. (1981). The enteric nervous system. Ann. Rev. Neurosci., 4: 227-272.
4. Ferguson, A. (1985). Immunological responses to food. Proc. Nutr. Soc., 44:73-80.
5. Harty, R.F. & Leibach, J.R. (1985). Immune disorders of the gastrointestinal tract and liver. Med. Clin. North America, 69: 675-704.
6. Pabst, R. & Trepel, F. (1975). Quantitative evaluation of the total number and distribution of lymphocytes in young pigs. Blut, 31: 77-86.
7. Schofield, G.C. (1968). Anatomy of muscular and neural tissues in the alimentary canal. In C.F. Code (Ed.), Handbook of physiology, Section 6: Alimentary canal, Vol. IV. Motility. American Physiological Soc., Washington, p. 1579-1627.
8. Gershon, M.D., Payette, R.F. & Rothman, T.P. (1985). Microenvironmental factors in phenotypic expression by enteric neurons: Parallels to lymphocytes. In G. Guillemin, M. Cohn & T. Melnechuk (Eds.), Neural modulation of immunity. Raven Press, N.Y., p. 221-242.
9. Buchan, A.M.J., Bryant, M.G., Polak, J.M., Gregor, M., Ghatei, M.A. & Bloom, S.R. (1981). Development of regulatory peptides in the human fetal intestine. In S.R. Bloom & J.E. Polak (Eds.), Gut hormones. Churchill Livingstone, N.Y., p. 119-124.
10. Gabella, G. (1979). Innervation of the gastrointestinal tract. Int. Rev. Cytol., 59: 130-193.
11. Henning, S.J. (1985). Ontogeny of enzymes in the small intestine. Ann. Rev. Physiol., 47: 231-245.

12. Johnson, L.R. (1985). Functional development of the stomach. Ann. Rev. Physiol., 47: 199-215.
13. LeDouarin, N.M. & Fontaine-Perus, J. (1981). The neural crest and the digestive tract: Developmental relationships. In S.R. Bloom & J.E. Polak (Eds.), Gut hormones. Churchill Livingstone, N.Y., p. 107-118.
14. Lipkin, M. (1985). Growth and dev lopment of gastrointestinal cells. Ann. Rev. Physiol., 47: 175-197.
15. Solcia, E., Capella, C., Buffa, R., Usellini, L. & Tenti, P. (1982). Morphological basis of gastrointestinal motility: Ultrastructure and histochemistry of endocrine-paracrine cells in the gut. In G. Bertaccini (Ed.), Mediators and drugs in gastrointestinal motility I. Morphological basis and neurophysiological control. Handbook of experimental pharmacology, Vol. 59/I. Springer-Verlag, N.Y., p. 55-78.
16. Costa, M. & Furness, J.B. (1982). Nervous control of intestinal motility. In G. Bertaccini (Ed)., Mediators and drugs in gastrointestinal motility I, Handbook of experimental pharmacology, Vol. 59/I. Springer-Verlag, N.Y., p. 279-382.
17. Oldfield, B.J. & McLachlan, E.M. (1981). An analysis of the sympathetic preganglionic neurons projecting from the upper thoracic spinal roots of the cat. J. Comp. Neurol., 196: 329-345.
18. Romagnano, M.A. & Hamill, R.W. (1984). Spinal sympathetic pathway: An enkephalin ladder. Science, 225: 737-739.
19. Baumgarten, H.G. (1982). Morphological basis of gastrointestinal motility: Structure and innervation of the gastrointestinal tract. In G. Bertaccini (Ed.), Mediators and drugs in gastrointestinal motility I, Handbook of experimental pharmacology, Vol.59/I. Springer-Verlag, N.Y., p. 7-53.
20. Krukoff, T.L., Ciriello, J. & Calaresu, F.R. (1985). Segmental distribution of peptide- and 5-HT-like immunoreactivity in nerve terminals and fibers of the thoracolumbar sympathetic nuclei of the cat. J. Comp. Neurol., 240: 103-116.
21. Smith, O.A. & DeVito, J.L. (1984). Central neural integration for the control of autonomic responses associated with emotion. Ann. Rev. Neurosci., 7: 43-65.
22. Krukoff, T.L., Ciriello, J. & Calaresu, F.R. (1985). Segmental distribution of peptide-like immunoreactivity in cell bodies of the thoracolumbar sympathetic nuclei of the cat. J. Comp. Neurol., 240: 90-102.
23. Hökfelt, T., Johansson, O., Ljungdahl, A., Lundberg, J.M. & Schultzberg, M. (1980). Peptidergic neurons. Nature, 284: 515-521.
24. Schultzberg, M. (1983). The peripheral nervous system. In P.C. Emson (Ed.), Chemical neuronanatomy. Raven Press, N.Y., p. 1-51.
25. Baron, R., Jänig, W. & McLachlan, E.M. (1985). The afferent and sympathetic components of the lumbar spinal outflow to the colon and pelvic organs in the cat. I. The hypogastric nerve. J. Comp. Neurol., 238: 135-146.
26. Baron, R., Jänig, W. & McLachlan, E.M. (1985). The afferent and sympathetic components of the lumbar spinal outflow to the colon and pelvic organs in the cat. III. The colonic nerves, incorporating an analysis of all components of the lumbar prevertebral outflow. J. Comp. Neurol., 238: 158-168.
27. Szurszewski, J.H. (1981). Physiology of mammalian prevertebral ganglia. Ann. Rev. Physiol., 43: 53-68.
28. Lundberg, J.M., Dahlström, A., Larsson, I., Petterson, G., Ahlman, H. & Kewenter, J. (1978). Efferent innervation of the small intestine by adrenergic neurons from the cervical sympathetic and stellate ganglia, studied by retrograde transport of peroxidase. Acta Physiol. Scand., 104: 33-42.
29. Burnstock, G. (1981). Physiology of the gastrointestinal nerves. In S.R. Bloom & J.M. Polak (Eds.), Gut hormones. Churchill Livingstone, N.Y., p. 482-486.
30. Lundberg, J.M., Hökfelt, T., Änggard, A., Terenius, L., Elde, R., Markey, K., Goldstein, M. & Kimmel, J. (1982). Organizational principles in the peripheral sympathetic nervous system: Subdivision by coexisting peptides (somatostatin-, avian pancreatic polypeptide-, and vasoactive intestinal polypeptide-like immunoreactive materials). Proc. Natl. Acad. Sci., 79: 1303-1307.
31. Lundberg, J.M., Terenius, L., Hökfelt, T., Martling, C.R., Tatemoto, K., Mutt, V., Polak, J. & Bloom, S. (1982). Neuropeptide Y (NPY)-like immunoreactivity in peripheral noradrenergic neurons and effects of NPY on sympathetic function. Acta Physiol. Scand., 116: 477-480.
32. Furness, J.B., Costa, M. & Keast, J.R. (1984). Cholinacetyltransferase and peptide immunoreactivity of submucous neurons of the guinea-pig small intestine. Cell Tiss. Res., 234: 71-92.

33. Bohlen, H.G. (Ed.) (1984). Regional vascular behavior in the gastrointestinal wall. Fed. Proc., 43: 7-15.
34. Guth, P.H. (1982). Stomach blood flow and acid secretion. Ann. Rev. Physiol., 44: 3-12.
35. Lundberg, J.M., Dahlström, A., Bylock, A., Ahlman, H., Petterson, G., Larsson, I., Hansson, H.-A. & Kewenter, J. (1978). Ultrastructural evidence for an innervation of epithelial enterochromaffine cells in the guinea pig duodenum. Acta Physiol. Scand., 104: 3-12.
36. Forte, J.G. (1985). Gastrointestinal physiology. Ann. Rev. Physiol., 47: 173-174.
37. Glazer, E.J. & Basbaum, A.I. (1981). Immunohistochemical localization of leucine-enkephalin in the spinal cord of the cat: Enkephalin-containing marginal neurons and pain modulation. J. Comp. Neurol., 196: 377-389.
38. Gwyn, D.G., Leslie, R.A. & Hopkins, D.A. (1985). Observations of the afferent and efferent organization of the vagus nerve and the innervation of the stomach in the squirrel monkey. J. Comp. Neurol., 29: 163-175.
39. Dennison, S.J., O'Conner, B.L., Aprison, M.H., Merritt, V.E. & Felten, D.L. (1981). Viscerotopic localization of preganglionic parasympathetic cell bodies with origin of the anterior and posterior subdiaphragmatic vagus nerves. J. Comp. Neurol., 197: 259-269.
40. Prechtl, J.C. & Powley, T.L. (1985). Organization and distribution of the rat subdiaphragmatic vagus and associated paraganglia. J. Comp. Neurol., 235: 182-195.
41. Kalia, M. & Mesulam, M.-M. (1980). Brain stem projections of sensory and motor components of the vagus complex in the cat: II. Laryngeal, tracheobronchial, pulmonary, cardiac, and gastrointestinal branches. J. Comp. Neurol., 193: 467-508.
42. Shapiro, R.E. & Miselis, R.R. (1985). The central organization of the vagus nerve innervating the stomach of the rat. J. Comp. Neurol., 238: 473-488.
43. Louis-Sylvestre, J. (1984). Meal size: Role of reflexly induced insulin release. J. Auton. Nerv. System, 10: 317-324.
44. Powley, T.L. & Berthoud, H.-R. (1985). Diet and cephalic phase insulin responses. Am. J. Clin. Nutr., 42: 991-1002.
45. Uvnäs-Moberg, K. (1983). Release of gastrointestinal peptides in response to vagal activation induced by electrical stimulation, feeding and suckling. In J.G. Kral, T.L. Powley & C. Mc. Brooks (Eds.), Vagal nerve function: Behavioral and methodological considerations. Elsevier, Amsterdam, p. 141-155.
46. Lundgren, O. (1983). Vagal control of the motor functions of the lower esophageal sphincter and the stomach. In J.G. Kral, T.L. Powley & C. Mc. Brooks (Eds.), Vagal nerve function: Behavioral and methodological considerations. Elsevier, Amsterdam, p. 185-197.
47. Lundberg, J.M., Hökfelt, T., Nilsson, G., Terenius, L., Rehfeld, J., Elde, R.P. & Said, S. (1978). Peptide neurons in the vagus, splanchnic and sciatic nerves. Acta Physiol. Scand., 104: 499-501.
48. Ahlman, H. & Dahlström, A. (1983). Vagal mechanisms controlling serotonin release from the gastrointestinal tract and pyloric motor function. In J.G. Kral, T.L. Powley & C.Mc. Brooks (Eds.), Vagal nerve function: Behavioral and functional considerations. Elsevier, Amsterdam, p. 119-140.
49. Gibbins, I.L., Furness, J.B., Costa, M., MacIntyre, I., Hillyard, C.J. & Girgis, S. (1985). Co-localization of calcitonin gene-related peptide-like immunoreactivity with substance P in cutaneous, vascular and visceral sensory neurons of guinea-pig. Neurosci. Letts., 57: 125-130.
50. Kai-Kai, M.A., Swann, R.W. & Keen, P. (1985). Localization of chromatographically characterized oxytocin and arginine-vasopressin to sensory neurons in the rat. Neurosci. Letts., 55: 83-88.
51. Leah, J.D., Cameron, A.A. & Snow, P.J. (1985). Neuropeptides in physiologically identified mammalian sensory neurons. Neurosci. Letts., 56: 257-263.
52. Kawatani, M., Erdman, S.L. & de Groat, W.C. (1985). Vasoactive intestinal polypeptide and substance P in primary sensory afferent pathways to the sacral spinal cord of the cat. J. Comp. Neurol., 241: 327-347.
53. Mei, N. (1985). Intestinal chemosensitivity. Physiol. Rev., 65: 211-237.
54. Rehfeld, J.F. (1983). Gastrin and cholecystokinin in the vagus. In J.G. Kral, T.L. Powley & C. Mc. Brooks (Eds.), Vagal nerve function: Behavioral and methodological considerations. Elsevier, Amsterdam, p. 113-118.
55. Uvnäs-Wallenstein, K. (1981). Peptides in metabolic autonomic nerves. Diabetologia, 20: 337-342.
56. Sawchenko, P.E. (1983). Central connections of the sensory and motor nuclei of the vagus nerve. In J.G. Kral, T.L. Powley & C. Mc. Brooks (Eds.), Vagal nerve function: Behavioral and methodological considerations. Elsevier, Amsterdam, p. 13-26.
57. Higgins, G.A., Hoffman, G.E., Wray, S. & Schwaber, J.S. (1984). Distribution of neurotensin-

immunoreactivity within barorecptive portions of the nucleus of the tractus solitarius and the dorsal vagal nucleus of the rat. J. Comp. Neurol., 226: 155-164.
58. Kalia, M., Fuxe, K., Hökfelt, T., Johansson, O., Lang, R., Ganten, D., Cuello, C. & Terenius, L. (1984). Distribution of neuropeptide immunoreactive nerve terminals within the subnuclei of the nucleus of the tractus solitarius of the rat. J. Comp. Neurol., 222: 409-444.
59. Van der Kooy, D., Koda, L.Y., McGinnity, J.F., Gerfen, C.R. & Bloom, F.E. (1984). The organization of the projections from the cortex, amygdala, and hypothalamus to the nucleus of the solitary tract. J. Comp. Neurol., 224: 1-24.
60. Mei, N. (1983). Recent studies on intestinal vagal afferent innervation. Functional implications. In J.G. Kral, T.L. Powley & C. Mc. Brooks (Eds.), Vagal nerve function: Behavioral and methodological considerations. Elsevier, Amsterdam, p. 199-206.
61. El Ouazzani, T. (1984). Thermoreceptors in the digestive tract and their role. J. Auton. Nerv. System, 10: 246-254.
62. Mei, N., Perrin, J., Crousillat, J. & Boyer, A. (1984). Comparison between the properties of the vagal and splanchnic glucoreceptors of the small intestine. Involvement in insulin release. J. Auton. Nerv. System, 10: 275-278.
63. Norgren, R. (1983). Afferent interactions of cranial nerves involved in ingestion. In J.G. Kral, T.L. Powley & C. Mc. Brooks (Eds.), Vagal nerve function: Behavioral and methodological considerations. Elsevier, Amsterdam, p. 67-77.
64. Smith, G.P., Jerome, C. & Norgren, R. (1985). Afferent axons in abdominal vagus mediate satiety effect of cholecystokinin in rats. Am. J. Physiol., 249: R638-R641.
65. Novin, D. (1983). The integration of visceral information in the control of feeding. In J.G. Kral, T.L. Powley & C. Mc. Brooks (Eds.), Vagal nerve function: Behavioral and methodological considerations. Elsevier, Amsterdam, p. 233-246.
66. Fantino, M. (1984). Role of sensory input in the control of food intake. J. Auton. Nerv. System, 10: 347-358.
67. Smith, G.P. & Jerome, C. (1983). Effects of total and selective abdominal vagotomies on water intake in rats. In J.G. Kral, T.L. Powley & C. Mc. Brooks (Eds.), Vagal nerve function: Behavioral and methodological considerations. Elsevier, Amsterdam, p. 259-271.
68. McHugh, P.R. (1983). The control of gastric emptying. In J.G. Kral, T.L. Powley & C. Mc. Brooks (Eds.), Vagal nerve function: Behavioral and methodological considerations. Elsevier, Amsterdam, p. 221-231.
69. Schwartz, T.W. (1983). Pancreatic polypeptide: A unique model for vagal control of endocrine systems. In J.G. Kral, T.L. Powley & C. Mc. Brooks (Eds.), Vagal nerve function: Behavioral and methodological considerations. Elsevier, Amsterdam, p. 99-118.
70. Jeanningros, R. (1984). Lateral hypothalamic responses to pre-absorptive and post-absorptive signals related to amino acid ingestion. J. Auton. Nerv. System, 10: 261-268.
71. Miolan, J.P. & Roman, C. (1984). The role of esophageal and intestinal receptors in the control of gastric motility. J. Auton. Nerv. Sytem, 10: 235-241.
72. Rousseau, J.P. & Falempin, M. (1984). Reinnervation of a striated muscle by vagal sensory axons. J. Auton. Nerv. System, 10: 217-223.
73. Smith, P.H. & Madson, K.L. (1981). Interactions between autonomic nerves and endocrine cells of the gastro-entero-pancreatic system. Diabetologia, 20: 314-324.
74. Wood, J.D. (1981). Intrinsic neural control of intestinal motility. Ann. Rev. Physiol., 43: 33-51.
75. Fujita, T. & Kobayashi, S. (1981). The endocrine cell. In S.R. Bloom & J.M. Polak (Eds.), Gut hormones. Churchill Livingstone, N.Y., p. 90-95.
76. Marangos, P.J., Schmechel, D.E. & Oertel, W.H. (1981). Neuron-specific enolase: A functional marker for the diffuse neuro-endocrine system. In S.R. Bloom & J.E. Polak (Eds.), Gut hormones. Churchill Livingstone, N.Y., p. 101-106.
77. Newson, B., Ahlman, H., Dahlström, A., Das Gupta, T.K. & Nyhus, L.M. (1979). Are there sensory neurons in the mucosa of the mammalian gut? Acta Physiol. Scand., 105: 521-532.
78. Keast, J.R., Furness, J.B. & Costa, M. (1985). Distribution of certain peptide-containing nerve fibers and endocrine cells in the gastrointestinal mucosa in five mammalian species. J. Comp. Neurol., 236: 403-422.
79. Clague, J.R., Sternini, C. & Brecha, N.C. (1985). Localization of calcitonin gene-related peptide-like immunoreactivity in neurons of the rat gastrointestinal tract. Neurosci. Letts., 56: 63-68.
80. Furness, J.B. & Costa, M. (1982). Identification of gastrointestinal neurotransmitters. In G. Bertaccini (Ed.), Mediators and drugs in gastrointestinal motility I. Morphological basis and neurophysiological control. Handbook of experimental pharmacology. Vol. 59/I. Springer-Verlag, N.Y., p. 383-460.

81. Costa, M., Furness, J.B., Cuello, A.C., Verhofstad, A.A.J., Steinbusch, H.W.J. & Elde, R.P. (1982). Neurons with 5-hydroxytryptamine-like immunoreactivity in the enteric nervous system: Their visualization and reactions to drug treatment. Neuroscience, 7: 351-363.
82. Wolter, H.J. (1985). Topography of cholinergic perikarya and nerve fibers as well as cholinergic vesicles in the rat duodenum. Brain Res., 399: 337-341.
83. Polak, J.M. & Bloom, S.R. (1981). Organization of the gut peptidergic innervation. In S.R. Bloom & J. M. Polak (Eds.), Gut hormones. Churchill Livingstone, N.Y., p. 487-494.
84. Schultzberg, M., Hökfelt, T., Nilsson, G., Terenius, L., Rehfeld, J.F., Brown, M., Elde, R., Goldstein, M. & Said, S. (1980). Distribution of peptide- and catecholamine-containing neurons in the gastrointestinal tract of rat and guinea-pig: Immunohistochemical studies with antisera to substance P, vasoactive intestinal polypeptide, enkephalins, somatostatin, gastrin/cholecystokinin, neurotensin, and dopamine B-hydroxylase. Neuroscience, 5: 689-744.
85. Wingate, D.L. (1985). The effect of diet on small intestinal and biliary tract function. Am. J. Clin. Nutr., 42: 1020-1024.
86. Hunter, J.C., Hannah, P.A. & Maggio, J.E. (1985). The regional distribution of kassinin-like immunoreactivity in the central and peripheral tissues of the cat. Brain Res., 341: 228-232.
87. Kandarakis, E.D., Iriuchijima, T., Prasad, C. & Wilber, J.F. (1985). Distribution and characterization of cyclo (HIS-PRO)-like immunoreactivity in the human gastrointestinal tract. Neuropeptides, 6: 21-25.
88. Aravich, P.F., Davis, B.J., Sladek, C.D., Felten, S.Y., Felten, D.L. & Sladek, J.R.Jr. (1986). Vasopressin in the gut: Neural and immune systems? Anat. Rec., 214: 5A.
89. Aravich, P.F. & Sladek, J.R.Jr. (1986). Aging of rodent vasopressin systems: Morphometric and functional considerations. In D.M. Gash & G.J. Boer (Eds.), Vasopressin: Principles and properties. Plenum, N.Y.
90. Janaky, T., Laszlo, F.A., Sirokman, F. & Morgat, J.T. (1982). Biological half-life and organ distribution of (^{3}H)8-arginine vasopressin in the rat. J. Endocr., 93: 295-303.
91. Bertaccini, G. (1982). Peptides: Other hormones. Vasopressin. In G. Bertaccini (Ed.), Mediators and drugs in gastrointestinal motility II. Endogenous and exogenous agents. Handbook of experimental pharmacology, Vol. 59/II. Springer-Verlag, N.Y., p. 161-165.
92. Richardson, D.I. & Withrington, P.G. (1982). Physiological regulation of the hepatic circulation. Ann. Rev. Physiol., 44: 57-69.
93. Winne, D. (1984). Role of blood flow in intestinal permeation. In T.Z. Csaky (Ed.), Pharmacology of intestinal permeation II. Handbook of experimental pharmacology, Vol. 70/II. Springer-Verlag, N.Y., p. 301-347.
94. Aravich, P.F. & Sladek, C.D. (in press). Vasopressin and glucoprivic-feeding behavior: A new perspective on an "old" peptide. Brain Res.
95. Aravich, P.F., Sladek, C.D., Forbes, G.B. & Gallagher, M.J. (in press). High-fat, high sucrose feeding and exercise: Relationship to vasopressin and oxytocin. Soc. Neurosci. Abs.
96. Aravich, P.F., Sladek, C.D. & Forbes, G.B. (1984). The dietary obesity syndrome and vasopressin secretion. Soc. Neurosci. Abs., 10: 651.
97. Johnson, H.M., Farrar, W.L. & Torres, B.A. (1982). Vasopressin replacement of interleukin 2 requirement in gamma interferon production: Lymphokine activity of a neuroendocrine hormone. J. Immunol., 129: 983-991.
98. Hunt, N.H., Perris, A.D. & Sandfort, P.A. (1977). Role of vasopressin in the mitotic response of rat bone marrow cells to haemorrahge. J. Endocr., 72: 5-16.
99. Geenen, V., Legros, J.-J., Franchimont, P., Baudrihaye, M., Defresne, M.-P. & Boniver, J. (1986). The neuroendocrine thymus: Coexistence of oxytocin and neurophysin in the human thymus. Science, 232: 508-510.
100. Castro, G.A. (1982). Immunological regulation of epithelial function. Am. J. Physiol., 243: G321-G329.
101. Mayrofer, G. (1984). Physiology of the intestinal immune system. In T.J. Newby & C.R. Stokes (Eds.), Local immune responses of the gut. CRC Press, Boca Raton, p. 1-96.
102. Bienenstock, J. (1984). Mucosal barrier functions. Nutr. Rev., 42: 105-108.
103. Johansson, S.G.O. (1984). Immunological mechanisms of food sensitivity. Nutr. Rev., 42: 79-84.
104. Levinsky, R.J. (1985). Factors influencing intestinal uptake of food antigens. Proc. Nutr. Soc., 44: 81-86.
105. Perdue, M.H., Forstner, J.F., Roomi, N.W. & Gall, D.G. (1984). Epithelial response to intestinal anaphylaxis in rats: Goblet cell secretion and enterocyte damage. Am. J. Physiol., 247: G632-G637.

106. Foucard, T. (1984). Developmental aspects of food sensitivity in childhood. Nutr. Rev., 42: 98-104.
107. Fortherby, K.J. & Hunter, J.O. (1985). Symptoms of food allergies. Clin. Gastroenterology, 14: 615-629.
108. Lessof, M.H. (1985). Food intolerance. Proc. Nutr. Soc., 44: 121-125.
109. May, C.D. (1984). Food sensitivity - Facts and fancies. Nutr. Rev., 42: 72-78.
110. Metcalfe, D.D. (1984). Diagnostic procedures for immunologically-mediated food sensitivity. Nutr. Rev., 42: 92-97.
111. Panush, R.S. & Webster, E.M. (1985). Food allergies and other adverse reactions to fo ds. Med. Clin. North America, 69: 533-546.
112. Bray, G.A. & York, D.A. (1979). Hypothalamic and genetic obesity in experimental animals: An autonomic and endocrine hypothesis. Physiol. Rev., 59: 719-809.
113. Corman, L.C. (1985). Effects of specific nutrients on the immune response. Med. Clin. North America, 69: 759-791.
114. Gershwin, M.E., Beach, R.S. & Hurley, L.S. (1985). Nutrition and immunity. Academic Press, N.Y.
115. Gross, R.L. & Newberne, P.M. (1980). Role of nutrition in immunologic function. Physiol. Rev., 60: 188-302.
116. Deutsch, J.A. (1985). The role of the stomach in eating. Am. J. Clin. Nutr., 42: 1040-1043.
117. Koopmans, H.S. (1985). Satiety signals from the gastrointestinal tract. Am. J. Clin. Nutr., 42: 1044-1049.
118. Koopmans, H.S., Sclafani, A., Fitchner, C. & Aravich, P.F. (1982). The effects of ileal transposition on food intake and body weight loss in VMH-obese rats. Am. J. Clin. Nutr., 35: 284-293.
119. Felten, D.L., Overhage, J.N., Felten, S.Y. & Schmedtje, J.F. (1981). Noradrenergic innervation of lymphoid tissue in the rabbit appendix: Further evidence for a link between the nervous and immune systems. Brain Res. Bull., 7: 595-612.
120. Jesseph, J.M. & Felten, D.L. (1984). Noradrenergic innervation of the gut-associated lymphoid tissues (GALT) in the rabbit. Anat. Rec., 208: 81A
121. Felten, D.L., Felten, S.Y., Carlson, S.L., Olschowka, J.A. & Livnat, S. (1985). Noradrenergic and peptidergic innervation of lymphoid tissue. J. Immunol., 135: 755s-765s.
122. Felten, D.L., Livnat, S., Felten, S.Y., Carlson, S.L., Bellinger, D.L. & Yeh, P. (1985). Sympathetic innervation of lymph nodes in mice. Brain Res. Bull., 13: 693-699.
123. Livnat, S., Felten, S.Y., Carlson, S.L., Bellinger, D.L. & Felten, D.L. (1985). Involvement of peripheral and central catecholamine systems in neural-immune interactions. J. Neuro-immunol., 10: 5-30.

Central Neurochemical Mechanisms in Experimental Stress Ulcer

Gary B. Glavin

Peptic ulcer is considered a "classic" psychosomatic disease. Many techniques have been employed for the induction of experimental ulcers in laboratory animals. These include administration of various drugs including non-steroidal anti-inflammatory agents; ethanol; steroids; dietary manipulations including starvation; brain lesion/stimulation and exposure to extreme environmental temperatures. As a result of the extensive use of these procedures, much information was gained regarding the pathogenesis and pharmacotherapy of peptic ulcer disease.

In the 1970s a new diagnostic category - stress ulcer - necessitated the inclusion of behavioral factors in the etiology of gut disease. The belief that there existed a behavioral or psychological component to the etiology of stress ulcer resulted in the search for effective animal models of this disease. Lee and Bianchi (1) proposed several criteria by which to assess the validity and efficacy of experimental stress ulcer models, including: minimization of pre-stress starvation, production of *true* ulcer (penetrating the *muscularis mucosa*) in the area of the gastrointestinal tract which is of interest and relevance, production of ulcers in a variety of animal species, response of the ulcers to current surgical and pharmacological treatment regimens, and the production of ulcers which did not spontaneously heal during the experimental observation period. The literature abounds with experimental ulcer models, however, to such models appear to satisfy most of the aforementioned criteria and also appear to be used more frequently than any others. These models are the immobilization or restraint technique (2) and the activity-stress ulcer model (3).

Immobilization

The use of acute immobilization or restraint to induce ulcers has been reviewed elsewhere (2, 4). Following is a brief description of the procedure used in our laboratory. Rats are food-deprived for 12 h and then placed into specially constructed restraint harnesses in the supine position. They are then placed into a cold (4°-6°C) environment (5) for 3 h. Following restraint the animals are immediately sacrificed, the stomach excised and examined for ulcers under a

---

Supported by NSERC, Manitoba Health Research Council, Health Sciences Centre, (Manitoba) Research Foundation.

dissecting microscope with an ocular micrometer, by an observer who is naive with respect to experimental conditions. The number and cumulative length (length plus width) in millimeters of any ulcers are recorded. In otherwise unmanipulated rats, this restraint regimen is reliably and consistently associated with ulcers (some of which penetrate the *muscularis*) in 95% to 100% of the animals so treated, and most rats exhibit an average of 20 to 40 mm of gastric glandular ulcers and erosions.

Our experience suggests that if careful consideration is given to choice of sex, strain, species, age, restraint method, restraint duration, circadian and circannual variation and diet (4), the restraint-stress-induced ulcer is a powerful, reliable, valid, and clinically relevant model of gut disease.

Activity-Stress

Pare and Houser (6) suggested the term activity-stress to account for the observation that if young adult male rats are housed in individual running wheel activity cages and fed only one h each day, they ate progressively less each day, exhibited markedly increased running activity, lost body weight, and died in 5-12 days. At autopsy, these animals exhibited massive gastric glandular ulcers (3, 7). It is important to note that food-yoked control rats (animals housed in standard laboratory cages *without* access to a running wheel but which are fed the *same* amount of food as activity-wheel rats) do not die and do not exhibit gastric ulcers or other stress responses. Interestingly, activity-stress ulcers appear to be associated with gastric *hyposecretion* and do not respond to histamine H_2 receptor blockade or to locallyacting antacids or anti-cholinergics (8, 9). However, centrally-acting agents such as imipramine and diazepam are effective in decreasing activity-stress gastric ulcers (9, 10). Activity-stress has seen extensive use in many laboratories investigating both central and peripheral mechanisms in gut disease and appears to be a reliable and reproducible model of relatively chronic stress-induced gastrointestinal disease.

Using both of these animal models, we have investigated the role of central neurotransmitters and aberrations therein, in the genesis and prevention of experimental stress ulcer in animals. Following is a summary of current work in our laboratory, with my colleagues Dr. Werner Westerberg, Dr. Frank LaBella, Dr. Gary Rockman, Dr. William Pare, Dr. Mark Hnatowich, Ms. Aisha Dugani and Ms. Kathleen Kiernan.

Noradrenaline

The role of brain noradrenaline (NA) in stress pathology has been recently reviewed (11). Brain NA appears to be markedly altered in both animal models of stress - up to 175% increases in NA turnover in many brain regions of re-straint stressed rats (12) and even greater changes in activity stress (13, 14, 15). Interestingly, centrally acting agents (e.g., desipramine, imipramine, chlorpromazine) are *more* effective in reducing activity stress ulcers than are peripherally acting agents such as anticholinergics, H_2 receptor blockers, and antacids (9, 10).

Table 1. Regional brain NA and MHPG-SO_4 levels (ng/g) for the NA depletion (FLA-63 + R04-1284) restraint stress study (mean ± S.E.M.).

Group:	Saline - no restraint		Saline - restraint		FLA-63 + R04-1284 - no restraint		FLA-63 + R04-1284 - restraint	
Region	NA	MHPG	NA	MHPG	NA	MHPG	NA	MHPG
Hypothalamus	1520.6	288.1	1611.1	333.1	97.7*	10.8*	101.3*	99.0*
	(61.0)	(21.2)	(120.3)	(9.2)	(8.0)	(7.7)	(6.0)	(6.1)
Thalamus	480.2	221.3	283.1*	520.0*	21.6*	115.1*	32.8*	131.3*
	(29.1)	(9.1)	(19.0)	(21.1)	(2.3)	(10.1)	(3.7)	(7.2)
Amygdala	411.9	181.0	390.3*	241.0*	11.6*	-	-	-
	(10.8)	(8.8)	(20.1)	(41.1)	(1.9)	-	-	-
Hippocampus	361.0	98.3	253.0*	121.3	9.6*	-	-	-
	(21.3)	(7.0)	(9.9)	(19.2)	(0.8)	-	-	-
Midbrain	488.8	220.0	422.3	288.0*	31.2*	117.0*	19.0*	121.2*
	(22.0)	(9.9)	(11.1)	(51.3)	(1.6)	(7.7)	(1.1)	(10.2)
Pons + med.	517.8	185.3	520.3	201.3	19.8*	90.0*	11.3*	111.7*
obl.	(19.7)	(11.0)	(31.3)	(19.8)	(1.1)	(7.7)	(2.2)	(8.3)
Cortex	191.1	99.1	208.6	160.1*	-	-	-	-
	(10.3)	(8.3)	(22.7)	(27.0)	-	-	-	-
Basal ganglia	228.5	173.1	201.1	411.8*	-	-	-	-
	(9.2)	(7.9)	(17.3)	(31.0)	-	-	-	-

- undetectable
* significantly different from saline control groups ($p < 0.05$)

In addition, we found a modest correlation between the degree of increase in NA turnover induced by stress and the development of gastric stress ulcers (12). Chronic but not acute pretreatment of rats with tricyclic antidepressants (sufficient to induce subsensitivity of central ß-adrenergic-receptor-coupled adenylate cyclase) attenuates subsequent stress-induced gastric pathology and corticosterone responses to stress. We thus support the work of Stone who suggests that chronic antidepressant drug treatment is a unique form of adaptation to stress (16, 17, 18).

Recently, we showed that rats given a regimen of the dopamine-ß-hydroxylase inhibitor, FLA-63, and the rapid vesicular NA depletor, R04-1284 (which depletes both the "functional" *and* "reserve" pools (19) of central NA) according to the method of Zolovick et al. (20), exhibited marked increases in their gastric ulcer and plasma corticosterone responses to restraint stress (21).

Table 2. Summary of stomach conditions[1] and plasma corticosterone levels for the NA-depletion (FLA-63 + R04-1284) restraint stress study (mean ± S.E.M).

Treatment	No. of rats	No. of rats with ulcers	No. of ulcers per rat		Cumulative ulcer length (mm)		Plasma cortico-sterone (CS)(μg/dl)	
Saline & restraint	10	10	4.1	(1.7)*	7.4	(3.4)*	68.3	(3.7)*
Saline - no restraint	10	0	0.0	(0.0)	0.0	(0.0)	31.2	(6.6)
FLA-63 + R04-1284 - restraint	10	10	11.6	(4.2)**	18.0	(3.9)**	77.1	(8.5)*
FLA-63 + R04-1284 - no restraint	10	0	0.0	(0.0)	0.0	(0.0)	36.6	(6.9)

1. glandular ulcers only
* significantly different from control ($p < 0.05$)
** significantly different from saline-restraint ($p < 0.05$)

Briefly, rats were given FLA-63 (10 mg/kg i.p.) followed 0.5 h later by R04-1284 (5.0 mg/kg). Eight hours later, brain NA was reduced to less than 5% of control (saline-treated) levels, while DA and 5-HT levels were within 90% of control values. Some animals were then given restraint stress and we observed marked exacerbation of stress pathology in NA-depleted rats.That this procedure was not in itself associated with stress responses and that it was a relatively specific (for NA) depletion, suggest that adequate central noradrenergic function is essential for the elaboration of coping responses to stress and that when such function is impaired, coping behavior is similarly impaired and exacerbated stress responses are observed. These observations are similar to those of Anisman et al. (22) and Weiss and his colleagues (23) who used electric shock and cold swim stress.

We also altered brain NA levels in a less direct fashion and observed subsequent stress responses in rats (24).

Table 3. Summary of ulcer and plasma corticostereone data for the restraint pre-treatment study (mean ± S.E.M.).

Group	No. of ulcers		Ulcer incidence	Plasma CS (μg/dl)	
Cold swim	19.8	(3.3)	8/8	39.75	(3.9)
Shock only	14.6	(4.0)	8/8	41.56	(9.1)
Shock & desipramin (10.0 mg/kg)	1.9	(0.4)*	6/8	33.56	(2.4)*
Methamphetamine (3.0 mg/kg)	4.6	(1.2)	6/8	38.50	(5.6)
No pre-treatment	10.3	(1.8)	8/8	45.88	(6.2)

* significantly less than no pre-treatment controls ($p < 0.05$)

Table 4. Summary of brain assay data for the restraint pre-treatment study (mean ± S.E.M.).

Group	NA (ng/g)	$MHPG-SO_4$ (ng/g)	DA (ng/g)
Cold swim	301.4 (19.5)**	259.6 (9.5)	1080.7 (101.9)
Shock only	347.6 (9.1)	233.2 (10.4)	923.1 (27.2)
Shock & desipramine (10.0 mg/kg)	388.6 (23.8)	191.5 (15.1)*	987.6 (28.7)
Methamphetamine (3.0 mg/kg)	356.5 (22.6)	184.9 (11.2)	1084.5 (64.4)
No pre-treatment	321.9 (12.5)	209.8 (18.6)	934.2 (18.5)

* significantly less than cold swim and shock groups ($p < 0.05$)
** significantly less than all other groups ($p < 0.05$)

Some animals were exposed to cold swim (5 min in 10° C water), to inescapable, uncontrollable electric shock (2.5 mA for 0.5 sec 12 times in 60 min), to the shock preceded by an injection of NA uptake inhibitor desipramine HCL, or to methamphetamine HCL (3.0 mg/kg s.c.) (to stimulate NA-containing cell bodies in the locus coeruleus and enhance NA release). All rats were then exposed to restraint-cold stress for three hours. Enhancing (methamphetamine group) or protecting (desipramine groups) brain NA prior to restraint stress exposure were associated with the least amount of stress gastric pathology.

Table 5. Summary of stomach pathology[1] for the methylphenidate-activity-stress study.

Group	No. of rats	No. of rats with ulcers	Mean (± S.E.M.) no. ulcers	Cumulative ulcer mean (± S.E.M.) length (mm)
Saline	15	15	8.9 (8.1)	16.3 (6.7)
Methylphenidate (5.0 mg/kg i.p.)	15	15	10.7 (9.6)	24.1 (7.1)*
Methylphenidate (10.0 mg/kg i.p.)	15	15	11.0 (9.8)	29.0 (8.3)*
Methylphenidate (20.0 mg/kg i.p.)	15	15	15.4 (10.9)	55.8 (8.8)*

1. glandular ulcers only
* significantly different from saline controls ($p < 0.05$)

Cold swim-exposed rats exhibited the greatest degree of restraint ulcer. A modest correlation ($r = 0.71$; $p < 0.05$) was observed between whole brain NA levels and the number of gastric ulcers occurring in response to restraint stress.

Again, the conclusion that disrupted (decreased) central noradrenergic function predisposes animals to exacerbated gastric responses to acute stress seems warranted.

Figure 1. Mean (± S.E.M.) 3-methyoxy-4-hydroxy-phenylethyleneglycol sulfate ($MHGP-SO_4$) levels in eight brain regions of wheel-housed (n = 15 per group) and home-cage-housed (n = 15 per group) rats.

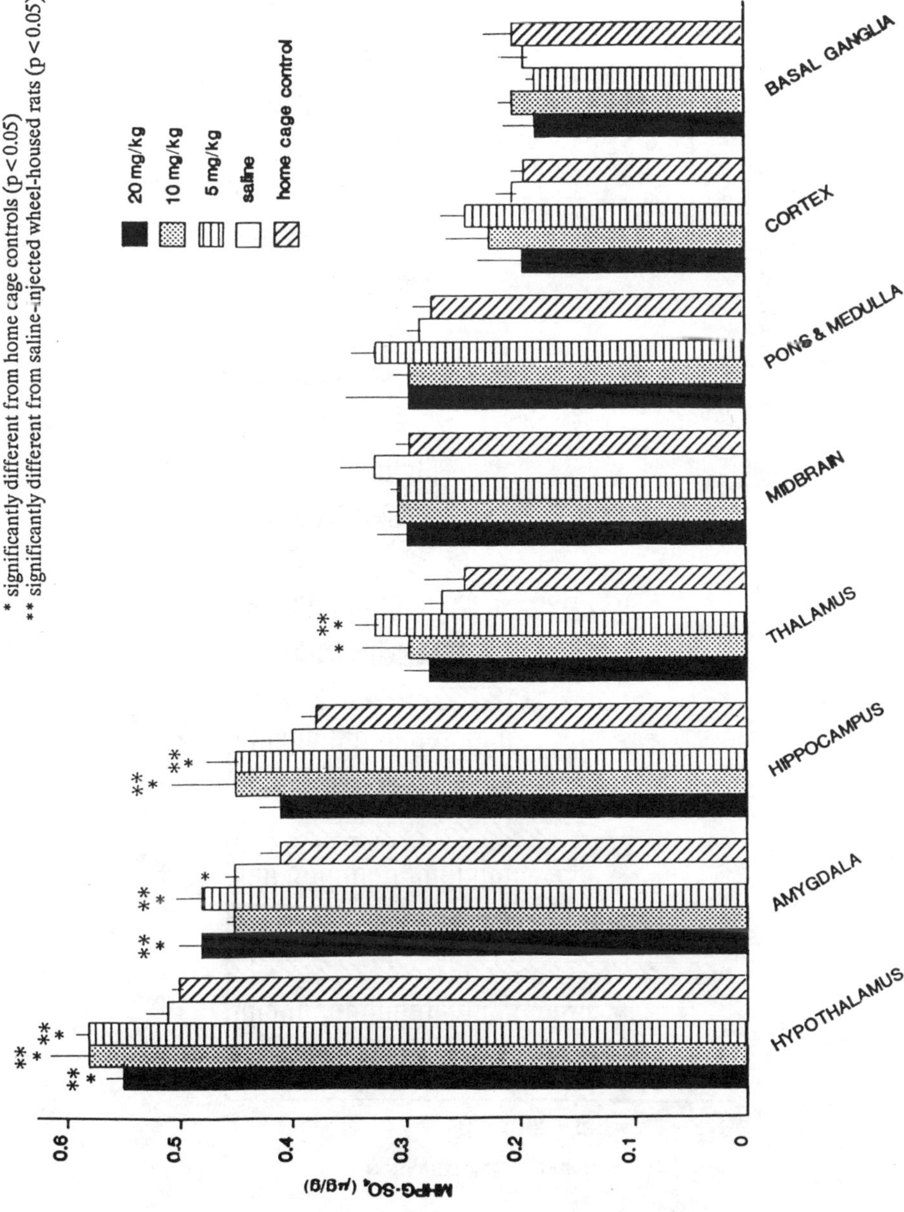

Figure 2. Mean (± S.E.M.) noradrenaline (NA) levels in eight brain regions of wheel-housed (n = 15 per group) and home-cage-housed (n = 15 per group) rats.

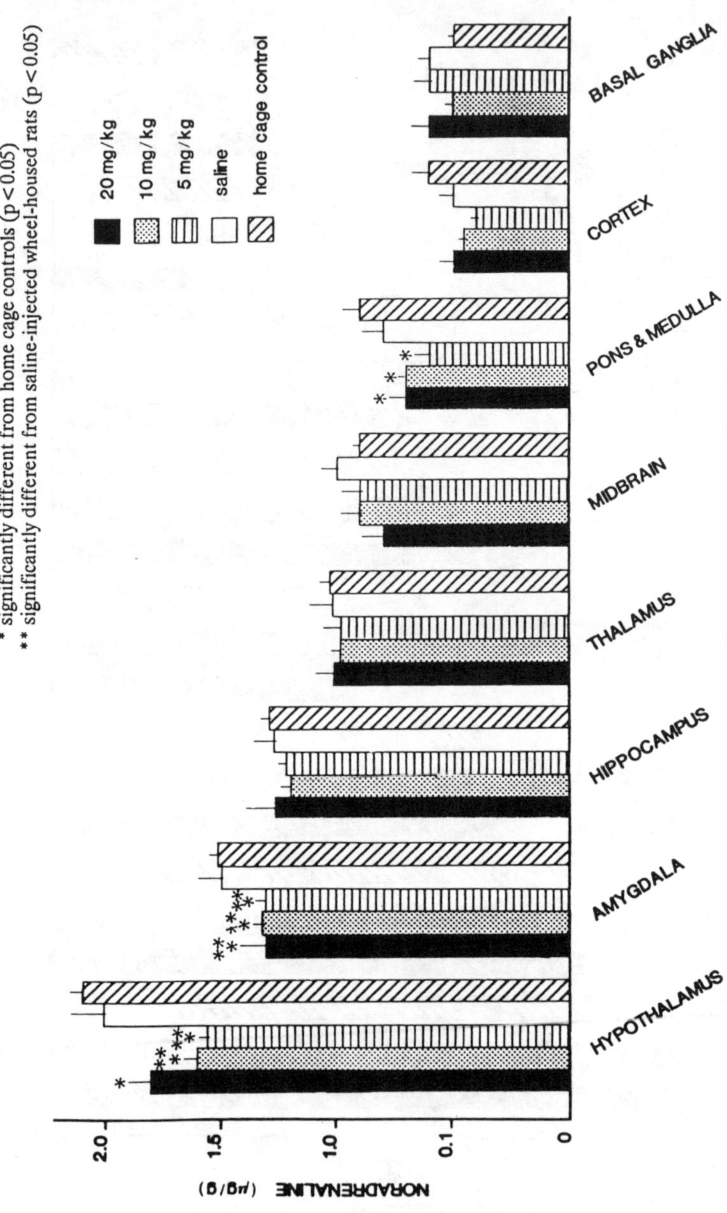

Finally we examined the effects of methylphenidate, believed to enhance brain noradrenergic activity and turnover through enhanced NA release, by stimulation of tyrosine hydroxylase activity (the rate-limiting enzyme in the biosynthesis of neural catecholamines), and by NA uptake inhibition, in the activity-stress ulcer paradigm (25). Methylphenidate i.p. (5.0, 10.0, or 20.0 mg/kg/day) did not influence either running wheel activity or daily food intake throughout the activity-stress period.

However, methylphenidate did produce dose-related increases in gastric ulcer severity paralleled by decreased NA and increased MHPG-SO_4 in the hypothalamus, hippocampus, and thalamus structures which have received considerable attention in terms of the regulation of gastric physiology and pathophysiology (26, 27).

Dopamine

Recent investigations have examined the relationship between central dopamine (DA) activity and gastric pathology. The elegant work of Szabo (28, 29) stems from his own research as well as his examination of the literature, both of which suggest that in disorders characterized by central DA deficiency, such as Parkinson's disease, duodenal ulcer incidence is relatively high, while schizophrenic disorders, believed to be due, in part, to excess brain DA function, are rarely associated with concomitant gastric disease. Szabo and his colleagues recently showed that the synthetic meperidine analog N-methyl-4-phenyl-1,2,3,6-tetrahydropyridine (MPTP) induced marked duodenal as well as gastric ulceration in addition to its well-known central DA toxicity (30).

Table 6. Effects of L-dopa on restraint-stress ulcer formation[1] and plasma corticosterone level.

Group	Mean (± S.E.M.) no. ulcers		Mean (± S.E.M.) ulcer length (mm)		Mean (± S.E.M.) plasma CS (μg/dl)	
1-dopa 0.5 mg/kg i.p.	7.4	(2.2)	22.8	(5.2)	66.2	(2.9)
1-dopa 1.0 mg/kg i.p.	2.8	(0.6)**	7.8	(2.8)**	47.4	(3.7)*
1-dopa 2.0 mg/kg i.p.	4.8	(1.0)	11.8	(2.4)	38.8	(2.6)*
Vehicle	4.7	(0.6)	16.0	(1.1)	68.6	(1.9)

1. glandular ulcers only
* significantly less than vehicle and 0.5 mg/kg groups ($p < 0.05$)
** significantly less than all other groups ($p < 0.05$)

Interestingly, MAO-A inhibition by 1-deprenyl (which attenuates MPTP-induced central DA toxicity) reduces MPTP-induced duodenal pathology (31). DA agonists also prevented cysteamine-induced duodenal ulcer formation (32). In addition, Hernandez and his colleagues (33) demonstrated a significant ulcer protective effect of peripherally-acting DA agonists and DA-releasing agents, suggesting that *peripheral* DA receptors mediate the observed gastric cytoprotection following dopamimetic treatment. In addition, we have preliminary data showing that peripherally administered DA agonists such as bromocriptine and bupropion reduce basal gastric acid secretion in rats. Conversely, the DA antagonists haloperidol and pimozide augment gastric acid output. Interestingly, L-dopa, given 1 h prior to cold-restraint stress (0.5, 1.0, or 2.0 mg/kg i.p.) resulted in decreased ulcer severity, but only at the higher doses and to the greatest extent at 1.0 mg/kg. Plasma corticosterone was reduced in a dose-related fashion by L-dopa.Domperidone, a *peripherally* acting DA antagonist was without effect in terms of antagonizing the ulcer protection afforded by the DA agonists bromocriptine or bupropion, nor did it augment haloperidol- or pimozide-induced exacerbation of restraint stress ulcers. These data suggest that central DA activity is important in determining the extent of stress-induced gastrointestinal pathology, in addition to any mediation by peripheral DA function. As early as 1976, Strocchi et al. (34) suggested that sulpiride, a DA pre-synaptic ("autoreceptor") antagonist reduced restraint-stress ulcers via restoration of *central* NA/DA balance and not via peripheral mechanisms. However, a very recent (and incomplete) study in our laboratory indicates otherwise and complicates matters somewhat. In rats given unilateral 6-OHDA lesions in the right substantia nigra according to the method of Ungerstedt and Arbuthnott (35), followed in 5 days of 3 hours of cold-restraint stress, ulcer severity was 50% of that seen in sham (saline infused) rats.

Table 7. Effects of unilateral 6-OH-DA stubstantia nigra lesions on restraint stress ulcer[1] formation.

Treatment	Mean (± S.E.M.) no. ulcers	Mean (± S.E.M.) ulcer length (mm)
6-OH-DA lesion (n = 8)	11.7 (0.6)*	22.7 (2.7)*
Vehicle (n = 8)	20.5 (3.8)*	40.5 (7.9)*

1. glandular ulcers only
* significantly less than control ($p < 0.05$)

However, a preliminary study in our laboratory using intracerebroventricularly (i.c.v.) administered DA agonists (bromocriptine and bupropion) and antagonists (haloperidol and pimozide) produced consistent effects; that is, agonists reduced and antagonists exacerbated stress pathology in the stomach. Clearly, the role of DA function in stress and stress responses is far from clear and must be extensively investigated.

Adenosine

The observation that caffeine, perhaps the most widely used psychotropic drug in the Western world, is associated with gastric distress and is a blocker of central adenosine receptors (36), prompted us to examine whether adenosine agonists might protect against stress-related gastric pathology (37). The metabolically stable adenosine agonist (-) phenylisopropyladenosine (-) PIA, at doses of 0.005, 0.10, and 0.25 mg/kg s.c. reduced the severity of restraint stress-induced gastric ulcers. Its stereoisomer (+) PIA reduced stress ulcer formation only at the highest dose examined (1.0 mg/kg). Interestingly, (-) PIA reduced the stress-induced rise in plasma corticosterone, but did so at higher doses than those required to attenuate ulcer formation. At higher concentrations of (-) PIA (1.0 mg/kg s.c.), a reversal of the agonist-induced protection was observed. Such a reversal may be mediated through A_2 sites which, when activated, stimulate adenylate cyclase in gut tissue and thus may increase gastric secretion and its pathological consequences.

Table 8. Effects of (-)Phenylisopropyladenosine (-PIA) restraint-induced ulcer[1] formation and plasma corticosterone levels.

Group	Mean (± S.E.M.) no of ulcers	Mean (± S.E.M.) ulcer length (mm)	Mean (± S.E.M.) plasma CS (µg/dl)
Vehicle	17.5 (0.7)	51.5 (3.7)	65.1 (4.3)
(-) PIA 0.01 mg/kg	15.3 (1.8)	41.0 (5.4)	61.0 (10.1)
(-) PIA 0.05 mg/kg	9.3 (1.6)*	18.2 (3.6)*	58.1 (1.2)
(-) PIA 0.10 mg/kg	10.3 (2.5)*	24.0 (5.6)*	37.4 (6.6)*
(-) PIA 0.25 mg/kg	12.7 (2.1)	23.5 (3.3)*	35.6 (1.8)*
(-) PIA 1.00 mg/kg	15.5 (6.3)	49.7 (16.9)	71.8 (6.0)
(+) PIA 0.01 mg/kg	15.1 (2.5)	37.9 (4.1)	70.3 (6.6)
(+) PIA 0.05 mg/kg	15.2 (2.6)	41.6 (6.6)	78.6 (2.8)
(+) PIA 0.10 mg/kg	18.2 (1.5)	50.3 (4.7)	77.6 (8.5)
(+) PIA 0.25 mg/kg	19.1 (0.9)	53.9 (7.5)	45.2 (3.1)*
(+) PIA 1.00 mg/kg	15.5 (1.2)	35.8 (10.5)*	80.0 (4.3)*

1. glandular ulcer only
* significantly less than (+) PIA at comparable dose, or vehicle ($p < 0.05$)

We wanted to clarify the nature of this apparent ulcer-protective effect of adenosine analogs. Accordingly, we administered the adenosine receptor blockers 8-phenyltheophylline (8-PT) which crosses the blood-brain-barrier and 8-sulphophenyltheophylline (8-SoPT), its polar derivative, which does not cross the blood-brain-barrier, but which has an affinity for blocking adenosine receptor-mediated processes similar to that of theophylline. At doses which did not affect ulceration, 8-PT, but not 8-SoPT administered 10 min prior to (-) PIA, completely blocked the ability of (-) PIA to reduce ulcer severity. In addition, 8-PT but not 8-SoPT, blocked the ability (-) PIA to attenuate the stress-induced rise in plasma corticosterone.

The finding that (-) PIA was approximately 20 times more potent than (+) PIA in reducing stress ulcer, suggests that adenosine A1 receptors were involved. In addition, the ability of 8-PT, but not 8-SoPT, to block the effects of (-) PIA strongly suggests that these are *central* adenosine receptors. It should be noted, however, that a recent report (38) showed exactly opposite results - adenosine A1 receptor stimulation was associated with *increased* stress ulcer formation. Nevertheless, it is provocative to speculate on the development of clinically efficacious central adenosine agonists which attenuate pathological responses to stress.

Table 9. Effets of addenosine receptor antagonists on ulcer[1] serverity and plasma corticosterone levels in stressed rats.

Group	Mean (± S.E.M.) ulcer length (mm)		Mean (± S.E.M.) plasma CS (μg/dl)	
Vehicle	39.8	(4.7)	64.8	(0.97)
(-) PIA (0.1 mg/kg) i.p.	20.6	(4.0)*	44.2	(0.91)*
(-) PIA + 8-phenyltheophylline (8-PT) (2.5 mg/kg) i.p.	38.7	(7.2)	61.4	(2.72)
8-PT (2.5 mg/kg) i.p.	37.6	(7.2)	61.4	(2.72)
(-) PIA + 8-sulphophenyltheophylline (8-SoPT) (30.0 mg/kg) i.p.	21.7	(1.5)*	34.0	(0.86)*
8-SoPT (30.0 mg/kg) i.p.	43.4	(2.5)	58.0	(1.82)

1. glandular ulcer only
* significantly less than vehicle ($p<0.05$)

Recently, however, Gerber et al. (39) noted that inhibitory adenosine A1 receptors exist in the canine gastric fundus and which apparently mediate acid secretory responses to cholinergic and histaminergic stimulation. Very recently, this group showed that such receptors appear to be located on parietal cells and may respond preferentially to inhibit histamine-stimulated cyclic AMP (40). Obviously, the locus of action of adenosine in modulating both basal and stress-perturbed gastric function needs to be more precisely determined.

Opiates

Much controversy exists surrounding the relationship between opiates and gastric pathology. Some workers report that opiate agonists (morphine, etorphine, loperamide) reduce (41), exacerbate (42) or produce no effect (43) on gastric function or stress pathology, while similar confusion exists regarding the opiate antagonists such as naloxone and naltrexone in terms of their effects on gastric pathophysiology. Whereas intestinal opiate receptors have been well characterized (indeed the guinea-pig ileum is a standard assay for opiate-like compounds), comparatively little is known about the existence, distribution, and subtypes, if any, of opiate receptors in the stomach. Recently, one group reported the existence of delta opiate receptors in the rat stomach using (^{3}H)-DADLE autoradiography (44), suggesting that at least some gastric processes might be mediated by peripheral opiate receptors. We recently attempted to locate mu opiate receptors in rat glandular stomach using a (^{3}H)etorphine radioligand binding assay, but were unable to obtain a sufficient degree of specific binding. Autoradiographic studies with the same ligand are in progress. We did, however, observe some interesting effects - both peripheral and central - of morphine and naloxone on stress pathology in rats. Morphine 4.0, 8.0, 16.0 and 32.0 mg/kg i.p. produced a dose-related decrease in restraint ulcer severity, with the maximum effect occurring at 16.0 mg/kg. Naloxone 12.5, 25.0, and 50.0 mg/kg i.p. produced a dose-dependent increase in stress ulcer formation. Naloxone 4.0 mg/kg i.p. given 15 min prior to morphine 8.0, 16.0 or 32.0 mg/kg i.p. antagonized the ulcer-protective effect of these doses of morphine. In morphine-dependent animals (twice daily injections of 25, 50, 75, 150, and 300 mg/kg over three days according to the method of Dua et al. (45)) allowed to withdraw spontaneously (two hours last morphine injection) or with naloxone-precipitated (4.0 mg/kg i.p. immediately after last morphine injection) withdrawal, restraint ulcer severity was extremely high, much more so than when either agent was given acutely. Animals with a comparable (three day) "history" of naloxone treatment (twice daily i.p. injections of 3.13, 6.25, 12.5, 25, and 50 mg/kg over three days), or naloxone "history" followed by morphine "antagonism" (16.0 mg/kg i.p.) exhibited a comparable degree of stress ulcer formation (46).

Table 10. Summary of ulcer* data (mean ± S.E.M.) in morphine and naloxone-treated rats given restraint stress.

Treatment	Mean (± S.E.M.) no. of ulcer	Mean (± S.E.M.) ulcer length (mm)
Vehicle only	5.80 (1.21)	8.80 (1.35)
Naloxone 12.5 mg/kg i.p.	4.50 (1.96)	6.70 (0.80)
Naloxone 25.0 mg/kg i.p.	4.30 (2.03)	6.80 (0.80)
Naloxone 50.0 mg/kg i.p.	5.40 (2.55)	7.20 (0.49)
Morphine 4.0 mg/kg i.p.	5.50 (1.91)	8.70 (3.34)
Morphine 8.0 mg/kg i.p.	2.50 (0.90)	2.60 (1.53)[1]
Morphine 16.0 mg/kg i.p.	1.50 (0.85)7	1.10 (0.66)[1]
Morphine 32.0 mg/kg i.p.	1.80 (0.70)[7]	2.50 (1.17)[1]
Nal. 4.0 mg/kg + morph. 8.0 mg/kg i.p.	5.24 (0.57)[7]	11.33 (2.60)[2]
Nal. 4.0 mg/kg + morph. 16.0 mg/kg i.p.	3.40 (0.67)	9.20 (2.80)[3]
Nal. 4.0 mg/kg + morph. 32.0 mg/kg i.p.	6.70 (1.76)[4]	10.30 (2.38)[4]
Morph. 32.0 mg/kg + nal. 4.0 mg/kg i.p.	4.70 (1.02)[4]	9.70 (1.41)[4]
Morphine dependent	7.20 (0.41)	23.00 (0.49)[5]
Morphine dependent-naloxone withdrawal	11.00 (2.22)[6]	35.00 (3.90)[6]
Chronic naloxone	11.00 (1.96)[6]	23.00 (6.17)[5]
Chronic naloxone-morphine 16.0 mg/kg i.p.	10.20 (1.01)[6]	23.00 (3.22)

* glanular ulcers only
1. significantly less than all other groups ($p<0.01$)
2. significantly greater than morphine 8.0 mg/kg alone ($p<0.01$)
3. significantly greater than morphine 16.0 mg/kg alone ($p<0.01$)
4. significantly greater than morphine 32.0 mg/kg alone ($p<0.01$)
5. significantly greater than all morphine alone, naloxone alone, and morphine naloxone groups ($p<0.01$)
6. significantly greater than all other groups ($p<0.01$)
7. significantly less than all naloxone groups ($p<0.01$)

Morphine inhibited basal gastric acid secretion in a dose-related fashion, while higher doses of naloxone augmented gastric secretion (conscious gastric collection in the chronic gastric cannula rat (47) unencumbered by other agents such as anesthetics, etc.).

Table 11. Effects of morphine and naloxone on basal gastric acid secretion in rats.

	Mean (± S.E.M.) gastric acid output (mEq/h)		
Treatment	Pre-injection	Injection	Post-injection
Morphine 4.0 mg/kg i.p.	23.45 (3.7)	1.05 (0.9)	0.00 (0.0)
Morphine 8.0 mg/kg i.p.	20.70 (2.9)	0.95 (0.7)	7.49 (1.1)
Morphine 16.0 mg/kg i.p.	19.46 (2.2)	1.19 (0.9)	0.70 (0.3)
Morphine 32.0 mg/kg i.p.	10.08 (1.9)	2.35 (1.1)	0.00 (0.0)
Morphine-dependent - vehicle	7.10 (3.1)	6.30 (2.2)	10.12 (4.3)
Morphine-dependent	5.95 (2.8)	3.78 (1.8)	10.23 (3.8)
Morphine-dependent - naloxone 4.0 mg/kg i.p.	9.12 (2.7)	7.70 (2.9)	37.80 (8.8)
Naloxone 5.25 mg/kg	21.04 (5.7)	31.43 (7.5)	24.60 (5.3)
Naloxone 12.25 mg/kg i.p.	12.60 (3.3)	26.37 (7.3)	63.32 (7.2)
Naloxone 25.00 mg/kg i.p.	30.21 (7.1)	38.12 (7.8)	97.79 (18.3)
Naloxone 50.00 mg/kg i.p.	18.62 (5.2)	74.20 (11.3)	30.45 (8.8)
Chronic naloxone - vehicle	12.92 (4.9)	10.85 (3.2)	17.61 (2.8)
Chronic naloxone	25.55 (4.3)	25.62 (4.8)	18.94 (3.3)
Chronic naloxone - morphine 16.0 mg/kg i.p.	12.99 (4.1)	0.00 (0.0)	0.00 (0.0)

Whole brain opiate radioligand binding assay data obtained using (^{3}H)-etorphine, revealed only an effect of stress and not of drug treatment. Stress produced a decrease in the number of opiate binding sites in the brain (lower Bmax) without changing the affinity (Kd) of the receptors, consistent with recent reports (48).

Other

Caffeine

We have also examined the effect of prenatal caffeine exposure on offspring responses to stress as adults (49). Pregnant rats were exposed to 0%, 0.017%, 0.034%, or 0.050% caffeine in their drinking water throughout the entire gestation period. All offspring were cross-fostered at birth to lactating but non-caffeine exposed dams. As adults (48, 68, or 196 days of age), caffeine-exposed rats did not differ from non-exposed animals in terms of open-field behavior (locomotion or "emotionality"). However, when subjected to restraint stress at 200 days of age, prenatal caffeine-exposed rats (especially in the 0.050% group) exhibited exacerbated gastric stress ulcer formation.

Table 12. Summary of restraint ulcer[1] data for the prenatal caffeine-treated rats[2].

Group	No. of rats	No. of rats with ulcers	Mean (± S.E.M.) no. of ulcers	Mean (± S.E.M.) ulcer length (mm)
Control	20	17	7.05 (1.68)	9.47 (4.16)
Caffeine 0.17 mg/ml	20	14	3.22 (0.59)	8.22 (2.07)
Caffeine 0.34 mg/ml	20	17	8.16 (3.30)	18.42 (6.45)*
Caffeine 0.50 mg/ml	20	15	14.00 (1.45)	16.42 (2.40)*

1. glandular ulcers only
2. pregnant rats were given water containing different amounts of caffeine throughout the entire gestation period

* significantly different from control ($p<0.05$)

It is suggested that prenatal caffeine exposure produces a sensitization or predisposition to stress ulcer in rats so treated and that early life alterations in brain adenosine receptor activity may have long-term consequences in terms of stress susceptibility.

Ethanol

In a somewhat similar paradigm, pregnant rats were exposed to ethanol in their drinking water (2.8 - 3.5 g/kg/day) during the first, second, third, all, or none of the trimesters of the gestational period (50). As adults, the offspring were subjected to a 40 day ethanol screening procedure designed to assess preference for ethanol over water (51). No differences among prenatal treatment groups were observed with respect to ethanol preference, however, among those offspring which preferred ethanol over water (>50% of total daily fluid intake was ethanol over the 40 day period), only those from the first trimester exposure demonstrated a significant decrease in their ethanol intake when given the 5-HT uptake blocker zimelidine as adults. Altered brain serotonergic activity has been proposed as one mechanism involved in the development and mainte-nance of ethanol dependence (52) and 5-HT uptake blockade with zimelidine, norzimelidine, and fluoxetine, has been associated with decreased voluntary ethanol consumption in ethanol-preferring rats (53) and humans (54). In addition, when given restraint stress as adults, first trimester-exposed rats exhibited exacerbated stress ulcer formation relative to all other groups.

Again, it appears that early exposure to a substance, in this case, ethanol, can produce long-lasting receptor/neurotransmitter aberrations, in this case, apparently 5-HT, as well as altered susceptibility to stress-effects which do not manifest themselves until adulthood. It is also of interest that Hellhammer et al. (55) reported that activity-stress (a model of *chronic* stress) produced decreased 5-HT levels in midbrain, cortex and hippocampus in rats which developed gastric lesions, further implicating central 5-HT in mediating stress-induced gastric pathology. We are examining regional brain 5-HT (as well as NA and DA) activity in animals prenatally exposed to ethanol in order to assess the role of central 5-HT in mediating this apparent predisposition to exacerbated stress pathology as adults.

Table 13. Effects of prenatal ethanol exposure[1] on adult responses to restraint stress.

Treatment	Mean (± S.E.M.) no. ulcers	Mean (± S.E.M.) ulcer length (mm)
1st trimester exposure	24.7 (5.1)	39.6 (6.3)*
2nd trimester exposure	18.9 (3.8)	26.2 (4.6)
3rd trimester exposure	22.3 (4.1)	21.6 (7.4)
continuous prenatal exposure	26.1 (5.6)	26.2 (6.2)
no prenatal exposure	21.2 (3.3)	35.6 (2.9)

1. pregnant rats were exposed to a free choise water or ethanol solution (3% v/v) throughout the entire gestation period. Ethanol intake averaged 2.8 to 3.5 g/kg/day.

* significantly greater than all other groups

Capsaicin

Capsaicin is a neurotoxin that can deplete sensory (myelinated afferent) nerves of substance P and interfere with certain sensory functions, including responses to noxious physical stimuli (56, 57). Capsaicin also interferes with the retrograde transport of nerve growth factor to the cell bodies of sensory nerves, resulting in decreased protein synthesis and decreased synthesis of substance P (58). Since capsaicin is commonly found in foods and is frequently used as a spice in middle Eastern countries, we were interested in its gastrointestinal effects.

Some rats were given a desensitizing dose regimen of capsaicin (25.0 mg/kg and 40.0 mg/kg i.p. over two days) and then examined for stress responses six days later. Responses to restraint stress for 1, 2, or 3 h indicated that ulcer severity was not different from control levels in capsaicin-treated rats while ulcer frequency (number of ulcers per rat) was higher at 3 h in capsaicin-treated rats. In all cases, however, plasma corticosterone responses to restraint stress were also much higher in capsaicin-treated rats.

Finally, capsaicin did not affect basal gastric acid secretion, but was associated with significantly *lower* pentagastrin-stimulated total acid output. It appears that capsaicin *may* exacerbate ulcer and corticosterone responses to stress, while not adversely affecting secretory function. We are examining this interesting dichotomy observed in the stress responses of capsaicin-treated rats.

Table 14. Effects of capsaicin[1] on gastric[2] and corticosterone response to restraint stress.

Treatment	Mean (± S.E.M.) no. ulcers	Mean (± S.E.M.) ulcer length (mm)	Mean (± S.E.M.) plasma CS (μg/dl)
Control 1 h	0.7 (0.2)	1.3 (0.9)	38.6 (3.9)
Control 2 h	4.7 (1.5)	7.7 (2.1)	38.5 (4.7)
Control 3 h	4.7 (1.5)	16.0 (1.8)	45.0 (3.4)
Capsaicin 1 h	1.3 (1.1)	2.7 (1.1)	74.4 (7.8)**
Capsaicin 2 h	2.3 (1.3)	6.3 (1.1)	64.9 (8.2)**
Capsaicin 3 h	13.0 (2.5)***	19.0 (2.1)*	66.2 (8.9)**

1. capsaicin was given at doses of 25.0 and 40.0 mg/kg s.c. over 2 consecutive days followed 6 days later by cold restraint stress
2. glandular ulcers only

* significantly greater than other capsaicin groups and controls of 1 and 2 h ($p < 0.01$)
** significantly greater than all control groups ($p < 0.01$)
*** significantly greater than all other groups ($p < 0.01$)

Table 15. Effects of capsaicin on basal and pentagastrin-stimulated gastric acid output.

	Mean (± S.E.M.) basal gastric secretion (μEQ/ml/hr)			Mean (± S.E.M.) pentagastrin-stimulated gastric secretion (μEQ/ml/hr)		
	1 h	2 h	3 h	1 h	2 h	3 h
Capsaicin	9.0 (1.1)	5.8 (0.8)	5.7 (0.9)	18.4 (2.2)*	15.9 (1.8)*	13.1 (2.3)
Control	12.2 (2.1)	9.7 (1.8)	5.9 (0.9)	32.6 (1.5)	25.9 (2.8)	20.7 (2.0)

* significantly less than controls ($p < 0.05$)

Conclusions

The data outline in this report clearly implicate several central nervous system neurotransmitters in initiating, maintaining, exacerbating, and reducing peripheral responses to stress challenge. That central nervous modulation is critical to the elaboration of responses to stress is at the core of the original stress-adaptation theory first proposed by Selye in the 1930s. In the decades since Selye's initial description and proposed mechanism of action of stress, research has alternated between emphasizing central and peripheral mechanisms. Evidence accumulated over the last decade, however, strongly suggests that stress, via as yet poorly defined central mechanisms, not only produces a syndrome in and of itself, but may also be involved in the pathogenesis of other diseases including immunodeficiency and psychiatric disorders such as depression. Recent research attention concentrating upon *multiple* neurotransmitter interactions and aberrations (neurotransmitter imbalance or "dysregulation" hypothesis) believed to be caused, in part, by stress, suggests an even greater role for central nervous mechanisms in stress and disease and, at the same time, presents both complication and intrigue to the stress researcher. It is hoped that the succeeding decades will see us not only meet, but solve the "challenge" of stress, best exemplified by Selye's words: "Even the grandeur of conquering the universe, or the fear that war may break out, or that our world may become overpopulated, seems to pale at the bedside of a patient who will die because we were remiss in our efforts to learn more about disease" (59).

References

1. Lee, Y. & Bianchi, R. (1971). Use of experimental peptic ulcer models for drug screening. In Pfeiffer, C. (Ed.), Peptic ulcer. Lippincott, Philadelphia.
2. Glavin, G. (1980). Restraint ulcer: History, current research and future implications. Brain Res. Bull., 5: 51-58.
3. Pare, W. (1980). Psychological studies of stress ulcer in the rat. Brain Res. Bull., 5: 73-79.
4. Pare, W. & Glavin, G. (1986). Restraint stress in biomedical research: A review. Neurosci. Biobehav. Rev., 10: 339-370.
5. Senay, E. & Levine, R. (1967). Synergism between cold and restraint for rapid production of stress ulcers in rats. Proc. Soc. Exp. Biol. Med., 124: 1221-1223.
6. Pare, W. & Houser, V. (1973). Activity and food-restriction effects on gastric glandular lesions in the rat: The activity-stress ulcer. Bull. Psychon. Soc., 2: 213-214.
7. Manning, J., Wall, H., Montgomery, C., Simmons, C. & Sessions, G. (1978). Microscopic examination of the activity-stress ulcer in the rat. Physiol. Behav., 21: 269-294.
8. Pare, W. (1977). Gastric secretion and activity-stress lesions in the rat. J. Comp. Physiol. Psychol., 91: 778-783.
9. Pare, W. (1976). The pharmaceutical management of gastric ulceration. Diss. Abst. Int., 37: 2521B.
10. Hara, C. & Ogawa, N. (1984). Effects of psychotropic drugs on the development of activity-stress ulcer in rats. Japan J. Pharmacol., 35: 474-477.
11. Glavin, G. (1985). Stress and brain noradrenaline: A review. Neurosci. Biobehav. Rev., 9: 233-243.
12. Glavin, G., Tanaka, M., Tsuda, A., Kohno, Y., Hoaki, Y. & Nagasaki, N. (1983). Regional rat brain noradrenaline turnover in response to restraint stress in rats. Pharmacol. Biochem. Behav., 19: 287-290.
13. Tsuda, A., Tanaka, M., Kohno, Y., Nishikawa, T., Iimori, K., Nakagawa, R., Hoaki, Y., Ida, Y. & Nagasaki, N. (1982). Marked enhancement of noradrenaline turnover in extensive brain regions after activity-stress in rats. Pharmacol. Biochem. Behav., 29: 337-341.
14. Tsuda, A., Tanaka, M., Kohno, Y., Ida, Y., Hoaki, Y., Iimori, K., Nakagawa, R., Nishikawa, T. & Nagasaki, N. (1983). Daily increase in noradrenaline turnover in brain regions of activity-stressed rats. Pharmacol. Biochem. Behav., 19: 393-396.
15. Rea, M. & Hellhammer, D. (1984). Activity-wheel stress: Changes in brain norepinephrine turnover and the occurrence of gastric lesions. Psychother. Psychosom., 42: 218-223.
16. Stone, E. (1981). Mechanism of stress-induced subsensitivity to norepinephrine. Pharmacol. Biochem. Behav., 14: 719-723.
17. Stone, E. & Platt, J. (1982). Brain adrenergic receptors and resistance to stress. Brain Res., 237: 405-414.
18. Stone, E., Slucky, A., Platt, J. & Trullas, R. (1985). Reduction of the cyclic adenosine, 3', 5',-monophosphate response to catecholamines in rat brain slices after repeated restraint stress. J. Pharmacol. Exp. Ther., 233: 382-388.
19. Thierry, A., Blanc, G. & Glowinski, J. (1973). Further evidence for the heterogeneous storage of noradrenaline in central noradrenergic terminals. Naunyn-Schmiedeberg's Arch. Pharmacol., 279: 255-256.
20. Zolovick, A., Rossi, J., Davies, R. & Panksepp, J. (1982). An improved pharmacological procedure for depletion of noradrenaline: Pharmacology and assessment of noradrenaline-associated behaviors. Eur. J. Pharmacol., 77: 265-271.

21. Glavin, G. (1985). Selective noradrenaline depletion markedly alters stress response in rats. Life Sci., 23: 461-465.
22. Anisman, H. & Zacharko, R. (1982). Depression: The predisposing influence of stress. Behav. Brain. Sci., 5: 89-137.
23. Weiss, J., Goodman, B., Losito, B., Corrigan, S., Charry, J. & Bailey, W. (1981). Behavioral depression produced by an uncontrollable stressor: Relationship to norepinephrine, dopamine, and serotonin levels in various regions of rat brain. Brain Res. Rev., 3: 167-205.
24. Glavin, G., Tanaka, M., Tsuda, A., Kohno, Y., Hoaki, Y. & Nagasaki, N. (1984). Effects of altered brain noradrenaline level on acute stress pathology in rats. Kurume. Med. J., 30: 31-34.
25. Glavin, G. (1985). Methylphenidate effects on activity-stress gastric lesions and regional brain noradrenaline metabolism in rats. Pharmacol. Biochem. Behav., 23: 379-383.
26. Henke, P. (1979). The hypothalamus-amygdala axis and experimental gastric ulcers. Neurosci. Biobehav. Rev., 3: 75-82.
27. Ossenkopp, K., Wiener, N. & Nobrega, J. (1980). Ventromedical hypothalamic lesions and stomach ulcers: Reduction by non-nutritive bulk ingested in the post lesion period. Physiol. Behav., 24: 1125-1131.
28. Szabo, S. (1979). Dopamine disorder in duodenal ulceration. Lancet, 2: 880-882.
29. Szabo, S., Sandrock, A., Nafradi, J., Maull, E., Gallagher, G. & Blyzniuk, A. (1982). Dopamine and dopamine receptors in the gut: Their possible role in duodenal ulceration. Adv. Biosci., 37: 165-170.
30. Szabo, S., Brown A. & Schnoor, J. (1984). Duodenal ulcer induction by a chemical that also causes Parkinson's disease. Fed. Proc., 43: 945.
31. Szabo, S. & Brown, A. (1985). The MPTP (1-methyl-4-phenyl-1,2,3,6-tetrahydropyridine)-induced duodenal ulcers are prevented by dopamine agonists or inhibitors of monoamine oxidase in the rat. Fed. Proc., 44: 733.
32. Neumeyer, J. & Szabo, S. (1983). (-)-10,11-methylenedioxy-N-propyl-norapomorphine, an orally effective dopamine agonist and duodenal antiulcerogen in the rat. Eur. J. Pharmacol., 88: 273-274.
33. Hernandez, D., Adcock, J., Orlando, R., Patrick, K., Nemeroff, C. & Prange, A. (1984). Prevention of stress induced gastric ulcers by dopamine agonists in the rat. Life Sci., 35, 2453-2458.
34. Strocchi, P., Gandolfi, O. & Montanaro, N. (1976). Effect of single and repeated administration of sulpiride on the restraint ulcer in the rat. Arzn. Forsch. (Drug Res.), 26: 419-421.
35. Ungerstedt, U. & Arbuthnott, G. (1970). Quantitative recording of rotational behavior in rats after 6-hydroxydopamine lesions of the nigrostriatal system. Brain Res., 24: 485-493.
36. Rall, T. (1985). Central nervous system stimulants: The methylxanthines. In A. Gilman, L. Goodman, T. Rall & F. Murad (Eds.), The pharmacological basis of therapeutics. MacMillan, N.Y., p. 589-603.
37. Geiger, J. & Glavin, G. (1985). Adenosine receptor activation in brain reduces stress-induced ulcer formation. Eur. J. Pharmacol., 115: 185-190.
38. Ushijima, I., Mizuki, Y. & Yamada, M. (1985). Development of stress-induced gastric lesions involves central adenosine A1-receptor stimulation. Brain Res., 339: 351-355.
39. Gerber, J., Fadul, S., Payne, N. & Nies, A. (1984). Adenosine: A modulator of gastric acid secretion in vivo. J. Pharmacol. Exp. Ther., 231: 109-113.
40. Gerber, J., Nies, A. & Payne, N. (1985). Adenosine receptors on canine parietal cells modulate gastric acid secretion to histamine. J. Pharmacol. Exp. Ther., 233: 623-627.
41. Glavin, G. (1985). Effects of morphine and naloxone on restraint-stress ulcers in rats. Pharmacol., 31: 57-60.
42. Ho, M., Dai, S. & Ogle, C. (1984). Decreased acid secretion and gastric lesion production by morphine in rats. Eur. J. Pharmacol., 102: 117-121.
43. Kitchen, I. & McEwan, A. (1983). Plasma corticosterone levels after i.c.v. injection of opioids in normal or ether stressed mice. Brit. J. Pharmacol., 79: 328P.
44. Nishimura, E., Buchan, A. & McIntoch, C. (1984). Autoradiographic localization of opioid receptors in the rat stomach. Neurosci. Lett., 50: 73-78.
45. Dua, A., Pinsky, C. & LaBella, F. (1985). Mu-and delta-opioid receptor-mediated epileptoid responses in morphine-dependent and non-dependent rats. EEG Clin. Neurophysiol., 61: 569-572.
46. Glavin, G., Kiernan, K., Hnatowich, M. & LaBella, F. (1986). Effects of morphine and naloxone on stress ulcer formation and gastric acid secretion. Eur. J. Pharmacol., 124: 121-127.

47. Pare, W., Isom, K., Vincent, G. & Glavin, G. (1977). A technique for chronic gastric fistula preparation in the rat. Lab. Anim. Sci., 27: 244-247.
48. Appelbaum, B. & Holtzman, S. (1985). Restraint stress enhances morphine-induced analgesia in the rat without changing apparent affinity of receptor. Life Sci., 36: 1069-1074.
49. Glavin, G. & Krueger, H. (1985). Effects of prenatal caffeine administration on offspring mortality, open-field behavior and adult gastric ulcer susceptibility. Neurobehav. Toxicol. Teratol., 7: 29-32.
50. Grace, G., Rockman, G. & Glavin, G. (1986). Effect of prenatal ethanol exposure on adult ethanol preference and response to zimelidine in rats. Alc. Alcoholism., 21: 25-31.
51. Rockman, G. & Glavin, G. (1984). Ethanol-stress interaction: Differences among ethanol-preferring rats responses to restraint. Alcohol, 1: 293-295.
52. Rockman, G., Amit, Z., Brown, Z., Bourque, C. & Ogren, S. (1982). An investigation of the mechanism of action of 5-hydroxytryptamine in the suppression of ethanol intake. Neuropharmacol., 21: 341-347.
53. Rockman, G., Amit, Z., Carr, G., Brown, Z. & Ogren, S. (1979). Attenuation of ethanol intake by 5-hydroxytryptamine uptake blockade in laboratory rats. I. Involvement of brain 5-hydroxytryptamine in the mediation of the positive reinforcing properties of ethanol. Arch. Int. Pharmacodyn. Ther., 241: 245-249.
54. Naranjo, C., Sellers, E., Roach, C., Woodley, D., Sanchez-Craig, M. & Sykora, K. (1984). Zimelidine-induced variations in alcohol intake by nondepressed heavy drinkers. Clin. Pharmacol. Ther., 35: 374-381.
55. Hellhammer, D., Hingtgen, J., Wade, S., Shea, P. & Aprison, M. (1983). Serotonergic changes in specific areas of rat brain associated with activity-stress gastric lesions. Psychosom. Med., 45: 115-122.
56. Nagy, J. (1982). Capsaicin: A chemical probe for sensory neuron mechanisms. In L. Iversen, S. Iversen & S. Snyder (Eds.), Handbook of psychopharmacology, Vol. 15. Plenum, N.Y., p. 185-235.
57. Nagy, J. & Van der Kooy, D. (1983). Effects of neonatal capsaicin treatment on nociceptive thresholds in the rat. J. Neurosci., 3: 1145-1160.
58. Burks, T., Buck, S. & Miller, M. (1985). Mechanisms of depletion of substance P by capsaicin. Fed. Proc., 44: 2531-2534.
59. Selye, H. (1964). From dream to discovery. McGraw-Hill, N.Y.

Control of Gastrointestinal Motility

Martin Wienbeck, Paul Enck and Joachim F. Erckenbrecht

Gastrointestinal motility closely interacts with other functions of the gut. The most important of these functions are absorption, secretion, and transit (Figure 1). Disturbances of one or several of these functions may lead to such common symptoms as diarrhea, constipation, and irritable bowel syndrome.

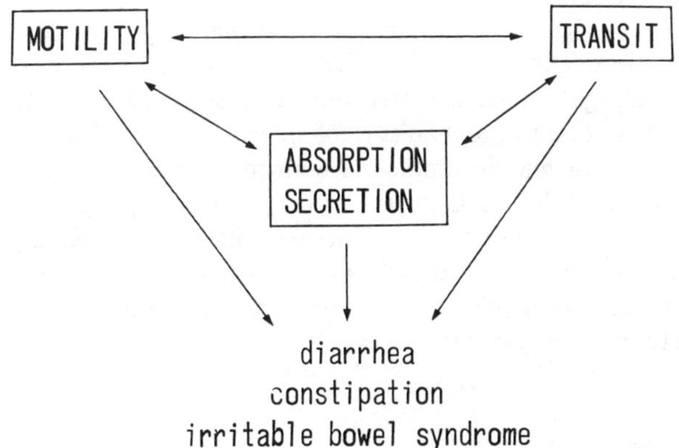

Figure 1. Functions of the gastrointestinal system.

Motility serves to propel, mix, store, and empty the contents in different parts of the gastrointestinal system. These functions are controlled by different types of motility.

Table 1. Types of motility and their effect on gut contents.

Propulsion	-	Transit, emptying
Segmentation	-	Mixing
Changes in tone	-	Storage

This work was supported in part by the Deutsche Forschungsgemeinschaft and by the Minister für Wissenschaft und Forschung des Landes Nordrhein-Westfalen.

Gastrointestinal motility also has to be coordinated between different parts of the gastrointestinal tract, in spite of the fact that patterns of motility vary from organ to organ according to their different functions (Table 2).

Table 2. Organs of the gastrointestinal tract and their major functions.

Esophagus	-	Propulsion, prevention of reflux
Stomach	-	Storage, secretion, mixing, controlled emptying
Small bowel	-	Absorption, mixing, propulsion
Large bowel	-	Absorption, mixing, storage, controlled emptying

Only highly integrated control mechanisms are able to coordinate these different functions in the gastrointestinal tract and to adapt to intervening variables, such as food intake or external stress.

Only since about 15 years ago have extrinsic nervous and humoral control of gastrointestinal functions been regarded as major mechanisms for the coordination of motility, secretion, and absorption. Although the existence of the intrinsic (or enteric) nervous system (ENS) was known of since the end of the last century (1), the detection of the mechanisms of neural transmission on the one hand and the description of gut hormones as neurotransmitters on the other hand were necessary to establish the importance of the ENS for gastrointestinal functioning. Gastrointestinal activity is maintained in isolated tissue, and vagotomy and sympathectomy have little effect on gut motility. Clearly, the CNS is incapable of affecting the gut in vitro; it therefore, must be connected to sensory and motor neurons to maintain its activity.

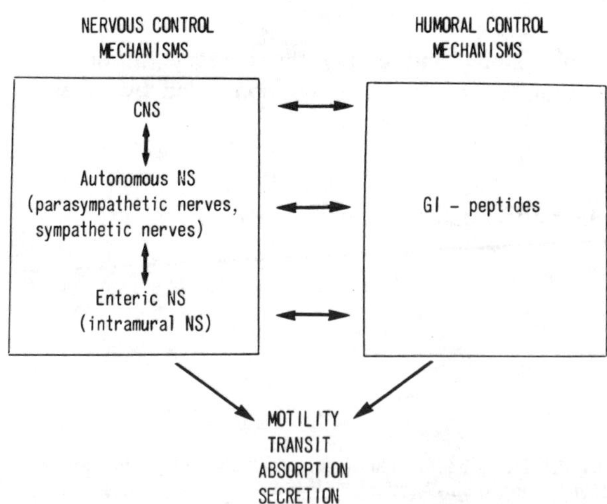

Figure 2. Control mechanisms of gastrointestinal motility.

On the other hand, aganglionic segments of the colon (as in Hirschsprung's disease) which still contain extrinsic adrenergic and cholinergic nerves do not adequately propel luminal contents. This leads to intestinal obstruction. An intact ENS, therefore, seems to be more critical to the bowel than are the brain and spinal cord.

Finally, the occurrence of common peptides in gut and brain, some of which have been shown to exert neural *and* endocrine actions in the gut, indicates that control of gastrointestinal motility is complex (Figure 2).

In the first part of this article, these different control mechanisms of gastrointestinal motility will be reviewed. The second part will describe the specific control of different parts of the gastrointestinal tract.

Control Mechanisms of Gut Motility

Central and peripheral neuronal control is maintained via sympathetic and parasympathetic nerves. In general, afferent pathways are at least as important in the autonomous nervous system as efferent pathways. This becomes evident by the anatomical observations that the number of afferent fibers in the vagus nerve surpasses those of the efferent fibers by more than 5:1. Inhibitory reflexes, such as a delay of gastric emptying following distension in the intestine, are mediated by adrenergic nerves (2). Reflex responses within the gut such as the response of the colon to food intake can be modulated by stimulation of the central nervous system (3). On the other hand, sympathectomy apparently has no major effect on bowel function under resting conditions (4). In the parasympathetic nerve supply, the vagus nerve exhibits both excitatory and inhibitory effects, depending on the site of action, while sacral parasympathetic nerves predominantly exert excitatory influences. In general, vagotomy produces little change in the gut beyond the level of the stomach (5).

The *enteric nervous system* (ENS) is at least as important for control of gastrointestinal motility as the extrinsic nerves. Enteric nerves are accumulated in two major networks or plexus of neurons, the submucosal or Meissner's plexus and the myenteric or Auerbach's plexus. These plexus serve as integrative centers for signal processing. They contain sensory, afferent neurons, motor neurons, and interneurons. The number of ganglion cells in the ENS is grater than 10^8 (6) and similar to the total number of neurons in the spinal cord, compared to 2×10^3 efferent fibers in the abdominal vagal nerves. "This organization eliminates the need for a large number of long-distance conducting pathways between the central nervous system and gut ... otherwise ... devoted to redundant information processing" (7).

Besides cholinergic and adrenergic transmitters the ENS contains a number of other neurotransmitters, mainly regulatory peptides, some of which have been found in the central nervous system as well.

These peptides are likely to act as neurotransmitters in the ENS. Some of them have also been shown to act as gastrointestinal hormones via release from epithelial cells in the gut wall. It is preferable, therefore, to use the more general term *regulatory peptides* (8).

Table 3. Regulatory peptides probably occurring in brain and gut.

Isolated and characterized in brain and gut:	
	CCK, Neurotensin, Secretin, Somatostatin, Substance P, Neuropeptide Y, Peptide YY
Isolated from gut, immunoreactive in brain:	
	Bombesin, Glucagon, Motilin, PP, VIP
Isolated from brain, immunoreactive in gut:	
	Endorphins, Enkephalins, TRH

Hormones are released into the blood and hence may interact with all specific receptors in the organism. In contrast, a neurotransmitter acts only by diffusion at receptors which are in the vicinity of the nerve endings. In addition to the classical endocrine or neuronal control system, these peptides may exert a paracrine action by diffusion from endocrine cells through the extracellular space to adjacent target cells. On the other hand, peptides from nerves may also have systemic actions if these peptides are released into the circulating blood.

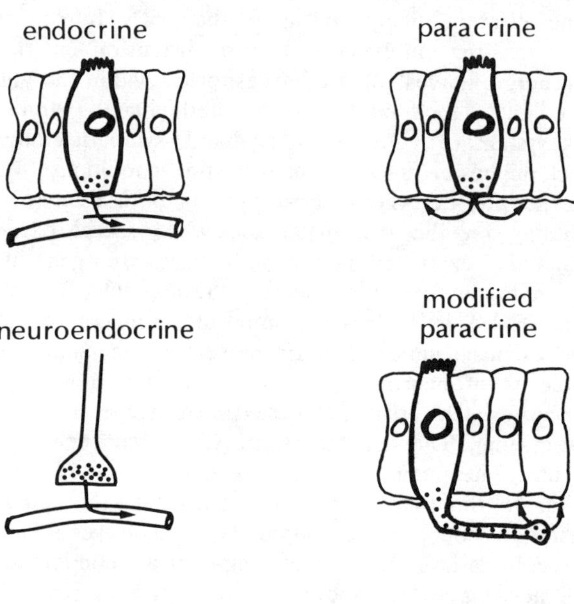

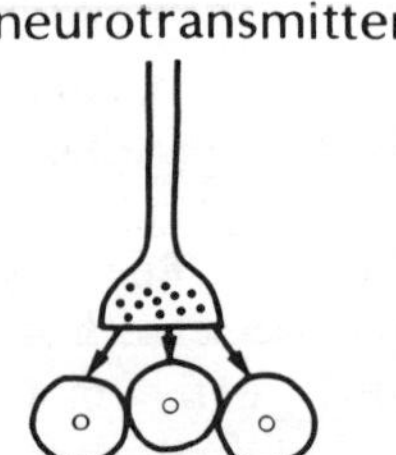

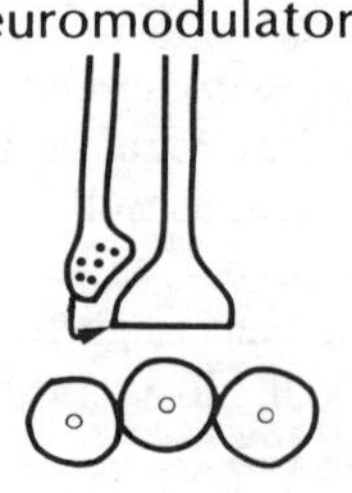

Figure 3. Schematic illustration of the different mechanisms of action of regulatory peptides in the neurohumoral control of gastrointestinal motility.

Furthermore, peptides may modulate the activity of other nerves in that they inhibit or promote the action of their neurotransmitters. These different mechanisms of peptide actions are illustrated in Figure 3.

Myogenic activity of gastrointestinal muscle interacts with the other control mechanisms of gastrointestinal motility. Muscle cells can send signals to each other via specific structures in their cell membranes. Thus, coordinated muscle activity is possible even over great distances. Myogenic activity is accompanied by myoelectrical signals. The basic electrical signals consist of slow wave or electrical control activity and spikes or electrical response activity (Figure 4).

ASCENDING COLON

SPONTANEOUS ELECTRICAL ACTIVITY

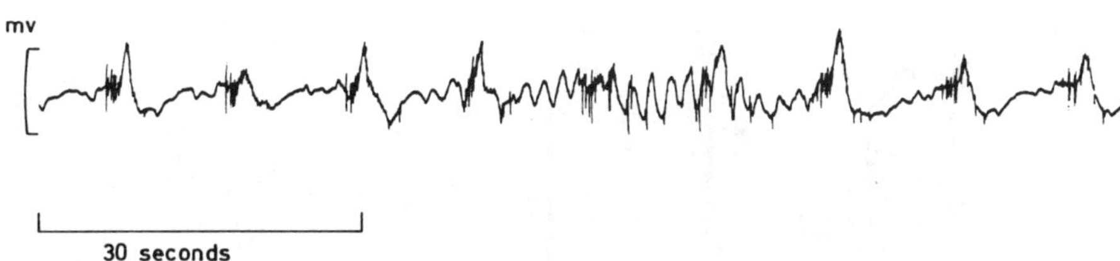

Figure 4. Example of recording of spontaneous myoelectrical slow wave and spike activity of the isolated circular muscle of the colon.

Isolated smooth muscle preparations of the gut usually maintain these basic activity patterns. Slow waves which are generated in the longitudinal muscle layer in the small intestine and in the circular muscle layer in the colon may generate coordinated activity even in a segment of the bowel in vitro (9).

Gastrointestinal motility, finally, is influenced by *intra-luminal contents* which act by their physical properties and via receptors in the gut wall which are sensitive to the amount and composition of the chyme. Ingestion of fat, for example, stimulates the release of CCK in man and impedes gastric emptying. Direct infusion of glucose into the duodenum enhances gastric emptying depending on the caloric content. The volume and viscosity of an ingested bolus affects gastric emptying, too.

Gastrointestinal Motility in Different Parts of the Gut

Esophageal motility is largely under nervous control. Extrinsic and intrinsic nerves induce peristaltic contractions in the body of the esophagus and simultaneous relaxations of the lower esophageal sphincter (LES). Stimulation of the cervical vagus nerve elicits these motor responses (10), and acoustic stress induces abnormal contractions of the esophagus (11). However, bilateral vagotomy does not eliminate esophageal peristalsis (12), indicating the presence of an additional myogenic and/or intrinsic nervous control. The LES receives stimulatory and inhibitory extrinsic and intrinsic nervous input (Figure 5).

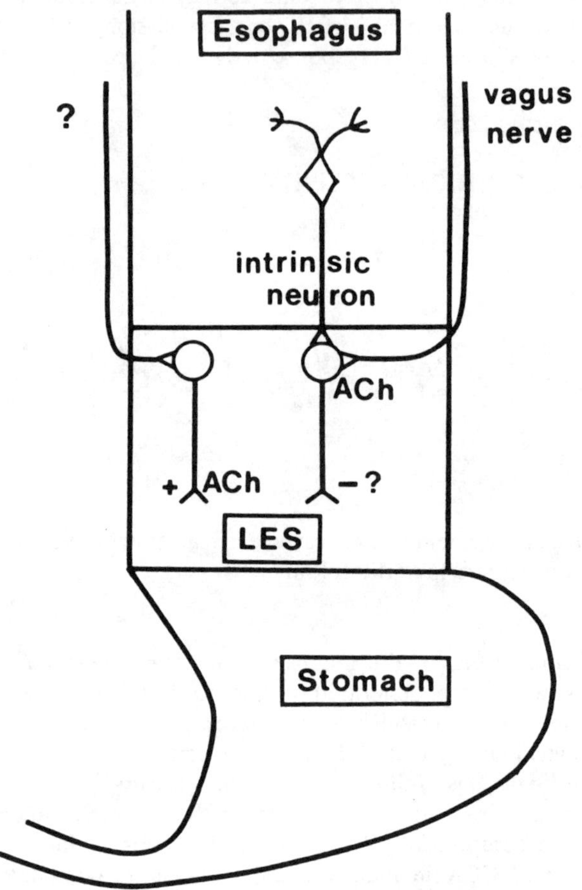

Figure 5. Schematic illustration of the neuronal control mechanisms of the lower esophageal sphincter.

VIP is a strong candidate as a neurotransmitter of the non-adrenergic non-cholinergic inhibitory innervation which mediates LES relaxation (13). Sensitivity of the LES to gastrointestinal peptides is altered in achalasia, apparently due to a denervation process. Therefore, the LES becomes supersensitive to gastrin, and paradoxically it contracts after the injection of CCK (14) (Figure 6).

A number of regulatory peptides have been shown to affect LES pressure (Table 4), but none of these actions have been proven to be physiological.

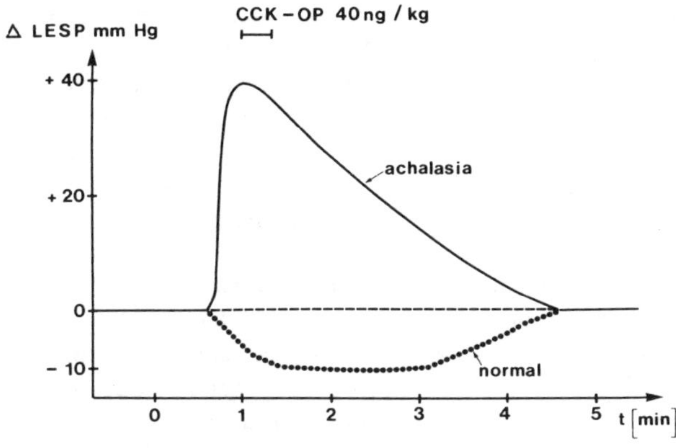

Figure 6. Changes in the lower esophageal sphincter pressure in achalasia and in normals after an intravenous injection of 40 ng CCK-octa-peptide/kg body weight.

Table 4. Regulatory Peptides Affecting the LES

Contractions	Relaxation
Gastrin	CCK (contractions in achalasia and opossum)
Motilin	Secretin (inhibits gastric stimulation)
Pancreatic polypeptides	Glucagon (contraction in cats) (in opossum)
Substance P	VIP (in animals only) (in opossum)
Bombesin (in opossum)	GIP (in cats)

Stomach motility and gastric emptying are controlled by nerves, too. The proximal part of the stomach, i.e., the fundus, mainly acts by changing its tone and, thus, adapting to different volumes. This process is under control of the vagus nerve; receptive relaxation is lost after vagotomy (Figure 7) (15).

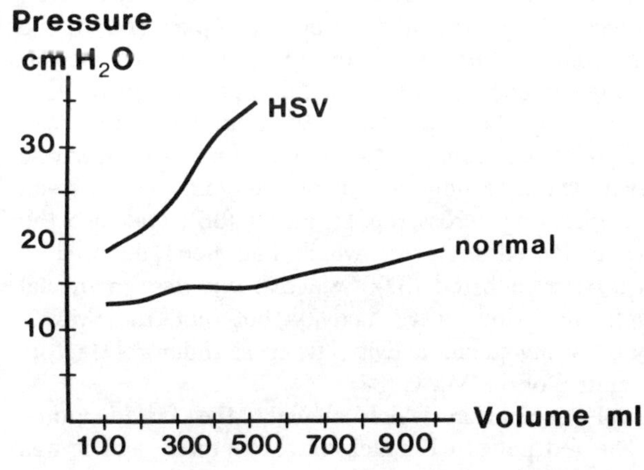

Figure 7. Pressure changes in the gastric fundus following distension under normal conditions and after highly selective vagotomy (HSV).

The distal part of the stomach or the antrum serves to mix and grind gastric contents. This process is not only under nervous, but also under humoral and myogenic control. Experimental stress by cold water, noise or labyrinthine stimulation increases the amplitude of gastric contractions (16) and changes its frequency (17). Peptides such as pentagastrin increase force and frequency of isolated human and canine antrum muscle contractions at a concentration which is below that stimulating gastric secretion (18), thus, indicating a physiological action. The only peptide that has been shown to influence motility when given in physiological doses is CCK (19) which inhibits proximal gastric contraction and stimulates antral contractions and spike potentials (20) even without extrinsic nerve supply (21). CCK is released by the presence of fat in the duodenum. It may delay gastric emptying (19). Motilin may act directly on the gastric muscle and increase contractions of the antrum and corpus (22). Motilin in low doses accelerates emptying of glucose, but not in that of fat (23).

Gastric emptying is controlled not only by gastric motility but also by gastro-duodenal coordination (24). Both are partly under sympathetic nervous control, since traumatic spinal cord transection above the level of sympathetic outflow to the gastrointestinal tract disturbs normal inter-digestive antral-duodenal motor coordination and may delay postprandial gastric emptying of liquid meals (25). Gastric emptying also varies depending on the composition and viscosity of the chyme: Liquids and semi-solid food are emptied faster than solid contents (26), and, the higher the caloric load of the meal the slower it is transported into the small bowel (27). Motility and absorption in the gastro-intestinal tract closely interact (28). Stress is a powerful stimulus in delaying gastric emptying (29) presumably via the release of endogenous enkephalins which have been shown to increase during experimental stress. In patients with rapid gastric emptying and in the dumping syndrome, neurotensin release was found to be increased (30).

In the *small bowel* the enteric nervous system becomes more important than extrinsic nervous control. Vagotomy has little effect on small bowel motility (31); those changes which have been observed (32) are probably mediated by an alteration of hormone secretion and hormone action. Motility in the small bowel differs between the fasted and the fed state. The fasting pattern is characterized by the periodic appearance of the migrating motor complex (MMC), a regular type of activity occurring about every two hours (33). Hormones such as motilin and somatostatin (34) may trigger a MMC, but this does not prove that this type of activity is controlled by these peptides. Experimental stress can interrupt this pattern (35). High transections of the spinal cord (25) decrease the number of MMCs; however, extrinsic denervation of segments of the small bowel did not prevent MMCs migrating across this segments (36), and also the initiation of MMCs in autotransplanted segments which had been denervated from central nervous input has been reported (37). Selective *myenteric* neuronal denervat[a]on, however, disrupts the slow wave activity but not the MMC, suggesting that the ENS controls myogenic activity, whereas humoral factors may be more important in the control of the MMC (38).

Feeding is the physiological mechanism which changes the fasted motor pattern into a fed one (39). The fed pattern is much more complex, and it was not well understood until now. It serves the needs of simultaneous mixing, propulsion and absorption of chyme. After vagotomy (40) and also after transplantation of a jejuno-ileal loop (41), feeding suppresses the fasting motor pattern only incompletely. These observations are in support of a neuronal control mechanism of small bowel motility. On the other hand pentagastrin also transfers the fasted into a fed-like pattern (42), and this pattern can be re-converted into the fasting one by the gastrin-antagonist proglumide (43).

Central nervous stimulation by noise accelerates intestinal transit (44), but the mechanism of this action is still unknown. Other types of central and also peripheral stimulation may cause reverse peristalsis and vomiting (45).

Spontaneous activity of the *colon* is under tonic nervous inhibition. The patterns of colonic motility are not yet well understood (46). Regulatory peptides such as enkephalins (47) and endorphins (48) play an important role, predominantly as neurotransmitters in the ENS. Enkephalins alter the motility of the colon in animal and man at very low concentrations (Figure 8) which presumably correspond to naturally occurring levels.

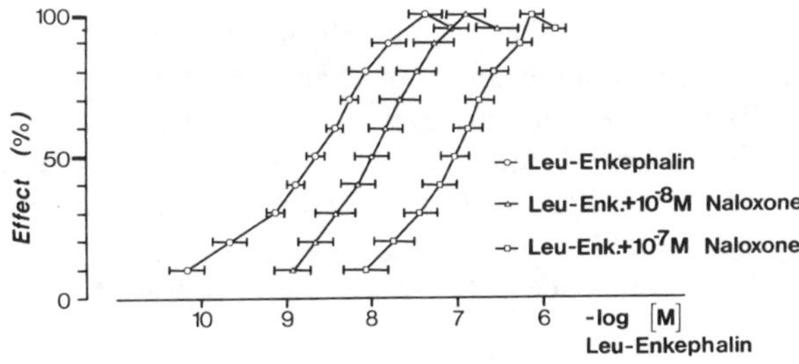

Figure 8. Concentration response relationship of the leucine-enkephalin action on the spontaneous contractile activity of the isolated circular muscle of the cat colon. The opiate receptor antagonist naloxone shifts the concentration-response curve to the right.

In contrast to the small intestine, the colon responds to opiates with a motor activation (49). This reaction is blocked by the specific opiate antagonist naloxone (50). Hence, enkephalins appear to act on specific receptors of the colon muscle. After food intake the distal colon responds with an increase in motor activity. This response has been related gastrin and CCK, since these hormones are released after food intake and both may also increase spike and motor activity of the rectosigmoid (51). However, the motor response of the colon is faster than the rise of the plasma levels of the hormones (51). Apparently, therefore, the initial postprandial stimulation of colonic motility is brought about by neural mechanisms involving cholinergic and opiate receptors. The late response may be due to a release of gastrointestinal hormones. A prominent late response of the sigmoid colon is seen in patients with the irritable bowel syndrome (52) and also in normals when they are subjected to external nervous stimulation by noise (53) (Figure 9).

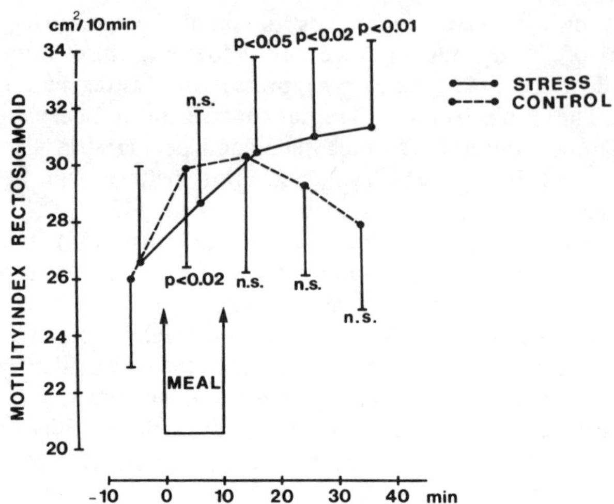

Figure 9. Colonic motility of the rectosigmoid during and after a meal in normal subjects exposed to stress (noise) and under resting conditions.

Changes in stool weight and frequency in normal subjects when exposed to mental stress (54) are not due to alterations in fluid absorption in the small bowel but presumably to motility changes in the small bowel and the colon (44).

Finally, the anal sphincter (IAS) is both under central and peripheral nervous control. Neuropathies, e.g., in diabetes, affect the internal and external sphincter function which frequently results in incontinence (55). However, the internal anal sphincter response could also be initiated by electrical field stimulation in vitro (56) suggesting an influence of the enteric nervous system.

Summary

Because of the multiple control mechanisms acting on gastrointestinal motility, only an integrated approach will enable us to fully understand normal motor activity and its disturbances. The major control mechanisms of motility and their interaction are illustrated in Figure 10.

It becomes evident that neuronal control of gastrointestinal motility is exerted not only by extrinsic nerves, i.e., the central and autonomous nervous system, but at least to a similar degree by intrinsic nerves of the enteric nervous system.

Parallel studies in vitro and in vivo including measurements of absorption and secretion serve to differentiate between the actions of extrinsic and intrinsic nerves, regulatory peptides, intraluminal contents, and myogenic activity. New models are sought which should help us to isolate the actions of these control mechanisms. The following models are currently used in our laboratory:

1) Measurement of the human gastrointestinal response to experimental stress (e.g., noise) by intraluminal recording of motor and myoelectrical activity, gut absorption, and transit times.

2) Response of the colon to environmental events in animals (cats) which carry implanted electrodes for recording of electrical activity.
3) Classical conditioning of gastrointestinal reactions such as reverse peristaltic activity in vivo (in dogs) and pharmacological manipulation of these reactions.
4) Classical conditioning of gastrointestinal reactions in isolated colon preparations (rats).

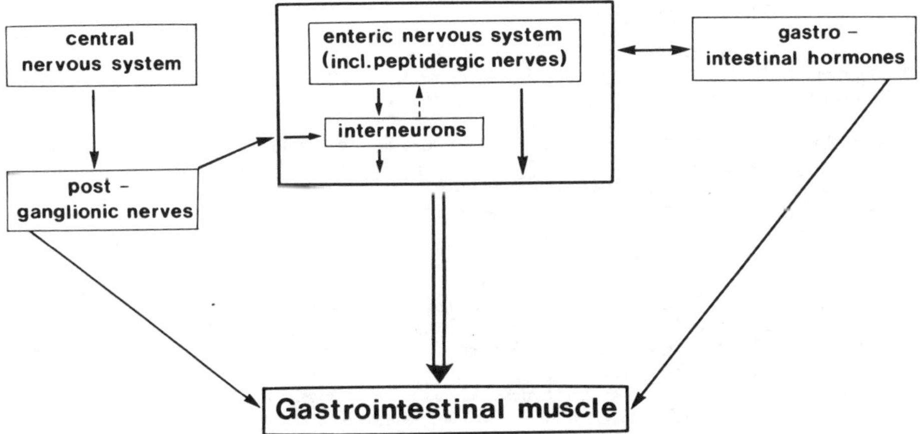

Figure 10. Schematic illustration of the different mechanisms acting on gastrointestinal motility. Biologically active regulatory peptides occur in the endocrine system, in the enteric nervous system, and also in postganglionic nerves.

It also becomes more and more evident that the enormous amount of data accumulating in these experiments can be handled only by a computer. Computer analysis, therefore, will become a prerequisite in motility research if complex models are used such as in studies of neuronal control of gastrointestinal motility.

References

1. Bayliss, W.M. & Starling, E.H. (1899). The movements and innervation of the small intestine. J. Physiol., 24: 99-143.
2. Cooke, A.R. & Clark, E.D. (1976). Effect of first part of duodenum on gastric emptying in dogs: Response to acid, fat, glucose, and neural blockade. Gastroenterology, 70: 555-565.
3. Erckenbrecht, J.F., Ziemer, B., Lesch, M., et al. (1984). Mental stress by noise alters the gastro-colonic reflex. Gut, 25: A 1314.
4. Furness, J.B. & Costa, M. (1974). The adrenergic innervation of the gastrointestinal tract. Ergebn. Physiol., 69: 1-51.
5. Rattan, S. (1981). Neural regulation of gastrointestinal motility: Nature of transmission. Med. Clin. North Am., 65: 1129-1147.

6. Furness, J.B. & Costa, M. (1980). Types of nerves in the enteric nervous system. Neurosience, 5: 1-20.
7. Wood, J.D. (1984). Enteric neurophysiology. Am. J. Physiol., 247: G 585-598.
8. Wienbeck, M. & Erckenbrecht, J.F. (1982). The control of gastointestinal motility by GI hormones. Clin. Gastroenterol., 11: 523-543.
9. Huizinga, J.D., Stern, H.S., Waterfall, W.E., El-Sharkawy, T.Y. & Diamant, N.E. (1985). Electrical activity apparently propagating in the circular muscle layer of the human colon. Dig. Dis. Sci., 30: 773.
10. Mukhopadhyay, A.K. & Weisbrodt, N.W. (1975). Neural organization of esophageal peristasis: Role of vagus nerve. Gastroenterology, 68: 444-447.
11. Stacher, G., Schmierer, G. & Landgraf, M. (1979). Tertiary esophageal contractions evoked by accoustical stimuli. Gastroenterology, 77: 49-54.
12. Diamant, N.E. & El-Sharkawy, T.Y. (1977). Neural control of esophageal peristalsis: A conceptual analysis. Gastroenterology, 72: 546-556.
13. Fahrenkrug, J. (1979). Vasoactive intestinal polypeptide: Measurement, distribution and putative neurotransmitter function. Digestion, 19: 146-169.
14. Dodds, W.J., Dent, J., Hogan, W.J., Patel, G.K., Toouli, J. & Arndorfer, R.C. (1981). Paradoxical lower esophageal sphincter contraction induced by cholecystokinin-octapeptide in patients with achalasia. Gastroenterology, 80: 327-333.
15. Thomas, G.E. & Baldwin, M.V. (1968). Pathways and mechanisms of regulation of gastric motility. In C.F. Code (Ed.), Handbook of physiology, Sec. 6, Vol. IV. American Physiological Society, Washington DC, p. 1937-1964.
16. Stanghellini, V., Malagelada, J.-R., Zinsmeister, A.R., Go, V.L.W. & Kao, P.C. (1985). Stress-induced gastroduodenal motor disturbances in humans: Possible humoral mechanisms. Gastroenterology, 83: 83-91.
17. Stern, R.M., Stewart, W.R., Lindblad, I.M. & Koch, K.L. (1985). Spectral analysis of tachygastria recorded during motion sickness. Dig. Dis. Sci., 30: 797.
18. Morgan, K.G., Schmalz, P.F., Go, V.L.W. & Szurszewski, J.H. (1978). Effects of pentagastrin, G 17 and G 34 on the electrical and mechanical activities of canine antral smooth muscle. Gastroenterology, 75: 405-412.
19. Debas, H.T., Farooq, O. & Grossman, M.I. (1975). Inhibition of gastric emptying is a physiological action of cholecystokinin. Gastroenterology, 68: 1211-1217.
20. Morgan, K.G., Schmalz, P.F., Go, V.L.W. & Szurszewski, J.H. (1978). Electrical and mechanical effects of molecular variants of CCK on antral smooth muscle. Am. J. Physiol., 235: E 324-329.
21. Scheurer, U., Varga, L., Drack, E., Bürki, H.-R. & Halter, F. (1983). Mechanisms of action of cholecystokinin octapeptide on rat antrum, pylorus, and duodenum. Am. J. Physiol., 244: G 266-272.
22. Strunz, U.T., Domschke, W., Mitznegg, P., et al. (1975). Analysis of the motor effects of 13-norleucine motilin on the rabbit, guinea pig, rat, and human alimentary tract in vitro. Gastroenterology, 68: 25-27.
23. Christofides, N.D., Long, R.G., Fitzpatrick, M.L., McGregor, G.P. & Bloom, S.R. (1981). Effect of motilin on the gastric emptying of glucose and fat in humans. Gastroenterology, 80: 456-460.
24. Schuurkes, J.A.J., Helsen, L.F.M. & van Nueten, J.M. (1982). Improved gastroduodenal coordination by the peripheral dopamine-antagonist domperidone. In M. Wienbeck (Ed.), Motility of the digestive tract. Raven Press, N.Y., p. 565-572.
25. Fearley, R.D., Szurszewski, J.H., Merrit, J.L. & di Magno, E.P. (1984). Effect of traumatic spinal cord transection on human upper gastrointestinal motility and gastric emptying. Gastroenterology, 87: 69-75.
26. Minami, H. & McCallum, R.W. (1984). The physiology and pathophysiology of gastric emptying in humans. Gastroenterology, 86: 1592-1610.
27. Brener, W., Hendrix, T.R. & McHugh, P.R. (1983). Regulation of the gastric emptying of glucose. Gastroenterology, 85: 76-82.
28. Lübke, H.J. & Wienbeck, M. (1985). Gastrointestinale Motilität und enterale Resorption beeinflussen sich gegenseitig. Klinikarzt, 14: 25-36.
29. Cann, P.A., Read, N.W., Cammack, J., et al. (1983). Physiological stress and the passage of a standard meal through the stomach and small intestine in man. Gut, 24: 236-240.
30. Blackburn, A.M., Christofides, N.D., Ghatei, M.A., et al. (1980). Elevations of plasma neurotensin in the dumping syndrome. Clin. Sci., 59: 237-243.
31. Gidda, J. & Goyal, R.K. (1980). Influence of vagus nerves on electrical activity of opossum small intestine. Am. J. Physiol., 239: G 406-410.

32. Weisbrodt, N.W., Copeland, E.M., Moore, E.P., et al. (1975). Effect of vagotomy on electrical activity of the small intestine of the dog. Am. J. Physiol., 228: G 650-655.
33. Szurszewski, J.H. (1969). A migrating electrical complex of the canine small intestine. Am. J. Physiol., 217: 1757-1763.
34. Lux, G., Femppel, J., Lederer, P., Rösch, W. & Domschke, W. (1980). Somatostatin induces interdigestive intestinal motor and secretory complex-like activity in man. Gastroenterology, 78: 1212.
35. McCrae, S., Younger, K., Thompson, D.G. & Wingate, D.L. (1982). Sustained mental stress alters human jejunal motor activity. Gut, 23: 404-409.
36. Itoh, Z., Aizawa, I. & Takeuchi, S. (1981). Neural regulation of interdigestive motor activity in canine jejunum. Am. J. Physiol., 240: G 324-330.
37. Sarna, S., Condon, R.E. & Cowles, V. (1983). Enteric mechanisms of initiation of migrating myoelectric complexes in dogs. Gastroenterology, 84: 814-822.
38. Fox, D.A. & Bass, P. (1984). Selective myenteric neuronal denervation of the rat jejunum. Differential control of the propagation of migrating myoelectric complex and basic electric rhythm. Gastroenterology, 87: 572-577.
39. Kerlin, P., Zinsmeister, A. & Phillips, S. (1983). Motor responses to food of the ileum, proximal colon, and distal colon of healthy humans. Gastroenterology, 84: 762-770.
40. Wingate, D.L. (1981). Backwards and forwards with the migrating complex. Dig. Dis. Sci., 26: 641-666.
41. Sarr, M.G. & Kelly, K.A. (1981). Myoelectric activity of the autotransplanted canine jejunoileum. Gastroenterology, 81: 303-310.
42. Peeters, T.L., Janssens, J. & Vantrappen, G.R. (1983). Somatostatin and the interdigestive migrating motor complex in man. Regul. Pept., 5: 209-217.
43. Erckenbrecht, J.F., Caspari, J. & Wienbeck, M. (1984). Penatagastrin induced motility pattern of the human upper gastrointestinal tract is reversed by proglumide. Gut, 25: 953-956.
44. Erckenbrecht, J.F., Ziemer, B., Lesch, M., et al. (1984). The effect of longterm mental stress by noise on transit of a meal through the small and large bowel. Gut, 25: A 1311.
45. Altaparmakov, I. & Kolev, O. (1985). Three mechanisms of vomiting induced by central stressful stimulation. Dig. Dis. Sci., 30: 757.
46. Enck, P. (1985). Psychological and psychophysiological investigations of motor and myoelectrical activity in patients with the irritable bowel syndrome (IBS), patients with lactose malabsorption, and normal subjects. Doctoral dissertation, Tübingen.
47. Wienbeck, M. & Dünzen, R.G. (1982). The effects of leucine-enkephalin on the spontaneous motility of the circular muscle of the cat colon. Gastroenterology, 20: 429-437.
48. Wienbeck, M. & Sperling, T. (1984). The effects of prostaglandins F_{2alpha} and E_2 on the motility of the cat colon in vitro. Gastroenterology, 22: 580-585.
49. Körner, M.M., Berger, W., Scholten, T. & Wienbeck, M. (1982). Differential effects of enkephalin analogue on the motility of the small and large intestine. In M.Wienbeck (Ed.), Moltility of the digestive tract. Raven Press, N.Y., p. 131-136.
50. Snape, W.J., Metarazzo, S.A. & Cohen, S. (1978). The effect of eating and gastrointestinal hormones on human colonic myoelectrical and motor activity. Gastroenterology, 75: 373-378.
51. Snape, W.J., Wright, S.H., Battle, W.M. & Cohen, S. (1979). The gastrocolic response: Evidence for a neural mechanism. Gastroenterology, 77: 1235-1240.
52. Sullivan, M.A., Cohen, S. & Snape, W.J. (1978). Colonic myoelectric activity in irritable bowel sydrome. Effect of eating and anticholinergics. N. Engl. J. Med., 298: 878-883.
53. Erckenbrecht, J.F. & Wienbeck, M. (1985). The effect of stress on the gastrointestinal tract. Paper, 15th Annual Meeting of the European Association for Behavior Therapy. Munich.
54. Erckenbrecht, J.F., Winter, H.J., Cicmir, I., et al. (1983). Recto-anal continence mechanisms in diabetes mellitus. Gastroenterology, 84: 1145.
55. Erckenbrecht, J.F., Schoepe-Stiller, A., Borgos, J., Rehm, S. & Wienbeck, M. (1985). The effect of mental stress by noise on motility and fluid absorption in the human upper small bowel. Dig. Dis. Sci., 30: 768.
56. Burleigh, D.E. & D'Mello, A. (1983). Neural and pharmacological factors affecting motility of the internal anal sphincter. Gastroenterology, 84: 409-417.

Perception of Gastrointestinal Events

William E. Whitehead

Neuroanatomical studies have established that most of the extrinsic nerves to the gastrointestinal tract are afferent or sensory nerves rather than efferent or motor nerves. It is estimated that 90% of the vagal fibers, 75% of splanchnic nerve fibers, and 50% of pelvic nerves are afferent (1). The parts of the gastrointestinal tract innervated by these nerve bundles are shown in Figure 1. The purpose of this paper will be to review what is known about the functional significance of this afferent information.

Types of Sensory Information Arising from the Gastrointestinal Tract

Three different approaches have been used to study the sensory innervation of the gastrointestinal tract: In one of them, stimuli are introduced into the gastrointestinal tract of a human observer and the subject is asked to report verbally whether he perceived the stimulus (2, 3). This is called the psychophysical approach. A second approach, used more often by Russian and Hungarian investigators, is to teach an animal subject by a process of Pavlovian (4) or instrumental (5, 6) conditioning to respond differentially to stimuli presented to the gastrointestinal tract. The third approach, which is used preferentially by neuroanatomists, is to record changes in the pattern of firing of exposed nerves when the gastrointestinal tract is stimulated (1, 7).

Psychophysical Method

Most of what we know about the subjective sensations which arise from the gastrointestinal tract was discovered by the psychophysical method at the end of the last century and summarized in the landmark book published by Hertz in 1911 entitled *Sensibility of the Alimentary Canal*. The types of stimuli which Hertz found subjects able to perceive are shown in Table 1, column a.

The list of stimuli which human subjects are unable to perceive is at least as important as the list of stimuli which they can perceive. There are several types of stimuli which have been shown to produce responses in nerves going to the CNS but which are apparently *not* available to subjective awareness (Table 1). These include the response of glucoreceptors, amino acid receptors, gastric pH receptors and osmoreceptors in the small intestine (1).

These discrepancies between the information which reaches the brain and what is available to awareness may provide clues to the role which such sensory information plays in behavioral self-regulation. Most of the stimuli available to awareness appear to be relevant to the learning of defensive or avoidance behaviors which prevent injury to the gastrointestinal tract (e.g., temperature sensors in the esophagus) or ingestion of toxic substances. Others, as we shall see, relate to the social control of defecation. On the other hand, the stimuli which are known to reach the brain but which are outside awareness appear to subserve homeostatic regulation but not to be directly relevant to the organism's interactions with the external environment.

Table 1. Gastrointestinal stimuli with afferent connection to CNS.

	Subjectively perceived[1]	Received but not perceived[2]
Esophagus	Distension	Light touch
	Hot & cold	Hydrochloric acid
	Alcohol	
Stomach	Distension, contraction	Hydrochloric acid
	Alcohol	Alkaline substances
	Glucose	
	Hot & cold	
Small Intestine	Distension	Light touch
	Glucose	
	Amino acids	
	Acids & alkali	
	Osmolarity	
Colon	Distension, contraction	Light touch
Rectum	Distension	Alcohol, glycerine
Anal canal	Distension	
	Alcohol	
	Glycerine	

1. Source: Hertz (2)
2. Sources: Mei (1), Hertz (2), Leek (7)

Psychophysical methods for the assessment of perception have evolved considerably since Hertz's observations were made 75 years ago. Primarily, these methodological advances consist of techniques for distinguishing between perceptual sensitivity, which might be thought of as the pure ability to perceive a stimulus, and response bias, which is the tendency for subjects to give one type of response over another for reasons having nothing to do with actual perception (8). These techniques have rarely been used in the assessment of gastrointestinal sensation, although there are exceptions: Both we (9) and Stunkard and Fox (10) have used signal detection theory to separate perceptual sensitivity from response bias in the detection of stomach contractions, and we have used forced-choice procedures to measure perception of rectal distension independently of response bias (11, 12). I have described these psychophysical techniques in greater detail in another context (13).

Conditioning Method

The conditioning technique whereby one teaches an animal to emit an overt response in the presence of a specific visceral stimulus, has so far yielded little new information about the types of sensations available from the gastrointestinal tract. This is perhaps due to the limited range of stimuli which have been investigated. However, two important points are made by this technique. First, the experiments of Adam (14) suggest that visceral stimuli may modulate ongoing motor behavior through their influence on affective tone or motivation. Adam's group has shown, e.g., that at low intensities electrical stimulation of the duodenum reduces aggressiveness in cats and elicits sleep, whereas more intense stimulation produces arousal and augments aggressive behavior (14-18).

The second important point made by conditioning methods of studying visceral perception is that through discrimination training, subjects may *learn* to perceive stimuli of which they were formerly unaware. Adam (5, 19), for example, was able to teach human subjects to detect and accurately report on distensions of the duodenum with very small volumes of air in a balloon which initially produced blocking of the α EEG (indicating that the sensory information was received in the CNS) but no subjective awareness.

This disparity between sensory information which the subject can accurately report on and the sensory information which is *potentially* available to awareness apparently arises because humans normally have no way of learning to accurately label visceral stimuli. Parents normally teach their children to attach verbal labels to events by pointing to the events and naming them. They also correct their children when they apply verbal labels inappropriately. However, such verbal learning is only possible when parents are able to observe the events themselves; this is not possible in the case for visceral stimuli from the gastrointestinal tract. Consequently, it may only be possible to adequately assess the ability for subjective perception of gastrointestinal responses by training people to the limits of their capacity. It is known, for example, that subjects who are unable to accurately report on the occurrence of heart beats can be taught in as few as 20 trials to discriminate these events quite accurat (20).

Recording from Dissected Nerves

The neuroanatomical technique for studying visceral afference is to isolate individual nerve fibers in the vagus or other nerves by dissection and then to record action potentials in the nerve during stimulation of the gastrointestinal tract. When a change in the pattern of firing - either an increase or a decrease - is consistently produced, there is a good basis for inferring that this is a specific afferent pathway to the CNS. This approach has shown that there are categories of sensory information which travel to the brainstem which appear not to be available to subjective awareness (Table 1, column b). However, there are inherent limitations to the technique: One may easily fail to detect the receptive field or the appropriate type of stimulus for a given fiber. Also, verbal reports provide much more detailed information about a sensory experience than do changes in firing rate in a nerve.

Another neuroanatomical technique which provides useful information about the neural pathways for afferent fibers from the gastrointestinal tract and the CNS location of their cell bodies is to paint the peripheral organ with horse-radish peroxidase. This stain is taken up by nerve endings and transported to the CNS where it can be indentified in slices of the brain, spinal cord, or ganglia. This technique demonstrates that most of the afferent fibers from the gastrointestinal tract terminate in the medulla oblongata of the brain stem in proximity to motor nuclei which control reflex vomiting and gastric acid secretion, among other gastrointestinal functions. However, a relatively small proportion of these fibers also travel to the cerebral cortex. Presumably, the later fibers contribute to subjective perception of gastrointestinal stimuli. For a more extensive review of the neuroanatomical localization of gastrointestinal afferent nerves, see Kalia (21) and Davison (22).

Gastrointestinal Sensations and Emotion

The James-Lange theory of emotion (23, 24) proposes that visceral sensations are the basis for attributing emotions to ourselves. This theory was modified by Schachter and Singer (25), who proposed that the perception of visceral sensations is a contributing factor to the self-attribution of emotion but that cognitive cues in the environment are an important second source of information about the specific emotion experienced. This theory has been generally supported in experimental studies (26). It is therefore necessary to ask what role the multitude of sensory information available from the gastrointestinal tract plays in the self-attribution of emotion.

There is a well-established association between affective states and gastrointestinal disturbances. Thus, Drossman, Sandler, McKee, and Lovitz (27), found that 70% of a sample of 789 students and hospital employees reported alterations in stool frequency and consistency in response to stress, and 54% reported that stress caused them to have abdominal pain. The association of depression with constipation has so impressed psychologists and psychiatrists that several psychometric tests of depression treat constipation as a soft sign of depression (e.g., *Zung Depression Scale*; 28). This association has become a part of everyday language in which affective reactions to events are often described metaphorically in terms of wanting to vomit or feeling that one will develop diarrhea. It is unclear, however, whether visceral sensations can cause or contribute to the development of affective responses or whether the association is always in the opposite direction - strong emotion secondarily causing gastrointestinal motor behavior.

Adam and his colleagues (14-18) found evidence in their animal studies that visceral afferent information might influence the motivational state and thus the affective state of an animal in opposite ways depending on the intensity of the stimulation. They found that low intensity electrical stimulation of a loop of bowel induced behavioral quiesence or sleep and reduced aggressive behavior in cats, whereas a higher intensity of the same stimulus produced behavioral arousal and motivated the animal to work to terminate the stimulation. They termed this opposite effect of gastrointestinal stimulation a Janus-effect after the two-faced god of Greek mythology. One can infer the same effects from the subjective sensations of pleasure and sleepiness produced by ingesting a good meal and the aversive effects of overdistending the stomach.

There is little direct evidence, however that gastrointestinal stimulation is interpreted as an affective experience. In various experiments over the last 15 years, I have asked subject to provide verbal descriptions after I stimulated the stomach, ilium, colon, and rectum with mechanical stimuli and after stimulating the stomach with hydrochloric acid. In no instances have subjects described the sensations produced by these stimuli in affective terms. Table 2, for example, summarizes the responses of 20 normal subjects when they were asked to describe how they detected contractions of their stomach. Most subjects described squeezing sensations in their abdomens. However, it is possible that the experimental setting mitigated against subjects ascribing emotions to the visceral sensations which they experienced in the gastroenterology laboratory.

Table 2. Cues used by 20 subjects to identify gastric contractions.

Cue	Frequency
Abdominal tension or pressure	16
Stomach sounds	13
Hunger pangs	3
Need to belch	3
Full feeling in throat	1

We (9) made an interesting observation in our study of how subjects perceive gastric contractions which is of relevance to the James-Lange theory of emotion (23, 24). Clearly this theory, and the associated attribution theory of emotion (25, 26) imply that subjects should have a generalized ability to perceive different visceral sensations. We, therefore, compared the ability to perceive spontaneously occurring stomach contractions to the ability to perceive heart beats, using a signal detection approach in both cases. We found heart beat perception to be significantly correlated with gastric contraction perception across subject ($r = 0.51$). This suggests that subjects who are good at perceiving one type of visceral arousal are also good at perceiving other types of visceral arousal.

Hunger and Satiety

The hypothesis that contractions of the stomach are interpreted as hunger signals originated with Cannon and Washburn (29). These investigators recorded stomach contractions by inflating a balloon in the stomach and connecting this to a smoked-drum kymograph. Their subjects reported that stomach contractions coincided with subjective reports of hunger. Stunkard's group (30, 31) later appeared to confirm this observation in measurements made with an open-tipped catheter. They made the interesting addtional observation that obese subjects seemed less likely to interpret gastric contractions as hunger, and it appeared for a time that the key to obesity had been found. However, subsequent work dashed these hopes. It was shown that teaching obese subjects to accurately discriminate stomach contractions did not improve their ability to regulate food intake (10). Additional research by this group using a signal detection approach showed that only 25% of subjects exhibited a significant correlation between hunger ratings and stomach contractions, and even in these subjects the relationship was not stable across different occasions of testing. The investigators suggested that the earlier results may have occurred as an artifact because both stomach contractions and reports of hunger increase in proportion to the length of time since the last meal.

Observations made by Drescher and myself (9) are consistent with this impression. When we asked subjects in open-ended questionnaires to describe the sensations they used to tell when their stomachs were contracting, only 3 of 20 mentioned hunger sensations (Table 2). Moreover, accuracy at detecting stomach contractions was not related to self-reports of sensing hunger waves. It appears from our data and the series of studies by Stunkard's group that the relationship between gastric contractions and hunger sensations is weak, if one exists at all.

Rather better support exists for the hypothesized relationship between gastric distension and subjective feelings of satiety. Hertz (2) appears to have been the first to describe this relationship between artificial filling of the stomach with a balloon and feelings of "repletion." Subsequent experiments by Deutsch, Young, and Kalogeris (32) and McHugh (33) in animals show that gastric distension is a potent inhibitor of eating which is reversible; withdrawing nutrient from the stomach after an animal has eaten to satiety causes the animal to resume eating and to replace the volume withdrawn. Control studies show that this effect is not mediated by pain. These experiments thus provide indirect evidence for the gastric distension - satiety hypothesis.

Experiments by Garfinkel, Moldofsky, Garner, Stancer, and Coscina (34) suggest that a disturbance of a different afferent-based satiety mechanism may contribute to the development of anorexia nervosa. They found that anorexics failed to develop an aversion to sucrose after repeated tastes of it. Moreover, this abnormality was stable over a year's observation and was not sensitive to increased food intake and weight gain (35). Similar observations were made by M. Hetherington and B. J. Rolls (personal communication) at our institution. She found that some bulimic patients did not show the normal decrease in ratings of hunger and of the pleasantness of a food when they ingested it in large amounts (during an eating binge), but instead showed a paradoxical increase in both. These provocative observations should be followed up, but it will be important to move towards experimental paradigms which differentiate perceptual sensitivity from response bias.

Stimulus Control of Defecation

The best evidence that sensations arising in the gastrointestinal tract have significance for behavioral interactions with the external world exists for sensations produced by rectal distension - the "call to stool."

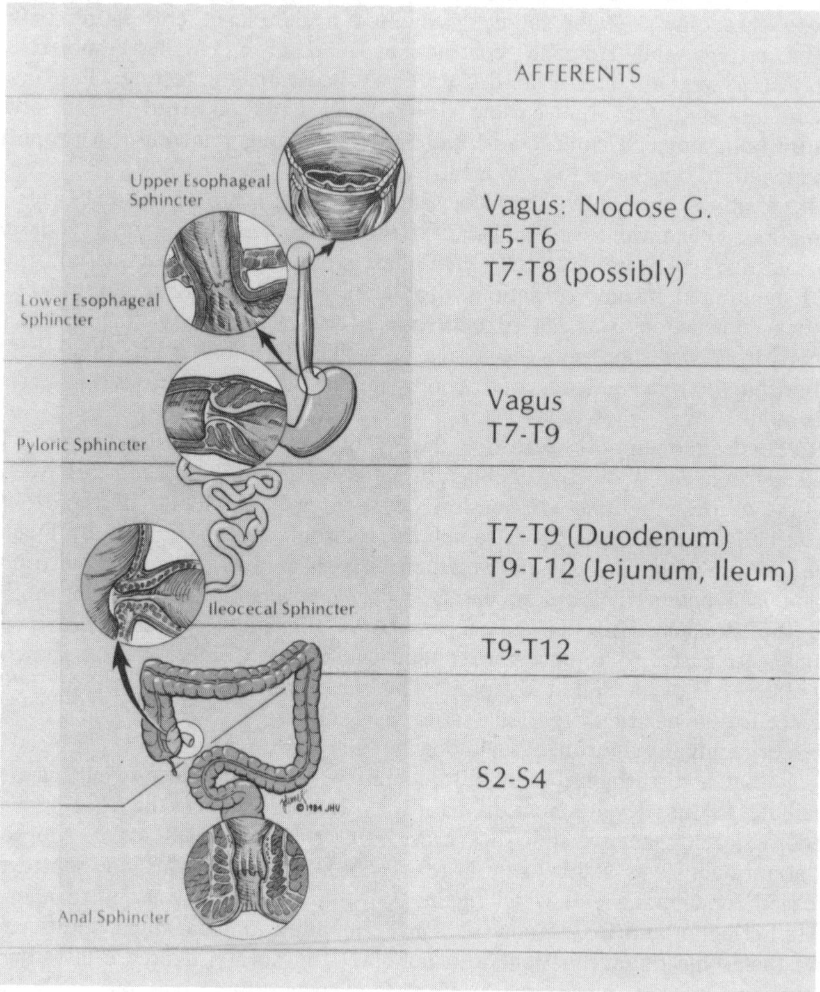

Figure 1. Schematic representation of the gastrointestinal tract showing its afferent innervation. The gastrointestinal tract can be divided into four compartments - esophagus, stomach, small intestine, and colon - that are separated from each other by sphincters. These compartments serve different functions and have different innervation (43; reproduced, with permission from Academic Press, New York, 1985).

The external anal sphincter response which normally follows rectal distension is critical to maintaining continence. This stimulus-response relationship was formerly viewed as a reflex (36, 37). However, a series of experiments done in my laboratory (38) showed that it is not a reflex but a learned, instrumental response which is under the stimulus control of rectal distension. The observations we made which support this point are that (1) the external anal sphincter response does not occur in children prior to toilet training; (2) it does not occur in half of chronically constipated individuals who have had no reason to learn and to practice the response; (3) it is much less likely to occur when the rectum is distended during sleep; and (4) the response can be produced or omitted on demand.

An obvious implication of the voluntary response hypothesis is that the inability to subjectively perceive rectal distension should lead to incontinence. Subsequent observations by our laboratory (39, 40) and by other investigators (41) confirm this. We found that as a group fecally incontinent patients had higher sensory thresholds than continent subjects and that subjects who were unable to discriminate distension of the rectum with 15 ml or less continued to be incontinent even when they had adequate strength in the external anal sphincter muscles (39). Wald and Tunguntla (41) reported that sensory impairment due to peripheral neuropathy is a frequent contributing cause of fecal incontinence in diabetic patients, and that training patients to discriminate smaller volumes of rectal distension improved their bowel control.

Figure 2 is an illustration of the importance of rectal sensation for bowel continence.

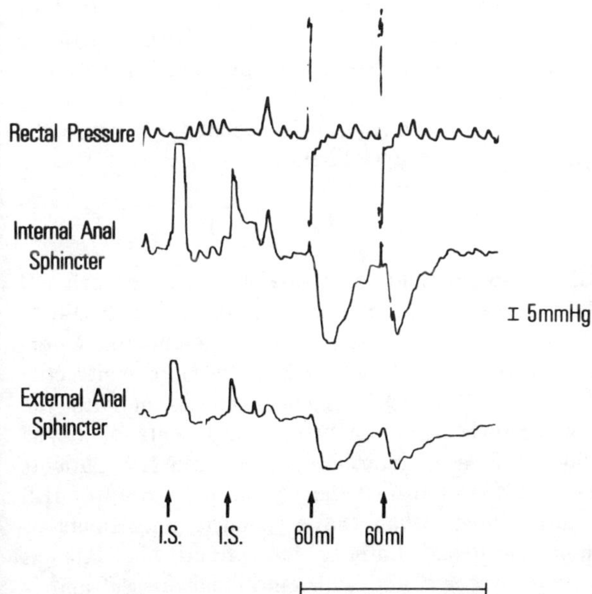

Figure 2. Sensory-loss incontinence in a 72-year-old patient with diabetes. When instructed to squeeze (labeled I.S.), she could contract the external anal sphincter appropriately. However, when the rectum was distended with a large 60-ml volume of air, she did not contract the external anal sphincter because she did not feel the stimulus (42; reproduced, with permission from Plenum Press, New York 1983).

This 72-year-old diabetic woman could contract the external anal sphincter muscles appropriately when instructed to do so (marked I.S. in the figure), but she failed to contract the sphincters in response to distension of the rectum with large, 60 ml volumes of air in a rectal balloon. As a result, she was incontinent 3-4 times per day. This woman was unable to learn to discriminate rectal distensions small enough to enable her to regain continence. However, she was significantly benefited by placing her on a habit training program in which she was instructed to voluntarily defecate at predetermined times three times a day to keep her rectum empty. This reduced the frequency of incontinence to an average of 3 times per week.

The nerve endings which subserve the perception of rectal distension appear not to be in the walls of the bowel but in the striated pelvic floor muscles which surround the rectum. This is suggested by the fact that rectal sensation thresholds are normal after surgical operations for imperforate anus in which the rectum is removed and proximal bowel is brought down to create a new rectum (43). However, it remains possible that patients who have had a pull-through operation learn to discriminate visceral afferents from the new segment of bowel and to relabel it as urgency to defecate.

Role of Visceral Perception in the Etiology of Functional Gastrointestinal Disorders

In recent years behavioral psychologists and psychophysiologists have suggested that perception of gastrointestinal events may play a role in the etiology of the irritable bowel syndrome (IBS) in one of two ways: Latimer (44) suggested that patients with the IBS may misperceive or mislabel the sensations produced by normal physiological activity in the bowel and may incorrectly attribute symptoms to themselves. We (45), on the other hand, have proposed that people may inadvertently use perceptions of gastrointestinalactivity to learn how to produce abnormal patterns of physiological activity, which secondarily cause the symptoms of IBS. These two hypotheses are reviewed below.

Misattribution Hypothesis

Latimer's misattribution hypothesis (46) depends on the results of an experiment which he and colleagues conducted (47). They compared 16 patients with IBS to 8 neurotic outpatients who did not complain of bowel symptoms and to 17 normal subjects. The IBS patients were found to have significantly more contractile activity in the colon than the normal subjects, which is consistent with the reports of previous investigators. However, the neurotic outpatients displayed amounts of physiological activity which were intermediate between IBS patients and normals, and not significantly different from either. Since this group of IBS patients tended also to be more neurotic than the psychiatric outpatients as measured by standard psychometric tests, Latimer interpreted his data as suggesting that colonic hyperactivity is correlated with emotional arousal and is not specific to IBS. He argued that what causes some patients to be labeled as having IBS while others are labeled as having other psychiatric disorders is that they selectively focus on and mislabel the same physiological activity which they have in common with psychiatric outpatients.

This misattribution hypothesis depends on there being no unique biological marker or mechanism for the symptoms of IBS. This remains a controversial question. Early experiments by Snape and Cohen's group (48, 49) suggested that IBS patients were distinguished from normal subjects by a greater ratio of very slow myoelectric slow waves (0-4 cpm) to all slow wave activity, and we found similar results for pressure waves (11). However, these results were achieved with visual scoring of polygraph records. Latimer's group (47) was unable to show any differences in frequency composition between normals and IBS patients when they used spectral analysis to evaluate their data. Thus, these different outcomes appear to depend on the method of data analysis. We have shown (50) that spectral analysis is an insensitive method of assessing slow wave activity in the colon because of instability in the frequency of such activity. A computer pattern recognition program which emulates visual scoring but does it more consistently than human scorers gives very different results from spectral analysis for the frequency decomposition of the same date.

Colonic Hyperalgesia in IBS

An implicit assumption of the misattribution hypothesis is that patients are more likely than normal subjects to report pain or bowel symptoms regardless of where in the bowel the activity occurs, i.e., pain reports are not specific to the site of stimulation. Latimer (51) has proposed that the tendency of IBS patients to over-report pain may not even be specific to the colon, but may reflect a neurotic tendency to over-report pain due to any type of stimulation. Recent studies by two groups of British investigators appear to refute this assumption by showing that there may be specific trigger points in the colon and small intestine from which the patient's typical clinical pain can be reproduced.

In the earliest study of pain due to distension of the colon, Ritchie (52) showed that when a balloon situated at 35 cm was inflated with 60 ml of air, a larger proportion of patients with IBS reported pain as compared to normal and constipated patients, and the pain was produced at a lower threshold of bowel wall tension than in normal subjects. These observations suggested a specific hyperalgesia in the colon in patients with IBS. This phenomenon of a lower threshold for pain reports due to colonic distension was replicated by Ritchie himself (53) and by Kullmann and Fielding (54); Whitehead, Engel, and Schuster (11); and Kroeger, Hoelzl, Fuenfgeld, Ottenjann, and Hoechter (55). However, Latimer et al. (51) failed to observe a difference in threshold between IBS patients and normals for unknown reasons.

Dawson's group (56, 57) has studied the localization of pain by inflating balloons in various parts of the colon and small intestine. They could reproduce the type of abdominal pain patients complained of at home in all but a small minority (15%), but the site of stimulation which reproduced the clinical pain varied greatly between patients. In one series of 20 patients, 11 had their pain reproduced by small intestinal stimulation, 3 by both small intestinal sites and colon sites, and in 3 of the remaining 6 patients, colonic distension reproduced their pain. In another series of 48 IBS patients, stimulation of some portion of the colon reproduced the patient's clinical pain in 29 cases. Dawson and his coworkers also noted that pain due to distension was poorly localized and was frequently referred to a site outside the colon such as the back or shoulder.

The most important finding from Dawson's studies was that clinical pain could be reproduced from specific sites in the gastrointestinal tract and that these sites varied among patients. This suggests the possibility that the pain associated with IBS may be due to specific areas of inflammation or tenderness. Further examination of these trigger sites may provide interesting new insights into the pathophysiology of IBS.

One ambiguity in the Dawson data is that the pain may not be due to balloon distension itself but to contractile activity which it induces. Ritchie (58) made radiological studies of the effects of balloon distension in the colon which led him to conclude that most of the pains observed in IBS patients in response to balloon distension were due to induced contractions which might be propagated along the bowel and that propagated contractions were associated with pain only in specific areas of the colon which might be at a distance from the balloon distension.

Another important implication of the Dawson studies is that many instances of abdominal pain associated with IBS arise from stimulation of and perhaps from contractions in, the small intestine. Dawson found that stimulation of the small intestine frequently produced pain which was referred to sites usually thought to represent colonic distension. Studies currently in progress at the Mayo Clinic by Kellow and Phillips (personal communication, 1985) similarly suggest that the small intestine may play a prominent role in the pain associated with IBS: Kellow and Phillips report that stepwise distension of a balloon in the small intestine produced reports of pain at a lower threshold and also larger amounts of contractile activity in IBS patients as compared to normal control subjects.

Learning of Pathophysiological Responses

It is now well established that human subjects can learn to modify gastrointestinal secretory (59, 60) and motor (61, 62) responses, when they are provided with biofeedback training, i.e., when they are provided with augmented sensory feedback and are motivated to learn. Neal Miller (63) was the first to point out that such learning of abnormal physiological responses might occur in the natural environment if sympathetic attention from parents or other people following somatic complaints were to substitute for the electronic feedback used in biofeedback experiments.

In a theoretical paper on psychosomatic etiology published in 1979 (45), we pointed out that this type of learning of physiological responses could only occur if the person is able to perceive the occurrence of the physiological event. The rationale is as follows: Operant learning can only take place if the person is able to associate the occurrence of rewards with the occurrence of responses and the non-occurrence of rewards with the non-occurrence of responses. There are indications that this association does not have to be "conscious," i.e., available to verbal report (64). However, there does have to be a reliable correlation between responses and rewards. In the case of covert visceral responses, the person delivering the reward cannot normally detect when the response occurs; he must depend on the patient's verbal report of symptom occurrence. Therefore, if patients are unaware of specific occurrences of the physiological response, they cannot complain in such a way that social rewards will be correlated with occurrences of the response, and learning will not occur.

This argument requires some additional speculation about mediating cognitive processes. One has to account for the effects of a patient telling others about his symptoms only some time after they have occurred. This is best understood in operant conditioning terms by conceptualizing thoughts about the probable reactions of others to symptoms and complaints as conditioned reinforcers which may support learning. The model for such learning is the token economy (65) in which plastic chips are first established as reinforcers by pairing them with food, after which these chips can be used to reinforce new responses. To continue to be effective, however, these chips must be exchangeable for primary reinforcers. Applying the model to the social learning of covert physiological responses, the speculation is that the patient perceives the occurrence of the physiological response and then imagines how others would react to these signs of illness if they only knew about them. Such thoughts act like the plastic chips in the token economy to bridge the temporal delay between the occurrence of the physiological responses and the occurrence of sympathetic attention or work avoidance for somatic complaints about these physiological responses.

Based on this reasoning, we (45) made two predictions: (1) that patients with a disorder will exhibit greater awareness of the associated physiological response (such as contractions of the colon in IBS) than will patients who do not have the disorder; and (2) that disorders such as IBS which result from easily-perceived pathophysiological responses will be more likely to come under the control of operant reinforcers than will disorders such as peptic ulcer which result from difficult-to-perceive pathophysiological responses.

The first prediction was tested by comparing the threshold for perception of balloon distension in the rectum in patients with irritable bowel syndrome and in normal control subjects. We used perception of balloon distension as an indicator of the likely ability to detect contractions of the colon because it is difficult to measure perception of naturally occurring contractions. This is a reasonable assumption of equality since stretch receptors in the wall of the colon are in series with muscle cells and respond to passive distension as well as to active contraction (7).

It is known that patients with irritable bowel syndrome have a lower threshold for reporting pain due to distension of the colon (see above). We wished to determine whether the threshold at which they first perceived nonpainful distension was also lower (11). We began by rapidly injecting 50 ml of air into a balloon and withdrawing it, and then asking the patients if they perceived this stimulus. If they responded affirmatively, the volume of the stimulus was reduced by 10 ml. This procedure was repeated until the patient denied sensation. The sensory threshold arrived at in this way (by the descending method of limits) was retested by a forced-choice procedure to eliminate response bias from estimates of sensory threshold. Forced choice meant thþt the subject was asked to choose between two periods of time in only one of which the stimulus was presented. The threshold was defined as the volume of distension below which the subject could not correctly identify the stimulus interval on at least 75% of trials.

When we compared 20 normal subjects to 19 IBS patients using this procedure, there were no differences between groups. All normals and 16 of 19 IBS patients could detect the weakest stimulus we were able to present (5 ml) on 100% of trials. Thus, although the predicted difference between IBS patients and normals was not seen, both patients and normals were able to detect such weak stimuli that differences between them were neither measurable nor physiologically meaningful. (It may be possible to make the balloon distension test more sensitive to individual differences by using gradual inflation since rate of inflation is known to be an important determinant of sensory threshold in the bowel.)

The second prediction we made was that patients with IBS would be more likely to exhibit learned illness behaviors which are maintained by social reinforcement than would patients with peptic ulcer disease. This prediction was tested in an epidemiological survey (66) in which 832 randomly selected people were telephoned and interviewed about their symptoms, the ways they responded to them, and their childhood experiences with illness. Sixty-seven people were designated as having IBS on the basis of their answering that they were often bothered by abdominal pain and constipation or diarrhea in the last year, and 84 people were designated as having peptic ulcer disease on the basis of their reports that they had been told by a doctor or nurse that they had an ulcer. The extent to which their medical self-care was maintained by social reinforcement was inferred from the questions given in Table 3. Patients with IBS reported that they had more colds and other illnesses per year, they believed their colds were more serious than those of other people, and they were more likely than the general population to go to a physician for treatment of a cold rather than to treat it themselves. Patients with IBS also had more disability days due to illness than the rest of the population. By contrast, patients with peptic ulcer disease were similar to the rest of the sample on these dimensions.

One possible explanation for the data shown in Table 3 was that patients with IBS were simply more anxious and depressed than others. To test this, we asked patients about the presence of anxiety and depression and also what types of medical care they were receiving. As shown in Table 4, both patients with IBS and patients with peptic ulcer disease reported more anxiety and depression than the general population, and a larger proportion of patients with peptic ulcer disease reported that they had a psychiatric disorder. Thus, differences between these two groups in the prevalence of nonspecific psychopathology did not account for the differences in illness behavior.

Table 3. Percent of males and females with IBS and PUD reporting chronic illness behavior.

	Males			Females			
	IBS	PUD	All Ss	IBS	PUD	All Ss	Statistical Differences*
Preoccupation with illness							
1) 2 or more colds/year	50.0	25.0	28.2	46.2	34.4	31.4	I, D
2) Colds more serious than those of other people	28.6	10.9	10.5	35.9	43.3	20.5	I, D
3) Go to doctor for colds	21.4	15.4	18.9	43.6	31.3	28.6	I
4) 2 or more acute physical illnesses/year	14.3	5.8	7.5	23.1	9.4	10.2	I, D
5) 2 or more doctor visits for acute physical illness/year	21.4	13.5	18.4	25.6	18.8	20.7	D
6) Hospitalization for acute physical illness in last year	17.9	9.6	8.0	17.9	15.6	11.5	I, D
7) Avoidance behavior: Miss work or change activities more than 4 days/year for acute physical illness	21.4	9.6	9.2	20.5	18.8	14.0	I

* I indicates that a significantly larger proportion of people with IBS responded yes to the question compared to people without IBS. P indicates that a larger proportion of people with PUD responded yes compared to people without PUD. D indicates that a larger proportion of people with IBS but not PUD answered yes compared to people with PUD but not IBS. Column labelled All Ss includes every subject interviewed.

Table 4. Psychopathology: Percent of males and females with IBS and PUD reporting anxiety, depression, and psychiatric illness.

	Males			Females			
	IBS	PUD	All Ss	IBS	PUD	All Ss	Statistical Differences*
Anxious	33.3	35.3	17.1	43.6	46.9	27.3	I, P
Depressed	35.7	34.6	20.3	56.4	59.4	40.1	I, P
Reported psychiatric illness	3.6	5.8	2.5	2.6	12.5	4.6	P

* Symbols defined as in Table 3.

Evidence that this pattern of illness behavior was due to learning came from responses to the question, "When you had a cold or flu as a child, did your parents show special consideration for you by giving you special foods, toys, or other gifts?" For the whole sample, people who answered yes to this question were significantly more likely to exhibit 4 of the 6 illness behaviors listed in Table 3. A significantly larger proportion of people with IBS (45%) answered yes to this question as compared to people with peptic ulcer disease (29%) or people in general (33%).

We have replicated these observations in two unpublished studies from our laboratory. In a dissertation study conducted by Paul Enck, we compared responses on the Pilowsky Illness Behavior Questionnaire in patients with IBS, patients with lactose malabsorption, and normal controls. Patients with IBS scored significantly higher on the scales for phobic health concerns and symptom preoccupation than normal subjects, and lactose malabsorbers scored in the middle. In the second study, we asked 452 women a series of questions about how their parents reacted when they had a cold as a child. As in our previous study, subjects whose parents reinforced somatic complaints during their childhood were significantly more likely than others to report bowel symptoms suggestive of IBS as adults. Sandler, Drossman, McKee, and Lovitz (67) made similar observations in their epidemiological study: They found that patients with bowel dysfunction who consulted a doctor had significantly more nongastrointestinal complaints and made more doctor visits per complaint than did normal subjects.

These findings suggest that a history of childhood reinforcement for somatic complaints contributes to the etiology of IBS but not to the etiology of peptic ulcer disease. However, they provide only indirect evidence that physiological responses in addition to verbal complaints were modified by such learning. To test this hypothesis directly, a prospective study is needed which includes measurement of gastrointestinal physiological activity and patterns of parental response to illness before such learning has occurred.

Summary and Implications for Future Research

The study of visceral afferent information from the gastrointestinal tract has been pursued in three independent traditions: the psychophysical approach, in which human subjects are asked to describe sensations produced by stimuli introduced through tubes; the conditioning approach, in which animal subjects are taught to make overt responses when a portion of the gastrointestinal tract is stimulated; and the neuroanatomical approach, in which recordings from cut nerves are used to indicate what afferent information is being conducted to the CNS. This review has shown that these techniques give different results and that the discrepancies between the types of information which are transmitted to the CNS and the types of information which are consciously perceived provides clues to the role of visceral afferent information in the organism's adjustment to its environment. It appears that the sensory information which is subjectively perceived enables us to avoid poisoning and to exercise social control over defecation, whereas the afferent information which is received by the CNS but not consciously perceived subserves primarily the homeostatic regulation of digestion.

There are already hints, however, that this is too simplistic an explanation. Hertz pointed out as early as 1911 that there are individual differences in the ability to perceive gastrointestinal stimuli, and he suggested that these differences may be due to learning. Clearly, we will be unable to complete anything like an adequate psychophysics of gastrointestinal afferent information unless we train subjects to the limits of their ability to discriminate gastrointestinal stimuli.

Various theories about the behavioral significance of perception of gastrointestinal events have been reviewed above. There is no compelling evidence that such perception plays a role in the self-attribution of emotion, although animal research summarized by Adam (14) suggests that gastrointestinal stimuli may modulate nonspecific motivational and affective states. The perception of gastric contractions appears to play little role in the self-attribution of hunger, but the feeling produced by gastric distension is apprently involved in saticty.

The most interesting speculations about the role of visceral perception relate to its possible significance for the etiology of gastrointestinal motility disorders. We have proposed (45) that patients may associate sympathetic attention for illness complaints with the physiological events which they perceive as causing those symptoms and may thereby learn inadvertently to emit abnormal motor behavior. Prospective longitudinal studies which involve the assessment of gastrointestinal motility and of family styles of responding to illness at several points during childhood and adolescence are needed to adequately test this hypothesis, which is so far supported only by indirect evidence. The implications of this hypothesis for the prevention of functional bowel disorders are considerable. If the hypothesis is supported, then education programs to teach parents appropriate ways of responding to the somatic complaints of their children may well result in a significantly lower incidence of functional gastrointestinal disorders, which today make up approximately half of all referrals to gastroenterologists (43).

References

1. Mei, N. (1985). Intestinal chemosensitivity. Physiol. Rev., 65: 211-237.
2. Hertz, A.F. (1911). The sensibility of the alimentary canal. Oxford University Press, London.
3. Jones, C.M. (1938). Digestive tract pain: Diagnosis and treatment. Macmillan, N.Y.
4. Bykov, K.M. (1957). The cerebral cortex and the internal organs. Chemical Publishing Company, N.Y.
5. Adam, G. (1967). Interoception and behavior. Academiai Kiado, Budapest.
6. Bardos, G. & Adam, G. (1977). Visceroceptive control of operant behavior in rats. Physiol. Behav., 20: 369-375.
7. Leek, B.F. (1972). Abdominal visceral receptors. In E. Neil (Ed.), Enteroceptors, Handbook of sensory physiology, Volume 3, No. 1. Springer-Verlag, N.Y., p. 113-160.
8. Swets, J.A. (1973). The relative operating characteristic in psychology. Science. 182: 990-1000.
9. Whitehead, W.E. & Drescher, V.M. (1980). Perception of gastric contractions and self-control of gastric motility. Psychophysiol., 17: 552-558.
10. Stunkard, A.J. & Fox, S. (1971). The relationship of gastric motility and hunger: A summary of the evidence. Psychosom. Med., 33: 123-134.

11. Whitehead, W.E., Engel, B.T. & Schuster, M.M. (1980). Irritable bowel syndrome: Physiological and psychological differences between diarrhea-predominant and constipation predominant patients. Digest. Dis. Sci., 25: 404-413.
12. Whitehead, W.E., Parker, L., Bosmajian, L., Morrill-Corbin, E.D., Middaugh, S., Garwood, M., Cataldo, M.F. & Freeman, J. (in press). Treatment of fecal incontinence in children with spina bifida: Comparison of biofeedback and behavior modification. Arch. Physic. Med. Rehab.
13. Whitehead, W.E. (1983). Interoception: Awareness of sensations arising in the gastrointestinal tract. In R. Hoelzl & W.E. Whitehead (Eds.), Psychophysiology of the gastrointestinal tract: Experimental and clinical applications. Plenum Press, N.Y., p. 333-350.
14. Adam, G. (1983). Intestinal afferent influence on behavior. In R. Hoelzl & W.E. Whitehead (Eds.), Psychophysiology of the gastrointestinal tract: Experimental and clinical applications. Plenum Press, N.Y., p. 351-380.
15. Kukorelli, T. & Juhasz, G. (1976). Electroencephalographic synchronization induced by stimulation of small intestine and splanchnic nerve in cats. Electroencephal. Clin. Neurophysiol., 41: 491-500.
16. Kukorelli, T. & Juhasz, G. (1977). Sleep induced by electrical stimulation in cats. Physiol. Behav., 19: 355-358.
17. Juhasz, G., Kukorelli, T. & Detari, L. (1980). Relationship between aggressive behavior, visceral afferentation and sleep in cats. Proceed. Intern. Union Physiol. Sci., 14: 497.
18. Bardos, G., Nagy, J. & Adam, G. (1979). Thresholds of behavioral reactions evoked by intestinal and skin stimuli in rats. Physiol. Behav., 24: 661-665.
19. Adam, G.P., Preisich, T., Kukorelli, T. & Keleman, V. (1965). Changes in human cerebral electrical activity in response to mechanical stimulation of the duodenum. Electroencephalogr. Clin. Neurophysiol., 18: 409-411.
20. Ross, A. & Brener, J. (1981). Two procedures for training cardiac discrimination: A comparison of solution strategies and their relationship to heart rate control. Psychophysiol., 18: 62-70.
21. Kalia, M. (in press). Brain stem nuclei involved in control of gastrointestinal afferents and efferents. In J. H. Szurszewski (Ed.), Proceedings of the Tenth International Symposium on Gastrointestinal Motility.
22. Davison, J. (in press). Central organization of gastrointestinal reflexes. In J. H. Szurszewski (Ed.), Proceedings of the Tenth International Symposium on Gastrointestinal Motility.
23. James, W. (1884). What is emotion? Mind, 19: 188-205.
24. Lange, C.(1922). The emotions (I.A. Haupt, Trans.). In K. Dunlap (Ed.), The emotions. Williams & Wilkins, Baltimore.
25. Schachter, A. & Singer, J.E. (1962). Cognitive, social, and psychological determinants of emotional state. Psychol. Rev., 69: 379-399.
26. Erdman, G. & Janke, W. (1978) Interactions between physiological and cognitive determinants of emotion: Experimental studies on Schachter's theory of emotions. Biol. Psychol., 6: 61-74.
27. Drossman, D.A., Sandler, R.S., McKee, D.C. & Lovitz, A.J. (1982). Bowel patterns among people not seeking health care: Use of a questionnaire to identify a population with bowel dysfunction. Gastroenterology, 83: 529-534.
28. Lyerly, S.B. (Ed.) (1978). Handbook of psychiatric scales, 2. NIMH, Rockville, Maryland.
29. Cannon, W.B. & Washburn, A.L. (1912). An explanation of hunger. Am. J. Physiol., 29: 441-454.
30. Stunkard, A.J. & Koch, C. (1964). The interpretation of gastric motility. I. Apparent bias in the reports of hunger by obese persons. Arch. Gen. Psychiat., 11: 74-82.
31. Griggs, R.C. & Stunkard, A.J. (1964). The interpretation of gastric motility. II. Sensitivity and bias in the perception of gastric motility. Arch. Gen. Psychiat., 11: 82-89.
32. Deutsch, J.A., Young, W.G. & Kalogeris, T.J. (1978). The stomach signals satiety. Science, 201: 165-167.
33. McHugh, P.R. & Moran, T.H. (1979). Calories and gastric emptying: A regulatory capacity with implications for feeding. Am. J. Physiol., 5: R254-260.
34. Garfinkel, P.E., Moldofsky, H., Garner, D.M., Starcer, H.C. & Coscina, D.V. (1978). Body awareness in anorexia nervosa: Disturbances in "body image" and "satiety." Psychosom. Med., 40: 487-498.
35. Garfinkel, P.E., Moldofsky, H. & Garner, D.M. (1979). The stability of perceptual disturbances in anorexia nervosa. Psychol. Med., 9: 703-708.
36. Schuster, M.M. (1968). Motor action of rectum and anal sphincter in continence and defecation. Handbook of Physiology, Section 6: Alimentary Canal, Volume IV: Motility. American Physiological Society, Washington, D.C., p. 2121-2140.

37. Schuster, M.M. (1975). The riddle of the sphincters. Gastroenterology, 69: 249-262.
38. Whitehead, W.E., Orr, W.C., Engel, B.T. & Schuster, M.M. (1981). External anal sphincter response to rectal distension: Learned response or reflex. Psychophysiology, 19: 57-62.
39. Whitehead, W.E., Engel, B.T. & Schuster, M.M. (1981). Perception of rectal distension is necessary to prevent fecal incontinence. In G. Adam, I. Meszaros & E. I. Banyai (Eds.), Advances in the Physiological Sciences, 17: 203-209.
40. Whitehead, W.E., Burgio, K.L. & Engel, B.T. (1985). Biofeedback treatment of fecal incontinence in geriatric patients. J. Am. Geriatr. Soc., 33: 320-324.
41. Wald, A. & Tunuguntla, A.K. (1984). Anorectal sensorimotor dysfunction in fecal incontinence and diabetes mellitus: Modification with biofeedback therapy. N. Engl. J. Med., 310: 1282-1287.
42. Whitehead, W.E. & Schuster, M.M. (1983). Manometric and electromyographic techniques for assessment of the anorectal mechanisms for continence and defectation. In R. Hoelzl and W.E. Whitehead (Eds.), Psychophysiology of the gastrointestinal tract: Experimental and clinical applications. Plenum Press, N.Y., p. 311-329.
43. Whitehead, W.E. & Schuster, M.M. (1985). Gastrointestinal disorders: Behavioral and physiological basis for treatment. Academic Press, N.Y.
44. Latimer, P. (1983). Functional gastrointestinal disorders: A behavioral approach. Springer-Verlag, N.Y.
45. Whitehead, W.E., Fedoravicius, A.S., Blackwell, B. & Wooley, S. (1979). Psychosomatic symptoms as learned responses. In J.R. McNamara (Ed.), Behavioral approaches in medicine: Application and analysis. Plenum Press. N.Y.
46. Latimer, P.R. (1981). Irritable bowel syndrome: A behavioral model. Behav. Res. & Ther., 19: 475-483.
47. Latimer, P., Sarna, S., Campbell, D., Latimer, M., Waterfall, W. & Daniel, E.E. (1981). Colonic motor and myoelectrical activity: A comparative study of normal subjects, psychoneurotic patients, and patients with irritable bowel syndrome. Gastroenterology, 80: 893-901.
48. Snape, W.J.Jr., Carlson, G.M. & Cohen, S. (1976). Colonic myoelectrical activity in the irritable bowel syndrome. Gastroenterology, 70: 326-330.
49. Snape, W.J.Jr., Carlson, G.M., Matarazzo, S.A. & Cohen, S. (1977). Evidence that abnormal myoelectrical activity produces colonic motor dysfunction in the irritable bowel syndrome. Gastroenterology, 72: 383-387.
50. Parker, R., Whitehead, W.E. & Schuster, M.M. (in press). Pattern recognition program for analysis of colon myoelectric and pressure data. Dig. Dis. Sci.
51. Latimer, P., Campbell, D., Latimer, M., Sarna, S., Daniel, E. & Waterfall, W. (1979). Irritable bowel syndrome: A test of the colonic hyperalgesia hypothesis. J. Behav. Med., 2: 285-295.
52. Ritchie, J. (1973). Pain from distension of the pelvic colon by inflating a balloon in the irritable colon syndrome. Gut, 14: 125-132.
53. Ritchie, J. (1977). The irritable bowel syndrome. Part II. Manometric and cineradiographic studies. Clin. Gastroenterol., 6: 622-631.
54. Kullmann, G. & Fielding, J.F. (1981). Rectal distensibility in the irritable bowel syndrome. Ir. Med. J., 74: 140-142.
55. Kroeger, C., Hoelzl, R., Fuenfgeld, M., Ottenjann, R. & Hoechter, W. (1985). Colonic motility and noziception in patients with irritable bowel syndrome. Paper presented at the 15th Annual Meeting of the European Association for Behavior Therapy. August 31, 1985, Munich, West Germany.
56. Swarbrick, E.T., Hegarty, J.E., Bat, L., Williams, C.B. & Dawson, A.M. (1980). Site of pain from the irritable bowel. Lancet, ii: 443-446.
57. Moriarity, K.J. & Dawson, A.M. (1982). Functional abdominal pain: Further evidence that the whole gut is involved. Brit. Med. J., 184: 1670-1672.
58. Ritchie, J. (1985). Mechanisms of pain in the irritable bowel syndrome. In N.W. Read (Ed.), Irritable bowel syndrome. Grune and Stratton, London, p. 163-171.
59. Whitehead, W.E., Renault, P.R. & Goldiamond, I. (1975). Modification of human gastric acid secretion with operant conditioning procedures. J. Appl. Behav. Anal., 8: 147-156.
60. Welgan, P.R. (1974). Learned control of gastric acid secretion in peptic ulcer patients. Psychosom. Med., 36: 411-419.
61. Bueno-Miranda, F., Cerulli, M. & Schuster, M.M. (1976). Operant conditioning of colonic motility in irritable bowel syndrome (IBS). Gastroenterology (Abstract), 70: 867.
62. Cerulli, M.A., Nikoomanesh, P. & Schuster, M.M. (1979). Progress in biofeedback conditioning for fecal incontinence. Gastroenterology, 76: 742-746.
63. Miller, N.E. (1973). Effect of learning on gastrointestinal functions. Clin. Gastroenterol., 6: 533-546.

64. Hefferline, A.F., Keenan, B. & Hartford, R.A. (1956). Escape and avoidance conditioning in human subjects without their observation of the response. Science, 130: 1338-1339.
65. Reynolds, G.S. (1968). A primer of operant conditioning. Scott Foresman, San Diego.
66. Whitehead, W.E., Winget, C., Fedoravicius, A.S., Wooley, S. & Blackwell, B. (1982). Learned illness behavior in patients with irritable bowel syndrome and peptic ulcer. Dig. Dis. Sci., 27: 202-208.
67. Sandler, R.S., Drossman, D.A., Nathan, H.P. & McKee, D.C. (1984). Symptom complaints and health care seeking behavior in subjects with bowel dysfunction. Gastroenterology, 87: 314-318.

Discussion:

Central Control of the Gastrointestinal System

Robert Murison

The presentations in the session on gastrointestinal function and disorders covered a wide area, and to some extent this diversity underlined the need for a more unified approach, even given the enormous complexity of the gastrointestinal system and its control mechanisms. The diversity was further enhanced by the wide range of psychosocial studies discussed, including psychophysiological methods, experimental Pavlovian methods, life event data, and experimental animal models.

Wienbeck discussed in detail the control mechanisms behind motility of the gut, together with the function of gut mobility, and the nervous control of it. He discussed also the effects of various stress procedures (e.g., acoustic stress) on motility. Care should be taken in interpretation of these psychophysiological data for two reasons. First, we are not clear over when our intended stressor is in fact a stressor, since most studies rely on only one dependent measure, with no endocrine measure to confirm the self-reported or inferred stressfulness of the manipulation. Secondly, different procedures, although deemed stressful, might have very different effects. For example, Thompson and Cann reported that oro-caecal transit time is delayed in a cold-pressure test (1), but hastened by acoustic (2) or dichotomous listening task (3) stress. What is clear from this presentation is that we are in no position to discuss the functional interactions between the central nervous system and the gut without first having a thorough understanding of the basic physiology of the gastrointestinal system.

This point is also born out by the studies reported by Felten. For this author at least, it seems that the reluctance (and downright hostility) to the field of psychoimmunology was partly because the critics could not see the hardware (endocrine and nervous connections) by which the CNS could influence the immune system. The role of the immune system in gastrointestinal function, and as a mediator between the brain and the gut is taken up by Felten. Presenting an enormous data collection, Felten described the innervation of the gut, and in particular of the gut-associated lymphoid tissues, thus laying an anatomical pathway for the central nervous system to directly modulate immune function in the gut, probably in association with classical hormones. Earlier, the field of psychoimmunology relied heavily on the known effects of endocrine (particularly adrenocortical) secretion on the immune system. In this and other work, Felten has shown with others that the brain-immune system is not solely an endocrine phenomenon, but also mediated by nervous tissue. Perhaps more than anything else, Felten's discussions showed us how little we know of the system we are dealing with, and that the only answer is in continued research, particularly in the interaction between hormones, nervous activity, immune system, immune-derived products, not only anatomical interactions, but also temporal. It is through the work of anatomists such as Felten that this hardware is coming to light, and this could lead to an easier understanding and greater acceptance of the evident influence of the brain on immune function. The functional significance of these nervous connections to GALT is unclear, but the possibilities are legion.

Some years ago, Goldmann and Rossoff (4) suggested that invasion of gut flora into the blood stream might have a direct contributory role in the development of gastric ulceration in animals, reporting that antibiotics such as polymyxin B reduced gastric pathology under stress. One might suppose that central effects on GALT via stress could effect gastric pathology by modulating the immune response to an invasion of such gut flora.

Whitehead reviews first the different methodologies employed in gastrointestinal research on the functional significance of the heavy preponderance of afferent (sensory) fibers in the innervation of the gut. In discussing these methodologies, and the data so collected, he repeatedly emphasizes the discrepancy between information from the gut which is available to the nervous system, and that which is perceived or results in conscious sensation. An important finding for the hypothesis set out later in his paper on the role of learning in gastrointestinal dysfunction is the apparent perception of distension of for example the rectum and lower bowel, in contrast to the apparent inability to perceive pH in the stomach.

Whitehead also discusses the correlation within individuals in their ability to perceive accurately afferent information from different organ systems, e.g., from the gut and cardiovascular system, tempting one to suggest that such psychological variability might also correlate to pathophysiological variability. Given the James-Lange model of emotional attribution, we might expect emotional variables to also correlate with such psychophysiological variability.

The major impetus of Whitehead's paper is in the use of what might be described as learning concepts in an analysis of gastrointestinal problems, specifically incontinence and the irritable bowel syndrome (IBS). Generally, the model suggest that (a) sickness behavior is reinforced in childhood and (b) that specific subgroups of individuals may come to reproduce the symptoms and sickness behavior in later life. The model requires a number of assumptions. First that the physiological event is availabl to consciousness, and can also lead to sickness behavior which can then be reinforced. Secondly, that the sickness behavior (e.g., IBS) in later life represents a true symptom, and not a sickness behavior per se. The model essentially claims, that when the gastrointestinal event is perceivable, it may become subject to conditioning, and thus directly influence behavior. Events, however, which are not available to consciousness will not be so easily conditioned. Thus peptic ulcer disease is less likely to be the result of childhood conditioning than is IBS or incontinence. At the same time we do know that in animal models of peptic ulcer disease, the development of symptoms is subject to conditioning in adult animals (5).

The model proposed by Whitehead elegantly allows for a number of factors to influence disease processes, including genetic predisposition (variability in perceptual skills and organ function), childhood learning, and the adult environment. The model and conceptual framework will however require empirical support, which, as stated by Whitehead, must come from longitudinal studies. We might also explore here the possibility of using Pavlovian conditioning in animals as a short-term solution to this problem area.

Glavin presented evidence that a number of centrally acting agents modulated the ulcerogenic response to stress in rats, concentrating on the two most common forms of ulcer-inducing stress, immobilization and activity stress. In his presentation, Glavin provided evidence for a role of a number of central substances in the ulcerative processes in animals: noradrenaline, dopamine, adenosine, opiates, caffeine, ethanol, and capsaicin. This work attempts to find the neurochemical basis of the demonstrated central influences on risk for or susceptibility to gastric ulceration.

There was some discussion again as to the significance of stress as a concept. Several workers use different types of stimulus situation to induce what is inferred as a state of stress. There is of course a need for those working with animal models to clearly define these stimulus situations, and perhaps even more so for those working with human stress. At the same time, there is much to be said for the definition proposed by Levine - stress is when my stomach hurts. In the case of the rat, stress is when my stomach bleeds.

Importantly, Glavin also presented data on effects of prenatal treatment with caffeine and alcohol on stress-induced ulcerations in adult animals. Together with the data reported by Ackerman and others some years ago (6), it is important to realize that the extent of the animals response to stress is heavily determined by events temporally far removed from the time of the stress itself.

In conclusion, these presentations covered a wide area, both anatomically and conceptually. The collection as a whole reminds us that the gastrointestinal system is complex and requires a more holistic approach than heretofore. To some extent also, one is taken with the question of what we mean by psychology in relation to psychological studies of gut function. These have varied from the psychophysiological approach, the classical experimental Pavlovian approach, to a more epidemiological approach.

Many participants commented later that since we know that the central nervous system and endocrine system effect gastrointestinal function, and that "stress," like all other psychological states, operates on the CNS and endocrine systems, the argument that any given disease state is totally unrelated to stress or psychosocial factors is both untenable, and unprovable.

The subject of animal models was taken up by Glavin in his discussion on effects of central nervous manipulations on susceptibility to gastric ulceration in animals. There was some lively discussion here and elsewhere as to the significance of gastric ulcerations (surface erosions) in rats. For the present purposes, leaving aside this imporatan debate, it is sufficient to point out that a number of both psychological and centrally-acting pharmacological manipulations are known to modulate the appearance of surface erosions in the animal stress models. That is, there is evidence of central control of bodily function, even though the significance of the model might remain unclear.

Finally, it should be restated that we are not arguing that psychological factors have a monopoly on disease initiation and prognosis, but that psychological factors may explain some of the variance, and that variance, although small in any one disease, may become highly significant when looking at the population at large with a multitude of possible disease states.

References

1. Thompson, D.G., Richelson, E. & Malagelada, J.-R. (1983). Perturbation of upper gastrointestinal function by cold stress. Gut, 24: 277-283.
2. Erckenbrecht, J.F., Ziemer, B., Lesch, M., Rehm, S., Kothe, W., Berger, W. & Wienbeck, M. (1985). Effect of long term mental stress by noise on transit of a meal through the small and large bowel. Gut, 25: A1311.
3. Cann, P.A., Read, N.W., Cammack, J., Childs, H., Holden, S., Kashman, R., Longmore, J., Nix, S., Simms, N., Swallow, K. & Weller, J. (1984). Psychological stress and the passage of a standard meal through the stomache and small intestine in man. Gut, 24: 236-240.
4. Rossoff, C.B. & Goldman, H. (1968). Effect of the intestinal bacterial flora on acute gastric stress ulceration. Gastroenterology, 55: 212-221.
5. Murison, R. & Overmier, J.B.: This volume.
6. Ackerman, S.H., Hofer, M.A. & Weiner, H. (1975). Age at maternal separation and gastric erosion susceptibility in the rat. Psychsom. Med., 37: 180-184.

3.

Central Control of the Cardiovascular System

The Function of the Autonomic System as Interface Between Body and Environment. Old and New Concepts: W.B. Cannon and W.R. Hess Revisited

Wilfrid Jänig

The peripheral autonomic nervous system is, according to anatomical criteria, divided into three parts: The thoraco-lumbar or sympathetic system, the cranio-sacral or parasympathetic system, and the enteric nervous system. This tripartition was proposed by Langley (1, 2) and he recommended restricting the terms "sympathetic" and "parasympathetic" to the efferent autonomic outflow from the neuraxis, thus *not* including the afferents in the autonomic nerves which innervate visceral organs, blood vessels, etc. These afferents should be generally called visceral afferents. We have no strong functional criteria enabling afferents which run in "sympathetic" nerves to be named "sympathetic" and "parasympathetic," respectively, though this point is not universally accepted (3-6).

The autonomic systems regulate, or participate in regulating various general and specific body functions such as supply of the organs with blood (cardiovascular system), regulation of body temperature, ingestion, transport and absorption nutrients, electrolytes and water (gastrointestinal tract), evacuation and continence of colon and urinary bladder, reproductive functions (reproductive organs), etc. Most of these functions, together with the neuroendocrine functions, are essential for the preservation of the inner milieu of the organism (homeostasis) and for the adaptation of this milieu when the organism is exposed to environmental challenges (7, 8). The diversity of the autonomic target organs, and the wide range of responses of these organs during the continuous regulations in the freely acting organism, requires a complex organization of the autonomic system, both in the periphery and in the central nervous system.

An organism can only perceive and act adequately in its environment according to the (neuronal, sensory, motor and higher-order) integrative programs it has in its brain. By way of these programs the brain analyzes the physical features of the environment and produces adequate motor reactions. Some simple motor programs are, for example, the spinal motor reflexes such as the monosynaptic stretch reflex and the flexor reflex; these programs are organized at the level of the spinal cord and include each several agonistically and antagonistically acting "final common motor paths," spinal interneurons and their synaptic connections with spinal afferents, and spinal descending command systems. The activation of these motor programs leads to coordinated (purposeful) changes in the force developed by the skeletal muscles. The neuronal programs in the brain are, so to speak, representations of the environment which is biologically relevant for the organism. The same reasoning may apply to the central organization of the autonomic system of the organisms. Each somatic action of the organism is accompanied by purposeful adaptive changes induced by the autonomic nervous and neuroendocrine systems. An increase in the complexity of the environment of the organism is associated with an increase in the complexity of the neuronal programs (sensory, motor, higher-order integrative) in the brain of that organism, entailing a wide repertoire of behavioral patterns. This in turn is probably associated with an increase in the complexity of the autonomic neuronal programs in the neuraxis, hypothalamus and limbic system, which enables the adaptation of the inner milieux to a wide range of environmental challenges. Organisms with a limited repertoire of behavioral patterns and a simple, stable environment probably also have less complexity organized autonomic systems," since they do not need more complex systems for the adaptation of the inner milieu." This is reflected in an increasing complexity of the morphology, pharmacology, and functioning of the peripheral autonomic nervous systems during phylogeny (9). It can be hypothesized that the central autonomic neuronal programs can also be seen as the central representations of the environmental challenges which are encountered by the organisms. The autonomic systems seem to be hierarchically organized in their neuronal programs, the highest programs being represented in telencephalic brain structures, the lower ones in the spinal cord (or even extracentrally in the prevertebral sympathetic ganglia).

The following article focusses on some features of the central organization of sympathetic systems. The point of reference will, as far as possible, be the lumbar sympathetic outflow to skin, skeletal muscle, pelvic organs and colon. The functional characteristics of the pre- and postganglionic neurons of this part of the sympathetic system have been thoroughly investigated (10, 11). Though there is a considerable gap in our knowledge concerning the central organization of these autonomic systems compared to what we know about the central organization of the motor and sensory systems, we can at least speculate about it along new neurobiological (behavioral, morphological, pharmacological, neurophysiological) data and indicate the conceptual frame of and future trends in research in this field.

W.B. Cannon and W.R. Hess: Two Forerunners

Cannon and Hess were very well aware of the complexity of the central organization of the autonomic nervous systems. Both of them believed that there is a high degree of order in these systems and that this order is laid down in the central nervous system. Both of them associated the terms sympathetic and parasympathetic with more generalized functions, the sympathetic system reacting more as a unitary system which is expressed in the term "sympathico-adrenal system" coined by Cannon (7, 8). Cannon believed that impulse activity spreads widely through the sympathetic channels in a diffuse fashion, whereas the parasympathetic divisions of the autonomic nervous system direct their discharges to specific organs.

Hess believed that the activation of the sympathetic nervous system increases the readiness of the organism to act in an emergency situation (*Leistungsbereitschaft*), whereas activity of the parasympathetic nervous system has a more protective function. Hess therefore named the sympathetic nervous system the "ergotropic" and the parasympathetic nervous system the "endophylactic-trophotropic system," implying the above-mentioned generalized functions. Hess transferred these functional terms and functional antagonism between the sympathetic and parasympathetic system to central structures, such as the hypothalamus (12-14).

Both Cannon and Hess considered the hypothalamus as the "head ganglion" of the autonomic nervous system. Cannon was a vigorous defender of the theory that the patterned autonomic, endocrine and somatic expressions of emotions lie in the diencephalon. Philip Bard, a pupil of Cannon, showed that diencephalic cats can display the full expression of aggressive emotional behavior, calling this "sham rage" (15, 16). When the hypothalamus, particularly its posterior part, is destroyed, the animals can no longer display the fully integrated pattern of this behavior, thus the integration of its different components resides in the hypothalamus. Pontine and mesencephalic cats can only display fractions of this behavioral pattern (17). They critically opposed the, by then famous, James-Lange's theory of emotions, which places the "origin" of the emotions in the periphery, in particular in the visceral and cardio-vascular domains, saying that emotions emerge when the afferents supplying these structures are excited (18, 19). Cannon created the so-called "thalamic theory of emotion." The important new message in this theory was that the diencephalon and, specifically, the hypothalamus contains the neuronal programs which are the neuronal representations of whole behaviors.

Hess showed that focal electrical stimulation of minute populations of neurons in the hypothalamus in awake, freely moving cats elicits well-known, well-coordinated behaviors. One of these is the (affective) defense reaction (*Abwehrverhalten*) which can be elicited from well-localized hypothalamic areas. This reaction can develop into attack or flight and is in its expression very similar to the naturally displayed behavior in the cat (Figure 1; 20, 21). Later, von Holst and von Saint Paul (22, 23) showed that the species-specific behavioral repertoire of the domestic chicken can be elicited by focal electrical stimulation of the diencephalic and adjacent brain areas.

The behavioral changes elicited by central electrical stimulation in anaesthetized animals are accompanied by affective experiences which are probably very similar to those produced by natural environmental stimuli and which are associated with neuronal activity in telencephalic (limbic and neocortical) brain structures. On the other hand, typical neuroendocrine changes occur in the organism which are mediated by the sympathetic nervous system (adrenal medulla) and by the hypothalamo-hypophyseal axis; some such changes are listed for the defense reaction in the lower part of Figure 1 (25).

These key experiments indicate that the hypothalamus is in a strategic position for integrating motor, sensory, neuroendocrine and autonomic systems into purposeful behavioral response patterns, the defense reaction (behavior) being one of them.

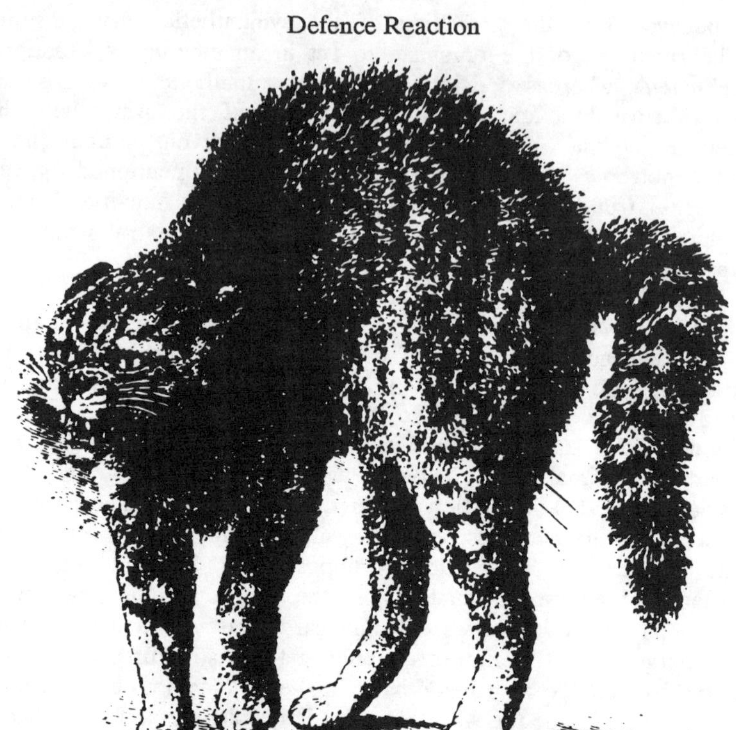

AUTONOMIC COMPONENTS (LUMBAR):

muscle vasodilator	MVD	↑	increase blood flow skeletal muscle	
muscle vasoconstrictor	MVC	↓		
cutaneous vasoconstrictor	CVC	↑	decrease blood flow skin	
sudomotor	SM	↑	sweating	
pilomotor	PM	↑	piloerection	
visceral vasoconstrictor	VVC	↑	decrease blood flow	gastroint. tr.
motility regulating	MR	↑	decrease motility	gastroint. tr.

ENDOCRINE COMPONENTS:

adrenal medulla	↑	release of catecholamines
anterior pituitary, adrenal cortex	↑	release of ACTH and cortisol
posterior pituitary	↑	release of vasopressin

Figure 1. Autonomic, endocrine and somatomotor components of the defense reaction. The reaction is organized by the hypothalamus (24). The lumbar sympathetic systems participating in this reaction are shown (Figure 13). The muscle vasodilatator system (MVD) which is cholinergic in the cat probably does not exist in human beings. The increase of blood flow through skeletal muscle is supported by the ß-adrenergic effect of adrenaline released from the adrenal medulla. Cat from Darwin (24).

The hypothalamus may also participate in the production of affective experiences associated with activity in suprahypothalamic brain structures of the limbic system and the neocortex.

Conditioned Emotional Responses and Autonomic Responses

An important experiment, combining measurements of cardiovascular parameters with those of somatomotor parameters during conditioned emotional responses, was conducted by Orville Smith and his group on male baboons. It was performed fully in the tradition of the work of the authors mentioned above, but they extended their work into modern neurobiology. In a first step, they asked the question whether the cardiovascular changes occurring during a conditioned emotional response are integrated in the hypothalamus and whether these autonomic changes can be abolished by locally controlled lesions in the hypothalamus without affecting the "emotionality" of the animal (as indicated by the somatic component of the conditioned emotional response), and other cardiovascular response patterns which can occur, e.g., during exercise and eating, and which are probably also organized by the hypothalamus. In a second step, Smith and coworkers determined the afferent and efferent connections of the hypothalamic area which integrates the cardiovascular responses of the conditioned emotional response (26-29).

The animals were first trained with operant techniques to perform mild dynamic exercise (turning a wheel with the legs) and to press a small lever. Then a conditioned emotional response was elicited in the animals by the classical conditioning paradigm: The procedure was begun by presenting the signal for lever pressing. After stable lever pressing was reached an auditory signal was applied for 1 min as a conditional stimulus. This stimulus was terminated by an unconditional stimulus consisting of electrical shocks of 7 to 15 mA, applied for 1 to 2 s to the abdominal skin. The command signal for lever pressing remained throughout the conditional stimulus and afterwards. Only one classical conditioning trial was made during a one day training period at intervals of 2 to 4 days. After the training procedures the animals were instrumented in order to measure heart rate, arterial blood pressure, renal blood flow and terminal aortic blood flow, the latter mainly as a measure of blood flow through the skeletal muscles of the hindlimbs. Furthermore, electrodes were stereotactically placed bilaterally in the perifornical regions of the hypothalamus for electrical stimulation and lesioning.

During the conditioning trial very characteristic cardiovascular changes occurred in the animal (Figure 2 left side, solid line curves): Heart rate, arterial blood pressure and renal resistance to blood flow increased whereas terminal aortic resistance decreased. The delayed increase of renal resistance and decrease of terminal aortic resistance were probably due to epinephrine released from the adrenal medulla. During the conditional stimulus the animal stopped pressing the lever; this was the somatic expression that the animal "felt emotional" (see upper curve in Figure 2 left side). This cardiovascular response was considerably different from those elicited by lever pressing (Figure 2

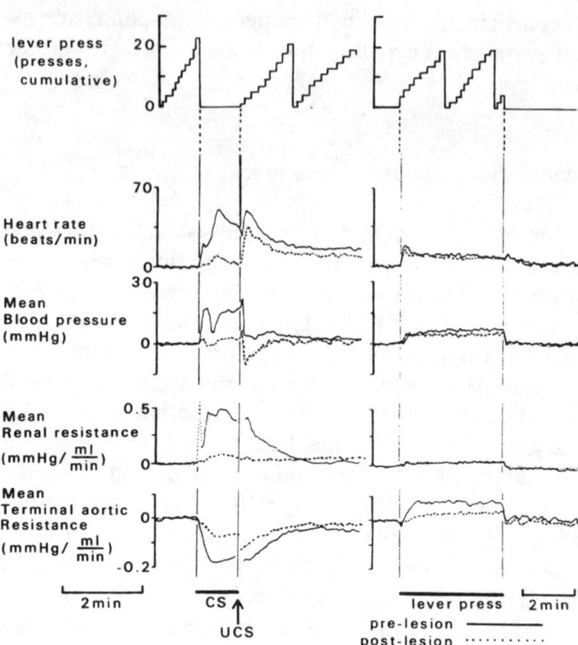

Figure 2. Cardiovascular responses during and after a conditioned emotional response (left side) and during pressing a lever before (solid line curves) and after (dotted line curves) bilateral electrolytical lesioning of the perifornical region in the hypothalamus of baboons. The conditioned emotional response was elicited by a conditional stimulus (CS, auditory signal of 2900 Hz, 80 dB interrupted 2.5 times per sec) and terminated by an unconditional stimulus UCS, electrical shock applied to the skin of the abdomen; 7-12 mA, duration 1 sec). Upper histograms: Rate of lever pressing; the cessation of the lever pressing during the CS indicates the somatic response showing that the monkey feels "emotional" (ordinate scale cumulative). This response is the same before and after the perifornical lesions. Ordinate scales of cardiovascular responses indicate the change from the preceding minute of lever pressing in the conditioned emotional response (left) or of rest (right). The data were averaged for five prelesion and five postlesion trials in six animals. Modified from Smith (27). Reproduced, with permission, from the Federation Proceedings, Vol. 29, 1980.

right side, solid line curves) and during exercise and eating (Figure 3, solid line curves).

After bilateral lesioning of the perfornical region in the hypothalamus (an area the electrical stimulation of which produced the same cardiovascular response pattern as that occurring during the conditioned emotional response), the cardiovascular changes during the conditional stimulus were largely abolished (see dotted line curves in Figure 2 left) whereas those occurring during lever pressing (Figure 2 right), exercise and eating (Figure 3) did not change significantly. Following the hypothalamic lesion, the animals continued to suppress the lever pressing during the conditional stimulus. Thus, they had not forgotten the significance of this stimulus and were still feeling "emotional" but this time without the characteristic changes of the cardiovascular parameters.

The following general conclusion can be drawn from this experiment: (1) The hypothalamus contains an area which controls the cardiovascular response pattern associated with emotional behavior.

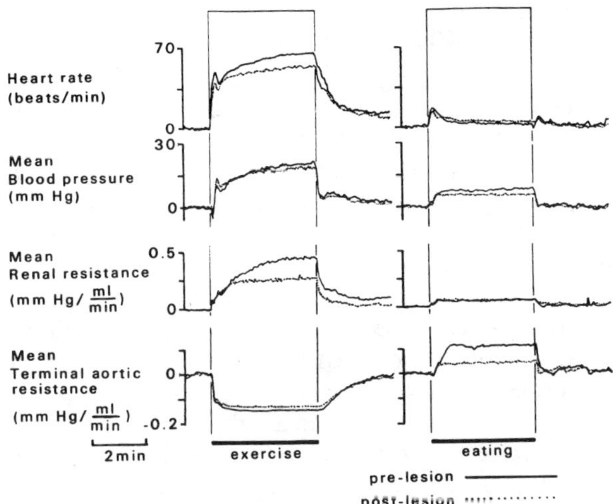

Figure 3. Cardiovascular responses during exercise (turning a wheel with the legs) and during eating before (solid line curves) and after (dotted line curves) bilateral electrolytical lesioning of the perifornical region of the hypothalamus of baboons. For details see legend of Figure 2. Modified from Smith et al. (27). Reproduced, with permission, from the Federation Proceedings, Vol. 39, 1980.

(2) Lesioning of this area abolishes this pattern but does not affect other patterns during other behaviors, such as exercise and eating. (3) After circumscribed destruction of the hypothalamic perifornical area the cardiovascular response pattern is abolished, though the animal is still feeling "emotional" during the conditional trial. Thus, two components of the conditioned emotional response have been separated by the lesion. (4) The cardiovascular response pattern is largely mediated by the sympathetic outflow. It is reasonable to assume that other autonomic processes occur in the body, such as a decrease in the motility of the gastrointestinal tract and contraction of its sphincters and activation of sweat glands and erector pili muscles, all these responses being mediated by the sympathetic nervous system; furthermore, certain neuroendocrine changes may occur via the anterior and posterior pituitary gland (see lower part of Figure 1).

A critical question is whether the cardiovascular response pattern which is associated with the conditioned emotional response is really organized by neurons in the perifornical region of the hypothalamus or whether nerve fibers transversing this area and having their cell bodies in other brain structures are important, implying that the interruption of these nerve fibers by the central lesion leads to the effects described above. This question can not at present be conclusively answered. The authors, however, have obtained strong evidence from their stimulation experiments and from their morphological investigations on efferent neurons projecting from and afferent neurons projecting to the perifornical area (see below) showing that the important integration of autonomic parameters occurs in this area (26-29). Furthermore, the results are fully consistent with the interpretation of the experiments of Bard, Cannon, Hess and Hilton (24).

The Hypothalamus as Interface Between Telencephalon, Neuraxis and Neuroendocrinium (Between Interior of the Body and Environment)

The hypothalamus is essential for homeostasis and as such it contains the neuronal mechanism for regulating various body functions such as the neuroendocrine processes, thermoregulation, regulation of osmolality and blood volume etc., including even more complex regulations such as defense behavior (see above). Practically, all these regulations include endocrine, autonomic and motor (behavioral) components. How these homeostatic regulations are brought about eludes our knowledge. However, experimental histological work with various modern techniques (tracer methods, double labelling of neurone populations, immunohistochemical methods, degeneration methods) has thrown some light on the miracle of the hypothalamic organization which allows us to speculate about the structural relation between hypothalamus and sympathetic outflow. It must, however, be kept in mind that the results obtained with these techniques allow only a limited understanding of the mechanisms of neural regulation of the physiological processes concerned.

The hypothalamus and, in particular, the perifornical-lateral hypothalamic region, which is important in integrating the conditioned emotional response pattern as described above, obtains various afferent inputs from rostral brain

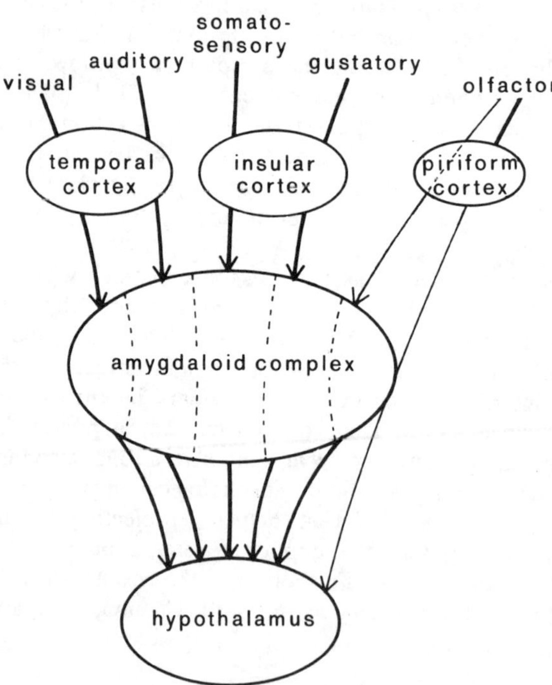

Figure 4. Influence of higher order sensory cortices on the hypothalamus via the amygdaloid complex. The amygdala is topically organized with respect to the afferent inflow from the temporal, insular and piriform cortices and therefore also with respect to the information from the five sensory systems. Monkey. Schematized after Turner et al. (30). The insular cortex appears to have a viscerotropic representation. Rat (31).

structures, which are involved in regulation of autonomic target organs, as well as from various regions of the brainstem. The rostral regions include limbic system structures such as the amygdala, septum (lateral septum, nucleus of diagonal band of Broca) and the preoptic area, all of which are possibly involved in the organization of emotional behavior. The input from the amygdaloid complex to the hypothalamus seems to be the most important one. This nuclear complex obtains its afferent inputs from various higher order sensory cortices via the temporal, insular and piriform cortex, from the prefrontal cortex and the subcallosal gyrus and from various regions of the hypothalamus, upper and lower brainstem. The cortical afferent inputs are topically organized; it is believed that the autonomic and endocrine regulations are particularly influenced by high-order cortical processes via these pathways (Figure 4).

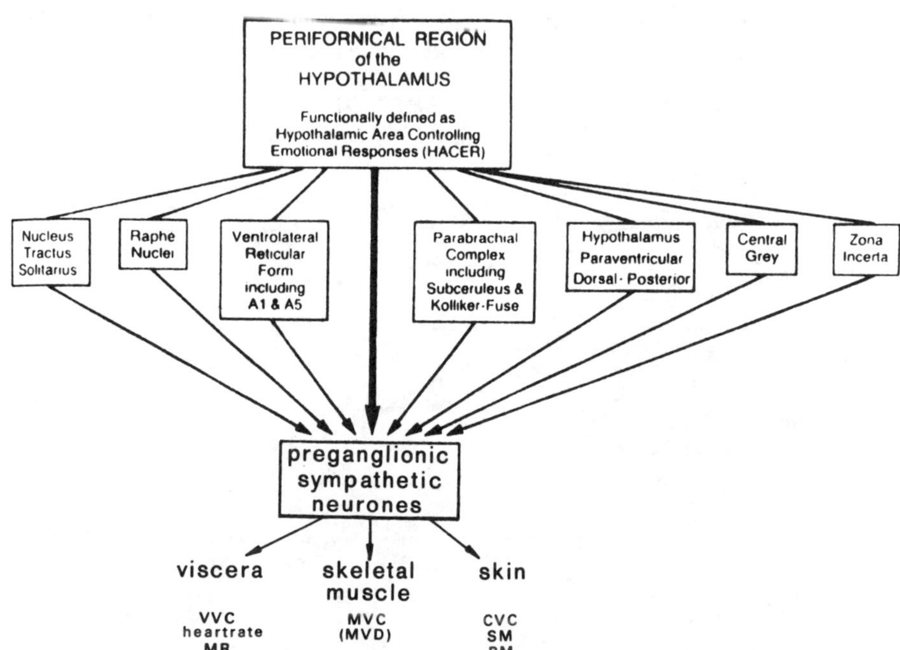

Figure 5. Anatomical basis for the integrative role of the perifornical region of the lateral hypothalamus controlling emotional responses. The efferent projections are shown to regions of the hypothalamus and brainstem, which project to the intermediate zone of the sympathetic preganglionic neurons themselves. The projections were determined his ologically by injecting horseradish peroxidase solution into the perifornical region. For abbreviations see Figures 1 and 10. Modified from Smith and De Vito (29). Reproduced, with permission, from the Annual Review of Neuroscience, Vol. 7. Copyright, 1984 by Annual Reviews Inc., 1984.

The output of the amygdaloid complex projects to the ventromedial region, of the frontal cortex, to various structures of the limbic system, to the hypothalamus via the stria terminalis and the ventral amygdalofugal path and to various regions in the upper and lower brainstem, most of which are involved in the regulation of autonomic processes and project to the region of the preganglionic sympathetic neurons in the thoraco-lumbar spinal cord (see Figure 5).

Efferent projections of a brain region can be tested by injecting radioactive labelled amino acids (e.g., leucine and proline) into the respective region. These amino acids are taken up by the cell bodies (not by axons) and transported in the axons to their synaptic terminals. Some efferent projections of the perifornical region of the hypothalamus traced in this way are illustrated in Figure 5. Most of these projections are to regions of the brainstem which project with part of their output to the intermediate zone of the thoracolumbar spinal cord where the sympathetic preganglionic neurons are situated; the perifornical area itself even seems to have some direct projections to the sympathetic pre-ganglionic neurons. This projection pattern clearly documents the integrative role of the perifornical hypothalamic area (28, 29).

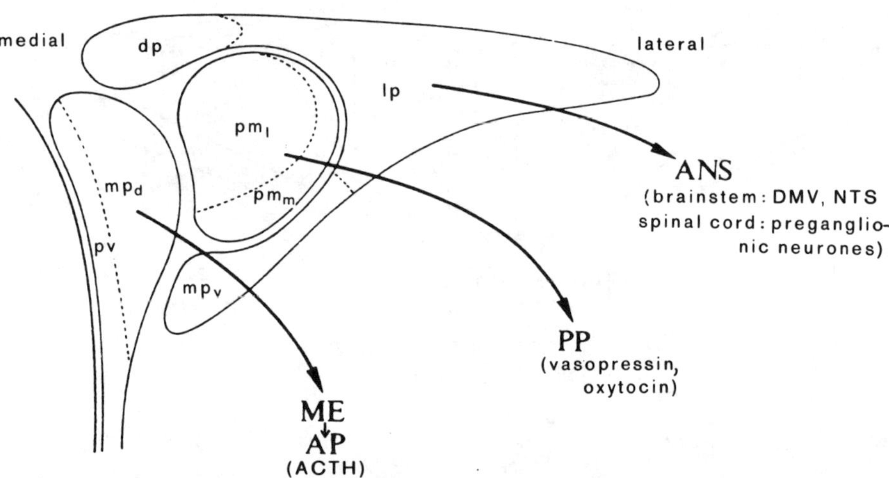

Figure 6. Integration of autonomic systems and endocrine systems by the paraventricular nuclei in the hypothalamus. ME, median eminence; AP, anterior pituitary gland; PP, posterior pituitary gland; DMV, dorsal vagal motor nucleus; NTS, nucleus tractus solitarii. Subdivisions of the PVH: dp, dorsal parvocellular part; lp, lateral parvocellular part; $mp_{d,v}$, dorsal and ventral subdivisions of the medial parvocellular part; $pm_{l,m}$, lateral (vasopressinergic) and medial (oxytocinergic) subdivisions of the posterior magnocellular part; pv, periventricular part. Rat. Modified from Swanson and Sawchenko (32). Reproduced, with permission, from the *Annual Review of Neuroscience*, Vol. 6. Copyright, 1983 by Annual Reviews Inc.

The paraventricular nuclei of the hypothalamus (right side of Figure 5) are probably also of the utmost importance for the integration of autonomic and endocrine systems. Elegant histological studies on the structure, projections, afferent inputs and putative neurotransmitters and neuromodulators of this nuclear complex of the rat have revealed that it consists of seven well-defined subnuclei, each receiving its characteristic input pattern from the lower and upper brainstem and from rostral brain structures, different subnuclei project to the posterior pituitary gland, to the median eminence (thus influencing the anterior pituitary gland), to autonomic nuclei within the lower brainstem and to the region of the sympathetic preganglionic neurons in the spinal cord (Figure 6). Up to 30 substances (monoamines, neuropeptides) have been shown to exist in characteristic chemotopic patterns in the neurons and synaptic terminals of this nuclear complex and may participate in the integrative processes (for review see 32). Thus, as seen from the cellular organization, the efferent projections and neural inputs and from the chemotopical organization, the paraventricular nucleus may be ideally suited for the integration of the autonomic, endocrine and somatomotor responses in drinking and feeding behavior, in the regulation of extracellular body fluid volume and composition, and possibly, in other complex adaptive functions (33-35). Again, it must be emphasized that the neurophysiological mechanism of these integrative processes are largely unknown.

The Brainstem and its Connections to the Sympathetic Preganglionic Neurons

The intermediate region of the thoraco-lumbar spinal cord where the sympathetic preganglionic neurons are located obtains several neural inputs from different nuclei in the brainstem and hypothalamus (Figure 5). These descending systems derive from nuclei which are probably important for the regulation of sympathetic activity to autonomic target organs, particularly to cardiovascular target organs. Illustrated on the left side of Figure 7 are the descending systems from the brainstem and hypothalamus which project to the region of the sympathetic preganglionic neurons. According to their origin and the peptides and the monoamines they contain, most of these systems are distinct; the serotonergic neurons may additionally contain a peptide, such as substance P. Furthermore, the intermediate zone of the sympathetic preganglionic neurons contains several substances (mostly peptide) which have been immunohistochemically identified in presynaptic terminals of unknown origin and in the preganglionic neurons (see left side of Figure 7; 36-47).

We have some evidence from pharmacological and physiological experiments (electrical and chemical stimulation and lesioning of the neurons of origin in the descending axons; iontophoretic application of monoamines and other substances onto preganglionic sympathetic neurons; recording of sympathetic activity and cardiovascular parameter such as heart rate and arterial blood pressure) that these descending systems are involved in regulation of sympathetic activity (48-53). However, with the possible exception of the neurons in the rostral ventrolateral medulla (see below), we have neither clearcut experimental evidence about the function of any descending system, nor about the relation of the descending system to functionally different types of preganglionic neurons (see below) nor whether any of the histochemically determined substances (monoamines, neuropeptides) are neurotransmitters or neuromodulators. It must be kept in mind that many descending axons to the preganglionic sympathetic neurons in the dorsolateral funiculus conduct at speeds of 2.5 to about 25 m/s (54), i.e., are myelinated. Do central neurons with myelinated axons contain monoamines and neuropeptides?

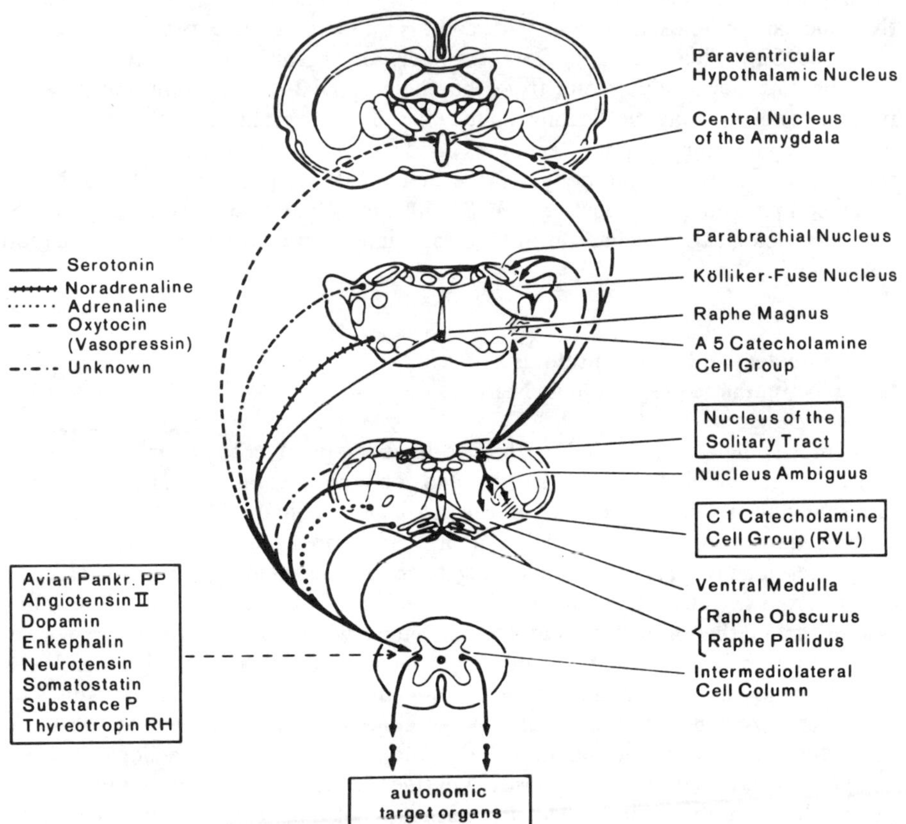

Figure 7. Descending neuronal systems from brainstem and hypothalamus to the intermediate region of sympathetic preganglionic neurons in the spinal cord (left side) and of projections from the nucleus tractus solitarii (right side). Rat. The substances listed in the box on the left side can be additionally shown to exist in the region of the preganglionic neurons and partly in synaptic terminals. Modified from Loewy (40, 41). Reproduced, with permission, from *Progress in Brain Research*, Vol. 57. Copyright, 1981/82 by Elsevier Biomedical Press.

Important for the regulation of the autonomic target organs is the visceral afferent inflow to the nucleus tractus solitarii from the arterial baro- and chemoreceptors, heart, trachea and lungs, esophagus, stomach, duodenum, small intestine and liver. This afferent input is viscerotopically organized (55-57). From the nucleus tractus solitarii neurons project to most areas in the brainstem and hypothalamus which in turn project to the region of the preganglionic sympathetic neurons in the spinal cord (see right side of Figure 7).

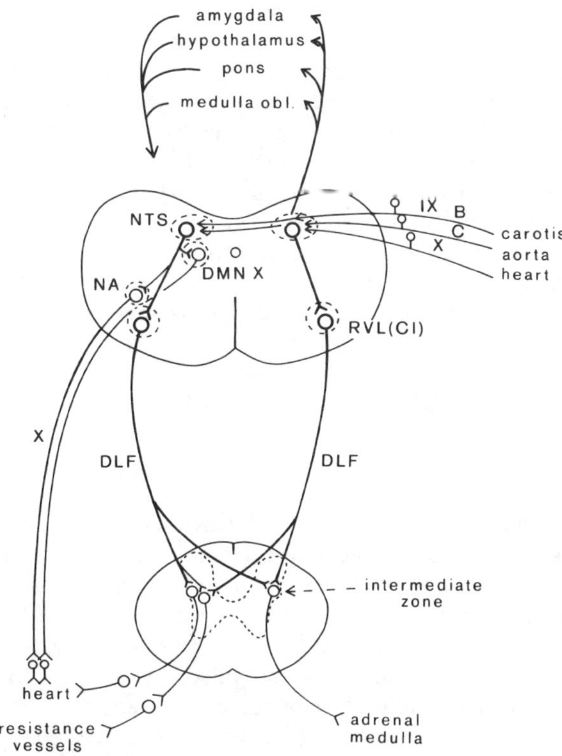

Figure 8. Possible "reflex" pathway for cardiovascular reflexes elicited from arterial baro- and chemoreceptors (B, C) and afferents from the heart in the rat. RVL, rostral ventrolateral region of the medulla oblongata which contains adrenergic neurons (C1 area). NTS, nucleus tractus solitarii; NA nucleus ambiguus; DMNX, dorsal motor nucleus of the vagus; DLF, dorsolateral funiculus. The pathways in the medulla oblongata are controlled by other regions of the brainstem, hypothalamus and limbic system which also receive afferent input from the NTS. These pathways are not necessary for the functioning of the homeostatic cardiovascular reflexes through the RVL, NA and DMNX. Schematized from Ross et al. (64, 65) and Granata et al. (67).

The neurons in the rostral ventrolateral area of the medulla oblongata (RVL in Figure 7) deserve a special comment. Many of the neurons in this area contain adrenalin, therefore it is called the C1 area. Recent experimental work on rats, cats and rabbits has shown convincingly that the neurons in the C1 region, which project to the sympathetic preganglionic neurons, are responsible for the ongoing activity in the sympathetic outflow to resistance vessels, in the adrenal medulla and to the heart (Figure 8). Electrical and chemical stimulation in this area lead to an increase in the heart rate and arterial blood pressure; electrolytical and chemical bilateral lesioning in this area lead to a similar drop in the arterial blood pressure as does complete transection of the cervical spinal cord, indicating that the activity in sympathetic neurons supplying the above-mentioned target organs drops virtually to zero. Furthermore, inhibitory reflexes induced by stimulation of the arterial baroreceptors in the carotid sinus, as well as inhibitory and excitatory reflexes elicited by stimulation of vagal afferents, are abolished after lesioning of the rostral ventrolateral medulla. The second-order baroreceptor neurons which relay the information from arterial baroreceptors to the neurons in the rostral ventrolateral medulla are probably situated in close vicinity to the medial border of the solitary tract with the long axis oriented in a dorsomedial to ventrolateral direction (58). Figure 8 illustrates the strategic position of the neurons in the rostral ventrolateral medulla between the nucleus tractus solitarii, which receives the visceral afferent input, and the sympathetic preganglionic neurons (59-68). Thus, neurons in the region of the rostral ventrolateral medulla, which may contain adrenalin, are esponsible for the resting activity in sympathetic neurons supplying resistance vessels, the heart and adrenal medulla and are probably involved in relaying baroreceptor and other homeostatic reflexes. Despite this impressive work, it is still not clear whether adrenaline is the transmitter in the spinal cord and whether the neurons from of the rostral ventrolateral medulla influence also neurons other than the preganglionic sympathetic cardiovascular type.

The Spinal Cord and the Final Common Sympathetic Motor Paths

The Final Common Sympathetic Motor Paths

The sympathetic outflow from the thoraco-lumbar spinal cord supplies various target organs in the cutaneous, deep somatic and visceral domains. Information from supraspinal brain structures and from the periphery is integrated by the sympathetic preganglionic neurons; in this sense these neurons are the final common sympathetic motor neurons of the central neuronal processes involved in the regulation of the target organs which are supplied by sympathetic postganglionic neurons (Figure 9). This notion needs some modification when compared to the concept of the "final common motor path" as described by Sherrington (69) for the spinal motorneurons. In the latter case the "effector" response depends only on the final common motor path. This is not necessarily the case for responses of the effector organs of the sympathetic nervous system and requires therefore some comments.

One possible site of integration in the periphery occurs in the sympathetic paravertebral and prevertebral ganglia. In these ganglia, preganglionic axons diverge and converge synaptically on postganglionic neurons. Synaptic mechanisms other than those which are cholinergic nicotinic may occur (70-72); in prevertebral ganglia; postganglionic neurons may integrate synaptic input from preganglionic neurons, spinal visceral afferents and afferents which have their cell bodies in the periphery (73, 74). Despite extensive investigations of synaptic processes in sympathetic ganglia, we have no consistent ideas about the significance of integrative processes in these ganglia during ongoing neural regulations of sympathetic target organs. From neurophysiological investigations of the discharge patterns of sympathetic pre- and postganglionic neurons, it appears that this activity is normally reliably transmitted in the separate sympathetic systems from the preganglionic to the postganlionic neurons (10, 11).

Another possible site of integration is at the level of the effector organ (Figure 9). The response of an autonomic target organ may not only depend on the neuronal influence but also on hormonal (e.g., circulatory catecholamines), local metabolic, mechanical (myogenic) and environmental (e.g., temperature) influences. These non-neural influences vary between different target organs. In the visceral domain, postganglionic sympathetic neurons (e.g. "motility-regulating" neurons, see below) may not influence effector organs directly but only indirectly, by controlling presynaptically the transmitter released from preganglionic parasympathetic axons.

FINAL COMMON SYMPATHETIC MOTOR PATH

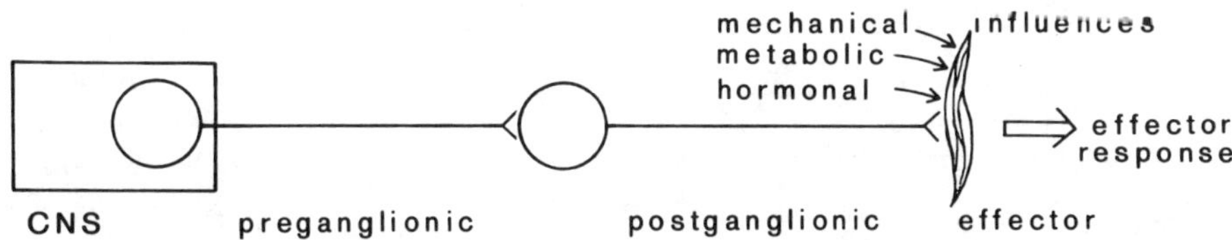

Figure 9. The final common sympathetic motor path as neuronal link between spinal cord and autonomic target organs. Some integrative processes may occur in the sympathetic ganglia, particularly the prevertebral ones. The target organs are not only under neuronal control but also influenced by other processes.

Functionally Identified Pre-Post-Ganglionic Sympathetic Channels

The variety of functionally different autonomic target organs supplied by the sympathetic outflow, the precision and range of responses of these target organs during ongoing regulations, and the potentially complex central organization of the sympathetic nervous system, leads one to assume that most types of target organ may each be supplied by a functionally separate pre-post-ganglionic sympathetic channel. This hypothesis has been tested for sympathetic neurons supplying target organs in skin and skeletal muscle and supplying pelvic organs and colon. The basic idea behind these experiments was that different target organs have different functions (see right side of Figure 9) and therefore functionally distinct innervations which include separate pre-post-ganglionic sympathetic channels and characteristic central organizations; sympathetic post- and preganglionic neurons influencing a particular target organ should, therefore, discharge in characteristic patterns upon natural stimulation of receptor populations on the body surface and in its interior, or upon central stimuli. Listening to the discharge patterns of the neurons of the individual peripheral sympathetic channels should not only give us information on the functional individuality of these channels but also on the central organization of the systems. Extensive neurophysiological work on the neurons of the lumbar sympathetic outflow supplying skeletal muscle, skin, pelvic organs and colon has revealed that this is indeed the case. Though this work is not yet finished, one can say that these tissues are supplied by at least nine sympathetic pre-post-ganglionic channels in the cat (Figure 10).

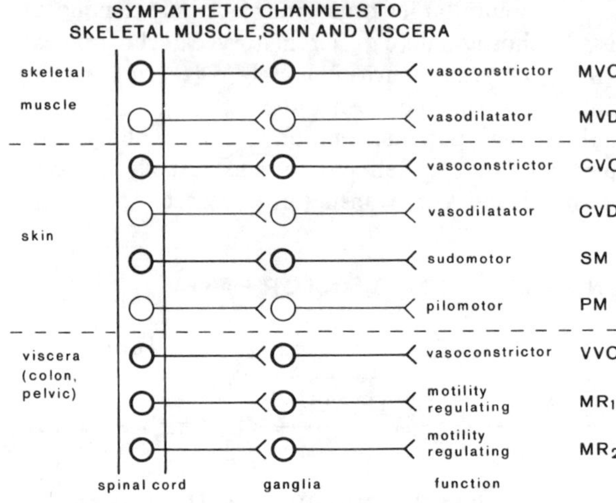

Figure 10. Sympathetic systems of the lumbar sympathetic outflow supplying the skeletal muscle and skin of hindlimb and tail and viscera (colon, pelvic organs) of the cat. The systems drawn heavily have ongoing activity in the anesthetized cat. The properties of the CVD neurons are not as well-established as those of the other systems (see 10, 80). SM neurons supply only sweat glands of the hairless skin of the paws PM neurons supply only erector pili muscles on the tail and back. The MR neurons consist probably of more than two types (76). Modified from Jänig (75). Reproduced, with permission, from *Clinical and Experimental Hypertension*. Copyright, 1984 by Elsevier.

Figure 11 illustrates typical discharge patterns in postganglionic vasoconstrictor neurons supplying skeletal muscle and hairy skin and Figure 12 a typical discharge pattern in a preganglionic "motility-regulating" neurone projecting in one lumbar splanchnic nerve. Details of the discharge patterns are described in the literature (10, 11, 75-79).

Figure 13 illustrates in a somewhat abstract form the discharge patterns of the neurons of the nine types of lumbar sympathetic pre-post-ganglionic channels. For the MVC, CVC, SM, VVC and the MR channels (for abbreviations see Figure 10), the essential information is available for the post- and preganglionic neurons. These patterns clearly indicate the functional individuality of the sympathetic systems. The systems have the following general features: (1) Most neurons of the MVC, CVC, SM, VVC and MR type have ongoing activity, the other systems do not. (2) MVC and VVC neurons are under strong inhibitory control of arterial baroreceptors. Their activity exhibits rhythmic changes with respiration, probably due to central coupling in the medulla oblongata between the neuronal system controlling respiration and the systems controlling the activity in vasoconstrictor neurons supplying resistance vessels (82-84). (3) Most CVC neurons are under inhibitory control of most afferent inputs.

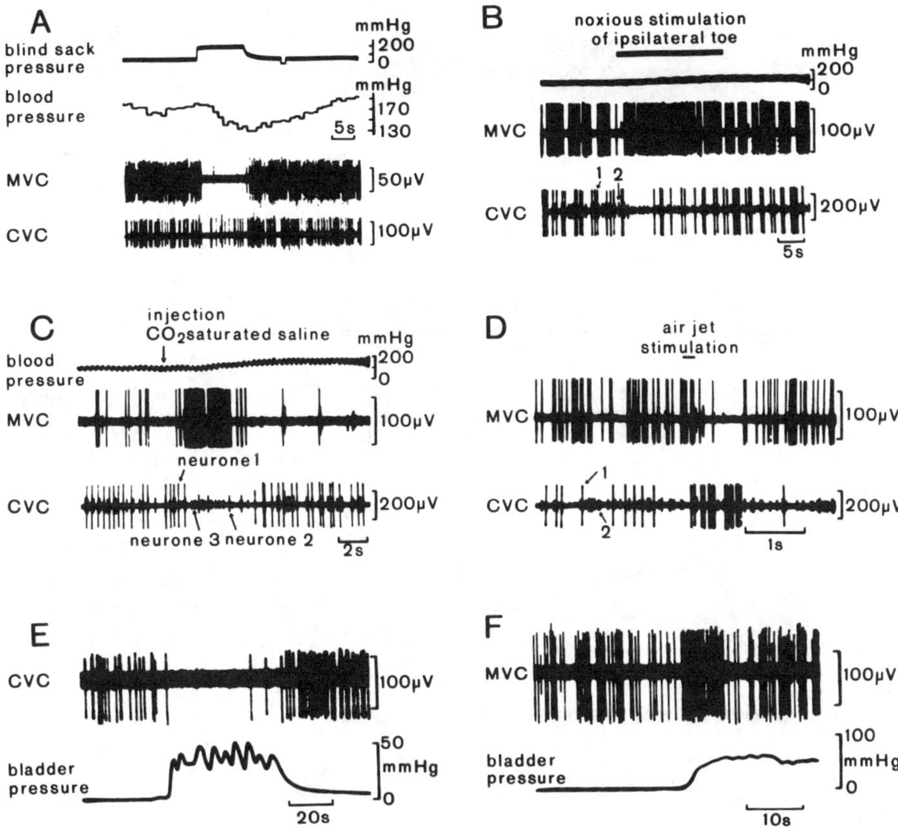

Figure 11. Reflex patterns in postganglionic vasoconstrictor neurons supplying skeletal muscle (MVC; deep peroneal nerve) and postganglionic vasoconstrictor neurons supplying hairy skin (CVC; superficial peroneal nerve) of the cat hindlimb. (A) Pressure increase applied in the left carotid blind sac. The carotid sinus nerve to the blind sac was left intact; right carotid sinus nerve and both cervical vagosympathetic trunks, including the aortic nerves, were cut. Both bundles from which the recordings were made contained several postganglionic axons. B-C. Simultaneous recordings from a single MVC neuron and a bundle with ttree CVC neurons (1-3). (B) Mechanical stimulation of cutaneous nociceptors in a toe of the ipsilateral hindpaw. Upper record, blood pressure. Note that CVC neurons *1* and *2* were inhibited. (C) Stimulation of arterial chemoreceptors by a bolus injection of CO_2-enriched saline solution (0.8 ml) through a catheter in the left lingual artery close to the glomus caroticum. Note that the CVC neurons *1* and *2* were inhibited and neuron *3* excited. (D) Short-lasting stimulation of hair follicle receptors on the trunk of the animal by air jets (10 trials superimposed). (E), (F) Reaction of a CVC neuron and an MVC neuron to isovolumetric contraction of the urinary bladder. (A) and (C) modified from Blumberg et al. (81); (B) and (D), Blumberg and Jänig, unpublished; (E) and (F), Hilbers and Jänig, unpublished.

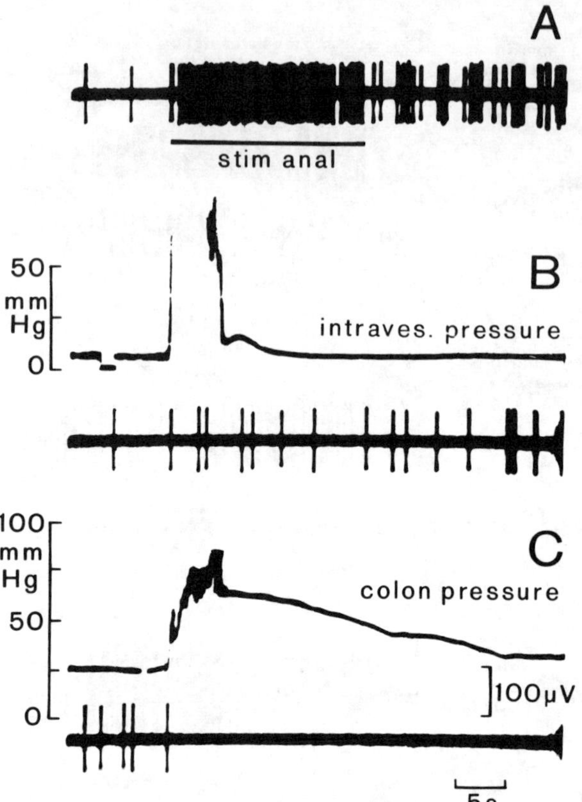

Figure 12. Response pattern of a preganglionic motility-regulating neuron (MR[1]) which projected in one lumbar splanchnic nerve of the cat. The neuron had some resting activity. (A) Activation of the neuron during mechanical shearing stimuli applied to the mucosal skin of the anus. The neuron exhibited afterdischarges.(B) Activation of the neuron by distension of the urinary bladder. Injection of 10 ml fluid in the balloon of the colon. See reflex pattern of MR1 neurons in Figure 13 (76). Reproduced, with permission, from *Journal of Autonomic Nervous System*. Copyright, 1986 by Elsevier.

The inhibitory control by arterial baroreceptors is weak or absent as is the coupling to the respiratory system. Some cutaneous vasocon-strictor neurons have a reflex pattern which is similar to that in MVC neurons (not shown in Figure 13). (4) The SM system is under excitatory control of the afferent inputs. The reflex excitation by stimulation of the Pacinian corpuscles in the paws (vibration) is unique. Arterial baroreceptors have no influence on SM activity. (5) Most MR neurons are largely under control of visceral afferents, e.g., from pelvic organs and colon, and not influenced by stimulation of arterial baro- and chemoreceptors. (6) PM, MVD and CVD neurons have no ongoing activity and can probably only be excited by very special stimuli under specific behavioral situations (see for example the activation of PM and MVD neurons during the defense behavior of the cat, Figure 1). The properties of CVD neurons are not well known: These neurons may be activated by central warm inputs (10, 80).

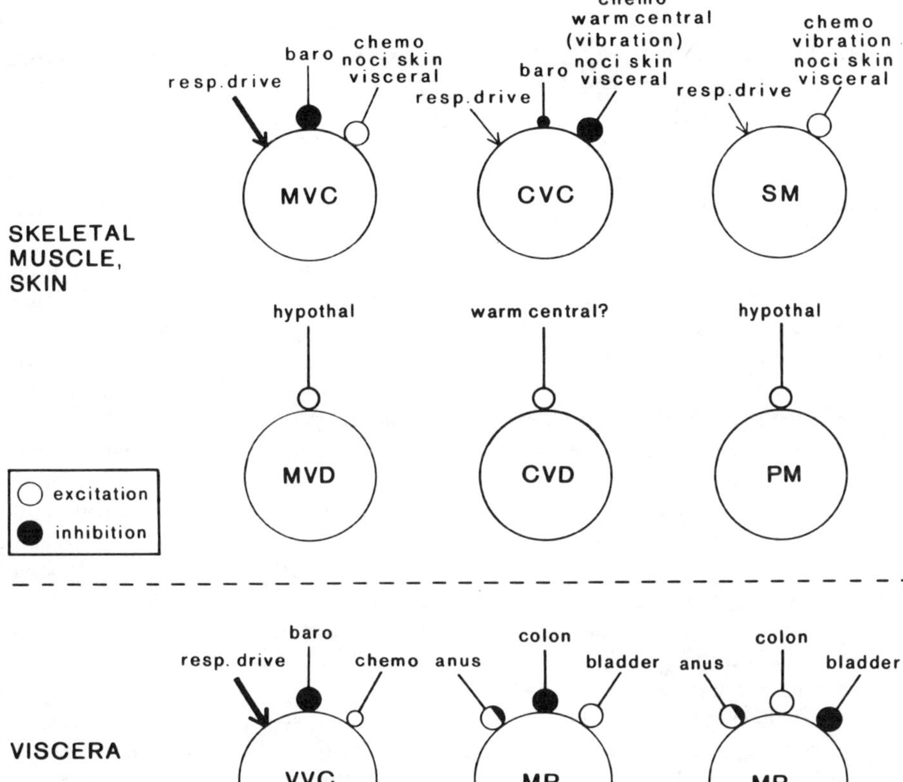

Figure 13. Reaction patterns of lumbar sympathetic systems supplying skeletal muscle (MVC, MVD) and skin (CVC, SM, PM, CVD) of the cat hindlimb and tail, and colon and pelvic organs (VVC, MR1, MR2) in animals with intact neuraxis. The open and closed small circles indicate excitatory and inhibitory actions, respectively, when the indicated afferent input is stimulated. Most neurons of the systems in the first and second row have ongoing activity. The neurons of the systems in the middle row are silent and influenced by very special stimuli only. Adequate stimulation of afferents: baro, arterial baroreceptors; chemo, arterial chemoreceptors; noci skin, cutanenous nociceptors of the ipsilateral hindpaw; visceral, visceral afferents from urinary bladder, colon and anus (distension, isovolumetric contraction, shearing stimuli); warm central, warm-sensitive neuronal structures in spinal canal and in hypothalamus; vibration, Pacinian corpuscles in hindpaw. Respiratory drive: grouping of discharges with respect to respiration pronounced in MVC and VVC neurons. Some CVC neurons behave like MVC neurons (not shown; see neuron 3 in Figure 11C). Some MR neurons are inhibited by mechanical shearing stimuli applied to the anus. Data from Jänig (10) and Baron et al. (80, 81). Reproduced, with permission, from *Journal of Autonomic Nervous System*. Copyright, 1980 by Elsevier.

The Integration in the Spinal Cord

Investigations of MVC, CVC and SM neurons in chronic spinal cats (spinalized at the low thoracic level; see 10) and of MR neurons in acutely spinalized cats (79) have revealed that most reflexes elicited from the skin and viscera remain qualitatively unchanged when compared to the reflexes in cats with intact neuraxis. These results and some other properties of the reflex patterns indicate that the spinal cord is an important level of integration for the sympathetic outflow and that this integration determines the specifity of the responses of the neurons of the sympathetic outflow. We have no idea how this integration of afferent activity from the three body domains, of activity in descending systems from the brainstem and hypothalamus and of interneuronal activity is brought about by the preganglionic neurons; we do not know what types of interneurons are involved. It could well be that the long, mostly rostrocaudally oriented dendrites of the preganglionic neurons (85) are important in this integration process. Generally one might speculate whether each sympathetic system is represented in the spinal cord by so-called "spinal sympathetic functional units," which consists of the preganglionic neurons, interneurons and synaptic connections of these neuron types with the spinal afferent inflow and the spinal descending systems (Figure 14). Functionally related "spinal sympathetic functional units" may share common interneuron pools and descending systems,etc. Though this is very speculative, it may serve as a reasonable working hypothesis for future neurobiological research on integrative processes of sympathetic activity in the spinal cord (10, 11).

The organization of the nine sympathetic systems supplying skeletal muscle, skin, pelvic organs and colon in the spinal cord and in the periphery is indicated schematically in Figure 14. Systems which are functionally related are positioned close together, such as the CVC and SM systems, the CVC and MVC systems, the MVC and VVC systems, and both MR systems. This functional relation is reflected in the similarity, but not necessarily in the identity of the discharge patterns of different types of neurons (see, e.g., MVC and VVC neurons; Figure 13) or in the reciprocity of the discharge patterns of functionally different types of neurons, with respect to the afferent inputs (e.g., in CVC and SM neurons, CVC and MVC neurons and in MR1 and MR2 neurons, see Figure 13). The "spinal sympathetic functional units" may be controlled by several descending systems from the brainstem and hypothalamus.

A further level of neuronal integration probably exists for the vasoconstrictor systems and the motility-regulating systems in the ganglia. In the prevertebral ganglia (MR systems, VVC system) activity in preganglionic neurons, in spinal afferents, which may synapse by collaterals with the postganglionic neurons, and in afferent neurons which have their cell bodies in the visceral organs is integrated. More than one transmitter may be involved in this integration and the prevertebral ganglia may relay extraspinal viscero-visceral reflexes. The functional significance of this integration during ongoing regulations of the visceral organs is unknown (for review see 73, 74). Synaptic long-term processes have been detected in paravertebral ganglia in vasoconstrictor systems supplying skeletal muscle and skin.

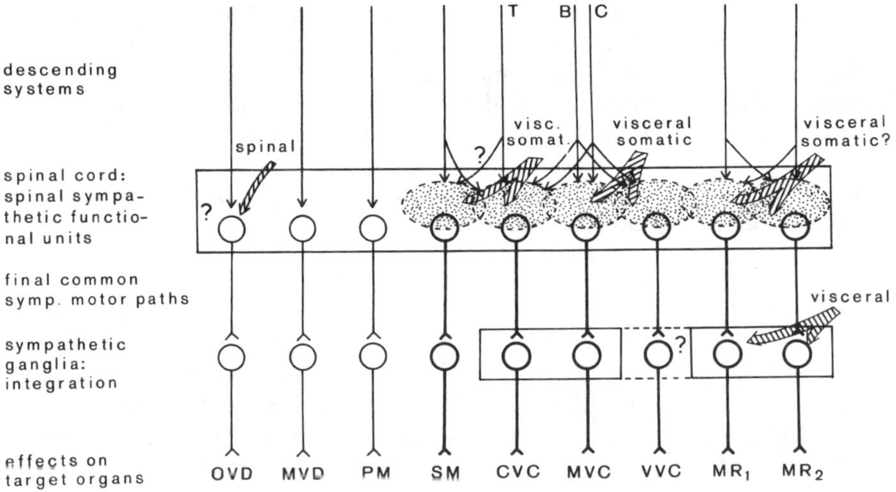

Figure 14. Idea about the spinal organization of the lumbar sympathetic systems supplying skeletal muscle, skin, distal colon and pelvic organs (systems projecting in the distal lumbar sympathetic trunk, distal to ganglion L_5 and in the lumbar splanchnic nerves). At the base of this organization are the sympathetic target organs which are supplied by the "final common sympathetic motor paths." The "target organs" of some MR neurons may be other neurons or the synaptic terminals on these neurons in the pelvic ganglia to the urinary bladder (86) and in the enteric nervous system of the colon. The transmission of information in the "final common sympathetic motor paths" from the pre- to the postganglionic neurons may be modified in the CVC and MVC systems in the ganglia of the sympathetic trunk (70-72) and in the inferior mesenteric ganglion (74). The stippled areas symbolize "spinal sympathetic functional units" which consist of preganglionic neurons, interneurons and their synaptic connections with the spinal primary afferent inputs from the somatic and visceral domains (shaded arrows) and with the descending systems. These spinal units may determine the characteristic discharge patterns of the sympathetic neurons which are drawn in thick lines (these systems also have ongoing activity). The other three systems (right side) are probably largely dependent on the activity in the descending systems. The existence of the CVD system is not as well established as that of the other systems (80, 87). The "spinal sympathetic functional units" are under control of various descending systems from brainstem and hypothalamus (T, thermo; B, baro; C, chemo). CVD, cutaneous vasodilator; MVD, muscle vasodilator; MR, motility-regulating. Modified from Jänig (10). Reproduced, with permission, from *Reviews of Physiology, Biochemistry and Experimental Pharmacology*. Copyright, 1985 by Elsevier.

The functional significance of these processes are also unclear (70-72). An important question concerning the organization of the sympathetic systems in the spinal cord (see Figure 14) is whether functionally different types of sympathetic preganglionic neurons are situated at different sites of the intermediate zone in the spinal cord. If this is the case one could query whether different types of descending systems from the brainstem and hypothalamus, which are involved in the regulation of sympathetic activity (see Figure 7), terminate in a topographical manner with respect to functionally similar preganglionic neurons. In a first approach to this problem functionally different groups of preganglionic neurons in the lumbar spinal cord of the cat have been labelled with horseradish peroxidase (HRP):

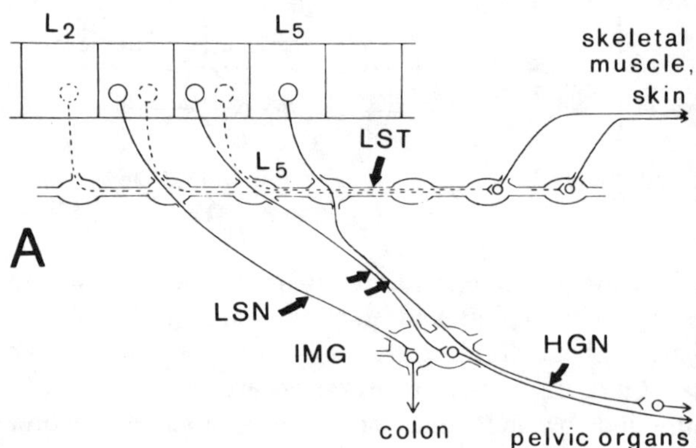

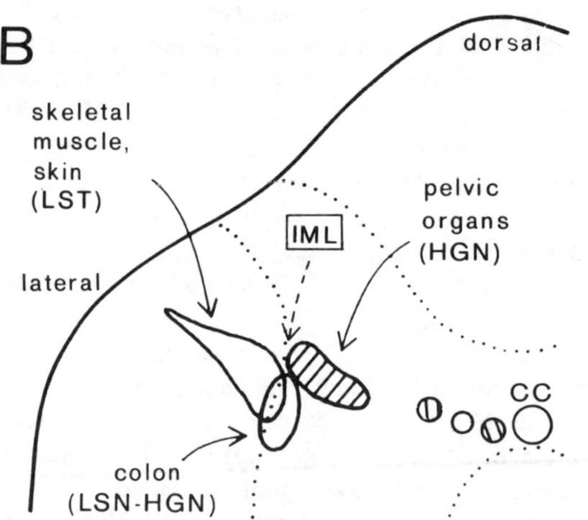

Figure 15. Location of functionally different sympathetic preganglionic neurons in the lumbar spinal cord. (A) Arrangement of lumbar splanchnic nerves (LSN), lumbar sympathetic trunk (LST) and hypogastric nerve (HGN) in the cat. The projections of different types of preganglionic neurons are indicated. Horseradish peroxidase (HRP) solution was applied to the central cut end of the LST (labelling of preganglionic neurons which influence target organs in skeletal muscle and skin), of the HGN (labelling of preganglionic neurons to pelvic organs) and of the LSN (labelling of preganglionic neurons which influence pelvic organs and colon). (B) Schematic outline of the main regions in which the labelled preganglionic neurons are found in a representative transverse section of the lumbar segment L4. Preganglionic neurons which synapse with postganglionic neurons in the inferior mesenteric ganglion (IMG) and which had no collaterals in the HGN were assumed to influence the colon. The location of these neurons deduced from the difference of the location of the LSN and the HGN labelled neurons. IML, nucleus intermediolateralis. Modified from Jänig and McLachlan (92).

First, lumbar pre-ganglionic neurons, which synapse with postganglionic neurons (which supply target organs in skeletal muscle and skin of the hindlimb and tail), projecting through the lumbar sympathetic trunk (LST) distal to the paravertebral ganglion L_5 (broken lines in Figure 15A); second, preganglionic neurons to the pelvic organs projecting in the lumbar splanchnic nerves (LSN) and hypogastric nerves (HGN in Figure 15A); third, preganglionic neurons which synapse with post-ganglionic neurons in the inferior mesenteric ganglion (IMG in Figure 15A) without having collaterals in the hypogastric nerve and which are probably involved in the regulation of the flow of blood through and the motility of the colon. The HRP was applied at the three different sites, as indicated by the arrows in Figure 15A, to the central stumps of the freshly cut nerves. The enzyme is taken up by the cut axons and transported to the preganglionic somata; three days after the HRP application the reaction product of the enzyme was made visible on horizontal longitudinal sections of the spinal cord. The computer reconstructions of the location of the labelled neurons on transverse sections (Figure 15B) show that most preganglionic neurons projecting in the distal LST are located in the "classical" nucleus inter-mediolateralis (IML in Figure 15B) at the border between white and gray matter, many of them being located in the white matter itself (pars funicularis). Most preganglionic neurons which project through the hypogastric nerves to the pelvic organs are situated medial to the LST neurons (almost no neurons can be found in the white matter). By comparing the location of the preganglionic neurons labelled from the LSN with those labelled from the HGN it is possible to give an idea as to the position of those preganglionic neurons probably involved in colon function. These neurons are located more ventrally but also largely medial to the "classical" nucleus intermediolateralis. Some of each type of neuron are located very far medial (88-92). This type of experimental morphological study shows quite clearly that functionally different types of lumbar sympathetic preganglionic neurons have distinct locations in the spinal cord. Whether this also applies to the individual types of preganglionic neurons (see Figure 10) awaits further functional and morphological studies.

Comments and Conclusions

The lumbar sympathetic innervation of skeletal muscle, skin and viscera is organized in functionally discrete pre-post-ganglionic channels. Each channel probably innervates a particular target organ and the pre- and postganglionic neurons of each channel discharge in a characteristic fashion upon peripheral and central stimuli. These discharges (reflex) patterns enable the neurons to be functionally recognized; they are also a mirror image of the central organization of the respective system. Though we always speak of "reflexes" and "reflex patterns" (see Figures 11-13), it must be kept in mind that these reflexes are the expression of the central organization, i.e., of the structure of the central neuronal programs, of the systems. These reflexes were elicited by adequate stimulation of receptor populations from the body surface and from its interior. The central neuronal programs "recognize" the afferent input as "meaningful" and create responses which can be observed in the neurons of the "final common sympathetic path." These reflexes are therefore isolated frag-ments of regulating systems and, as such, "experimental artifacts." Thus, the responses seen in the neurons are not "caused" by the afferent input, but instead excitation of a specific set of afferent induces the central program(s) to react in the manner as observed at the output system and the response is determined by the intrinsic structure of that program. This is quite obvious for the arterial "barometer reflex," an important element of nervous control of autonomic cardiovascular regulation. The pathway "arterial baroreceptor - nucleus tractus solitarii - rostral ventrolateral (CL) region in the medulla oblongata - dorsolateral spinal funiculus - preganglionic sympathetic neurons" as outlined in Figure 8, may be called "baroreceptor reflex pathways." However, in reality, we are dealing with a complex neuronal program in the medulla oblongata, which includes the neurons in the nucleus tractus solitarii, those in the rostral ventrolateral medulla, the cardiac preganglionic motor neurons in the nucleus ambiguus and in the dorsal motor nucleus of the vagus, and the excitatory and inhibitory synaptic connections among and between these neurons and other neurons in the medulla oblongata. This program, which serves the phasic regulation of the arterial pressure, is under control of other programs in the brainstem, hypothalamus and amygdala (see Figure 7) and is closely coupled with respiratory neurons in the lower brainstem (neuronal networks which control respiration); the result of this coupling can be seen as the rhythmic changes of the discharges in the vasoconstrictor neurons supplying resistance vessels (see MVC and VVC neurons in Figure 13) and in sympathetic neurons supplying the heart.

A second interesting example which can be reasonably well understood may be the "vibration reflex" in the sympathetic outflow of the sweat glands (sudomotor neurons, SM) and blood vessels (cutaneous vasoconstrictor neurons, CVC) of the hairless skin of the cat hindpaw (see Figure 13): Stimulation of Pacinian corpuscles in the cat hindpaw by vibration leads to activation of the SM neurons and to inhibition of activity in some CVC neurons; the activation of sweat glands is accompanied by an increase in cutaneous blood flow and in this way supplies plasma for sweat production. The neuronal program which organizes the particular response pattern of sudomotor and cutaneous vasoconstrictor neurons exists in the spinal cord; the same pattern can also be elicited in chronic spinal cats (87, 93).

The principles of the peripheral and central organization of the sympathetic systems, as outlined here for the lumbar sympathetic outflow, probably also applies to the thoracic sympathetic outflow to the abdominal and thoracic viscera and to the head. Sympathetic preganglionic neurons, which project through the cervical sympathetic trunk to the superior cervical ganglion, supplying various effector organs of the head and should also exhibit distinct reflex patterns (94).

Cannon and Hess saw the sympathetic nervous system more or less as a system which reacts in a diffuse fashion as a unit. They connected the activation of the system with certain functional states of the organism and observed it from the high-order programs, which are organized in the brainstem, hypothalamus and limbic system. Modern neurobiological research shows that these autonomic systems are highly differentiated. They are organized in a hierarchical fashion: the elementary neuronal programs of the autonomic systems in the spinal cord and medulla oblongata are at the base (e.g., for regulation of the cardiac output, peripheral resistance to blood flow, continence and evacuation of urinary bladder and colon). These elementary programs are used by higher order programs in the upper brainstem and, particularly, in the hypothalamus (e.g., for thermoregulation, regulation of extracellular fluid volume and composition, regulation of the gastrointestinal tract, regulation of emotional expression). In the hypothalamus autonomic functions are coupled with endocrine functions and motor functions. The limbic system, which contains the highest neuronal representation of the inner environment, is the liaison brain to the programs representing the external world. However, it must be kept in mind that also, at each level of organization, integration occurs between autonomic systems and other (sensory, motor) systems. Thus, there is not only a vertical but also a horizontal organization.

It may appear, on the one hand, that generally nothing new has been added to the traditional concepts about the functioning of the autonomic systems created by Cannon, Hess and others; on the other hand, the traditional views are going to have to be atomized in view of the vast amount of new data. However, we are plainly converging in our conceptual thinking towards more differentiated models of the autonomic systems. These newly developed and advanced concepts will replace or modify older concepts which hide behind terms such as "sympathico-adrenal system," "homeostasis," "sympathetic and parasympathetic reaction patterns," etc. It is to be hoped that this new development will also give us new access to the understanding of the autonomic systems in the diseased state of humans, such as, for example, in various forms of psychosomatic illness, in hypertension and in certain types of pathological pain (5, 95-98).

Summary

The sympathetic nervous system is organized in a hierarchical fashion. The periphery consists of the final common sympathetic pathways (the pre-post-ganglionic channels) which are largely separated with respect to the target organs. These pathways transmit the product of neuronal integration in the central nervous system to the target organs which each receive a characteristic reflex (reaction) pattern. These pattern may be modified in certain sympathetic systems by integrative processes in the sympathetic ganglia. A further integrative step may occur in the periphery at the level of the target organs. Many organs are not only under neuronal control but also under local metabolic, myogenic, local hormonal and distant hormonal control.

The reflex pattern of a particular type of sympathetic pre- or postganglionic neuron enables the neuron to be recognized functionally, with respect to the target organs, and this pattern is an expression of the central organization of the respective system. The reflex patterns are, so to speak, the "functional fingerprints" of the sympathetic systems.

Spinal cord, lower and upper brainstem, hypothalamus and suprahypothalamic telencephalic brain structures contain the central neuronal programs which organize the discharge patterns in the sympathetic output system. At the base are the "spinal sympathetic functional units," which consist of preganglionic neurons, putative interneurons and the connections of these parasympathetic neurons with the spinal afferent input and the descending spinal systems. These units coordinate the discharge patterns of the sympathetic systems at the lowest level of central integration. They are connected with the brainstem and hypothalamus by descending systems.

The brainstem contains many regions which project directly or indirectly to the intermediate region of the sympathetic preganglionic neurons of the spinal cord and which are involved in the regulation of the autonomic target organs. Many of these projecting systems can be characterized biochemically as being peptidergic and/or monoaminergic. Whether and in which way any of these monoamines and peptides function as neurotransmitter or neuromodulator in the region of the sympathetic preganglionic neurons, has still to be established. Most of the brainstem systems receive synaptic inputs from the nucleus tractus solitarii which itself obtains its main afferent input from internal organs in a organotropic manner. We are aware that these brainstem systems contain the programs which enable various autonomic, homeostatic and other regulations to take place; however, we are more or less ignorant of how the regulations are brought about. The most well-known pathway consists of the cardio-vascular afferents (baro- and chemoreceptive, heart) which project to the nucleus tractus solitarii, then from here to the rostral ventrolateral area of the medulla oblongata and, finally, to the region of the sympathetic preganglionic neurons. This pathway may "relay" information from cardiovascular afferents to preganglionic neurons involved in the regulation of resistance vessels, the heart and catecholamine release from the adrenal medulla. Acute bilateral lesioning of the rostral ventrolateral area of the medulla oblongata has the same effect on the arterial pressure as high cervical spinalization, indicating that the activity in the sympathetic systems to heart, resistance vessels and adrenal medulla decreases close to zero.

The hypothalamus organizes elementary behavioral patterns, consisting of motor, autonomic and endocrine components. It is the liaison brain region between autonomic and neuroendocrine systems and the telencephalon, i.e., between the neuroendocrine regulation of the processes in the body and the higher brain functions which occur in the telencephalon. Focal lesioning of small areas in the hypothalamus may lead to uncoupling of neuroendocrine adaptive processes and motor components in behavioral patterns. This applies, for example, to conditioned emotional responses in monkeys of which the cardiovascular adaptive processes can be abolished by small bilateral perifornical lesions in the hypothalamus, without affecting the motor responses or the "emotionality" (emotional state) of the animal. The hypothalamus has very close reciprocal connections with all brainstem areas which are involved in the regulation of autonomic functions. The way in which different behavioral and different complex adaptive-regulating patterns are organized by the hypothalamus eludes our knowledge.

Summarizing, it can be assumed that there is a high differentiation in sympathetic systems supplying different target organs, this reflecting a high degree of differentiation in the neuraxis and hypothalamus. On the other hand, we are aware - last but not least from Cannon and Hess - that the sympathetic systems function as a unity in the freely acting organism, this being an expression of the organization in the hypothalamus and suprahypothalamic structures. Both points of view are not exclusive, but only complement one another.

References

1. Langley, J.N. (1903). Das sympathische und verwandte nervöse Systeme der Wirbeltiere (autonomes nervöses System). Ergn. Physiol. 2/II: 818-872.
2. Langley, J.N. (1921). The autonomic nervous system. Part 1. W.Heffer, Cambridge.
3. Malliani, A. (1982). Cardiovascular sympathetic afferent fibers. Rev. Physiol. Biochem. Pharmacol., 94: 11-74.
4. Mei, N. (1983). Sensory structures in the viscera. Progress in sensory physiology, Vol. 4. Springer-Verlag, Berlin, Heidelberg, p. 1-42.
5. Jänig, W. (1985). Systemic and specific autonomic reactions in pain: Efferent, afferent and endocrine components. Europ. J. Anaesthesiol., 2: 319-346.
6. Jänig, W. & Morrison, J.F.B. (1986). Functional properties of spinal visceral afferents supplying abdominal and pelvic organs, with special emphasis on visceral nociception. In F. Cervero & J.F.B. Morrison (Eds.), Visceral sensation. Progress in Brain Research, Vol. 67. Elsevier Biomedical Press, Amsterdam, N.Y., Oxford, p. 87-114.
7. Cannon, W.B. (1929). Organization for physiological homeostasis. Physiol. Rev., 9: 399-431.
8. Cannon, W.B. (1939). The wisdom of the body. W.W. Norton & Co. The Norton Library, N.Y., revised and enlarged edition of 1932.
9. Nilsson, S. (1983). Autonomic nerve function in the vertebrates. Springer-Verlag, Berlin, Heidelberg, N.Y.
10. Jänig, W. (1985). Organization of the lumbar sympathetic outflow to skeletal muscle and skin of the cat hindlimb and tail. Rev. Physiol. Biochem. Pharmacol., 102: 119-213.
11. Jänig, W. (1986). Spinal cord integration of visceral sensory systems and sympathetic nervous system reflexes. In F. Cervero & J.F.B. Morrison (Eds.), Visceral sensation. Progress in Brain Research, Vol. 67. Elsevier Biomedical Press, Amsterdam, N.Y., Oxford, p. 255-277.
12. Hess, W.R. (1948). Die funktionelle Organisation des vegetativen Nervensystems. Schwabe, Basel.
13. Hess, W.R. (1949). Das Zwischenhirn. Schwabe, Basel.
14. Akert, K. (Ed.) (1981). Biological order and brain organization. Selected works of W.R. Hess. Springer-Verlag, Berlin, Heidelberg, N.Y.
15. Bard, P. (1928). A diencephalic mechanism for the expression of rage with special reference to the sympathetic nervous system. Am. J. Physiol., 84: 490-515.
16. Bard, P. & Rioch, D.Mc.K. (1937). A study of four cats deprived of neocortex and additional portions of the forebrain. Bull. Johns Hopk. Hosp., 60: 73-147.
17. Bard, P. & Macht, M.B. (1958). The behaviour of chronically decerbrate cats. In G.E.W. Wolstenholme & C.M. O'Connor (Eds.), Neurological basis of behaviour. Ciba Foundation Symposium. Little, Brown & Co, Boston, p. 55-71.
18. Cannon, W.B. (1927). The James-Lange theory of emotions: A critical examination and an alternative theory. J. Psychol., 39: 106-124.
19. Bard, P. (1934). An emotional expression after decortication with some remarks on certain theoretical views. Part I. Psychol. Rev., 41: 309-329; Part II. Psychol. Rev., 41: 424-449.
20. Hess, W.R. & Brügger, M. (1943). Das subcorticale Zentrum der affektiven Abwehrreaktion. Helv. Physiol. Pharmacol. Acta 1:33-52.
21. Hunsperger, R.W. (1956). Affektreaktionen auf electrische Reizung im Hirnstamm der Katze. Helv. Physiol. Pharmacol. Acta 14: 70-92.
22. Von Holst, E. & von Saint Paul, U. (1960). Vom Wirkgefüge der Triebe. Naturwissenschaften, 47: 409-422.
23. Von Holst, E. & von Saint Paul, U. (1962). Electrically controlled behaviour. Sci. Am., 206: 50-60.

24. Darwin, C. (1872). The expression of the emotions in man and animals. John Murray, London.
25. Hilton, S.M. (1982). The defense-arousal system and its relevance for circulatory and respiratory control. J. Exp. Biol., 100: 159-174.
26. Smith, O.A., Hohmer, A.R., Astley, C.A. & Taylor, D.J. (1979). Renal and hindlimb vascular control during acute emotion in the baboon. Am. J. Physiol., 236: R198-R250.
27. Smith, O.A., Astley, C.A., DeVito, J.L., Stein, J.M. & Walsh, K.E. (1980). Functional analysis of hypothalamic control of the cardiovascular responses accompanying emotional behavior. Fed. Proc., 39: 2487-2494.
28. Smith, O.A., DeVito, J.L. & Astley, C.A. (1984). Organization of central nervous system pathways influencing blood pressure responses during emotional behavior. Clin. Exp.Hypertens. - Theory and Practice, A6: 185-204.
29. Smith, O.A. & DeVito, J.L. (1984). Central neural integration for the control of autonomic responses associated with emotion. Annu. Rev. Neurosci., 7: 43-65.
30. Turner, B.H., Mishkin, M. & Knapp, M. (1980). Organization of the amygdalopetal projections from modality-specific cortical association areas in the monkey. J. Comp. Neurol., 191: 515-54
31. Saper, C. (1982). Convergence of autonomic and limbic connections in the insular cortex of the rat. J. Comp. Neurol, 210: 163-173.
32. Swanson, L.W. & Sawchenko, P.E. (1983). Hypothalamic integration: Organization of the paraventricular and supraoptic nuclei. Annu. Rev. Neurosci., 6: 269-324.
33. Swanson, L.W. & Sawchenko, P.E. (1980). Paraventricular nucleus: A site for the integration of neuroendocrine and autonomic mechanisms. Neuroendocrinology, 31: 410-417.
34. Swanson, L.W. & Mogenson, G.J. (1981). Neural mechanisms for the functional coupling of autonomic, endocrine and somatomotor responses in adaptive behaviour. Brain Res. Rev., 3: 1-34.
35. Sawchenko, P.E. (1982). Anatomic relationships between the paraventricular nucleus of the hypothalamus and visceral regulatory mechanisms: Implications for the control of feeding behavior. In B.G. Hoebel & D. Novin (Eds.), Neural basis of feeding and reward. M.E. Haer Inst., Brunswick, p. 259-274.
36. Amendt, K., Czachurski, J., Dembowsky, K. & Seller, H. (1979). Bulbospinal projections to the intermediolateral cell column; a neuroanatomical study. J. Auton. Nerv. Syst., 1: 103-117.
37. Loewy, A.D. & McKellar, S. (1980). The neuroanatomical basis of central cardiovascular control. Fed. Proc., 39: 2495-2503.
38. Loewy, A.D. & Neil, J.J. (1981). The role of descending monoaminergic systems in the central control of blood pressure. Fed. Proc., 40: 2778-2785.
39. Dampney, R.A.L. (1981). Functional organization of central cardiovascular pathways. Clin. Exp. Pharmacol. Physiol., 8: 241-259.
40. Loewy, A.D. (1981). Descending pathways to sympathetic and parasympathetic preganglionic neurons. J. Auton. Nerv. Syst., 3: 265-275.
41. Loewy, A.D. (1982). Descending pathways to the sympathetic preganglionic neurons. In H.G.J.M. Kuypers & G.F. Martin (Eds.), Anatomy of descending pathways to the spinal cord. Progress in Brain Resaerch, Vol. 57. Elsevier Biomedical Press, Amsterdam, N.Y., Oxford, p. 267-277.
42. Blessing, W.W., Goodchild, A.K., Dampney, R.A.L., & Chalmers, J.P. (1981). Cell groups in the lower brain stem of the rabbit projecting to the spinal cord, with special reference to catecholamine-containing cells. Brain. Res., 221: 35-55.
43. Bowker, R.M., Westlund, K.N., Sullivan, M.C. & Coulter, J.D. (1982). Organization of descending serotonergic projections to the spinal cord. In H.G.J.M. Kuypers & G.F. Martin (Eds.), Anatomy of descending pathways to the spinal cord. Progress in Brain Research, Vol. 57. Elsevier Biomedial Press, Amsterdam, N.Y., Oxford, p. 239-265.
44. Holstege, G. & Kuypers, H.G.J.M. (1982). The anatomy of brain stem pathways to the spinal cord in cat. A labeled amino acid tracing study. In H.G.J.M. Kuypers & G.F. Martin (Eds.), Anatomy of descending pathways to the spinal cord. Progress in Brain Research, Vol. 57. Elsevier Biomedical Press, Amsterdam, N.Y., Oxford, p. 145-175.
45. Westlund, K.N., Bowker, R.M., Ziegler, M.G. & Coulter, J.D. (1982). Descending noradrenergic projections and their spinal terminations. In H.G.J.M. Kuypers & G.F. Martin (Eds.), Anatomy of descending pathways to the spinal cord. Progress in Brain Research, Vol. 57. Elsevier Biomedial Press, Amsterdam, N.Y., Oxford, p. 219-238.
46. Krukoff, T.L., Ciriello, J. & Calaresu, F.R. (1985). Segmental distributions of peptide-like immunoreactivity in cell bodies of the thoracolumbar sympathetic nuclei of the cat. J. Comp. Neurol., 240: 90-102.

47. Krukoff, T.L., Ciriello, J. & Calaresu, F.R. (1985). Segmental distribution of peptide-like and 5-HT-like immunoreactivity in nerve terminals and fibers of the thoracolumbar sympathetic nuclei of the cat. J. Comp. Neurol., 240: 103-116.
48. Coote, J.H. & MacLeod, V.H. (1974). The influence of bulbospinal monoaminergic pathways on sympathetic nerve activity. J. Physiol. (London), 241: 453-475.
49. Coote, J.H., MacLeod, V.H. & Martin, J.L. (1978). Bulbospinal tryptaminergic neurones: A search for the role of bulbospinal tryptaminergic neurones in the control of sympathetic activity. Pflügers Arch., 377: 109-116.
50. Coote, J.H., MacLeod, V.H., Fleetwood-Walker, S. & Gilbey, M.P. (1981). The response of individual sympathetic preganglionic neurones to microelectrophoretically applied endogenous monoamines. Brain Res., 215: 135-145.
51. Mraovitch, S., Kumada, M. & Reis, D. (1982). Role of the nucleus parabrachialis in cardiovascular regulation in the cat. Brain Res., 232: 57-75.
52. Neil, J.J. & Loewy, A.D.(1982). Decrease in blood pressure in response to L-glutamate injections into the A5 catecholamine cell group. Brain Res., 241: 271-278.
53. Howe, P.R.C., Kuhn, D.M., Minson, J.B., Stead, B.H. & Chalmers, J.P. (1983). Evidence for a bulbospinal serotonergic pressor pathway in the rat brain. Brain Res., 270: 29-36.
54. Dembowsky, K., Czachurski, J. & Seller, H. (1985). An intracellular study of the synaptic input to sympathetic preganglionic neurones in the third thoracic segment of the cat. J. Auton. Nerv. Syst., 13: 201-244.
55. Kalia, M. & Mesulam, M.-M. (1980). Brain stem projections of sensory and motor components of the vagus complex in the cat: I. The cervical vagus and nodose ganglion. J. Comp. Neurol., 193: 435-465.
56. Kalia, M. & Mesulam, M.-M. (1980). Brain stem projections of sensory and motor components of the vagus complex in the cat: II. Laryngeal, tracheobronchial, pulmonary, cardiac, and gastrointestinal branches. J. Comp. Neurol., 193: 467-508.
57. Spyer, K.M. (1981). Neural organization and control of the baroreceptor reflex. Rev. Physiol. Biochem. Pharmacol., 88: 23-124.
58. Czachurski, J., Lackner, K.J., Ockert, D. & Seller, H. (1982). Localization of neurones with baroreceptor input in the medial solitary nucleus by means of intracellular application of horseradish peroxidase in the cat. Neurosci. Lett., 28: 133-137.
59. Dampney, R.A.L., Goodchild, A.K., Robertson, L.G. & Montgomery, W. (1982). Role of ventrolateral medulla in vasomotor regulation: A correlative anatomical and physiological study. Brain Res., 249: 223-235.
60. McAllen, R.M., Neil, J.J. & Loewy, A.D. (1982). Effects of kainic acid applied to the ventral surface of the medulla oblongata on vasomotor tone, the baroreceptor reflex and hypothalamic autonomic responses. Brain Res., 238: 65-76.
61. Granata, A.R., Ruggiero, D.A., Park, D.H., Joh, T.H. & Reis, D.J. (1983). Lesions of epinephrine neurons in the rostral ventrolateral medulla abolish the vasodepressor components of baroreflex and cardiopulmonary reflex. Hypertension 5, Suppl., 5: 80-84.
62. Hilton, S.M., Marshall, J.M. & Timms, R.J. (1983). Ventral medullary relay neurones in the pathway from the defence areas of the cat and their effect on blood pressure. J. Physiol., 345: 149-166.
63. Ross, C.A., Ruggiero, D.A., Joh, T.H., Park, D.H. & Reis, D.J. (1983). Adrenaline synthesizing neurons in the rostral ventrolateral medulla: a possible role in tonic vasomotor control. Brain Res., 273: 356-361.
64. Ross, C.A., Ruggiero, D.A., Joh, T.H., Park, D.H. & Reis, D.J. (1984). Rostral ventrolateral medulla: Selective projections to the thoracic autonomic cell column from the region containing C1 adrenaline neurons. J. Comp. Neurol., 228: 168-185.
65. Ross, C.A., Ruggiero, D.A., Park, D.H., Joh, T.H., Sved, A.F., Fernandez-Pardal, J., Saavedra, J.M. & Reis, D.J. (1984). Tonic vasomotor control by the rostral ventrolateral medulla: effect of electrical or chemical stimulation of the area containing Cl-adrenaline neurons on arterial pressure, heart rate, and plasma catecholamines and vasopressin. J. Neurosci., 4: 474-494.
66. Farlow, D.M., Goodchild, A.K. & Dampney, R.A.L. (1984). Evidence that vasomotor neurons in the rostral ventrolateral medulla project to the spinal sympathetic outflow via the dorsomedial pressor area. Brain Res., 298: 313-320.
67. Granata, A.R., Ruggiero, D.A., Park, D.H., Joh, T.H. & Reis, D.J. (1985). Brain stem area with C1 epinephrine neurons mediates baroreceptor vasodepressor responses. Am. J. Physiol., 248: H547-H567.
68. Ruggiero, D.A., Ross, C.A., Anwar, M., Park, D.H. & Reis, D.J. (1985). Distribution of neurons containing phenylethanolamine N-methyltransferase in medulla and hypothalamus of rat. J. Comp. Neurol., 239: 127-154.

69. Sherrington, C. (1906). The integrative action of the nervous system. Yale University Press, New Haven.
70. Blumberg, H. & Jänig, W. (1983). Enhancement of resting activity in postganglionic vasoconstrictor neurones following short-lasting repetitive activation of preganglionic axons. Pflügers Arch., 396: 89-94.
71. Jänig, W., Krauspe, R. & Wiedersatz, G. (1982). Transmission of impulses from pre- to postganglionic vasoconstrictor and sudomotor neurons. J. Auton. Nerv. Syst., 6: 95-106.
72. Jänig, W., Krauspe, R. & Wiedersatz, G. (1983). Reflex activation of postganglionic vasoconstrictor neurons supplying skeletal muscle by stimulation of arterial chemoreceptors via non-nicotinic synaptic mechanisms in sympathetic ganglia. Pflügers Arch., 396: 96-100.
73. Szurszewski, J.H. (1981) Physiology of mammalian prevertebral ganglia. Annu. Rev. Physiol., 43: 53-68.
74. Simmons, M. (1985). The complexitiy and diversity of synaptic transmission in the prevertebral sympathetic ganglia. Prog. Neurobiol., 24: 43-93.
75. Jänig, W. (1984). Vasoconstrictor systems supplying skeletal muscle, skin, and viscera. Clin. Exp. Hypertens.- Theory and Practice A 6: 329-346.
76. Bahr, R., Bartel, B., Blumberg, H. & Jänig, W. (1986). Functional characterization of preganglionic neurons projecting in the lumbar splanchnic nerves: Neurons regulating motility. J. Auton. Nerv. Syst., 15: 109-130.
77. Bahr, R., Bartel, B., Blumberg, H. & Jänig, W. (1986). Functional characterization of preganglionic neurons projecting in the lumbar splanchnic nerves: Vasoconstrictor neurons. J. Auton. Nerv. Syst., 15: 131-140.
78. Bahr, R., Bartel, B., Blumberg, H. & Jänig, W. (1986). Secondary functional properties of lumbar visceral preganglionic neurons. J. Auton. Nerv. Syst.,15: 141-152.
79. Bartel, B., Blumberg, H. & Jänig, W. (1986). Discharge patterns of motility-regulating neurons projecting in the lumbar splanchnic nerves to visceral stimuli in spinal cats. J. Auton. Nerv. Syst.,15: 153-163.
80. Bell, C., Jänig, W., Kümmel, H. & Xu, H. (1985). Differentiation of vasodilator and sudomotor responses in the cat paw pad to preganglionic sympathetic stimulation. J. Physiol. (London), 364: 93-104.
81. Blumberg, H., Jänig, W., Rieckmann, C. & Szulczyk, P. (1980). Baroreceptor and chemoreceptor reflexes in postganglionic neurones supplying skeletal muscle and hairy skin. J. Auton. Nerv. Syst., 2: 223-240.
82. Richter, D.W. (1982). Generation and maintenance of the respiratory rhythm. J. Exp. Biol., 100: 93-107.
83. Richter, D.W. & Ballantyne, D. (1983). A three phase theory about the basic respiratory pattern generator. In M.E. Schläfke, H.P. Koepchen & W.R. See (Eds.), Central neurone environment and the control system of breathing and circulation. Springer-Verlag, Berlin, Heidelberg, N.Y., Tokyo, p. 164-174.
84. Bainton, C.R., Richter, D.W., Seller, H., Ballantyne, D. & Klein, J.P. (1985). Respiratory modulation of sympathetic activity. J. Auton. Nerv. Syst., 12: 77-90.
85. Dembowsky, K., Czachurski, J. & Seller, H. (1985). Morphology of sympathetic preganglionic neurones in the thoracic spinal cord of the cat: an intracellular horseradish peroxidase study. J. Comp. Neurol., 238: 453-465.
86. De Groat, W.C. & Booth, A.M. (1980). Inhibition and facilitation in parasymapathetic ganglia in the urinary bladder. Fed. Proc., 39: 2990-2996.
87. Jänig, W. & Kümmel, H. (1981). Organization of the sympathetic innervation supplying the hairless skin of the cat's paw. J. Auton. Nerv. Syst., 3: 215-230.
88. Baron, R., Jänig, W. & McLachlan, E.M. (1985). On the anatomical organization of the lumbosacral sympathetic chain and the lumbar splanchnic nerves of the cat - Langley revisited. J. Auton. Nerv. Syst., 12: 289-300.
89. Baron, R., Jänig, W. & McLachlan, E.M. (1985). The afferent and sympathetic components of the lumbar spinal outflow to the colon and pelvic organs in the cat: I. The hypogastric nerve. J. Comp. Neurol., 238: 135-146.
90. Baron, R., Jänig, W. & McLachlan, E.M. (1985). The afferent and sympathetic components of the lumbar spinal outflow to the colon and pelvic organs in the cat: II. The lumbar splanchnic nerves. J. Comp. Neurol., 238: 147-157.
91. Jänig, W. & McLachlan, E.M. (1986). The sympathetic and sensory components of the caudal lumbar sympathetic trunk in the cat. J. Comp. Neurol., 245: 62-73.
92. Jänig, W. & McLachlan, E.M. (1986). Identification of distinct topographical distributions of lumbar sympathetic and sensory neurons projecting to end organs with different functions in the cat. J. Comp. Neurol., 246: 104-112.
93. Jänig, W. & Kümmel, H. (1977). Functional discrimination of postganglionic neurones to the

cat's hindpaw with respect to the skin potentials recorded from the hairless skin. Pflügers Arch., 371: 217-225.

94. Jänig, W. & Schmidt, R.F. (1970). Single unit responses in the cervical sympathetic trunk upon somatic nerve stimulation. Pflügers Arch., 314: 199-216.
95. Blumberg, H. & Jänig, W. (1983). Changes of reflexes in vasoconstrictor neurons supplying the cat hindlimb following chronic nerve lesions: A model for studying mechanisms of reflex sympathetic dystrophy? J. Auton. Nerv. Syst., 7: 399-411.
96. Jänig, W. & Kollmann, W. (1984). The involvement of the sympathetic nervous system in pain. Possible neuronal mechanisms. Arzneim-Forsch./Drug Res., 34 (II): 1066-1073.
97. Blumberg, H. & Jänig, W. (1985). Reflex patterns in postganglionic vasoconstrictor neurons following chronic nerve lesions. J. Auton. Nerv. Syst., 14: 157-180.
98. Jänig, W. (1985). Causalgia and reflex sympathetic dystrophy: In which way is the sympathetic nervous system involved? Trends Neurosci., 8: 471-477.

Socio-Emotional Inputs to Central Neuronal Regulation of the Cardiovascular System

Johannes Siegrist, Herbert Matschinger and Karin Siegrist

To the outsider it seems that during the last few years an important development has taken place in the neuroscience which facilitates communication between neuroscientists and sociobehavioral scientists. Previously, nervous, endocrine and immune systems were considered largely as independent, autonomous phenomena. However, increasing evidence during the last few years suggest significant interrelationships between these systems. As William Ganong pointed out during the last meeting: "It is inappropriate to talk about separate nervous and endocrine systems. Instead there is a system of neuroendocrine cells that secrete chemical messengers with morphological specialization into neurons, gland cells, and structures inbetween" (1). And it is now well known, especially through elegant studies of David Felten and his group (2) that cell-mediated immune response can be modulated not only by the central nervous system via noradrenergic fibers but also via peptides such as thymosins, lymphokines (3), and endorphins (4). Thus, higher nervous activity seems to be systematically involved in integrated bodily processes in health and disease. But when talking about higher nervous activity we have to take into consideration sensory, cognitive and emotional input since the brain acts in a significant way as a mediator between body and environment. It has become fashionable to interpret human disease in the framework of a "bio-psycho-social" model (5). Yet, as will be shown later in this paper, basic theoretical concepts linking the three phenomena in a clear way arc still poorly developed, and such a task may provide an intellectual challenge to the dialogue between neuroscientists and sociobehavioral sciences.

The present paper consists of three parts. First, conceptual clarifications in the field of social stress experiences as candidates for centrally mediated cardiovascular dysfunction are developed, and a set of testable hypothesis is derived. In the second part, empirical results from our own research, mainly from an ongoing prospective study on cardiovascular risk in several hundred middle-aged blue-collar workers, are presented which refer to these hypotheses. Limitations and future prospects of the approach are shortly discussed. The final part of the paper outlines in a very preliminary way a model in which

The authors wish to thank Ingbert Weber, Gudrun Hess, Angelika Simon-Sebastian, Ruth Grünewald, Daniela Klein, and Brigitte Fischer-Feuerstein for their assistance in the common research project of the department. Special support was given by Prof. D. Seidel and Dr. H. Cremer from the Department of Clinical Chemistry, University of Göttingen in the analysis of blood lipids. This research is supported by Deutsche Forschungsgemeinschaft (Si 236/5).

pathways between experiences of socioemotional distress, activation of the limbic system and of related neuroendocrine messengers are supposed to impair bodily and especially cardiovascular function.

No doubt, the study of social stressors, psychological coping processes and centrally mediated impairment of bodily function is a difficult and controversial area. Nevertheless, progress has been made in the recent past due to a closer cooperation between relevant disciplines as well as due to the availability of more valid and more specific markers of the organism's stress response. It seems now that three developments were of special interest in this regard. First the replacement of the Selye type of general stress paradigm by a more sophisticated model focussing on different patterns of neurohormonal dysbalance according to different patterns of stimuli (6); second the recognition of the crucial role of cognitive appraisal in modulating individual control over adverse conditions (7); and third the notion that in addition to classical clear-cut stressors such as disaster, injury, death of a close family member, more subtle longlasting stressors may be harmful, acting as a "bias" with the potential of functional dysregulation (8). Most importantly, this latter development has allowed the establishment of models of synergistic interaction between pre-existing organic lesions and stress-induced dysfunction and thus has brought this field of research close to clinical medicine (9, 10).

Let us ask now whether we can specify the term "stressful experience" in a scientifically meaningful way. In accordance with Ursin we consider stress a specific form of activation caused by a threatening situation with "high response demand." By "threat" we mean a situation which endangers an individual's basic reward system (in terms of achievement, success, continuity of social status, integrity of one's body, etc.). By "high response demand" we mean that external or internal standards urge the individual to meet the challenging situation. Situations with high response demand however can be faced actively or passively. The term "coping" refers to efforts to obtain a positive response outcome and thus implies active handling of response demand (11).

In addition to Ursin's general definition we propose to concentrate on a specific subtype of stressful experience that we call "active distress." "Active distress" is supposed to occur if a threatening or demanding situation which is faced by coping efforts nevertheless ends with poor pay-off. In other words: Active distress is the experience of high coping in demanding situations, high expectancy but low probability of positive response outcome (which is identical with low control over outcome) (12).

But why does an individual continue to cope, to maintain a positive response expectancy if at the same time he or she experiences a low pay-off? Two answers must be given to this question. First, the individual may be exposed to coercion and may be unable to escape from the situation or to face it in a passive way. Although experience of active distress may be restricted to several underprivileged groups it nevertheless is a probable reaction towards a number of restrictive working conditions in industrialized societies (e.g., 13, 14; for details see below). The second answer relates to an individual's appraisal of demanding situations and of his own coping potential. David Glass (15) has suggested that characteristics such as increased irritability, hostility and inability to withdraw from imposed demands should be interpreted as an interpersonal strategy of individuals who are markedly afraid of losing their sense of control. Enhanced need for control over one's immediate social environment is realized not only at the behavioral but also at the perceptual level. This is our crucial point in addition to Glass: Individuals with these behavioral characteristics tend towards unrealistic appraisal of demanding situations and of their related internal coping potential. Fear of losing control is thought to stimulate overcommitment, either in the form of underestimation of demands and associated overestimation of coping potential, or in the form of overestimation of demands and underestimation of resources. Underestimation of challenging situations and overestimation of one's coping potential is more likely to occur. This misperceptual bias allows one to maintain or even to expand a territory of supposed own control (16). Maintenance of positive response expectancy is highly probable in individuals with high need for control even in situations which in realistic terms give poor pay-off. Filtered positive feedback from significant others in these situations may reinforce unrealistic appraisal.

So far we can summarize as follows: Sustained activation experienced as "active distress" is likely to occur in situations with high response demand, positive response expectancy and low control over the outcome. Individuals with behaviors and cognitions indicating enhanced "need for control" are at special risk for this type of sustained activation.

Before developing a set of testable propositions from these specifications we would like to point out that active distress probably involves the simultaneous arousal of the sympatho-adrenomedullary and the pituitary-adrenocortical axis (17) as well as the pituitary-sex-steroid axis (18). It is thought that their sustained synergistic activation may create neuro-hormonal dysbalance and by doing so may trigger cardiovascular pathology (19). The final part of the paper tries to establish some evidence along these lines including a centrally mediated development of some conditions of essential hypertension and some conditions of hyperlipidemia as early markers of cardiovascular dysfunction.

Control-limiting situations with high response demand can be found at the work place where time urgency, responsibility or high work-load are combined with limited decision-making. Recurrent threats are experienced in occupations with low job-security, with experiences of cut-down in personnel and forced downward mobility. Interpersonal conflicts and severe life-changes also may confront an individual with threatening or demanding situations where expected responses are out of personal control. Our *first proposition* is as follows: Individuals in middle-adulthood are more likely to develop cardiovascular risk (i.e., hypertension, hyperlipidemia) if they face recurrent control-limiting conditions and if they respond to these conditions with a coping style "enhanced need for control."

The *second proposition* gives an additional specification: Effects of "need for control" on indicators of cardiovascular risk (e.g., blood lipids) are more pronounced if the respective system is already impaired (e.g., if hypercholesterolemia is already established). This proposition is related to synergistic interaction between somatic conditions and centrally-mediated socio-emotional inputs to cardiovascular dysfunction.

The *third proposition* deals with the dynamics of an individual's coping career and therefore needs further explanation.

NEED FOR CONTROL

CONCEPT:

- Attitudes of excessive work commitment, need for social approval, competitiveness and latent hostility in demanding situations.—
- Learned during childhood (imitation or compensation); learned as coping technique during secondary socialization.—
- Mechanism: unrealistic appraisal of demanding situations (under—or overestimation of demands and/or coping potential).—
- Experiences of active distress under control-limiting social circumstances.—

MEASUREMENT:

- Trait-oriented measurement (questionnaire) with 44 dichotomous items measuring 6 aspects of attitudes mentioned.—
- Uni-dimensionality of dimensions (probabilistic test-model).—
- 2 underlying factors (confirmatory factor analysis)
  I Vigor
  II Immersion.—
- Short version (17 items): adequate representation of the 2 factors.—

Figure 1. The concept "need for control."

As can be seen from Figure 1, the concept "need for control" consists of two theoretically meaningful factors called "vigor" and "immersion." The demonstration of the basic latent structure of the concept by means of a congeneric measurement model is based on 44 items representing 6 relevant dimensions of excessive need for control (20). "Vigor" summarizes behaviors associated with overcommitment and coping efforts. "Immersion" summarizes behaviors, cognitions, and emotions associated with experiences of irritation, frustration and inability to withdraw from obligations. Our basic assumption states that the location of an individual on the two factors changes over time and that this change is a valid indicator of a change in an individual's coping career. As experiences of high commitment are at the very beginning of an individual's coping career, especially so in occupational life during early and middle adulthood, behaviors associated with "vigor" are thought to exert an influence on early markers of cardiovascular risk. Yet, this effect is restricted to those risk constellations where adverse social conditions sustain experiences of active distress. Positive response expectancy due to underestimation of demands may be experienced as rewarding over a certain time. But if this cognitive and motivational pattern is maintained under aggravating social conditions and under conditions of objectively impaired coping potential, sustained active distress is likely to occur. Thus, it is under conditions of sustained active distress that the coping characteristic "vigor" must strikingly impairs the cardiovascular system.

At a later stage, when underestimation of demands cannot be maintained any longer, due to aggravating conditions (e.g., impact of age), attitudes associated with "immersion" become relevant predictors of cardiovascular vulnerability. "Immersion" indicates a more realistic assessment of coping resources. As can be seen from Figure 2 the typical coping career consists of three roughly idealized stages. At an early stage, "vigor" is the latent factor which has the potential to explain variation of indicators of cardiovascular risk, mainly blood pressure and blood lipids to some degree.

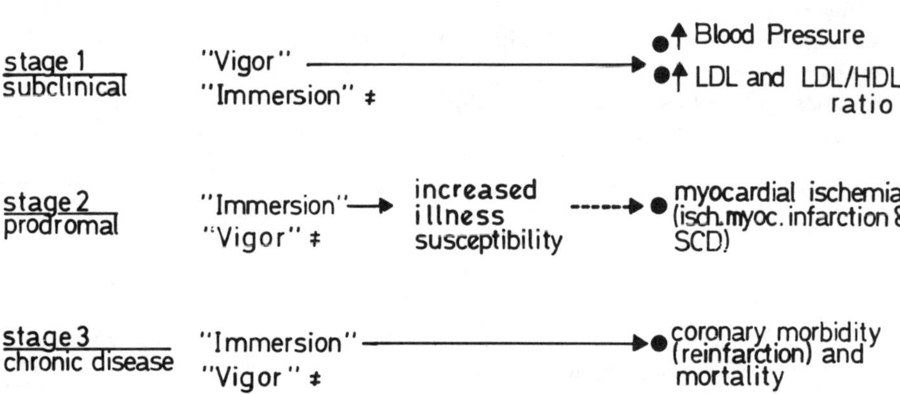

Figure 2. Stages of a typical cardiovascular coping career.

The second stage characterizes groups of highly vulnerable individuals who, in addition to, somatic risk factors and longterm exposure to social stressors, experience an increased susceptibility to cardiovascular disease. This increased susceptibility is manifested, in our view, in recurrent unexplained disruption of nocturnal sleep as well as in feelings of anger and hopelessness which persist over months. In this prodromal stage, the latent factor "immersion" has better predictive power than "vigor" although the two latent factors are consistently positively correlated.

The third stage is that of overt chronic coronary disease where "immersion" continues to be the critical component (20).

Thus, our final proposition states (1) that high levels of "immersion" in these groups are associated with high frequency of unexplained recurrent sleep disturbances and high scores on "feelings of irritation and hopelessness" as indicators of an increased susceptibility; and (2) that individuals who on the basis of these indicators are located at stage II of a cardiovascular coping career are at higher risk of manifest cardiovascular disease onset, especially ischemic heart disease such as acute myocardial infarction and sudden cardiac death.

Materials and Methods

We present some empirical findings on the first and second stage of a cardiovascular coping career. Most of the findings result from an ongoing prospective study of cardiovascular risks in 416 blue-collar metal workers (age 25-55) who were initially free from overt coronary heart disease. The study started in 1982. In the meantime three panel waves have been conducted including medical examination (blood pressure, ECG, blood lipids, weight) and careful assessment of a wide range of subjective psychosocial conditions.

Blood pressure readings by sphygmography were taken according to WHO criteria at standardized diurnal time. Cholesterol, triglycerides, low-density lipoproteins, high-density lipoproteins, and very-low density lipoproteins were assessed by the department of Clinical Chemistry at the University of Göttingen under the direction of Prof. D. Seidel. Body weight and height were registered and a structured interview of about 40 minutes took place. This latter contained information on cardiovascular risk factors, sleep, work stressors, occupational career, interpersonal difficulties, social support, and negative life events.

- t 1 / 1982 — (N=416) = 100% — BP, ECG, Weight/H. - Psych./Soz. I
- t 2 / 1983 — (N=356) = 86% — BP, BLip., Weight/H. - Psych./Soz. I +)
- t 3 / 1985 — (N=317) = 76% — BP, BLip., ECG, Weight/H. - Psych./Soz. I +) PS Stress Test (HR, BP, VPB)

+) as well as special screenings in selected subgroups

Figure 3. Longitudinal study design: Cardiovascular risk of male blue-collar workers (age 25-55) initially free from overt CHD.

Finally a paper-and-pencil-test measuring "need for control" (44 dichotomous items) was applied. Figure 3 summarizes the design.

Additional measurements were conducted in selected subgroups as shown in Figure 4. On the basis of repeated severe recent sleep disturbances individuals were invited to undergo ambulant polysomnographic registration as well as selected clinical examinations such as echocardiography, Holter ECG, exercise ECG, and catheterization.

- t 2 N=20 (representative sample of 78 subj. with severe recent sleep disturbances): ambulant polysomnographic registration (Holter ECG, thoracic and abdominal respiration activity; transcutaneous oxygen tension)
  (clinical screening of sleep apnea positive subj.)
- t 3 N=35 (majority of subj. with untreated borderline hypertension): echocardiographie
  N=12 (subj. with most serious sleep disturbances): Holter ECG (Oxford 4000)

Figure 4. Additional screenings.

Results

Results related to the first proposition are presented in Figure 5, which shows part of a linear structural model which is applied in order to estimate the relative weight of the coping characteristic "vigor" in explaining blood pressure level. Linear structural models provide a combination of factor analysis and path analysis operating with latent variables as well. It is interesting to note that "vigor" exerts a significant influence (see respective γ-coefficients) on the level of systolic blood pressure only under adverse social conditions such as forced piecework (the upper model in Figure 5).

This is a typical example of what we call a psychosocial risk constellation. We need information on both, individual coping characteristics and micro-social environments in order to make meaningful predictions. As can be seen such a contextual model is able to explain much more of the observed blood pressure variation (namely 44%) than a model which includes vigorous persons under non-adversive, non-challenging social conditions (14% of blood pressure variation explained). Finally, what may be striking from the Figure is the fact that the γ-coefficient of "vigor" in metal workers with forced piecework is much higher than coefficients of well-established medical risk factors such as age and overweight (20).

Aggravated working conditions:
metal workers with forced piecework (N = 89)

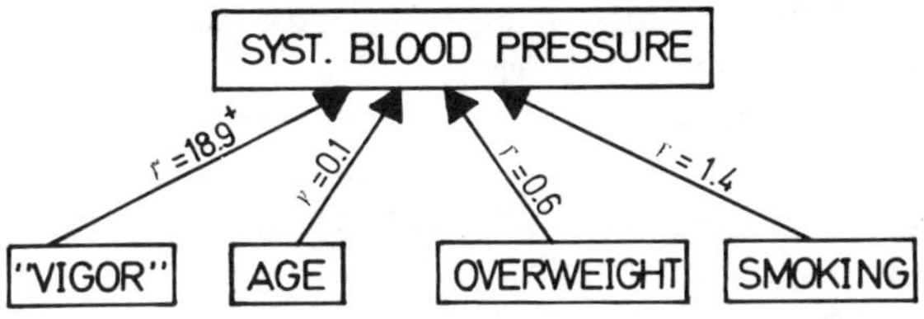

The total model explains 44 % of BP variance

Normal working conditions:
metal workers without forced piecework (N = 199)

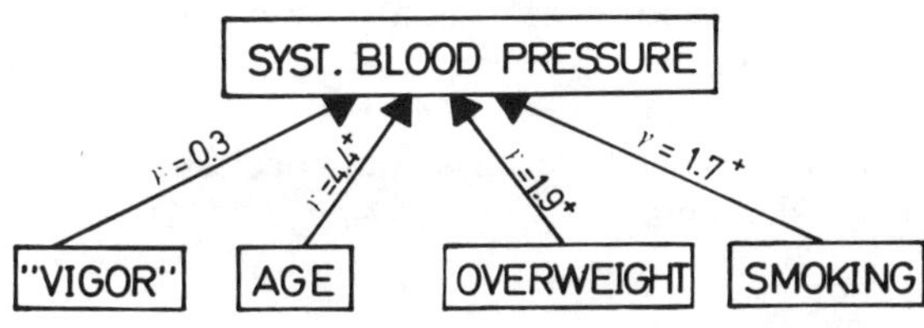

The total model explains 14% of BP variance

+) $p < .05$

Figure 5. Linear structural model (part) in healthy blue-collar workers with (upper part) or without (lower part) forced piecework: Effects of "vigor" on systolic blood pressure (for details see 20).

A second linear structural model has been tested for two subgroups of metal workers: "Medium-to-high-status group" (skilled workers) and "low-status group" (unskilled workers) using the same exogenous and endogenous variables. Here again, a significant effect of "vigor" on the level of systolic blood pressure can be found in the low-status group only, where 54% of blood pressure variation is explained by the model, as compared to 27% in the more privileged group of workers (20).

In order to test the second proposition a linear structural model has been applied to estimate levels of low-density-lipoproteins (LDL) as a critical cardiovascular risk factor. A significant effect of "vigor" on LDL has been demonstrated in the group of workers with already established mild hypercholesterolemia but not in men with normal values (see Figure 6).

The respective γ-coefficient of "vigor" on LDL is about ten times as high in the clinically vulnerable group as compared to the normo-cholesterolemic group. Again, mean LDL level is significantly higher in low-status-workers (after controlling for age, overweight, and cigarette smoking) (20). The same results - but in the opposite direction - were obtained in this model if high-density lipoprotein was selected as the most endogenous variable. This result strengthens the validity of the former findings since opposite biological effects of LDL and HDL are well established.

Further evidence on interactive effects between conditions of active distress and marked hyperlipidemia has been found in studying relationships between severe recent sleep disturbances and level of low-density lipoprotein. The probability of an association between the categories "most severe sleep disturbances" and "low-density lipoprotein-level which needs definite medical treatment" (LDL > 180 mg/100 ml) is significantly beyond chance ($z = 1.64$; $p = 0.05$).

But before presenting results on relationships between sleep disturbances and cardiovascular risk, let us explore psycho-social circumstances of increased illness susceptibility. We pointed out that in a later stage of a coping career the individual recognizes and admits that his capacity to regulate obligations, to keep external demands at a certain distance, has disappeared. Signs of increased illness susceptibility become apparent together with high scores on the latent factor "immersion." Systematic relations between degree of "immersion" and frequency of disrupted sleep as well þs frequency of prolonged feelings of anger and helplessness are expected. Table 1 shows data related to this proposition. Linear regression analysis using data of the first panel wave has been applied in order to estimate effects of "immersion" and of age (as a relevant predictor of sleep disturbances) on frequency of waking up during the night. In addition, effects of "immersion" on two other indicators of increased susceptibility (sustained feelings of anger and sustained feelings of hopelessness) are calculated, again taking age into consideration.

Men with (mild) hypercholesterolemia (N=90)

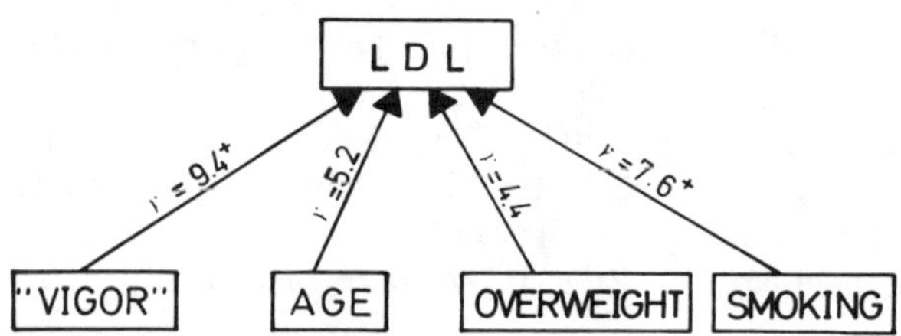

Men with hormocholesterolemia (N =168)

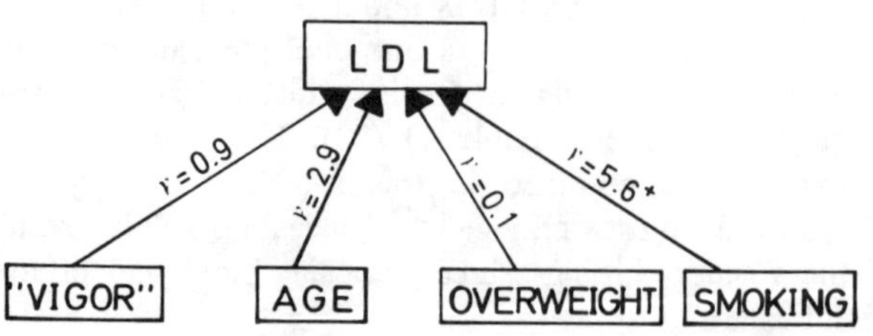

Figure 6. Linear structural model (part) healthy blue-collar workers with (upper part) or without (lower part) hypercholesterolemia: Effects of "Vigor" on low-density lipoprotein (LDL).

Table 1. Linear regression analysis of the latent factors "immersion" and "vigor" of "need for control" and as well as of "age" on: (a) frequency of waking up during night, (b) "sustained feelings of anger" (c) "sustained feelings of hopelessness" in a cohort of healthy blue-collar workers (N=381).

	a) frequency of waking up		b) feelings of anger		c) feelings of hopelessness	
	ß	F	ß	F	ß	F
"immersion"	0.29	28.10**	0.21	14.30*	0.25	19.90**
"vigor"	-0.12	5.20	-0.02	0.10	0.01	0.01
"age"	0.22	21.10**	-0.06	1.80	-0.01	0.01

* $p<0.001$, ** $p<0.0001$

As can be seen, "immersion" exerts a significant effect on frequency of nocturnal sleep disturbances (with a ß-coefficient higher than age). "Immersion" is also significantly related to "sustained feelings of anger" and to "sustained feelings of hopelessness" whereas age does not exert any remarkable effect. The same holds true for "vigor," which is in accordance with our theoretical concept.

These results have been replicated with data from the second panel wave of the same cohort (N=334) where ß-coefficients were somewhat lower although still statistically significant. In a more sophisticated newly developed statistical technique using multiple logistic regression analysis, H. Matschinger and M. Grünewald from our department have demonstrated that the individual's probability of experiencing severe sleep disturbances is highly correlated to the score of "immersion" (as measured by a unidimensional scale) only in a subgroup of workers who can be characterized as living under aggravated socio-economic circumstances (e.g., experience of increased workload during the last year). No such linear relationship is found in workers where stressful social contexts seem to be absent (21) (see Figure 7).

This finding again supports the relevance of an interactive approach in studying psychosocial cardiovascular risk constellations.

The second part of the third proposition, that is the relationship between indicators of increased susceptibility and imminent ischemic heart disease is still under consideration in our prospective study. Figure 8 demonstrates that the three year incidence of hard coronary events (lethal and no±-lethal acute myocardial infarction) is critically increased in our blue-collar population as compared to an age-matched male population where all occupational groups are represented.

The relative risk of 3.2 reflects both higher levels of somatic coronary risk factors and higher levels of experienced active distress due to unfavorable coping conditions.

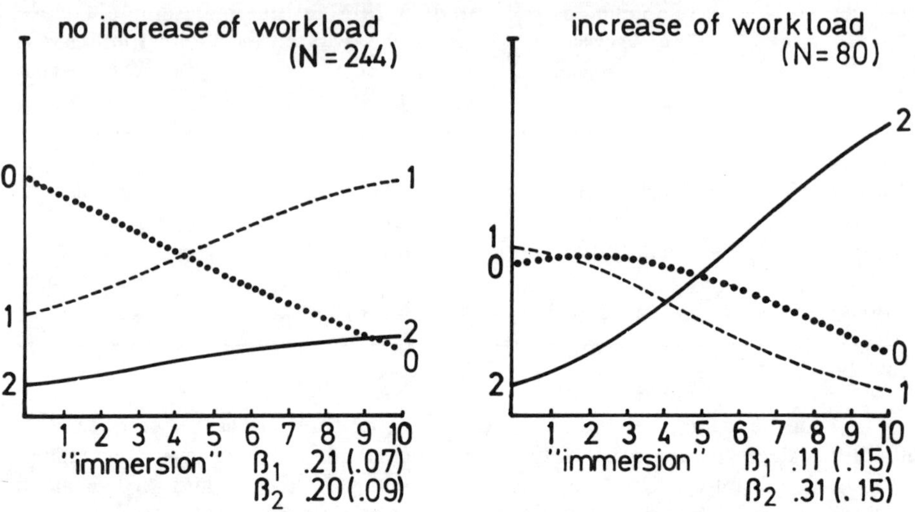

Figure 7. Multiple logistic regression analysis: Relationship between frequency of disrupted nocturnal sleep and score on "immersion" under adverse (right) vs. non-adverse (left) working conditions (for details see 21).

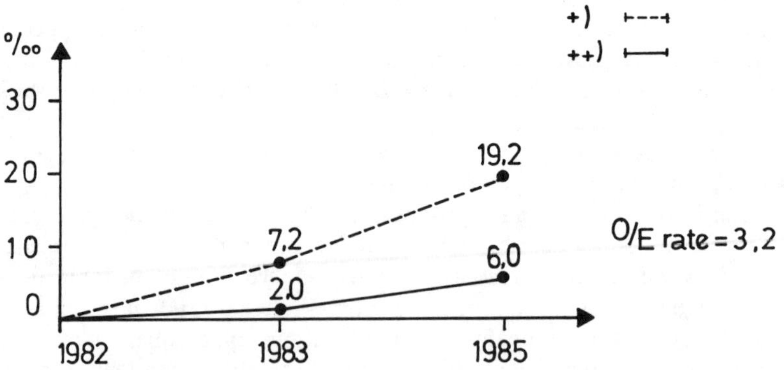

Figure 8. 3-year incidence of acute myocardial infarction (lethal and non-lethal; ICD 410-414) in 365 male blue-collar workers (25-55 y) [+] as compared to the male population (20-64 y) of the WHO myocardial register Heidelberg[++] (in %).

Elsewhere we have shown a marked profile of increased susceptibility due to active distress in the first few victims of hard coronary events (22). After completing the third panel wave, we now can see that 50% of the future victims of lethal or non-lethal myocardial infarction experienced a high frequency of waking up during the night, as compared to 20% in the total sample. 83% of future victims as compared to 43% experienced high or moderate frequency of waking up too early in the morning.

Some further results related to this proposition are restricted to less severe indicators of cardiovascular risk. We mention them rather briefly as they are based on selected subgroups of the total sample.

During the second panel wave we invited a representative sample of all those workers who said they suffered from recurrent unexplained disruption of nocturnal sleep to undergo poly-somnographic registration at least during one night. Very surprisingly, 40% of the sample of apparently healthy men suffering from sleep disturbances exhibited clear signs of sleep apnea (e.g., more than 50 episodes of apnea during more than 10 seconds - most of them more than 20 seconds - in a single night). The only obvious characteristic was obesity (mean: 21% overweight), whereas mean blood pressure was in the upper limit of normal values. Clinical examination demonstrated the presence of marked left ventricular hypertrophy in the sleep apnea-positive persons and an increased risk of arrhythmias (23).

Very recent findings are now available from the third panel wave, inviting a subsample of 12 otherwise healthy blue-collar workers who said they suffered from unexplained severe disruption of nocturnal sleep during the last month to undergo Holter ECG (system Oxford 4000) for one night. Cardiac arrhythmias Lown type 3B were found in two subjects, Lown type 4A in one subject and evidence for a disturbed conductive system of the heart was present in a fourth subject.

Results indicate that unexplained disruptions of nocturnal sleep may serve as an indicator of increased cardiovascular risk although they clearly show different causes: There are somatic conditions such as sleep apnea with its own cardiovascular risk; in rare cases there may even be somatic conditions indicating nocturnal unstable angina, and there is the majority of psychosocial conditions where disrupted sleep is understood as a sign of increased susceptibility to cardiovascular dysfunction.

In our framework it seems worth noting that blue-collars without sleep apnea exhibit significantly increased cyclic variation of heart rate during the night, as compared to men with undisturbed sleep ($T=3.33$; $z=-2.84$; $p<0.01$). They also showed higher values on some of the indicators of psychosocial stress. Elevated heart rate during the night as a consequence of severe daily stress has been reported in experimental animal studies (24). In our approach, we can illustrate this by several case studies, as for example in Figure 9.

The upper part of the Figure shows the typical pattern of mean nocturnal heart rate in a normal subject. This contrasts with the lower part where no obvious difference in heart rate between waking and sleeping can be seen. The subject has reported severe sleep disturbances, marked feelings of helplessness and anger, he has been suffering from increased workload, and in addition he has experienced severe recent life events, among others death of a close family member.

Preliminary conformation of the validity of the indicator "recurrent disruption of nocturnal sleep" for increased susceptibility to imminent overt ischemic heart disease comes from a retroperspective study on men and women who during the last six months experienced an acute myocardial infarction. This shows that every third subject was aware of aggravated sleeping problems during the weeks preceding disease onset (N=44). In their own view 50% of them were primarily due to socioemotional distress, 25% to nocturnal unstable angina and 25% to other somatic complaints.

HOLTER-ECG (Oxford 4000)

a) Normal subject (Nr. 279)

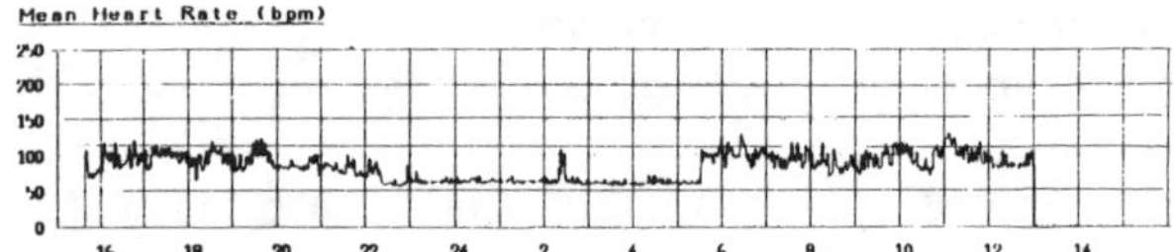

b) Subject with lowered coping threshold (severe unexplained sleep disturbances, marked feelings of helplessness and anger); severe life events (Nr. 196)

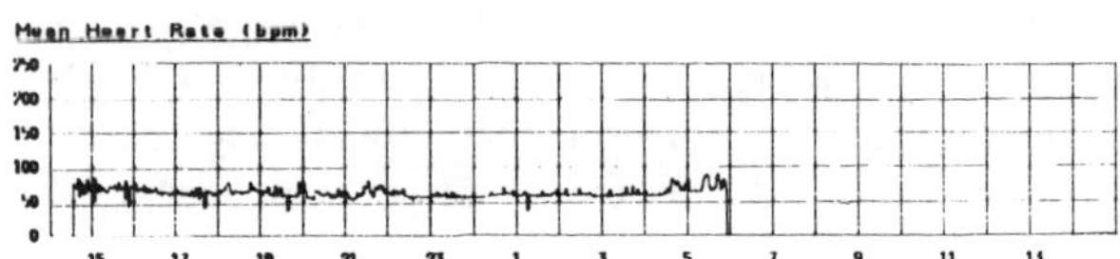

Figure 9. Holter ECG (mean heart rate) during night in two healthy workers: a) without distress, b) with distress.

So far a theoretical model in social epidemiology has been presented which analyses cardiovascular risk in the framework of a coping career, and selected empirical results were demonstrated which gave some support to this approach. The assumption was stated that active distress acts as a crucial link between socioemotional inputs and centrally-mediated cardiovascular dysfunction. The final part of this paper is concerned with major implications of this latter statement.

Activation in the form of active distress is supposed to provoke neural, neuroendocrine and neuroimmune reactions. The most prominent neuroendocrine reactions are the release of pituitary and adrenal hormones where at least three stress axes are involved: The sympatho-adrenomedullary axis, the pituitary-adrenocortical axis and the pituitary-sex-steroid axis (25). Amygdaloid, hippocampal and hypothalamic areas play a decisive role in triggering this release, and it is of special interest to see increasing evidence of a structural and functional role of several neurotransmitters and especially of neuropeptides in regulating pituitary function at the CNS-level. Or, as Bohus has put it: "Stress hormones, particularly neuropeptides belonging to the second generation, modulate brain processes that organize specific and non-specific adaptive behavior" (26). More recently, Brown and Fisher have argued that peptides are likely candidates for mediating the coordinated endocrine and autonomic responses essential for homeostasis of the organism (27), and they have shown respective functions for thyrotropin releasing factor, corticotropin releasing factor, angiotensin II and other peptides.

Expertise and time is actually lacking to demonstrate intimate relations between these second generation stress hormones and the classical monoaminergic and serotonergic systems, but two facts seem to justify a prominent role of the peptidergic system in health and disease: First the fact that central and peripheral existence of receptors for peptide-hormones including in the gut, the cardiovascular system and the immune system, is now well established (28), and secondly the fact that peptides seem to be responsible for effects with a slow onset and a long duration (29).

This latter fact fits with Herbert Weiner's notion that higher nervous activity caused by distress acts as a "bias" which gradually impairs the respective peripheral - e.g., cardiovascular - system (30). We would like to elaborate this point to some degree as it is essential for an interpretation of our epidemiologic findings in terms of possibly underlying pathophysiology.

A better understanding of molecular biology of the cell has opened new vistas on maladaptive receptor function due to sustained hormonal activation. It is well known that hormones initiate a biologic action by binding to specific cellular recognition sites (receptors). At least for two types of receptors, ß-adrenergic receptors (31) and hepatic LDL receptors (32), it has been shown that alterations in receptor-coupling do occur not only as a function of structural (e.g., genetic) deficiency but also as a function of hormonal overstimulation. Lefkowitz et al. recently presented convincing data on a bifunctional nature of adrenergic receptors, i.e., binding and activation. Longlasting or excessive hormonal stimulation impairs binding capacity of the receptor and thus induces desensitization of subsequent activation. A major pathway leading to such receptor desensitization has already been identified as "down-regulation" or loss of receptors from cell surface (31).

In patients with congestive heart failure it has been demonstrated that the density of ß-adrenergic receptors in the failed left ventricles of heart-transplant recipients was 50% lower than that in control tissue taken from transplant donors (33). The role of receptor desensitization in the development of primary hypertension is still controversial. One group has postulated that a reduction in vascular ß-adrenergic receptors, with no chance in α-adrenergic receptors in the face of increased sympatho-adrenal-drive, could lead to unchecked vasoconstriction and hypertension (34).

Very recently Muranaka et al. found decreased vascular sensitivity to noradrenaline in coronary-prone type A subjects, perhaps due to down-regulation secondary to chronically high catecholamine secretion during stress (35). The centrally-mediated neurohormonal mechanisms which facilitate the development of some forms of primary hypertension are a matter far too difficult to be touched by this paper. These few suggestions nevertheless show that observed epidemiologic relationships between indicators of sustained active distress and high levels of blood pressure are in accordance with recent concepts of biased coupling between hormones and adrenergic receptors. Goldstein et al., in studying relationships between defective lipoprotein receptors and arteriosclerosis (32) have admitted that a variety of non-genetic exogenous factors raise LDL-levels in part by suppressing the synthesis of hepatic LDL-receptors. No study until now has demonstrated neurohormonal influences on this chain of events. Such influences nevertheless are highly probable. Epinephrine-mediated increase in plasma cholesterol has been documented in humans by Dimsdale et al. (36), and Manuck et al. could demonstrate that under conditions of atherogenic diet only social stress resulted in a significant increase of coronary artery arteriosclerosis (9). Thus epidemiologic associations between indicators of sustained active distress and lipid levels might be in accordance with recent developments in basic and clinical research.

More data are already available on influences of the peptidergic system on sleep regulation. For example the delta-sleep-inducing peptide (DSIP) has shown anti-stress properties in animal studies, and peptides may also be involved in the disturbance of a functional balance between serotonergic and catecholaminergic systems and subsequently in the disruption of regular sleep pattern (37).

Finally, the role of neural and neurohormonal processes in triggering cardiac arrhythmias, thrombosis, and ischemia leading to acute myocardial infarction is beyond the scope of this paper and has been elaborated in a series of recent publications (38-40).

In conclusion, we can state that observed statistical relationships in socioepidemiologic research support the concept of neuronal control of bodily function, at least if markers of cardiovascular risk are taken into consideration.

The basic question whether we are ready to consider human adaptive diseases as "biopsychsocial phenomena" is still unanswered. What is the relation of social to biological processes in disease? Only rarely has this question been raised (18) as psychosomatics, psychoneuroendocrinology and psychoneuroimmunology focus on the single person and its organism rather than on networks of inter-depending individuals. Yet, the social dimension of an individual's life is crucial as far as development, learning, and brain organization is concerned (41, 42). Animal studies suggest that the limbic system, and more specifically the amygdaloid and the septo-hippocampal systems act as a kind of target site for socio-environmental input into neocortical areas. For example, the corticomedial amygdala is involved in aggressive and flight-motivated agonistic behavior in rats and, thus, is likely candidate for neural structures involved in the more general processing of social experiences (43, 44). The septo-hippocampal system has been related to the storing of spatial memory, and this may include an individual's social space as well (18, 45). Threats to one's acquired social status, disruption of intimate social bonds, continuous frustration of expectations (as in the case of active distress) can evoke powerful neurohormonal dysbalance and by doing so impair peripheral organ systems. Clearly such a system of hierarchial relationships between social environment, brain function and adaptive disease has to be explored in much more detail in future work. It is only on the basis of such work that a clear-cut concept of adaptive human disease as a bio-psychosocial phenomenon can be expected.

References

1. Ganong, W.F. (in press). The neuroendocrine system. First Annual International Symposium Neuronal Control of Bodily Function.
2. Felten, D.L. & Felten, S.Y. (in press). Overview of the autonomic nervous system. First International Symposium Neuronal Control of Bodily Function.
3. Hall, N., McGillis, J., Spangelo, B., et al. (1984). Immune regulation of the hypothalamic-hypophyseal-adrenal axis: A role for thymosins and lymphokines. In R.E. Ballieux (Ed.), Breakdown in human adaptation to stress. M. Nijhoff, p. 722-731.
4. Mehrishi, J.N. & Millcs, J.H. (198?). Opiate receptors on lymphocytes and platelets in men. Clin. Immunol. Immunopathol., 27: 240.
5. Engel, G.E. (1977). The need for a new medical model: A challenge for biomedicine. Science, 196: 139.
6. Mason, J.W. (1971). A reevaluation of the concept of "Nonspecificity" in stress theory. J. Psychiat. Res., 8: 323.
7. Hamilton, V. & Warburton, D.M. (1979). Human stress and cognition. Wiley, Chichester, N.Y.
8. Weiner, H. (1977). Psychobiology in human disease. Elsevier, N.Y.
9. Manuck, S.P., Caplan, J.R. & Clarkson, T.B. (1983). Social instability and coronary artery arteriosclerosis in cynomolgus monkies. Neurosci. Biobehav. Rev., 7: 485.
10. Tapp, W.N., Levin, B.E. & Natelson, B.H. (1983). Stress induced heart failure. Psychosom. Med., 45: 171.
11. Ursin, H. (1984). Expectancy and activation: An attempt to systematise stress theory. Unpubl. manuscript.
12. Siegrist, J., Dittmann, K.H., Rittner, K. & Weber, I. (1982). The social context of active distress in patients with early myocardial infarction. Soc. Sci. Med., 16: 443.
13. Karasek, R., Russell, S. & Theorell, T. (1982). Physiology of stress and regeneration in job related cariovascular illness. J. Hum. Stress, 8: 29.
14. Weber, I. (1984). Berufstätigkeit, Belastungserfahrung und koronares Risiko. Minerva, München.
15. Glass, D.C. (1977). Behavior pattern, stress and coronary disease. Erlbaum, Hillsdale.
16. Siegrist, J., Dittmann, K.H., Rittner, K. & Weber, I. (1980). Soziale Belastungen und Herzinfarkt. Enke, Stuttgart.
17. Henry, J.P. & Stephens, P.M. (1977). Stress, health and the social environment. Springer-Verlag, Berlin, N.Y., Heidelberg.
18. Henry, J.P. (1982). The relation of social to biological processes in disease. Soc. Sci. & Med., 16: 369.
19. Dembroski, T., Schmidt, P. & Blümchen, G. (Eds.) (1983). Biobehavioral bases of coronary heart disease. Karger, Basel.
20. Matschinger, H., Siegrist, J., Siegrist, K. & Dittmann, K.H. (1986). Type A as a coping career - towards a conceptual and methodological redefinition. In T.H. Schmidt, T.M. Dembroski & G. Blümchen (Eds.), Biological and psychological factors in cardivascular disease. Springer-Verlag, Berlin, p. 104-126
21. Siegrist, J. & Peter, J.H. (1986). Schlafstörungen und cardiovaskuläres Risiko. Medizinische Klinik, 81: 429.
22. Siegrist, J. (1984). Threat to social status and cardiovascular risk. Psychother. Psychosom., 42: 90.
23. Peter, J.H., Siegrist, J., Podszus, T., Mayer, J., Selzer, K. & von Wichert, P. (1985). Prevalence of sleep apnea in healthy industrial workers. Klin. Wochenschr., 63: 807.
24. Van Holst, D. (1986). Psychosocial stress and its pathophysiological effects in free shrews. In T.H. Schmidt, T.M. Demborski & G. Blümchen (Eds.), Biological and physiological factors in cardiovascular disease. Springer-Verlag, Berlin, p. 476-490.

25. Henry, J.P. (1983). Coronary heart disease and arousal of the adrenal cortical axis. In T. Dembroski, P. Schmidt & G. Blümchen (Eds.), Biobehavioral bases of coronary heart disease. Karger, Basel, p. 365-381.
26. Bohus, B. (1984). Endocrine infuence on disease outcome: Experimental findings and implication. J. Psychosom. Res., 28: 429.
27. Brown, M.R. & Fisher, L.A. (1984). Brain peptides as intercellular messengers. JAMA 251, 1310.
28. Krieger, D.T. & Martin, J.B. (1982). Brain peptides. N. Engl. J. Med., 304: 876.
29. Hökfelt, T. (in press). Neuropeptides and their possible role as auxiliary messengers. In First Annual International Symposium Neuronal Control of Bodily Function.
30. Weiner, H. (1984). The prospects for psychosomatic medicine: Selected topics. Psychosom. Med., 44: 491.
31. Lefkowitz, R.J., Caron, N.G. & Stiles, G.L. (1984). Mechanisms of membrane receptors regulation. N. Engl. J. Med., 310: 1570.
32. Goldstein, J.L., Kita, T. & Brown, M.S. (1983). Defective lipoprotein receptors and artherosclerosis. N. Engl. J. Med., 309: 288.
33. Bristow, M.R., Ginsburg, R., Minobe, W., et al. (1982). Decreased catecholamine sensitivity and ß-adrenergic receptor density in failing human hearts. N. Engl. J. Med., 307: 205.
34. Woodcock, E.A., Olsson, C.A. & Johnston, C.I. (1980). Reduced vascular ß-adrenergic receptors in DOCA salt hypertensive rats. Biochem. Pharmacol., 29: 1645.
35. Muranaka, M., Monou, H. & Suzuki, J. (1985). Family history of hypertension and type A behavior pattern modulate cardiovascular responses to isoproterenol and norepinephrine. Paper presented at the 8th World Congress of Psychosomatic Medicine Chicago.
36. Dimsdale, J.E., Herd, J.A. & Hardly, L.H. (1983). Epinephrine-mediated increases in plasma cholesterol. Psychosom. Med., 45: 227.
37. Monnier, M. (1983). Functions of the nervous system, Vol. 4. Elsevier, Amsterdam, N.Y., Oxford, p. 161-220.
38. Lown, B., DeSilva, R.A. & Lenson, R. (1978). Roles of psychologic stress and autonomic nervous system changes in provocation of ventricular premature complexes. Am. J. Cardiol., 41.
39. Bull, J.C. & Elliot, R.S. (1980). Psychosocial and behavioral influences in the pathogenesis of acquired cardiovascular disease. Am. Heart J., 100: 723.
40. Deanfield, J.E., Kensett, M., Wilson, R.A., et al. (1984). Silent myocardial ischemia due to mental stress. Lancet, 3: 1001.
41. Mead, G.H. (1962). Mind, self and society. Chicago.
42. Changeux, P. (1983). Der neuronale Mensch. Rowohlt, Hamburg.
43. Bolhuis, J.J., Fitzgerald, R.E., Dijk, D.J. & Koolhaas, J.M. (1984). The corticomedial-amygdala and learning in an agonistic situation in rat. Physiol. Behav., 32: 575.
44. Fokkema, D.S. (1985). Social behavior and blood pressure, a study of rats. Groningen (unpublished manuscript).
45. Gray, J.A. (1985). Emotional behavior and the limbic system. In M.R. Trimble (Ed.), Interface between neurology and psychiatry. Karger, Basel, München, p. 1-25.

Sympathetic Afferents

and Positive Feedback Mechanisms

Federico Lombardi, Tomaso Gnecchi Ruscone,
Gabriella Malfatto and Alberto Malliani

As a result of extensive electrophysiological studies it has been demonstrated that afferent sympathetic nerve fibers with cardiac and aortic receptors, in the anesthetized animal under apparently normal resting conditions, display a tonic impulse activity in response to normal and specific hemodynamic stimuli (1, 2). In different experimental models sympathetic cardiovascular afferent fibers were also found to be sensitive to chemical and mechanical events, a characteristic that makes them particularly suited to signal physiological and pathophysiological events. Their reflex function was investigated in response to electrical (3, 4), mechanical (4-6) and chemical (7, 8) stimuli. The overall result was that the activation of sympathetic cardiovascular afferent fibers was mainly associated to excitatory reflexes possessing positive feedback characteristics, as discussed in the following sections.

In vagotomized cats with both carotid arteries occluded, stretching the wall of the thoracic aorta with a special cannula without obstructing the flow, thus simulating an increase in mean arterial pressure, was associated to a reflex increase in heart rate, in blood pressure and in myocardial contractility (9). These experiments, in which supraspinal inhibitory mechanisms were not operative, were the first evidence of spinal excitatory reflexes exhibiting positive feedback characteristics.

In conscious dogs with intact innervation, the stretch of a segment of the thoracic aorta was also accompanied by an increment of mean arterial pressure, left ventricular pressure, left ventricular dP/dt and heart rate (10). These reflexes, which were independent of pain, confirmed the occurrence of sympathetic excitatory reflexes also in conscious and fully innervated animals and suggested that the excitatory mechanisms mediated by the cardiovascular sympathetic afferents could participate in the control of cardiovacular functions in different physiological and pathophysiological conditions.

In particular, we have recently advanced the hypothesis that excitatory sympathetic reflexes may play an important role in the genesis of arterial hypertension (11, 12). It has been previously suggested that hypertension can be considered as a disease of regulation (13): It is a common opinion that such a disturbance could be caused by an increased sympathetic tone. According to our positive feedback hypothesis, this increase may be related not only to an augmented central command but also to the peripheral action of sympatho-sympathetic circuits (12).

An indirect support to this concept may be derived by considering the mechanisms of action of ß-adrenergic blocking agents in the treatment of hypertension. The progressive decrease in total peripheral resistance that occurs with chronic administration despite a reduction of cardiac output is difficult to explain (14). It is interesting what has been proposed by Lewis (15) and Vaughan Williams (16) as a determinant component of the antihypertensive effects of ß-blockers: According to their hypothesis an attenuation of the sensory input from the cardiovascular system to the supraspinal structures could result in a diminished sympathetic outflow directed back to the cardiovascular system. However, it is clear that a reduced sensory input in a negative feedback model should correspond to an increase of activity in the output.

We have recently evaluated the effects of propranolol on the firing rate of aortic and pulmonary vein sympathetic afferent fibers (17). The study was restricted to this specific population of fibers capable of mediating excitatory sympathetic reflexes (1, 2).

Experiments were carried out in vagotomized cats anesthetized with chloralose, paralyzed and artificially ventilated. After removing the heads of the second and third ribs, the stellate ganglion and its branches were exposed on the left side. Afferent neural impulse activity was recorded from filaments isolated under a dissection microscope from the cut peripheral end of the third and fourth left thoracic sympathetic rami communicantes. Filaments were split until discharge from a single active unit was present.

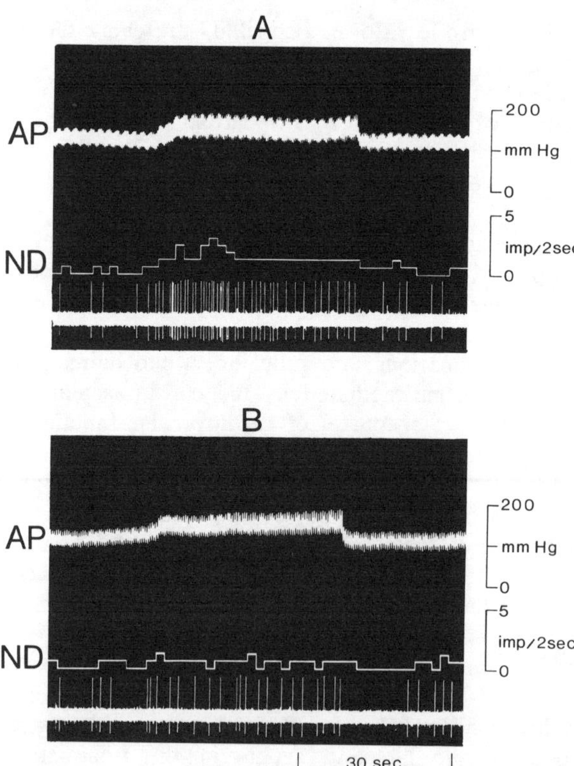

Figure 1. Effects of a brief occlusion of the thoracic aorta on the impuls activity of an afferent sympathetic fiber with sensory field in the aorta before (A) and after (B) d-l propanolol administration. AP = arterial pressure; ND = neural discharge; presented as histogram of neural activity and as analogue recording (17; unpublished).

A preliminary localization of the endings was performed at the beginning of the recording phase by light mechanical probing of the aorta or the pulmonary veins. A definite localization was always obtained at the end of the experiment by repeating the probing procedure. The mechanical properties of aortic and pulmonary vein fibers were assessed by their response to increases in aortic pressure produced by distal thoracic aortic constrictions. After 2-3 control occlusions propranolol (0.2-0.4 mg/kg) was injected intravenously over a five-minute period and the constrictions were repeated.

Results and Discussion

The data in Figure 1A show that aortic occlusion caused a significant increase in the firing rate of sympathetic afferents, that persisted throughout the rise in pressure.

NEURAL DISCHARGE DURING AORTIC OCCLUSION

(Aortic fibers , n =11)

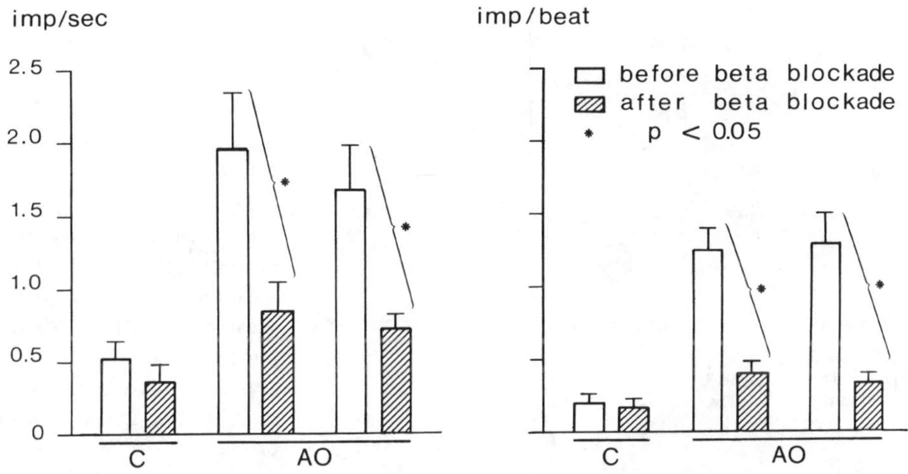

Figure 2. Effects of aortic pressure rises on the neural discharge of 11 sympathetic afferent fibers with sensory field in the aorta, before and after d-l propranolol administration, during the early phase of the pressure rise as well as during the stable phase. Neural discharge is presented both in impulses/sec and in impulses/beat, thus taking into account the bradycardia induced by ß-adrenergic blockade. Notice the markedly different responses before and after drug injection.

Propranolol administration did not significantly modify the resting firing rate of the sympathetic units under study but markedly blunted their response to a similar mechanical stimulus (Figure 1B). These effects were evident during the early and late phases of the occlusion and were already evident when the firing rate of the fibers were expressed in impulses every cardiac beat (Figure 2). From these experiments we concluded that ß-adrenergic receptor blockade can reduce the responsiveness to similar increases in arterial blood pressure of cardiovascular sympathetic afferent fibers thus modifying the afferent component of the excitatory reflexes.

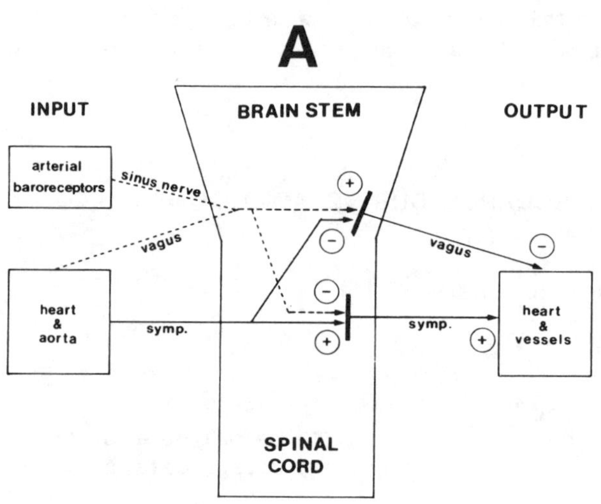

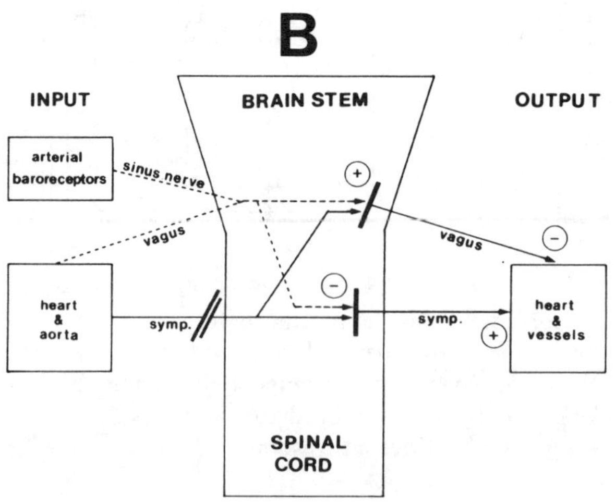

Figure 3. Schema of the interaction between the reflexes mediated from the heart and aorta by cardiovascular and sympathetic afferents possessing positive feedback characteristics, and supraspinal reflexes with negative feedback properties (A). By interrupting sympathetic afferents from the heart and aorta (B) by cutting the dorsal roots from C8 to T6, the inhibitory influence of supraspinal reflexes becomes more evident.

The different concept of neural regulation of cardiovascular functions consisting in an interaction of negative and positive feedback reflex mechanisms is further emphasized by more recent ongoing experiments.

Hemodynamic events, such as arterial pressure rises, constitute a stimulus capable of activating mechanoreceptive endings of both vagal and sympathetic afferent fibers, impinging upon either supraspinal or spinal structure and mediating inhibitory and excitatory reflexes (1, 2). Thus, also the reflex bradycardia which accompanies arterial pressure rises and which is traditionally interpreted as arising from a single reflexogenic area (i.e., carotid and aortic arterial baroreceptors) (19) is likely to be the result of a complex interplay of opposite mechanisms. We therefore compared the effect of interrupting the excitatory influences mediated by sympathetic afferents, in the reflex bradycardia induced by arterial pressure rises.

As illustrated in the schema of Figure 3, the interruption of a large part of cardiovascular sympathetic afferents was obtained by sectioning the spinal dorsal roots from C8 to T6. After rhizotomy, only afferents inpinging upon supraspinal structure mediating inhibitory reflexes were operative. Preliminary results, obtained in chloralose anesthetized as well as in some decerebrate cats (19), indicate that the heart rate reduction induced by similar arterial pressure rises was enhanced after dorsal root section. Thus, the interruption of excitatory influences mediated by cardiovascular sympathetic afferent fibers can produce a further prevalence of the inhibitory baroreceptive mechanisms.

Conclusion

Experimental data support the concept that the neural control of circulation is likely to operate through an integration of opposite mechanisms. Sympathetic afferents, which are tonically active, not only mediate reflexes with positive feedback properties, but also modulate the supraspinal negative feedback mechanisms.

References

1. Malliani, A. (1982). Cardiovascular sympathetic afferent fibers. Rev. Physiol. Biochem. Pharmacol., 94: 11-74.
2. Bishop, V.S., Malliani, A. & Thoren, P. (1983). Cardiac mechanoreceptors. In J.T. Shepherd, F.M. Abboud & S.R. Geiger (Eds.), Handbook of physiology, section 2: The cardiovascular system. Vol. III, Peripheral circulation and organ blood flow. Bethesda, American Physiological Society.
3. Schwartz, P.J., Pagani, M., Lombardi, F., Malliani, A. & Brown, A.M. (1973). A cardiocardiac sympathovagal reflex in the cat. Circ. Res., 32: 215-220.
4. Uchida, Y., Kamisaka, K., Murao, S. & Ueda, H. (1974). Mechanosensitivity of afferent cardiac sympathetic nerve fibers. Am. J. Physiol., 226: 1088-1093.
5. Lombardi, F., Malliani, A. & Pagani, M. (1976). Nervous activity of afferent sympathetic fibers innervating the pulmonary veins. Brain Res., 113: 197-200.
6. Casati, R., Lombardi, F. & Malliani, A. (1979). Afferent sympathetic unmyelinated fibers with left ventricular endings in cats. J. Physiol., 292: 135-148.
7. Kaufman, M.P., Baker, D.G., Coleridge, H.M. & Coleridge, J.C.G. (1980). Stimulation by bradykinin of afferent vagal C-fibers with chemosensitive endings in the heart and aorta of the dog. Circ. Res., 46: 476-484.

8. Lombardi, F., Della Bella, P., Casati, R. & Malliani, A. (1981). Effects of intracoronary administration of bradykinin on the impulse activity of afferent sympathetic unmyelinated fibers with left ventricular endings in the cat. Circ. Res., 48: 69-75.
9. Lioy, F., Malliani, A., Pagani, M., Recordati, G. & Schwartz, P.J. (1974). Reflex hemodynamic responses initiated from the thoracic aorta. Circ. Res., 34: 78-84.
10. Pagani, M., Pizzinelli, P., Bergamaschi, M. & Malliani, A. (1982). A positive feedback sympathetic pressor reflex during stretch of the thoracic aorta in conscious dogs. Circ. Res., 50: 125-132.
11. Malliani, A., Lombardi, F., Pagani, M., Recordati, G. & Schwartz, P.J. (1975). Spinal sympathetic reflexes in the cat and the pathogenesis of arterial hypertension. Clin. Sci. Mol. Med., 48: 259s-267s.
12. Malliani, A., Pagani, M. & Bergamaschi, M. (1979). Positive feedback sympathetic reflexes and hypertension. Am. J. Cardiol., 44: 860-865.
13. Page, I.H. (1974). Arterial hypertension in retrospect. Circ. Res., 34: 133-142.
14. Tarazi, R. & Dustan, H.P. (1972). ß-adrenergic blockade in hypertension. Am. J. Cardiol., 29: 633-640.
15. Lewis, P. (1960). The essential action of propranolol in hypertension. Am. J. Med., 60: 837-852.
16. Vaughan Williams, E.M. (1977). Adaption of the heart and sympathetic system to prolonged adrenoreceptor blockade. Proc. Soc. Med., 70 (suppl.II): 49-59.
17. Lombardi, F., Casalone, C., Malfatto, G., Gnecchi Ruscone, T., Casati, R. & Malliani, A. (1986). Effects of propranolol on the impulse activity of cardiovascular sympathetic afferent fibers. Hypertension, 8: 50-55.
18. Heymans, C. & Neil, E. (1958). Reflexogenic areas of the cardiovascular system. Churchill, London.
19. Gnecchi Ruscone, T., Lombardi, F., Malfatto, G., Di Mattia, D., Canesi, M. & Malliani, A. (1986). Modulation of baroflexly mediated bradycardia by sympathetic afferents. Eur. J. Clin. Invest., 16 (II): 71

Hypertension and the Brain

Herbert Weiner

The idea that the brain participates in the etiology, pathogenesis, pathophysiology, or maintenance of high blood pressure (BP) in man has had a checkered history. Its status has received desultory support ever since Goldblatt (1) showed that constriction of one renal artery in a dog raised its BP. Over the next two decades the mechanism of this effect was elucidated: A fall in intravascular pressure in the artery releases renin. This enzyme converts angiotensinogen into angiotensin II, a potent vasoconstrictor, and an agonist that promotes the release of mineralocorticoid, aldosterone, from adrenal cortical cells. Aldosterone controls the renal reabsorption of the sodium ion and thus of water. During the decade when this mechanism was elucidated, it was also demonstrated that the administration of desoxycorticosterone acetate (DOCA) and the feeding of salt to rats could produce high BP. And thus the matter stood; the focus of hypertension research was on the pathogenetic role of the kidney, the sodium ion and its regulation and, therefore, on blood volume. These themes were, of course, played with some variations: Increased intracellular (cytosolic) sodium is still a fashionable candidate for causing high BP, or investigators have sought for a chemically - unidentified substance produced by the kidney that incited high BP in normotensive animals when they were transfused with the blood of hypertensive animals or human beings.

However, several lines of evidence did not fit into this scheme; for example, some hypertensive patients could be "cured" by lumbo-sacral sympathectomy; other patients had low levels of plasma renin activity (PRA), or high levels of blood norepinephrine (NE). It has only recently been realized that the control of renin release was not only controlled by the pressure within the renal artery, but by beta-adrenergic sympathetic activity (2). Furthermore, an isorenin-angiotensin system is resent in the hypothalamus (3, 4). Finally, there is increasing evidence that human ("essential") hypertension is not a uniform disease, but is a syndrome (5, 6): It is unlikely that a single "cause" accounts for its various forms.

The Secondary Role of the Brain in Experimental High BP

A major revision in thinking about experimental high BP came about with the demonstration that the brain is also involved in raising BP when the two

Supported in part by a grant from the John D. & Catherine C. Marthur Foundation: "Health-damaging and Health-promoting Behavior."

methods - renal artery constriction, and DOCA-salt administration - were used to incite it. These experiments showed that:

1) The brain participates at some stage in the initiation and maintenance of high BP.
2) The brain stem mechanisms are different during the initial induction phase versus the subsequent sustaining phase of experimental high BP.

The development of high BP in animals subjected to renal artery constriction was averted by pretreatment with 6-hydroxydopamine (6-OHDA) instilled into the fourth ventricle. But once high BP levels were established in these animals, 6-OHDA treatment no longer lowered BP (7, 8). The sequence of events was as follows: Constricting the renal artery released renin whereby angiotensin II was produced. Angiotensin II entered the brain via the *area postrema* (8, 9) to produce powerful pressor effects that are in turn mediated by sympathetic discharge and norepinephrine (10-12). Angiotensin II, when infused in very small amounts intervertebrally, significantly increased BP. Its effects could be blocked by pretreatment with reserpine (12), and by destruction of inhibitory brain stem catecholaminergic neurons. The increase in centrally mediated sympathetic activity not only produced vasoconstriction but released more renin from the kidney (13).

Desoxycorticosterone-salt hypertension in rats was associated with an increase in the activity of peripheral sympathetic nerves and of the adrenal medulla (14, 15). While peripheral sympathetic activity increased, a decrease occurred in NA turnover rates in the medulla oblongata (15). Sympathetic ganglionic blocking agents lowered the BP of pretreated rats but did not increase NA turnover rates in the medulla oblongata. The lowered turnover rates in the medulla oblongata were related to the increased peripheral sympathetic activity. If NA neurons in the medulla oblongata were destroyed by the prior intraventricular installation of 6-OHDA, high BP levels and the increased peripheral sympathetic activity were prevented from occurring in rats (7). Once high BP levels were established in these rats, 6-OHDA treatment did not lower them (7, 16).

Desoxycorticosterone-salt hypertension in rats is, therefore, mediated through the participation of the brain stem. Once high BP levels are established, some other mechanisms sustain them, because destruction of NA neurons in the medulla oblongata only prevents the development of hypertension but does not "cure" it. Thus a dual brain mechanism is involved: One initiates (is pathogenetic) and the other sustains increased BP levels. To those with a "peripheralist" bias for explaining high BP, this work must be disconcerting.

The Primary Role of the Brain in Experimental High BP

Experiments in animals underscore the fact that high BP may be initiated and maintained by a variety of ways. In one rat model - the Kyoto Wistar strain (SHR) - the brain plays a primary role in initiating the rise in BP, in other related animal strains, it plays a secondary role. This principle is illustrated by related animal strains, it plays a secondary role. This principle is illustrated by comparing the two closely related strains. In the Milan Wistar strain, the origins of the high BP seem to reside in the kidney (17, 18). By contrast, the primary pathogenetic factors in the SHR strain are mediated both by enhanced sympathetic outflow and by adrenocorticotrophic hormone (ACTH), and possibly thyrotropin (TSH) (19). Subsequent changes in the resistance vessels, the kidney, and the chemical composition of the heart occur to sustain high BP (18). However, environmental influences interact with genetic predisposition in such animals: The development of high BP may be slowed by socially isolating very young animals of this strain (20), and may be accelerated by shocking them with electricity (21).

Research on the SHR illustrates the thesis that the initiation and maintenance of high BP are mediated through different brain mechanisms. To illustrate: Injections of 6-OHDA (which causes degeneration of noradrenergic and dopaminergic nerve endings in the brain and depletion of their transmitter stores), into the lateral ventricles of young rats of this strain prevented the development of elevated BP levels (18). But the intraventricular injections of 6-OHDA, did not lower high BP levels once established (16, 22). Therefore, NA and dopaminergic neurons in the brain play a role in the initiation, but do not seem to play a role in the maintenance of high BP. Once established, the high BP levels are maintained by serotonergic neurons in the brain since parachlorphenylaline, which depresses serotonin synthesis, reduced high systolic BP in this rat strain (23).

But additional factors in other regions of the brain sustain high BP in the SHR. The intraventricular injection of a competitive antagonist of angiotensin lowered BP levels in SHR's after bilateral nephrectomy. The brain isorenin-angiotensin systems apparently maintain high blood pressure. In addition, angiotensin levels are high in the cerebrospinal fluid of these rats before they develop high BP (24). Angiotensin excites neurosecretory neurons in the cat's brain and stimulates catecholaminergic release (3, 4, 25, 26).

The formulation that high BP in the SHR is due to the unfolding of a genetic program, and that it is "spontaneous" is an oversimplification. It is clear that BP levels can be manipulated by prior social experience or shocking these animals with electricity.

A wide variety of smells, sounds, and social behaviors play a role in altering BP levels in other models of experimental high BP. When the milieu of a dog's brain was altered by infusion of angiotensin II into the vertebral arteries (27), or when the nucleus of the tractus solitarius in the cat's brain was lesioned (28), mean BP levels were raised and BP lability was much increased, especially during the day. Everyday sounds were particularly prone to produce such BP fluctuations, as were the act of eating, grooming behavior, the sight and smell of food, touch, and novel and conditioning stimuli. Reis (28) concluded that brain stem baroreceptor mechanisms (whose neurotransmitter is thought to be L-glutamic acid) usually buffer sympathetically mediated vasoconstrictor discharge (and thus phasic BP increases) against sensory and conditioning stimuli and aroused emotions. The source of the vasoconstrictor discharge lies rostral to the medulla in the anterior basal hypothalamus.

Thus these experimental procedures not only alter the regulation of tonic levels and phasic increases of BP levels, but also alter the response of the BP to sensory input of various kinds. They change the animal's behavior and circulatory responses to the environment.

Evidence for the Role of the Nervous System in Hypertension Derived from the Action of Anti-Hypertensive Agents

The pharmacological action of a drug does not permit inferences about the etiology or pathogenesis of disease (congestive heart failure is not due to a lack of digitalis). Yet the action of a drug suggests that a particular system is involved at some stage in a disease's unfolding (see above).

The fact is that all of the drugs used in the treatment of human hypertension - with the exception of diuretic agents - act upon the central nervous system or its autonomic extensions into the body. Reserpine, alpha-methyl dopa, clonidine and even propranolol act centrally. Propranolol (a "beta blocker") and hexamethonium (a "ganglionic blocker") also act on one or other aspect of sympathetic neural mechanisms. That is not to say that they work in all persons. But the argument could well be advanced that they would have no value in the therapy of hypertension, if neural and neuronal mechanisms did not participate at some stage in its development.

Experimental High BP in Animals: Evidence for the Participation of the Brain

Above three methods for producing high BP in animals were described. Many other techniques have been used to promote high BP (29), for example by :

1) Conditioned responses: Classical, operant, avoidant and emotional.
2) Sensory stimulation: Loud sounds, blasting animals with air.
3) Brain stimulation, and lesions.
4) Crowding animals together.
5) Restraining animals.
6) Breeding specific strains of rats.
7) Social "stimulation."

Three lessons may be learned from such procedures. These are:

1) The effects are mediated indirectly or directly by the brain.
2) High BP may come about by a variety of ways; there probably is no single "cause" of the high BP.
3) High BP comes about by interactive processes.

The basis for the last statement is from Forsyth (30), who showed that Rhesus monkeys, trained on a Sidman avoidance schedule, increased their cardiac output (CD), heart rate (HR) and blood flow through the heart, skeletal muscle and liver. Eventually, peripheral resistance increased. (This sequence of circulatory events is also seen early in the course of one form of human hypertension). However, this avoidance schedule did not produce high BP levels in monkeys immediately; it took six or more months for them to do so (31). When training sessions were discontinued the monkey's BP returned to normal levels.

The aversive conditioning of dogs has to be combined with the infusion of a salt solution to produce sustained BP increases (32). In rats, foot-shock together with eating salt, but not separately, had the same effects (33).

The genetic predisposition to high BP interacts with other factors which I have already mentioned. Furthermore, heterozygous SHR's did not develop high BP unless they were exposed to electric shocks (34).

The experimental model developed by Henry and his colleagues (35) is also an interactive one. Male mice, isolated after weaning, became the socially dominant animals in a colony, and developed systolic BP elevations. Presumably, this effect was mediated by an increased production and secretion of catecholamines by the adrenal medulla (35). However, castration of these males averted the development of high BP.

There is, therefore, abundant evidence to suggest that experimentally-produced high BP is not the result of any single factor or mechanism.

The Relationship of Behavior to Experimental High BP

The brain not only monitors and regulates every bodily function but is the raison d'être for behavior. What then is the relationship of behavior to high BP in animals?

In Henry's experiment, just cited, dominance behavior eventuates in high systolic BP. In the SHR, which develops high BP at about 40 weeks, muricidal behavior was observed during the period when BP levels were rising, but not before or after (36). These data do not necessarily mean that one (behavior or high BP) "causes" the other (high BP or behavior). They might both be the result of a third process; for example, the muricidal behavior and the rising BP levels might be the result of high concentrations of angiotensin II in the cerebrospinal fluid of these animals. Angiotensin II stimulates the release of norepinephrine from peripheral and central neurons. In turn, amphetamine administration to rodents can produce muricide.

Evidence for the Participation of the Brain in Human Hypertension

Because human hypertension early in its course is usually asymptomatic, one has no means of knowing when BP levels cross over an arbitrarily drawn line (e.g., 140/90 mm Hg), and, therefore, how long it has been present. To make the matter even more vexing, BP values in man vary constantly by as much as 25%. These pressures are affected by the settings in which they are taken, and whether the patient is upright or recumbent. Further, circadian BP patterns occur in everyone, the subject's weight, age, sex, the thickness of the upper arm - relative to cuff size - and degree of arterial sclerosis influence recorded BP levels.

In the past few years, a new research strategy has been developed. It consists of studying patients as early as possible in the hypertensive process, and before (mal)adaptive changes to high BP levels occur in the kidney and arteriolar tree. When this strategy has been employed, patients with "borderline" hypertension[1] are diagnosed.

Patients with borderline hypertension seem not to have uniform profiles of cardiovascular patterns. One pattern, however, clearly reveals the influence of the brain: It consists of an increased BP, CO, and HR. Plasma renin activity and serum NA levels are elevated. Plasma volume is decreased, being unevenly distributed so that it is mainly located in the cardiopulmonary bed. Total peripheral resistance (PR) is calculated to be inappropriately normal. Propranolol reduces HR, CO, and Plasma renin activity but BP and serum NA levels still remain elevated; they can be reduced by alpha-adrenergic blocking agents. Therefore these patterned changes are the product of increased sympathetic activity emanating from brain stem centers and are not the product of a primary renal mechanism (37-39). These patients also have a characteristic psychological profile; they are constantly prepared to fight (38, 40, 41). They seem to be the ones who respond best to relaxation (42). Other "borderline" hypertensive patients have other circulatory profiles but the participation of the brain in their production is by no means established.

Two additional arguments favor the contention that the brain plays a role in human hypertension (or in some of its forms): The first is a physiological one, the second a social one. The basis for the former statement is that circadian patterns of BP occur in everyone. Remarkably enough, during sleep some hypertensive patients have BP levels within the normal range (43). The nadir of systolic or diastolic BP levels in normotensive subjects is usually at midnight but in some hypertensive patients it is phase-shifted to 0400 hours (44). In view of the fact that sleep patterns and stages are centrally elaborated by a series of oscillators, the phase-shift implies a disturbance in the central regulation of BP rhythms.

---

1. Borderline hypertension is usually equated with labile hypertension and is defined as a phase of hypertension (or of pre-hypertension), in which some BP determinations are above the arbitrary cut-off point and some are below it. Given the lability of hypertension in any patient it is obvious that good operational definitions are required so that research may be carried out. For instance, a patient with moderate, established hypertension, will at some time during the day have a (momentary) normal BP. If enough measurements are made such a pressure can be recorded, making the patient a "borderline." Conversely, even normotensive patients may react to environmental contingencies by having momentary acute elevations in BP; if BP measurements are continually recorded such a patient (or person or control) could also be classified (or misclassified) as a borderline hypertensive. If only one BP measurement is made, a person who is actually a "true" borderline hypertensive (about half the measurements being above, and about half below the arbitrary cut-off) could be classified as either a "normotensive" or a "hypertensive" depending upon the single BP measure obtained. However, not all patients with "borderline" hypertension go on to sustained hypertension or suffer its complications.

The evidence that social factors play a role is based on the fact that:

1) a clear-cut increase prevalence of hypertension occurs in Black compared to White Americans;
2) in some societies BP levels do not increase with age.

In the case of the former, it is of some interest that Black persons tend to have a greater incidence of low plasma renin activity (42%) than do white persons (26%) (45, 46). However, these data were obtained in hypertensive patients, and not in populations of normotensive subjects. Thus there is as yet no proof that there is a genetic reason (expressed phenotypically as low plasma renin activity) for the increased prevalence of hypertension in Black Americans.

What other reasons could there be? The evidence is that these are social ones operating on the predisposed. In Harburg and his colleague's (47) work associations were obtained between raised BP levels in Black men living in the unpredictable environment of the inner city, low socio-economic status, a high rate of crime and violence, crowding, and marital disruption. The BP levels of Black men living in a more salubrious, nearby environment were lower. Furthermore, the arbitrary violence of the ghetto police engendered unexpressed rage in some but not in others, which could further be related to BP levels (48). But not every Black man living in this social environment developed high BP levels. If these associations are meaningful then the opposite should also be true; and indeed that is the conclusion arrived at by Henry and Cassell (49). When a society is stable, when its customs, traditions, and institutions are structured, well-established and slow to change - when the environment is predictable and the adaptive tasks of its residents are small - then BP levels in population do not rise with age.

How could social factors not operate through the mind-brain? The task of the future is to determine how perceived danger, violence, and social discord are translated into behavior and changes in BP levels.

Future Directions in Hypertension Research

The suggestions that follow are based on three lines of evidence that:

1) Changes in cardiovascular patterns are integrated and differentiated according to the situation or the behavior with which they are coordinated: For example, when normotensive subjects take important examinations, systolic and diastolic BP, PR, and left atrial pressure rise but there is no change in stroke volume, CO or HR (50). During exercise, systolic and diastolic BP, HR, and CO increase, but PR falls and muscle blood flow is enhanced. The orthostasis response consists of an enhancement of mean BP, HR, PR, myocardial contractility, PRA and serum aldosterone levels, but SV falls and CO remains unaltered. At the same time, blood flow is brisker in the carotid arteries but diminishes in the iliac vessels (51). Conditioned emotional responses in monkeys are associated with another pattern, integrated with bar-pressing

motor behavior (52). Preparing to fight and actual fighting are associated with quite specific and discriminated cardiovascular patterns in cats, which differ from each other and all of the above (43).

2) In some hypertensive patients, the integrated cardiovascular patterns differ from normotensive ones in degree, in other patients certain situations and tasks are associated with cardiovascular responses that are excessive but other ones are not. No one has systematically studied patients, belonging to clearly-defined subforms of the syndrome, across various situations, tasks or behaviors. In support of this idea is the observation that patients with that subform of "borderline" hypertension, described previously (with increased HR, BP, NA, and PRA but normal PR) seem to respond to orthostasis by excessively raising their BP and plasma NA levels.

In other borderline hypertensive patients, not further characterized, mental arithmetic (53-55), shock avoidance (56), and color-word interference tasks (57), provoked acute and excessive increases in HR and (especially systolic) BP. Yet isometric and isotonic exercises (58-60), tilting the patient, the cold pressor test (57) elicited no excessive BP responses.

The discrepancy between the responses to these various tasks, maneuvers or behaviors is curious, because, mental arithmetic, isotonic exercises and tilting all tend to promote an increase in plasma NA levels due to increased peripheral sympathetic discharge.

The excessive BP responsiveness seem to be elicited in some borderline hypertensive patients by tasks of a "psychological" nature and not by those designed mainly to perturb the physiology of the body.

3) The integrated cardiovascular patterns described in (1) (above) are subserved by discrete circuits in the brain. The evidence for this statement is based on the fact that in anticipation of, and at the start of exercise, HR and CO increase, vasodilation and an increased blood supply to muscle occurs. These anticipatory responses may be abolished by lesioning the fields (H_2) of Fore - a section of the circuit that is believed to begin in the motor cortex and passes via the subthalamus, posterior hypothalamus, and ventral brain stem (61).

The integrated circulatory response elicited by orthostasis is subserved by a neural circuit activated by vestibular stimulation, which passes via the eighth nerve to the cerebellum, the paramedian reticular nucleus and medullary vasomotor nuclei (50).

Separate pathways are involved in the conditioned cardiac responses (62) and in the "defense reaction" (61), each of which also subserve different integrated cardiovascular adjustments. Phasic BP changes are moderated by the baroreceptor - nucleus tractus solitarius system. A serotonergic system emanating from the raphe system is involved in the modulation of heart rate.

Advances in our knowledge of the neural circuits subserving integrated cardiovascular responses might be applied to further our understanding of (some forms) of hypertension. One might ask: Are certain neural circuits more "active" to produce excessive responses? Conversely, are inhibitory circuits which modulate responses less so? Is there an "imbalance" between the activities of some circuits (mediating "psychological" tasks) and those that subserve exercise? What is the meaning of such an imbalance?

To answer such questions, it is proposed that representative patients, carefully characterized in the manner outlined, be tested on various tasks and behaviors - orthostasis, mental arithmetic, exercises, etc., - in order that inferences might be made - from the integrated circulatory changes produced- about the function and activities of the neural circuits that subserve them.

References

1. Goldblatt, H. (1947). Renal origins of hypertension. Physiol. Rev., 27: 120.
2. Ganong, W.F. (1972). Effects of sympathetic activity and ACTH on renin and aldosterone secretion. In J. Genest & E. Koiw (Eds.), Hypertension. Springer-Verlag, Berlin.
3. Ganten, D., Marquez-Julio, A., Granger, P., Hayduk, K., Karsunsky, K.P., Boucher, R. & Genest, J. (1971). Renin in dog brain. Am. J. Physiol., 221: 1733.
4. Ganten, D., Schelling, P. & Ganten, V. (1977). Tissue isorenins. In J. Genest, E. Koiw & O. Kuchel (Eds.), Hypertension (1st ed.). McGraw-Hill, N.Y., Ch. 6.10, p. 240.
5. Laragh, J.H., Baer, L.H., Brunner, H.R., Buhler, F.R. & Sealey Vaughan, E.D.Jr. (1972). Renin, angiotension and aldosterone in pathogenesis and management of hypertensive vascular disease. Am. J. Med., 52: 633.
6. Julius, S., Randall, O.S., Esler, M.D., Kashima, T., Ellis, C.N. & Bennett, J. (1975). Altered cardiac responsiveness and regulation in the normal cardiac output type of borderline hypertension. Circ. Res., 199: 36-37 (Suppl. 1).
7. Finch, L., Haeusler, G. & Thoenen, H. (1972). Failure to induce experimental hypertension in rats after intraventricular injection of 6-hydroxydopamin. Br. J. Pharmacol., 44: 356.
8. Lewis, P.J., Reid, J.L., Chalmers, J.P. & Dollery, C.T. (1973). Importance of central catecholaminergic neurons in the development of renal hypertension. Clin. Sci. Mol. Med., 45: 1156.
9. Joy, M.D. & Lowe, R.D. (1970). The site of cardiovascular action of angiotensin II in the brain. Clin. Sci. Mol. Med., 39: 327.
10. Ferrario, C.M., Dickinson, C.J., Gildenberg, P.L. & McCubbin, J.W. (1969). Central vasomotor stimulation by anigiotensin. Fed. Proc., 28: 394.
11. Gildenberg, P.L. (1971). Site of angiotensin vasopressor activity in the brain. Fed. Proc., 30: 432.
12. Sweet, C.S. & Brody, M.J. (1971). Arterial hypertension elicited by prolonged intravertebral infusion of angiotensin in the conscious dog. Fed. Proc., 30: 432.
13. Bunag, R.D., Page, I.H. & McCubbin, J.W. (1966). Neural stimulation of release of renin. Circ. Res., 19: 851.
14. De Champlain, J. (1972). Hypertension and the sympathetic nervous system. In S.M. Snyder (Ed.), Perspectives in neuropharmacology. Oxford Unitiversity Press, N.Y., p. 215.
15. De Champlain, J. & van Amerigen, M.R. (1973). Role of symathetic fibers and of adrenal medulla in the maintenance of cariovascular homeostasis in normotensive and hypertensive rats. In E. Usdin & S.M. Snyder (Eds.), Frontiers in catecholamine research. Pergamon Press, N.Y., p. 951.
16. Haeusler, G., Finch, L. & Thoenen, H. (1972). Central adrenergic neurons and the initiation and development of experimental hypertension. Experientia, 28: 1200.
17. Bianchi, G., Fox, U., DiFrancesco, G.F., Bardi, U. & Radice, M. (1973). Hypertensive role of the kidney in spontaneously hypertensive rats. Clin. Sci. Mol. Med., 45: 1355.
18. Folkow, B.U.G. & Hallbäck, M.I.L. (1977). Physiopathology of spontaneous hypertension in rats. In J. Genest, E. Koiw & O. Kuchel (Eds.), Hypertension (1st ed.). McGraw-Hill, N.Y., Ch. 11, p. 507.
19. Okamoto, K. (1972). Spontaneous hypertension. Igaku Shoin, Tokyo.
20. Hallbäck, M.I.L. (1975). Consequences of social isolation on blood pressure, cardiovascular reactivity and design in spontaneous hypertensive rats. Acta Physiol. Scand., 93: 455.
21. Yamori, Y., Matsumoto, M., Yamabe, H. & Okamoto, K. (1969). Augmentation of spontaneous hypertension by chronic stress in rats. Jpn. Circ. J., 33: 3019.

22. Haeusler, G., Gerold, J. & Thoenen, H. (1972). Cardiovascular effects of 6-hydroxydopamin injected into a lateral brain ventricle of the rat. Naunyn Schmiedberg's Arch. Pharmacol., 274: 211.
23. Jarrot, B., McQueen, A. & Louis, W.J. (1975). Serotonin levels in vascular tissues and the effects of a serotonin synthesis inhibitor on blood pressure in rats. Clin. Exp. Pharmacol. Physiol., 2: 201.
24. Scroop, G.C. & Lowe, R.D. (1968). Central pressure effect of angiotensin mediated by the parasympathetic nervous system. Nature (London), 220: 331.
25. Nicholl, R.A. & Barker, J.L. (1971). Excitation of supraoptic neurosecretory cells by angiotensin II. Nature (London), 233: 172
26. Phillips, M.I., Mann, J.F.E., Haebara, H., Dietz, R., Schelling, P. & Ganten, D. (1977). Lowering of hypertension by central saraladin in the absence of plasma renin. Nature (London), 270: 445.
27. McCubbin, J.W. (1967). Interrelationship between the sympathetic nervous system and the renin-angiotensin system. In P. Kezdi (Ed.), Baroceptors and hypertension. Pergamon Press, N.Y., p. 327.
28. Reis, D.J. (1981). Brain stem mechanisms in experimental hypertension. In H. Weiner, M.A. Hofer & A.J. Stunkard (Eds.), Brain, behavior and bodily disease. Raven Press, N.Y., p. 229.
29. Weiner, H. (1979). Psychobiology of essential hypertension. Elsevier, N.Y.
30. Forsyth, R.P. (1971). Regional blood-flow changes during 72-hour avoidance schedules in the monkey. Science, 173: 546.
31. Forsyth, R.P. (1969). Blood pressure responses to long-term aviodance schedules in the restrained rhesus monkey. Psychosom. Med., 31: 300.
32. Anderson, D.E. (1982). Behavioral conditioning and experimental hypertension. In 1981 Joint USA-USSR Symposium, Hypertension: Biobehavioral and epidemiological aspects. U.S. Department of Health and Human Services, Bethesda, MD.
33. Friedman, R. & Iwai, J. (1977). Dietary sodium, psychic stress, and genetic predisposition to experimental hypertension. Proc. Soc. Exp. Biol. Med., 155: 449.
34. Lawler, J.E., Barker, G.F., Hubbard, J.W. & Schaub, R.G. (1981). Effects of stress on blood pressure and cardiac pathology in rats with borderline hypertension. Hypertension, 3: 496.
35. Henry, J.P., Meehan, J.P. & Stephens, P.M. (1967). The use of psychosocial stimuli to induce prolonged systolic hypertension in mice. Psychosom. Med., 29: 408.
36. Rifkin, R.J., Silverman, J.M., Chavez, F.T. & Frankl, G. (1974). Intensified mouse killing in the spontaneously hypertensive rat. Life Sci., 14: 985.
37. Julius, S. & Esler, M. (1975). Autonomic nervous cardiovascular regulation in boderline hypertension. Am. J. Cardiol., 36: 685.
38. Esler, M.D., Julius, S., Zweifler, A., Harburg, E., Gardiner, H. & DeQuattro, V. (1977). Mild high-renin essential hypertension. New Engl. J. Med., 296: 405.
39. Esler, M.D., Julius, S., Randall, O.S., Ellis, C.N. & Kashima, T. (1975). Relation of renin status to neurogenic vascular resistance in borderline hypertension. Am. J. Cardiol., 36: 708.
40. Thailer, S.A., Friedman, R., Harshfield, G.A. & Pickering, T.G. (1985). Psychologic differences between high-, normal-, low-renin hypertensivness. Psychosom. Med., 47: 294.
41. Von Uexküll, T. (1963). Grundfragen der Psychosomatischen Medizin. Rowohlt, Reinbek bei Hamburg.
42. Agras, W.S., Southham, M.A. & Taylor, C.B. (1983). Long-term predictors of relaxation-induced blood pressure lowering during the work day. J. Consult. Clin. Psychol., 51: 193.
43. Zanchetti, A. & Bartorelli, C. (1977). Central nervous mechanisms in arterial hypertension: Experimental and clinical evidence. In. J. Genest, E. Koiw & O. Kuchel (Eds.), Hypertension, Chap. 5.1 (1st Ed). McGraw-Hill, N.Y., p. 59.
44. Schmidt, T.H., Schäfer, N. & Marth, H. (1974). Vergleich tagesperiodischer Schwankungen blutig gemessener Blutdruckwerte bei Normotonikern und Hypertonikern. Verhandlungen der Deutschen Gesellschaft der Inneren Medizin. 80th Congress, Bergmann, München, p. 298.
45. Crane, M.G., Harris, J.J. & Johns, V.J. (1972). Hyporeninemic hypertension. Am. J. Med., 52: 457.
46. Mroczek, W.J., Finnerty, F.A. & Catt, K.J. (1973). Lack of association between plasma renin and history of heart attack or stroke in patients with essentiell hypertension. Lancet, 2: 464.
47. Harburg, E., Erfurt, J.C., Hauenstein, L.S., Chape, C., Schull, W.J. & Schork, M.A. (1973). Socio-ecological stress, suppressed hostility, skin color, and black-white male blood pressure. Psychosom. Med., 35: 276.
48. Harburg, E., Blakelock, E.N. & Roeper, P.J. (1979). Resentful and reflective coping with arbitrary authority and blood pressure. Detroit. Psychosom. Med., 41: 189.

49. Henry, J.P. & Cassel, J.C. (1969). Psychosocial factors in essential hypertension. Recent epidemiologic and animal experimental evidence. Am. J. Epidemol., 90: 171.
50. Von Uexküll, T. (1982). Zur Psychosomatik der essentiellen Hypertonie - Die Situation als Krankheitsfaktor. In K. Kohle (Ed.), Zur Psychosomatik von Herz-Kreislauf-Erkrankungen, Vol. 8. Forum Galenus, Mannheim, p. 54.
51. Doba, N. & Reis, D.J. (1974). Role of the cerebellum and the vestibular apparatus in regulation of orthostatic reflexes in the cat. Circ. Res., 34: 9.
52. Smith, A.O., Astley, C.A., DeVito, J.L., Stein, J.M. & Walsh, K.E. (1980). Functional analysis of hypothalamic control of the cardiovascular responses accompanying emotional behavior. Fed. Proc., 39: 2487.
53. Baumann, R., Ziprian, H., Gödicke, W., Hartrodt, W., Naumann, E. & Läuter, J. (1973). The influence of acute psychic stress situations on biochemical and vegetative parameters of essentiell hypertensives at the early stage of the disease. Psychother. Psychosom., 22: 131.
54. Brod, J., Fencl, V., Hejn, Z. & Zirka, J. (1959). Circulatory changes underlying blood pressure elevation during acute emotional stress (mental arithmetic) in normotensive and hypertensive subjects. Clin. Sci., 18: 269.
55. Nestel, P.J. (1969). Blood-pressure and catecholamine excretion after mental stress in labile hypertension. Lancet, 1: 692.
56. Light, K. & Obrist, P. (1980). Cardiovascular reactivity to behavioral stress in young males with and without marginally elevated causal systolic pressures. Comparison of clinic, home and laboratory measure. Hypertension, 2: 802.
57. Eliasson, K., Hjemdahl, P. & Kahan, T. (1983). Circulatory and sympathoadrenal responses to stress in borderline and established hypertension. J. Hypertens., 1: 131.
58. Julius, S. & Conway, J. (1968). Hemodynamic studies in patients with borderline blood pressure elevation. Circulation, 38: 282.
59. Lund-Johnson, P. (1967). Hemodynamics in early essential hypertension. Acta Med. Scand. Suppl., 482: 1.
60. Sannerstedt, R. (1960). Hemodynamic responses to excercise in patients with arterial hypertension. Acta Med. Scand. Suppl., 458: 1.
61. Uvnäs, B. (1960). Central cardiovascular control. In J. Field (Ed.), The handbook of physiology, Sec. I. American Physiological Society, Washington, DC, Ch. 40, p. 1131.
62. Cohen, D.H. (1982). Cardiovascular neurobiology: The substrate for biobehavioral approaches to hypertension. In 1981 Joint USA-USSR Symposium. Hypertension: Biobehavioral and epidemiological aspects. Department of Health and Human Sevices, Bethesda, MD.

Discussion:

Central Control of the Cardiovascular System

Dieter Vaitl

In the last two decades, a considerable scientific and public interest in the impact of environmental factors on the physiology of the living organisms has been developed. In this connection, the influences of socio-psychological factors on the pathogenesis and persistance of cardiovascular diseases are of particular importance. In spite of our present knowledge and the wealth of information available, it still remains to be demonstrated in which way the central nervous system interacts with the cardiovascular system and transfers changes in the environment to the heart and to the vessels. Furthermore, it is under debate which pathological alterations of the cardiovascular system can be attributed to changes in the individual's environment.

In previous chapters, various aspects of the brain-circulation interaction have been addressed in a very profound and subtle manner. Their common denominator appeared to be that cardiovascular responses are viewed as integral components of behavior. Besides this general and somehow trivial aspect, it seems worthwhile to emphasize in the following part a more specific aspect which is that cardiovascular responses can be conditional. Instead of being pure reflexes arising from innate genetic programs (see the article by Jänig for discussion of the reflex notion) they can be modulated and elicited according to environmental demands and be emitted in anticipation of consequences (1). This, however, requires specific and fine-grained brain-circulation interactions.

As Lombardi (in this chapter) has demonstrated, the sympathetically and vagally mediated positive and negative feedback mechanisms for hemodynamic regulation are tonically active. They interact continually in order to achieve the most adequate neural regulation of cardiac performance. Spinal integrity is apparently sufficient for the existence and interaction of these regulatory reflexes. According to this notion, states of increased sympathetic excitation do not result from an increased sympathetic outflow stimulated by central commands or decreased buffering mechanisms, but from a peripheral reinforcement as well as from positive feedback mechanisms.

It is commonly accepted that these excitatory reflexes may play an important role in cardiovascular disorders, such as hypertension, myocardial ischemia, and cardiac arrhythmias. However, until now the question has not yet been answered as to how these reflexes are modulated by higher nervous processes. With regard to this issue, the competence of the Milan group should be mentioned (2). Reviewing their own work on the role of the sympathetic nervous system in congestive heart failure, the authors suggested that in cases of increased volume load both vagal and sympathetic afferent fibers are excited and that the power of the reflexes depends upon the "central excitatory state." They assume that the "gain" of either reflex circuit is selectively modified by such central excitatory states. Similar findings concern other reflexes. It is well known that baroreceptor reflexes can be altered by exercise (3), and "emotion" (4). Conversly, Billman (5) has pointed out that responses to environmental stimuli can both modify and be modified by cardiovascular reflexes. Experiments on this issue originated from the expectation that the simultaneous activation of passive reflexes evoked by aversive stress (during classical conditioning) and excitatory reflexes stimulated by anterior wall ischemia would lead to an algebraic summation of the two reflexes (6). However, this was not the case. The consistent cardiovascular response pattern elicited by aversive stress is attenuated while anterior wall ischemia is induced by the occlusion of the left anterior descending coronary artery. This unexpected result has been interpreted by Billman as an adaptive response during ischemia which reduces the metabolic strain and conserves the oxygen the tissue still receives.

Even if one does not favor "teleologic" interpretations the interaction of cardiovascular reflexes and their susceptibility to central commands appears to be dynamic in nature and changes considerably to meet the environmental demands.

In this context, the question must be raised as to whether and to what extent the modifiability of cardiovascular regulation is influenced by learning processes. Since this aspect has not yet been touched on in the symposium, some statements on this topic should be made.

As in many areas of biology, advances in understanding complex phenomena frequently follow the development of simpler model systems. A particularly effective experimental model for studying the relationship between external events, behavior, and cardiovascular activity is Pavlovian conditioning. In the last decade, many attempts have been made to explore the physiological processes involved in associative learning (cf. excellent review articles by Cohen & Randall (7) and Engel (8)).

Briefly, the cardiovascular responses are unlikely to be mechanically elicited in a reflex-like fashion by adequate stimuli; they are at least in part conditional both to the stimuli applied and to the contingencies prevailing during conditioning. If, for example, an innocuous conditional stimulus such as a light signal or a sound is paired with a nociceptive stimulus, after a series of pairings the conditional stimulus by itself is capable of eliciting a set of responses which are associated with escape or avoidance behavior, including increases in cardiac output, blood pressure, blood flow in the active striated musculature. The same light or sound, however, may elicit exactly the opposite response pattern when escape or avoidance behavior is blocked. There are numerous examples of the phenomenon that responses to the conditional signals are controlled by the central nervous system in a different way than are the responses to the aversive signal. This has been observed in chronotropic and dromotropic cardiac responses as well as in the responses of the coronary and renal vascular beds (for critical review see (8)). Thus, the properties of the external milieu seem to exert a differential influence on the cardiovascular response pattern.

With respect to the basic issue of this symposium on the central control of cardiovascular regulation, it is tempting to speculate about the possible pathways involved in the transmission of sensory signal input to the conditional cardiovascular response patterns. The only vertebrate model existing which would ultimately allow the cellular analysis of long-term associative learning as in Pavlovian conditioning is largely restricted to conditioned heart rate changes in pigeons. Cohen (9) has described a descending neural pathway from the avian homologue of the amygdala to preganglionic neurons. Given this descending pathway, the pigeon model also implies ascendent visual pathways that transmit the conditional stimulus information. It could be shown that these pathways are not merely input channels but that they exhibit training-dependent modification of the discharges evoked by conditional stimuli during heart-rate conditioning experiments. Modifications did occur primarily in the avian lateral geniculate nucleus. Cohen (9) assumes that the pathways which mediate conditional cardiovascular changes may show training-induced modification at most, if not all, of their central relays. At present, there is no model available which might be adopted similarly for conditional cardiovascular responses in humans.

A small diversion into the realm of theories and models might be permitted through information provided by clinical observation in humans. The article by Siegrist has addressed an interesting point which seems worthwhile to focus on: The close relationship between sleep disturbances and cardiac arrhythmias. Given that this observation in postmyocardial infarction patients is correct, it is possible that higher neural relay stations are involved and are functioning as either filter or trigger mechanisms. Recently, Skinner (10) has proposed a model for arrhythmogenesis in pigs which might contribute to this issue. He started his research work by answering the question: Which intervention can prevent the lethal consequences of coronary artery occlusion in the psychologically stressed pig? Three independent interventions appeared to be possible: (1) Behavioral adaption to the stressful events, (2) the intracerebral injection of ß-blockers, and (3) the blockade of the frontocortical-brainstem pathway.

This latter invention led him to formulate the hypothesis that precipitating events (environmental stressors) evoke specific electrical and chemical perturbations in frontal lobes which determine whether or not the frontocortical brainstem pathway is activated. The triggered activity results in an increase of both sympathetic and vagal outflow ("dual autonomic tone") and inhibits homeostatic reflexes. When coronary arteries are partially occluded this projected autonomic imbalance may trigger the initiation of ventricular fibrillation. Since coronary artery occlusion is neither necessary nor sufficient to cause ventricular fibrillation, the influence from frontal lobes may play an important role as a central trigger mechanism. There is evidence to suggest that slow wave sleep is accompanied by dual autonomic tone and that during this sleep stage the rates of ventricular arrhythmias in the infarcted heart are also high. This led to the speculation that increased dual autonomic outflow during sleep might also be triggered by frontal cortex activity.

In this context, one might ask: Are sleep disorders, as reported by Siegrist, valuable and reliable clinical signs for neurovegetative imbalance? If so, can they be considered as prodromal symptoms which signal precisely - like an early warning system - that environmental stress and strain sequences are starting to exert their deleterious influence upon one's cardiovascular system?

This might provide specific information about the critical phase of the onset of serious neurovegetative imbalance and could, therefore, be used as a guideline for specific client-centered medical and behavioral analyses as well as clinical interventions. This has also been proposed by Weiner (see his article in this chapter) with respect to the heterogeneous cardiovascular response profiles in hypertensives (see also the recent meta-analysis of the literature on the response specificity issue by Frederikson (11)).

In order to determine the onset of neurovegetative imbalance, however, very sensitive and reliable techniques are needed, which indicate, for instance, acute changes in sympathetic and parasympathetic predominance ("dual tone" according to Skinner's model of arrhythmogenesis (10)) in patients. Recently, a non-invasive assessment of sympatho-vagal interaction has been proposed by Pagani (12) which is primarily based on spectral power analyses of heart rate variability and can be done with relatively small samples of heart beats. Given the validity of this assessment, it will allow detection of one's proneness to neurovegetative imbalance prior to excessive alterations of cardiovascular responses in both patients and persons at risk.

According to this, an approach based on single case studies and n=1 experimentation might be an additional research tool and an alternative to the large-scale nation-wide intervention trials which have been criticized in the past for various reasons.

References

1. Barry, R.J. (1984). Stimulus emission and the orienting response. Psychophysiology, 21: 535-540.
2. Malliani, A. & Pagani, M. (1983). The role of the sympathetic nervous system in congestive heart failure. Eur. Heart J., 4: 49-54.
3. Walgenbach, S.C. & Donald, D.E. (1983). Inhibition by carotid baroreflex of exercise: Induced increases in arterial pressure. Circ. Res., 52: 253-262.
4. Engel, B.T. & Joseph, J.A. (1982). Attenuation of baroreflexes during operant conditioning. Psychophysiology, 19: 609-614.
5. Billman, G.E. (1986). Behavioral stress and myocardial ischemia: An example of conditional response modification. Behav. Brain Sci., 9: 295-296.
6. Billman, G.E. & Randall, D.C. (1980). Classic aversive conditioning of coronary blood flow in mongrel dogs. Pavlovian J. Biol. Sci., 15: 93-101.
7. Cohen, D.H. & Randall, D.C. (1984). Conditioning of cardiovascular responses. In R.M. Berne & J.F. Hoffman (Eds.), Annual review of physiology.
8. Engel, B.T. (1986). An essay on the circulation as behavior. Behav. Brain Sci., 9: 285-318.
9. Cohen, D.H. (1980). The functional neuroanatomy of a conditioned response. In R.F. Thompson, L.H. Hicks & V.B. Shvyrkov (Eds.), Neural mechanisms of goal-directed behavior and learning. Academic Press, N.Y.
10. Skinner, J.E. (1985). The regulation of cardiac vulnerability by the cerebral defense. J. Am. Coll. Cardiol., 88B-94B.
11. Frederikson, M. (1986). Behavioral aspects of cardiovascular reactivity in essential hypertension. In T.H. Schmidt, T.M. Dembroski & G. Blümchen (Eds.), Biological and psychological factors in cardiovascular disease. Springer-Verlag, Berlin.
12. Pagani, M., Lombardi, F., Guzzetti, S., Rimoldi, O., Furlan, R., Pizzinelli, P., Sandrone, G., Malfatto, G., Dell'Orto, S., Piccaluga, E., Turiel, M., Baselli, G., Cerutti, S. & Malliani, A. (1986). Power spectral analysis of heart rate and arterial pressure variabilities as a marker of sympatho-vagal interaction in man and conscious dog. Circ. Res., 59: 178-193.

4.

Recent Approaches in Psychobiological Research

Research Directions in Behavioral Medicine

Fritz A. Henn, Emmeline Edwards and Joel Johnson

Behavioral medicine appears to divide from psychosomatic medicine and in America grew out of the psychobiology of Adolf Meyer (1). This orientation was holistic and led to an integration of various influences in shaping disease. Soon after, psychoanalysis became dominant and Alexander's work (2) set the stage for the founding of psychosomatic medicine. There was a great enthusiasm for psychological forces in specific medical diseases and the emphasis was on psychogenesis of some medical illnesses. This was the source of much activity and speculation. Unfortunately these hopes did not reach fruition and the enthusiasm of physicians changed into doubt and finally rejection. The danger of unreachable promises in this area of psychiatry was real and costly and gradually fewer and fewer physicians were interested in psychosomatic questions. As psychiatry moved into general hospitals, liaison psychiatry began to emerge and once again questions of psychological influences on medical illness became fashionable (3). In this climate behavioral psychologists and biologists began to work on the ways in which psychological stimuli could influence bodily function and Behavioral Medicine was born.

For me the excitement of the research findings is tempered by the oversell of the new psychosomatics. While I see great potential for clinical applications, I feel they will have to be built up systematically on a foundation of solid basic research. The model for clinical advances is that of a liaison service as opposed to a consult service. As Hackett (4) says "a consultation service is a rescue squad ... (while) liaison is setting up fire prevention programs ..." Thus using the knowledge of behavioral medicine, the field must get into preventive programs, which while unspectacular may have great impact on the level of health in the community. This is essential to maintain the growth in both basic and applied research in the area.

The area of research which is most exciting to me is the specification of the CNS mechanisms which mediate between psychological events and altered bodily functions. This may also help explain some areas of psychopathology such as depression secondary to a medical illness. Thus, any studies which address the CNS mechanisms which result in lasting functional changes in brain or body secondary to environmental or psychological input, appears to me to be of major importance. The chain between psychological input --> brain --> body is clearly a two way street and an understanding of the mechanisms of adaptation may help us to understand several aspects of psychopathology as well as medical illnesses. As an example, let me briefly review two rodent studies involving stress. The first deals with immunological changes and the second with depressive illness, common mechanistic elements will be seen in both.

The first involves the studies of Riley (5), which examine the effects of stress on the immune system. The basic finding is that controlled stress can46 have profound effects on immunocompetence. For example, using tumor growth as an assay of immunological competence in a strain of mice capable of controlling tumor growth, they found a 4-fold difference in tumor size in 30 days after exposing mice to mild rotational stress. The mechanism appears to be mediated through corticosterone release which causes a decrease in T cell and NK cells and an involution of the thymus. This finding is obviously both exciting and potentially dangerous as the next fact quickly brings out. Looking at a closely related strain of mice far greater differences in tumor viability are found attributable to strain differences, so genetics must clearly play a role in deferring the response. My point is that we are probably dealing with complex multi-factorial phenomena and the quick head line "stress reduction can cure cancer" may harm the field more than anything else. On the other hand, detailing the mechanism of psychoendocrine control of immune function and analysis of the role of genetic susceptibility to the phenomena are valid and fundable directions to proceed.

Looking at another aspect of stress and its effects may help us not only understand bodily functions, but mental function and disfunction as well. I am referring to stress models of psychopathology.

Seligman and his associates (6), demonstrated that exposure to uncontrollable shock produces a behavioral deficit described as "learned helplessness." This phenomenon transfers across different aversive training and testing contexts and the apparent development of an escape deficit seems to depend on factors such as the nature of the aversive stimulus (7, 8), the parameters of the presentation of that stimulus (9, 10) and the nature of the escape response (6, 11).

The mechanism by which exposure to uncontrollable shock produces this behavioral deficit remains undefined. However, we have established a psychobiological concept of "learned helplessness" including a distinct behavioral and neurobiological mechanism. Our laboratory has been studying a modified version of Seligman's "learned helplessness" model where our experimental animals are only exposed to mild uncontrollable shock. With this approach we have compared two distinct groups of rats which emerge when subjected to a mild course of uncontrollable shock. The selection is from two different groups of animals: (1) those that show no deficit in subsequent shock escape test and (2) those that show a profound learning deficit. This has provided a better medium for behavioral and pharmacological manipulations.

Establishment of Model

Sprague-Dawley rats are used in our experiments. These rats are obtained from Charles River Breeding laboratories and are delivered to the Division of Animal Resources where they are kept under standard conditions. Upon arrival, these rats, weighing 150-200 g, are maintained on an ad libitum food and water schedule. Behavioral training and testing sessions are scheduled during the light phase of a twelve hour light/dark cycle.

The critical element of our behavioral biochemical studies is the consistency and accuracy with which the behavior can be quantified. After exposure to uncontrollable shock there have been numerous reports of a learning deficit which only show a degree of internal consistency within each investigator's paradigm. Researchers from various laboratories have agreed that there is a behavioral difference between response deficient rats and rats that have received identical shock and still respond at control levels (12). There is a high degree of variability in obtaining the behavioral deficit after inescapable shock training. Therefore, in our studies a revised "learned helplessness" model is used. In our experimental set up the rats are placed in an experimental chamber with an electrified grid floor. Each chamber is 12 x 18 x 12 cm. Side and ceilings are constructed of aluminum and plexiglas. The floor is constructed of stainless steel rods spaced 1.9 cm apart. During the shock escape test, a lever is mounted 7 cm off the grid floor on one wall. A yellow cue light is placed 5 cm above the lever. Shock is delivered to each chamber by a Coulborn solid state shock source (model E13-16).

Shock Training

Training consists of placing the rats in the experimental chamber where they receive intermittent inescapable 0.8 mA footshock. Each training session lasts forty minutes. The onset and offset of the shock being established by a probability generator result in an average schedule of 20 minutes of shock with a minimum time of 1.5 seconds between on and off events.

Shock Escape Testing

Twenty-four hours after training, each rat is individually tested in an escape situation where footshock can be eliminated by a single bar press. Shock is delivered at the intensity of 0.8 mA in a pulsating schedule of 35 msec on/ 35 msec off, with the yellow cue light being on during the shock period. Shock onset begins one trial and pressing the lever or the end of 60 seconds shuts off the shock. Intertrial intervals of 24 seconds begin with the yellow cue light out. Fifteen trials are given in each testing session. Latencies up to 20 seconds before the lever is pressed and the shock terminated are considered a successful escape to shock. 20- to 60-second latencies are recorded as failures. Scores are recorded automatically. Non-specific effects of footshock are eliminated by including internal controls in the testing paradigm. Behavioral, pharmacological and biochemical determinations are carried out for these internal controls. These rats are only subjected to the shock escape test, enabling us to determine the effects of shock per se. From past experiments in our laboratory, these controls routinely do not show significant changes both behaviorally and biochemically from non-deficient or naive rats.

Behavioral Deficit

Behavioral deficits are measured as the number of failures using the following criteria:

1) Rats scoring 1-5 failures in a 15-trial testing session are not response deficient (ND) and learn the shock escape test as quickly as controls.
2) Rats scoring 11-15 failures in a 15-trial testing session are considered response deficient (RD).

In a typical experiment where a total of 40 rats are used (10 internal controls, 30 trained and tested in shock paradigm), 25% of the trained and tested rats are response deficient (RD) while another 35% are non-deficient and respond at a level similar to control rats in the shock escape test. Rats scoring in the range of 6-10 failures are not considered in subsequent analysis. Behavioral and biochemical determinations performed on rats falling into the 6-10 failures group revealed a high degree of heterogeneity within the group. In addition, a large percentage of the 6-10 failures group exhibit improved shock escape score when subjected to additional shock treatment (repeated training session).

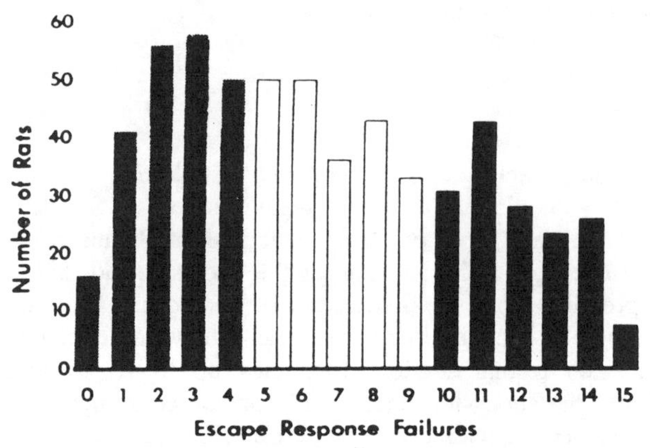

Figure 1A. Features of escape responding after exposure to inescapable shock and control responding. Failures to escape in rats trained 24 h previously. Dark shading indicates the subpopulation defined as having severe response deficits (RD), while the lighter shading denotes animals having no deficit (ND) after undergoing identical treatment. The total number of animals involved was 592, with 27% falling in the range of 10-15 failures, and 37% between 0-4 failures.

The behavioral deficit exhibited after exposure to uncontrollable shock is reversed with time. When deficient rats are again tested in a shock escape situation, three weeks later, their behavior parallels the behavior of controls.

We noted that the percentage of rats developing the shock induced behavioral deficit is dependent on the strain of rats used. Routinely, 30% of the Sprague Dawley rats (Charles River breeding laboratories) trained and tested, developed a behavioral deficit in a shock escape test, while with the Biolabs strain only 21% of response deficient rats are obtained. Rats obtained from Taconic Farms and Simonsen labs only yielded 11% response deficient rats the standard training and testing paradigm.

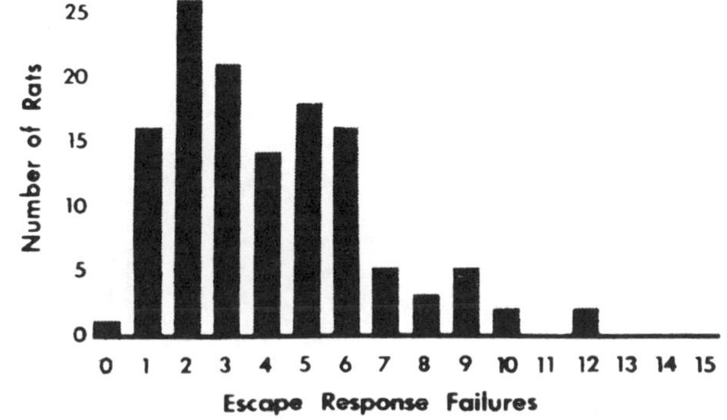

Figure 1B. Testing of naive rats; animals are exposed to the escape paradigm with no prior training, 60% of these animals score 0-4.

This suggested that the behavioral deficit emerging after exposure to mild uncontrollable shock may involve a genetic component. Our laboratory has undertaken the selective breeding of response deficient rats (RD), non deficient rats and controls. With data of only three generations of each group, hereditary differences between our selected lines are becoming evident. Litters from response deficient rats have produced under identical conditions of shock training and testing, 44% of escape response deficient rats. Conversely, litters from non-deficient rats have produced less than 2% of animals with a shock escape deficit. However, the effect of hereditary differences on behavior must be characterized thoroughly by biochemical analysis.

Neurobiological Changes

We have identified some neurobiochemical differences between the two groups emerging after a mild course of uncontrollable shock. These differences may pinpoint the anatomical locus of the behavioral deficit.

Neurotransmitters

Various brain regions were analyzed for their concentrations of DA, NE, 5-HT. These neurotransmitter levels were analyzed by simultaneous assays performed by reverse phase high performance liquid chromatography (HPLC) with electrochemical detection. HPLC determinations of the biogenic amines in various brain regions did not reveal any significant changes in norepinephrine, epinephrine, dopamine, and their metabolites in response deficient rats when compared to non-deficient rats. However, in the hippocampus, the serotonin/norepinephrine ratios (5-HT/NE) disclosed some differences between response deficient rats, non-deficient rats, and controls. In general, small consistent increases in 5-HT and decreases in NE levels are observed.

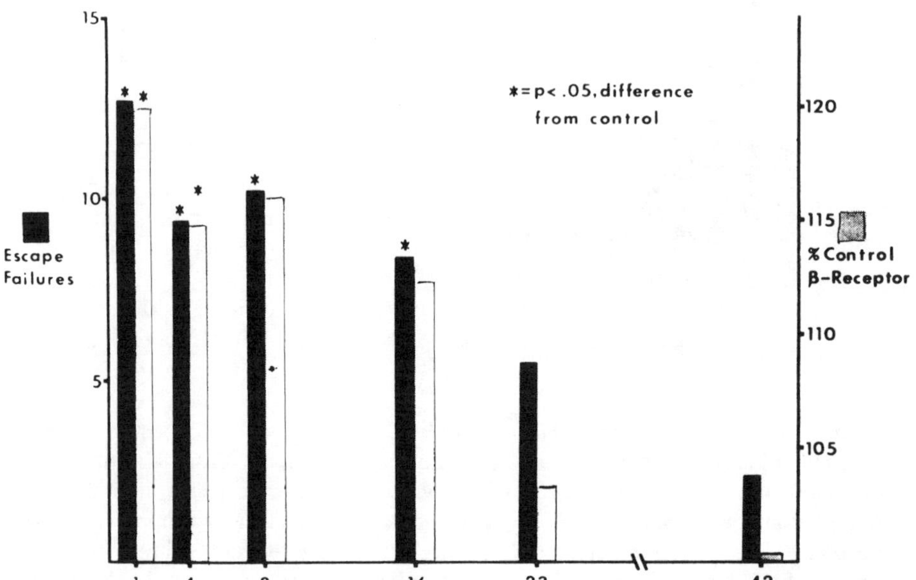

Figure 2. Behavioral and ß-receptor changes with time after exposure to inescapable shock. Rats were trained and tested as described in the text. Cohorts of animals were subsequently retested at 4, 8, 16, 23, and 42 days. Control values throughout the experiment remained at 4 ± 2 failures. n's for each group are given below in parentheses. Hippocampal ß-receptor measurements were determined using ^{125}ICYP as the ligand. Binding saturation curves were analyzed using an Eadi-Hofstee transformation and B_{max} obtained through extrapolation. Data are expressed as percent of control values, actual B_{max} values are as follows: Day 1: control (31) 55.0 ± 13.6 fmol/mg protein, learning deficient (12) 64.9 ± 13.4 fmol/mg protein; Day 4: control (8) 54.8 ± 3.5 fmol/mg protein, learning deficient (8) 63.5 ± 6.5 fmol/mg protein; Day 8: control (6) 58.9 ± 9.1 fmol/mg protein, learning deficient (6) 69.4 ± 14.7 fmol/mg protein; Day 16: control (6) 56.1 ± 13.7 fmol/mg protein, learning deficient (6) 63.4 ± 9.4 fmol/mg protein; Day 23: control (6) 156.1 ± 18.2 fmol/mg protein; learning deficient (6) 151.6 ± 27.2 fmol/mg protein; Day 42: control (6) 62.1 ± 7.0 fmol/mg protein, learning deficient (6) 62.3 ± 6.5 fmol/mg protein. Actual failure values are as follows: Day 1 (8) 12.8 ± 1.0, Day 4 (8) 9.6 ± 3.4, Day 8 (6) 10.5 ± 2.0, Day 16 (6) 8.3 ± 3.3, Day 23 (6) 4.8 ± 2.3, Day 42 (4) 3.8 ± 1.7. Significance is determined with a two-tailed Student's t-test evaluating differences between means.

Receptors

ß-adrenergic and serotonin receptors were studied in response deficient rats, non-deficient rats and controls. The various brain regions analyzed, include the cerebellum, hippocampus, hypothalamus, septum, and anterior neocortex. Major differences in ß-adrenergic receptors were seen in the hippocampus of response deficient rats.

The status of ß-adrenergic receptors was assessed by a filtration assay using ^{125}I-cyanopindolol (^{125}I-CYP) as the probe. Briefly, hippocampal membrane preparations were incubated for 55 minutes at 37° C with increasing concentrations of ^{125}I-CYP (0-240 pm) in the presence or absence of 10^{-6} M propanolol used for non-specific binding determination (13).

In response deficient rats, the ß-adrenergic receptor is up regulated in the hippocampus but not in the anterior neocortex nor the septum. Changes in hippocampal ß-receptors follow a time course similar to the shock escape deficit and a strong correlation between ß-adrenergic receptor status and shock escape deficit scores has been established for the response deficient rats. Within three weeks following the shock escape test, both failure scores and ß-adrenergic receptor status of response deficient rats were comparable to controls. Adenylate cyclase responsiveness to norepinephrine was determined in response deficient, non-deficient, and control rats. Basal and stimulated cyclic AMP levels were measured using the protein binding assay of Gilman (14) in kit forms as provided by Amersham, Inc. Response deficient rats exhibit a large increase in Adenylate cyclase activity in hippocampal slices, indicating that an amplification of the noradrenergic receptor Adenylate cyclase system may be linked to the behavioral changes seen in our model of shock-induced deficit. Modifications at the receptor level in response to environmental conditions attest to the plasticity of the central nervous system and to the involvement of neurochemical mechanisms in some behavioral responses. In our modified version of "learned helplessness," there is a biochemical modulation of the brain in response to a purely environmental manipulation. This suggests that certain stimuli, obviously drugs among them, can lead to altered behavioral patterns driven by altered CNS structures.

Pharmacology

Pharmacological interventions produce a time dependent reversal of both the shock-induced behavioral deficit and the ß-adrenergic receptor up regulation characteristic of response deficient rats. In our drug studies we followed the schedule of training and testing of our regular paradigm, but shock escape testing was followed by a five day drug treatment. Tested controls were divided into two groups: Drug treated and vehicle treated. Simultaneously trained and tested rats were first divided into response deficient and non-deficient rats. Each of these two groups were further divided into a drug treated group and a vehicle treated group.

To date, drug studies performed with our model of shock-induced deficit have focused on compounds known to interact with either noradrenergic or serotonergic systems. Imipramine (10 mg/kg x 5 days) a relatively non-specific catecholamine uptake inhibitor reversed the behavioral deficit. The shock escape score of response deficient rats improved in 80% of the rats retested after the Imipramine treatment (11.6 ± 1.8 --> 4.2 ± 3.6 failure scores). A number of tricyclic antidepressants, monoamine oxidase inhibitors, and second generation antidepressants were tested. All clinically effective drugs reversed the learning deficit, non-specific drugs, such as neuroleptics, sedatives or stimulants, do not appear to reverse the learning deficit. Among the drugs tested were the relatively specific 5-HT uptake inhibitor fluvoxamine and the novel compound mianserin thought to act mainly through the 5-HT system. Both of these compounds caused behavior reversal of the deficit.

Interestingly, the reversal shock-induced learning deficit was accompanied by a significant down regulation of the ß-adrenergic receptor in the response deficient rats. This was expected for the TCA's such as Imipramine which have previously been shown to down regulate ß-receptors. It was surprising that the behavioral changes and down regulation of ß-receptors induced by Imipramine appear to be similar and faster than the down regulation caused by this compound in naive animals. Even more unexpected, mianserin lowers the up regulation of the ß-receptor in response deficient animals while causing no change in the hippocampal ß-receptor of non-deficient rats. Mianserin had previously been shown not to down regulate the ß-adrenergic receptors in behaviorally naive rats (15). Hence the up regulated receptor seen in our animal model may be either more sensitive to presynaptic influences or under the exquisite control of a postsynaptic regulatory process. So specific drugs may have an exclusive effect on a pathologic transmitter system while exhibiting no control over receptors in a normal or naive animal.

Drug	ß-receptor	Effect on escape reversal
Imipramine	down-regulated 25%	reversal
Mianserin	down-regulated 28%	reversal

Neuroregulatory Role of 5-HT

Studies with mianserin and fluvoxamine suggested that a serotonergic mechanism may also be involved in the mediation of the deficit produced by mild uncontrollable shock. The decrease of serotonin levels prevents the development of the shock induced behavioral deficit seen in our model. Sprague Dawley rats pretreated with PCPA, a known 5-HT synthesis inhibitor exhibited shock escape scores similar to non-deficient and control rats (3.0 ± 0.17, PCPA-treated vs. 7.6 ± 3.3, saline treated, $t=5.96$, $p<0.001$).

Bilateral lesions of serotonergic tracts with 5,7 dihydroxy-tryptamine (5,7 DHT) also prevented the development of shock-induced behavioral deficit after the training and testing paradigm. Receptor binding assays for S_2

receptors (^{3}H-spiroperidol binding) and S_1 receptors (^{3}H-serotonin binding) in the anterior neocortex and the hippocampus did not reveal any significant differences in both the affinity and the maximum number of sites in response deficient, non-deficient and control rats. However, a normal level of 5-HT activity is necessary to maintain ß levels in the hippocampus. Recent experiments in our laboratories revealed a significant down regulation of hippocampal ß-receptors after various treatments known to influence 5-HT levels and 5-HT transmission (B_{max} in fm/mg protein 116.5 ± 9.2, response deficient rats vs. 62.8 ± 5.7 and 5-HT depleted rats). These studies suggest that a feed-back mechanism between noradrenergic and serotonin systems could act as a mediator of the behavioral and biochemical characteristics of our response deficient rats. Such an hypothesis would support the work of Sulser (16) who has suggested that an intact serotonergic input is necessary for the down regulation of ß-receptors by various therapeutic drugs.

Our current data do not disclose a simple relationship between drug-induced alterations in the 5-HT system, uncontrollable shock and behavioral deficits. However, we are focusing our research efforts on the following anatomical circuit for our "learned helplessness" model:

Anterior neocortex	--> Hippocampus	--> Fornix	--> Septum
GABA	NE	GABA	5-HT
5-HT			

This partial limbic circuit including the hippocampus and the septum is modulated by neurotransmitter and neurohormonal inputs. This complex functional "lobe" receives serotonergic, adrenergic, cholinergic and peptidergic input in addition to the local circuitry.

The study of this model illustrates that the brain is plastic and can adapt, with behavioral consequences, to environmental manipulations which appear psychological in nature. They also point to the complexity of the response and the interplay of genetic effects with these phenomena.

In summary, the thrust of the research appears to be in CNS mechanisms and the promise is indeed large, especially if we remain systematic in our basic investigations and careful of our clinical claims.

References

1. Lidz, T. (1966). Adolf Meyer and the development of American Psychiatry. Am. J. Psychiat. 123: 320-322.
2. Alexander, F. (1936). The medical value of psychoanalysis. Norton, N.Y.
3. Oken, D. (1983). Liaison Psychiatry (Liaison medicine). Adv. Psychosom. Med., 11: 23-51.
4. Hackett, T.P. (1978). Beginnings liaison psychiatry in general hospital. In Hackett & Cassen (Eds.), Handbook of general hospital psychiatry. Mosby, St. Louis, p. 1-14.
5. Riley, V. (1981). Psychoneuroendocrine influences on immunocompetence and neoplasia. Science, 212: 1100-1109.
6. Seligman, M.E.P. & Beagley, G. (1975). Learned helplessness in the rat. J. Comp. Physiol. Psychol., 88: 534-541.

7. Goodkin, F. (1976). Rats learn the relationship between responding and environmental events: An expansion of the learned helplessness hypothesis. Learn. Motivat., 7: 382-393.
8. Weiss, J.M. & Glaser, H.I. (1975). The effects of acute exposure to stressors on subsequent avoidance behavior. Psychosom. Med., 37: 499-521.
9. Anderson, D.C., Koehn, C., Crowell, C. & Lupo, J.V. (1976). Different intensities of unsignalled inescapable shock treatments as determinants of nonshock motivation open field behavior: A resolution of disparate results. Physiol. Behav., 17: 391-394.
10. Rosellini, R.A. & Seligman, M.E.P. (1978). Role of shock intensity in the learned helplessness paradigm. Anim. Learn. Behav., 6: 143-146.
11. Wilson, W.J. & Butcher, L.L. (1980). A potential shock reducing contingency in the back shock technique: Implications for learned helplessness. Anim. Learn. Behav., 8: 435-440.
12. Katz, R.J. (1981). Animal models and human depressive disorders. Neurosci. Biobehav. Rev., 5: 231-246.
13. Engel, G., Hoyer, D., Berthold, R. & Wagner, H. (1981). ± ^{125}Iodocyanopindolol, a new ligand for ß-receptors: Identification and quantification of subclasses of ß-adrenoreceptors in guinea-pig. Naunyn-Schmiedberg's Arch. Pharmacol., 317: 277-285.
14. Gilman, A.G. (1970). A protein binding assay adenosine 3', 5'-monophosphate. Proc. Natl. Acad. Sci. USA., 67: 305-312.
15. Mishra, R., Janowsky, A. & Sulser, F. (1980). Action of mianserin and zimelidine on the norepinephrine receptor coupled adenylate cyclase system in brain: Subsensitivity without reduction in ß-adrenergic receptor binding. Neuropharm., 19: 983-987.
16. Sulser, F., Manier, D.H., Janowsky, A.J. & Okada, F. (1983). Regulation of the noradrenergic receptor systems in brain that are coupled to adenylate cyclase. J. Neural. Trans. Suppl., 18: 121-130.

Recording of Postganglionic Impulse Traffic in Man. What Can it Tell Us About Health and Disease?

B. Gunnar Wallin

The sympathetic nervous system regulates a large number of functions in the body, and these functions are often altered in the diseased state. Much work has been devoted to elucidating how the sympathetic influence is brought about. Since the sympathetic system has an integrative function, and since it is influenced by wakefulness, emotions, intellect, psychological make-up, etc., many problems can be studied only in the awake state and preferably in conscious man. The most common approach is to try to draw conclusions from recordings of sympathetic effector organ activities (e.g., variations of heart rate, blood flow, sweating, blood pressure). It is, however, complicated to translate effector organ activities into neural terms, both because effector organs react slowly to variations in autonomic neural drive and because they react also to chemical, hormonal and mechanical stimuli.

Around 1966 Hagbarth and Vallbo developed a microelectrode technique for recording action potentials from individual nerve fibers in man and it was soon discovered that the method could be used to measure also sympathetic activity (1). With this important methodological advancement it became possible to record sympathetic action potentials directly as they appeared unobscured by the sluggishness of the effector organs. One could distinguish between sympathetic outflows to skin and muscle, the strength of the activity could be studied both at rest and during various manoeuvres and variations of activity could be correlated to the experiences and thoughts of the subject.

Anatomical Background and Recording Technique

The majority of postganglionic sympathetic fibers to skin and muscles in the extremities run in the peripheral nerves. Each nerve comprises a number of well-isolated fascicles in which the unmyelinated C-fibers are found, not diffusely distributed but aggregated in groups in Schwann cells. Distally, each nerve fascicle contains fibers connected only to a skin area or only to a muscle, thus providing the possibility of making selective recordings from either skin or muscle fibers. The recording microelectrode is made from insulated

---

Supported by Swedish Medical Research Council Grant No B86-04X-03546-158.

tungsten, with an uninsulated tip a few microns in diameter. The electrode is inserted manually through the intact and unanesthetized skin into the underlying nerve in an alert and co-operating subject. The reference electrode is placed subcutaneously 1-2 cm away. Usually multiunit activity is obtained (and indeed preferred), but occasionally, single unit activity is encountered. Most recordings are made in large nerves such as median, tibial or peroneal nerves, but smaller cutaneous nerves have been used. Recordings cause only minimal discomfort and no permanent after-effects have been reported, although paraesthesia may occur in 10-20% of the subjects for a few days after the experiment. In most experiments ECG and respiratory movements are recorded and sometimes intraarterial blood pressure is monitored. Changes of electrical skin resistance (evoked by sweating) and a finger or toe pulse plethysmogram (photoelectric) are often included. For detailed descriptions of the recording technique and the evidence for the sympathetic nature of the recorded impulses see Vallbo (2).

Sympathetic Outflow in Human Extremity Nerves

In both muscle and skin fascicles, sympathetic outflow is seen as multiunit volleys of impulses with interposed intervals of neural silence; there is no evidence of continuous activity. The temporal pattern of activity, however, is entirely different in the two types of nerves. In muscle nerves the activity is made up of vasoconstrictor impulses grouped in the cardiac rhythm. In contrast, sympathetic discharges in skin nerves (containing a mixture of vasoconstrictor and sudomotor impulses) occur in a more irregular pattern without obvious cardiac rhythmicity (3).

Muscle Sympathetic Activity (MSA)

When MSA and intraarterial blood pressure are recorded at rest there is a close inverse correlation between variations of nerve activity and pressure: The bursts occur predominantly during reductions and disappear during increases of blood pressure (4, 5). A blood pressure fall during a prolonged diastole is followed by a particulary strong MSA burst (6). Electrical stimulation of the carotid sinus nerves inhibits MSA with accompanying reduction of muscle vascular resistance (7). The findings suggest that the cardiac rhythmicity is due to arterial baroreceptors modulation of the neural outflow. With each systolic blood pressure peak, sympathetic activity is inhibited, but reappears when diastolic blood pressure falls below a certain level. Bilateral local anaesthesia of glossopharyngeal and vagus nerves in the neck evoked a pronounced increase of MSA (accompanied by high blood pressure and tachycardia), and the pulse synchrony was replaced by a 0.4-0.7 Hz irregular rhythm (similar to but not identical with sympathetic activity in skin nerves; see below) (8). Thus it seems that central sympathetic outflow to muscles consists of irregular discharges and that the characteristic temporal pattern is brought about by recurrent baroreceptor inhibition entraining the bursts in the cardiac rhythm.

A detailed analysis of the relationship between MSA and blood pressure shows that the outflow of impulses correlates with fluctuations of diastolic blood pressure, but not with the long-term level of blood pressure (5). This relationship between MSA and diastolic blood pressure variations follows from the fact that the baroreflex is inhibitory and since systolic inhibition of sympathetic activity is complete, diastolic blood pressure variations are the basis of regulation. The reflex influence from arterial baroreceptors on MSA has dynamic properties. For example, at a given value of diastolic blood pressure, sympathetic discharges are stronger and more common during the falling phase of a blood pressure change than during the rising phase. If afferent baroreceptor nerve traffic is altered by step changes of transmural carotid pressure there is only a transient change of MSA; adaptation is more or less complete after 1-2 sec even if the stimulus is maintained (9, 10). Since aortic baroreceptors are uninfluenced by the stimulus, static arterial baroreceptor effects on MSA cannot be excluded but together with the lack of correlation between mean levels of MSA and diastolic blood pressure the findings suggest that arterial baroreflex effects on MSA are more important for buffering changes of arterial blood pressure than for setting the long-term blood pressure level.

Besides the arterial baroreceptors other receptors influence the strength of MSA. When subatmospheric pressure was applied around the lower part of the body thereby reducing central blood volume, there was a static increase in MSA. The intimate relationship to transient blood pressure fluctuations was preserved (11). Since there were no changes in diastolic pressure which could explain the increase in MSA, it was concluded that effects from other receptors, presumably intrathoracic volume receptors, must have occurred.

Recent evidence suggest that MSA is influenced also from chemoreceptors. Generalized hypercapnea (7% CO_2) and hypoxia (8% O_2) both increased MSA and the effect was potentiated during simultaneous hypercapnea and hypoxia (Blumberg, personal communication). Also local muscle ischaemia developed during isometric handgrip induced an increase of MSA which quickly subsided when the ischaemia relieved (12), suggesting a reflex effect evoked by chemo-sensitive afferent nerve endings in the contracting muscles.

A poorly understood feature of MSA is the profound difference in strength of activity between individuals. In a given subject the pattern of outflow of sympathetic impulses shows a high degree of similarity in different extremity nerves and the level of activity at rest (expressed as number of bursts/100 heart beats or bursts/minute) is reproducible from day to day even with years between recordings (13). Between individuals, however, the level of activity at supine rest ranges from below 10 to more than 90 bursts/100 heart beats and as mentioned above the differences are not related to differences in arterial blood pressure (5, 14).

Skin Sympathetic Activity (SSA)

The outflow of sudomotor and vasoconstrictor impulses in skin nerves is important for thermoregulation. For example, if room temperature is lowered there is an increase of SSA and since at the same time there are plethysmographic signs of vasoconstriction (and absence of electrodermal responses indicative of sweating) one has to conclude that the increase of activity is due to a selective activation of vasoconstrictor impulses. Also when room temperature is increased there is an increase of SSA but now associated with vasodilatation and electrodermal signs of sweating (15). Thus, in this situation there must have been a selective activation of sudomotor impulses. SSA is not influenced only by thermal stimuli but both a sudden deep breath and a variety of arousal stimuli regularly elicit a strong burst of SSA (16), and the reflex delay correlates with conduction time in postganglionic fibers (17). Emotional excitement usually induces more long-lasting increase of outflow in both vasoconstrictor and sudomotor neurons. Thus SSA is involved in emotional reactions, and stress-induced long-lasting simultaneous activation of sudomotor and vasoconstrictor fibers constitutes the neurophysiological basis of cold sweat.

The Concept of Sympathetic Tone

The different properties of sympathetic activity in skin and muscle nerve fascicles, and even of sudomotor and vasoconstrictor activity in skin nerves, emphasize that there is no common overall sympathetic tone. Instead the sympathetic nervous system should be regarded as a number of functionally separate subdivisions, each of which is modulated by its own central connections and afferent influences. This view is in agreement with the finding of different contributions of individual organs to total noradrenaline release (18). For MSA an individual, characteristic resting tone can be defined, which seems to be similar for all extremity muscles. For SSA the term "tone" is of little value in view of the profound variations according to environmental circumstances.

Relationship Between MSA and Plasma Noradrenaline

At rest, plasma levels of noradrenaline, the transmitter released from postganglionic sympathetic neurons, vary markedly between individuals, but in a given subject the level is fairly stable from one day to another. Similarly MSA tends to be stable in an individual and vary markedly between individuals. Moreover, a significant correlation between levels of MSA at rest and plasma noradrenaline from antecubital venous blood was found in normotensive subjects (19) and in patients with essential hypertension (20). A possible explanation for this finding could be that striated muscles, comprising 40% of total body weight, contain such a large number of sympathetic terminals that spillover from these will be a major contribution to plasma noradrenaline, especially when blood is sampled from an antecubital vein, where 45% of the noradrenaline is estimated to derive from local release from the forearm (21). If other sympathetic outflows (e.g., to the kidneys) are similar to that of muscle, the correlation would be strengthened.

Pathophysiological Studies

In pathological states sympathetic outflow can change by different mechanisms.

1) *Peripheral efferent lesions* such as degeneration of efferent postganglionic fibers will reduce the number of impulses reaching the effector organs. Qualitatively, however, reflex patterns remain normal. This abnormality has been demonstrated in polyneuropathy (22).
2) *Peripheral afferent lesions*. Altered function in afferent fibers may have different effects if the sensory input is excitatory or inhibitory. For example, impaired sensation may give impaired responses to arousal stimuli in SSA. Increased sensation may give rise to increased reflex effects. This occurs in glossopharyngeal neuralgia with syncope (23). In this rare condition the syncope is due to exaggerated baroreflex inhibition of MSA and heart rate. Presumably, this occurs because of an ephapse with abnormal impulse transmission from afferent fibers from the throat to afferent fibers from carotid baroreceptors (both travelling in the glossopharyngeal nerve); each pain attack will then induce exaggerated baroreflex inhibition. In contrast, impaired afferent activity from baroreceptors (impaired inhibition) may give a pathological increase of MSA. This may explain an increased MSA in some patients with the Guillain-Barré syndrome (24).
3) *Central lesions* may interrupt excitatory or inhibitory pathways and may also cause qualitative changes of sympathetic reflexes. In patients with spinal cord lesions sympathetic outflow below the lesion exhibits several abnormalities: (1) resting sympathetic activity is abnormally low, (2) reflex discharges occur in parallel in MSA and SSA in response to bladder stimuli and cutaneous stimuli below the lesion, (3) sympathetic reflex discharges cause prolonged cutaneous vasoconstrictions, (4) baroreflex influence on MSA is absent. These abnormalities may be contributing factors behind episodes of hypertension in patients with spinal cord lesions (25, 26).

References

1. Hagbarth, K.-E. & Vallbo, A.B. (1968). Pulse and respiratory grouping of sympathetic impulses in human muscle nerves. Acta Physiol. Scand., 74: 96-108.
2. Vallbo, A.B., Hagbarth, K.-E., Torebjörk, H.E. & Wallin, B.G. (1979). Somatosensory, proprioceptive and sympathetic activity in human peripheral nerves. Physiol. Rev., 59: 919-957.
3. Wallin, B.G. (1983). Intraneural recording and autonomic function in man. In R. Bannister (Ed.), Autonomic failure. Oxford University Press, p. 36-51.
4. Delius, W., Hagbarth, K.-E., Hongell, A. & Wallin, B.G. (1972). General characteristics of sympathetic activity in human muscle nerves. Acta Physiol. Scand., 84: 65-81.
5. Sundlöf, G. & Wallin, B.G. (1978). Human muscle nerve sympathetic activity at rest. Relationship to blood pressure and age. J. Physiol., 274: 621-637.
6. Wallin, B.G., Delius, W. & Sundlöf, G. (1974). Human muscle nerve sympathetic activity in cardiac arrhythmias. Scand. J. Clin. Lab. Invest., 34: 293-300.
7. Wallin, B.G., Sundlöf, G. & Delius, W. (1975). The effect of carotid sinus nerve stimulation on muscle and skin nerve sympathetic activity in man. Pflügers Arch., 358: 101-110.
8. Fagius, J., Wallin, B.G., Sundlöf, G., Nerhed, C. & Englesson, S. (1985). Sympathetic outflow in man after anaesthesia of the glossopharyngeal and vagus nerves. Brain, 108: 423-438.
9. Bath, E., Lindblad, L.-E. & Wallin, B.G. (1981). Effects of dynamic and static neck suction on muscle nerve sympathetic activity, heart rate and blood pressure in man. J. Physiol., 311: 551-564.
10. Wallin, B.G. & Eckberg, D.L. (1982). Sympathetic transients caused by abrupt alterations of carotid baroreceptor activity in man. Am. J. Physiol., 242: H185-H190.
11. Sundlöf, G. & Wallin, B.G. (1978). Effects of lower body negative pressure on human muscle nerve sympathetic activity. J. Physiol., 278: 525-532.

12. Mark, A.L., Victor, P.G., Nerhed, C. & Wallin, B.G. (1985). Microneurographic studies of the mechanisms of sympathetic nerve responses to static exercise in humans. Circ. Res., 57: 461-469.
13. Sundlöf, G. & Wallin, B.G. (1977). The variability of muscle nerve sympathetic activity in resting recumbent man. J. Physiol., 272: 383-397.
14. Wallin, B.G. & Sundlöf, G. (1979). A quantitative study of muscle nerve sympathetic activity in resting normotensive and hypertensive subjects. Hypertension, 1: 67-77.
15. Bini, G., Hagbarth, K.-E., Hynninen, P. & Wallin, B.G. (1980). Thermoregulatory and rhythm-generating mechanisms governing the sudomotor and vasoconstrictor outflow in human cutaneous nerves. J. Physiol., 306: 537-552.
16. Hagbarth, K.-E., Hallin, R.G., Hongell, A., Torebjörk, H.E. & Wallin, B.G. (1972). General characteristics of sympathetic activity in human skin nerves. Acta Physiol. Scand., 84: 164-176.
17. Fagius, J. & Wallin, B.G. (1980). Sympathetic reflex latencies and conduction velocities in normal man. J. Neurol. Sci., 47: 433-448.
18. Esler, M., Wilett, I., Leonard, P., Hasking, G., Johns, J., Little, P. & Jennings, G. (1984). Plasma noradrenaline kinetics in humans. J. Autonom. Nerv. System, 11: 125-144.
19. Wallin, B.G., Sundlöf, G., Eriksson, B.-M., Dominiak, P., Grobecker, H. & Lindblad, L.-E. (1981). Plasma noradrenaline correlates to sympathetic muscle nerve activity in normotensive man. Acta Physiol. Scand., 111: 69-73.
20. Mörlin, C., Wallin, B.G. & Eriksson, B.-M. (1983). Muscle sympathetic activity and plasma noradrenaline in normotensive and hypertensive man. Acta Physiol. Scand., 119: 117-121.
21. Hjemdahl, P., Freyschuss, U., Juhlin-Dannfelt, A. & Linde, B. (1984). Differentiated sympathetic activation during mental stress evoked by the Stroop Test. Acta Physiol. Scand. Suppl., 527: 25-29.
22. Fagius, J. & Wallin, B.G. (1980). Sympathetic reflex latencies and conduction velocities in patients with polyneuropathy. J. Neurol. Sci., 47: 449-461.
23. Wallin, B.G., Westerberg, C.-E. & Sundlöf, G. (1984). Syncope induced by glossopharyngeal neuralgia: Sympathetic outflow to muscle. Neurology (Cleveland), 34: 533-524.
24. Fagius, J. & Wallin, B.G. (1983). Microneurographic evidence of excessive sympathetic outflow in the Guillain-Barré syndrome. Brain, 106: 589-600.
25. Wallin, B.G. & Stjernberg, L. (1984). Sympathetic activity in man after spinal cord injury. Outflow to skin below the lesion. Brain, 107: 183-198.
26. Stjernberg, L., Blumberg, H. & Wallin, B.G. (1986). Sympathetic activity in man after spinal cord injury. Outflow to muscle below the lesion. Brain, 109: 695-715.3

Pathophysiology as a Guide to Drug Development in Tissue Hypoxia

Thies Peters

Drug treatment of atherosclerotic disorders still poses major problems for the patient and for the physician. Although many drugs - probably too many - are available, convincing progress in this field is lacking. This is regrettable particularly because life expectancy grows and because of the high incidence of these disorders in the elderly population and their impact on quality of life, morbidity and mortality. These conditions require long term or even life long treatment with safe and target orientated drugs.

It has frequently been experienced in the past that knowledge of the pathophysiology underlying a certain disease has allowed the development of a specific type of drug which is able to interrupt a pathophysiologic sequence of events. An action of this kind may have the advantage of being directed to pathologic processes rather than involving and disturbing physiologic events. During recent years knowledge concerning the molecular pathophysiology of arteriosclerotic disorders has increased mainly as a result of improved technology and of new pharmacologically active compounds, which can be used as tools to discover so far unknown interrelations. Among the mechanisms involved in atherosclerotic disorders major attention has been focussed upon ionic events occurring during early phases of ischemia. Most investigators centered their interest upon one particular ion, the calcium-ion (1), and especially upon its intracellular compartmentalization, concentration, and regulatory properties for cell function.

What were the reasons? Practically all physiologic processes involve the presence of ions like sodium, potassium, magnesium, and calcium. However, calcium appears to be the most critical ion, because it can function as an ionic messenger and fine tune a great number of cellular processes. Whereas an alteration of intracellular sodium- or potassium-ions by several millimoles is of minor importance for cell function, the decrease or increase of micromolar amounts of calcium-ions determines whether a cell rests or performs its typical physiologic function or even dies. A cell type well investigated in this respect is the cardiac muscle cell. At calcium-ion-concentrations below 0.1 μm the cell is relaxed. In between 0.1 and 1 μm it develops tension. In between 1 and 10 μm relaxation becomes progressively impaired, the membrane depolarizes, ionic permeabilities increase, aberrations of cell metabolism develop and eventually the cell dies.

Similar observations have been made for red blood cells, vascular smooth muscle cells, neuronal cells, to give only a few examples. The principal sequence of events is very similar in all cell types: Below 1 μm calcium ions fulfil physiological requirements; above 1 μm they initiate a cascade of pathologic consequences which involve loss of function and cell death.

In conclusion, it seems to be of vital importance to keep the intracellular free calcium concentration properly within physiologic limits.

Connection Between Decreased Oxygen Supply and Intracellular Calcium-Ion Concentration

An early, almost immediate, reaction of tissue exposed to oxygen lack is lactic acid production as a consequence of anaerobic glycolysis. Concomitant acidification concerns both the intra- and the extracellular environment. The change in pH proceeds slowly but may be rather pronounced (2). Among the intracellular calcium-binding structures some acidic lipids, especially phosphatidyl-serine molecules, display a pH-dependent affinity for calcium (3, 4, 5). These lipids are located at the internal surface of the plasmalemma (6) and seem to play a role in physiological regulation of intracellular calcium-ion release and sequestration (4). Increasing the proton concentration reduces their binding affinity for calcium and, as a consequence, calcium ions are slowly released into the cytosol. For cardiac muscle cells it could be demonstrated that another important store, the sarcoplasmic reticulum, releases calcium upon acidification (7). Since pools of calcium involved in physiological regulation are thus emptied, a loss of physiological function should be the result. This postulate is in accordance with the observation that after cessation of blood flow specific functions like consciousness or cardiac concentration are lost within less than half a minute (consciousness 10 sec, see (8); heart beat 30 sec, own observations).

Another effect of an intracellular increase of ionized calcium consists of a gating of potassium efflux. This calcium-induced increase of potassium permeability has been demonstrated for a variety of excitable and nonexcitable cells (for review see 9). As a result, in ischemic tissues the extracellular potassium concentration should increase.

By means of ion-selective electrodes it can be demonstrated that during the phase of declining pH after the loss of function the extracellular potassium concentration rises initially slowly from a value of 4 mM up to a threshold of about 13 mM. Thereafter, it abruptly increases to values of about 80 mM. Concomitantly cell depolarization occurs (10-13). The depolarized membrane loses its function as a permeability barrier for ions. According to the high gradient for calcium ions from the extra- to the intracellular space a net influx of this ion can be observed, e.g., in neuronal tissues, when the external potassium concentration exceeds 10 to 15 mM (14). In fact, as soon as the extracellular potassium concentration exceeds the values mentioned, calcium-ion concentration in the extracellular space drops which is, at least in part, a reflection of net movement of calcium through the plasmalemma (13, 15). In neuronal tissues one of the immediate consequences of calcium-influx should be a release of neurotransmitters which was proven by Govoni et al. (16) and by Akerman and Heinonen (14). Additionally, potassium is a very potent vasoconstricting agent in that it allows entry of calcium due to depolarization (for review see 17).

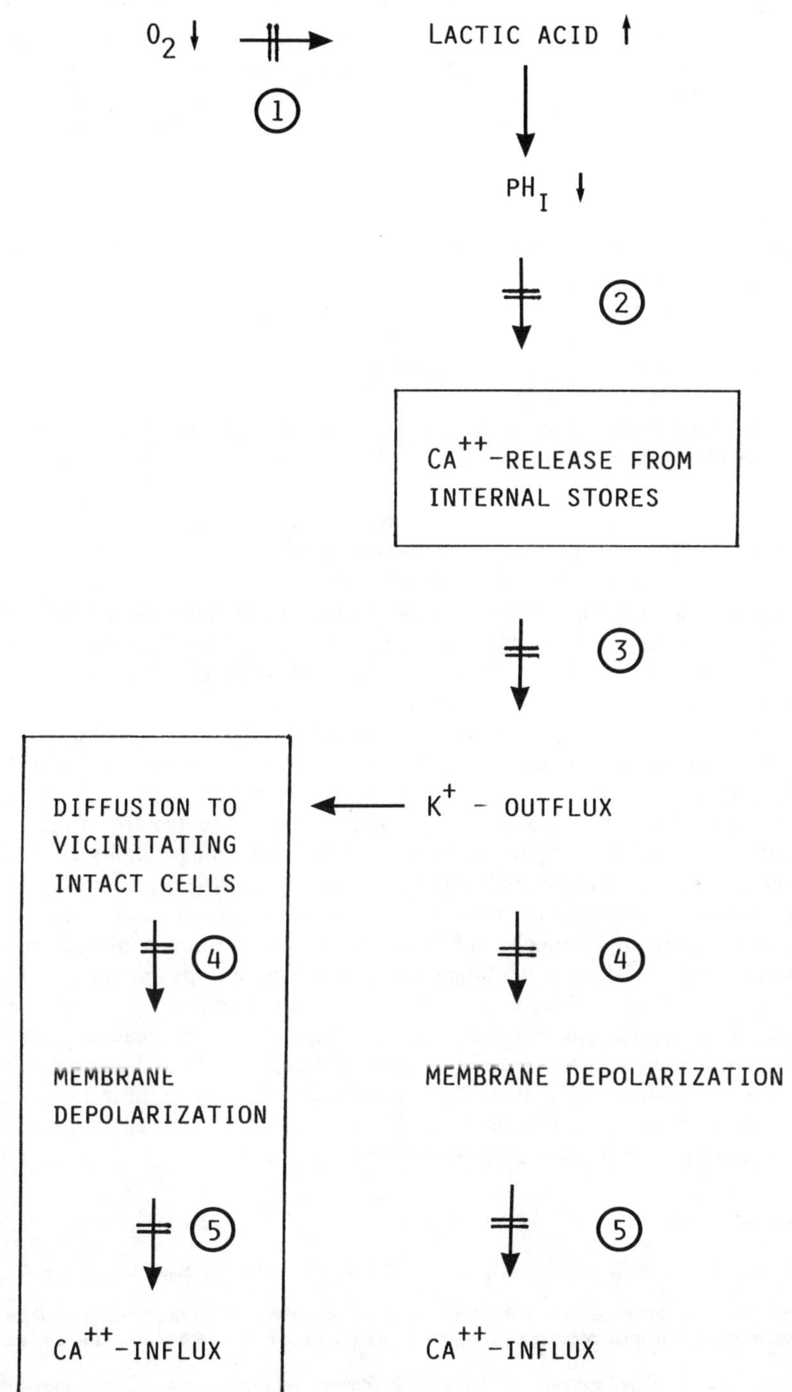

Figure 1. Ionic events involved in early ischemia.

A hypothesis was forwarded, which suggests that a regional ischemic damage is amplified by diffusion of potassium to vicinitating parenchymal and smooth muscle cells. Subsequently, depolarization of both, parenchymal and smooth muscle cells, should aggravate the ischemic damage. Under these aspects potassium would be the mediator and calcium the effector in the spread of ischemic events like in stroke or cardiac infarction (5).

In Figure 1 the ionic events involved in early ischemia are schematically depicted, with the aim to outline possible pharmacologic interventions. As can be obtained it appears desirable to interfere with events particularly restricted to pathology by means of drugs which specifically inhibit calcium-induced potassium efflux or drugs which specifically prevent from depolarization-induced calcium influx, preferably from calcium leaks.

Schematic presentation of proven and hypothetical (framed) steps involved in early regional ischemia and the respective possibilities of intervention.

1) Drugs which more or less specifically decrease physiologic activity will reduce metabolism and thus the production of lactic acids (e.g., narcotics).
2) Drugs which inhibit calcium release from physiologic stores should more specifically inhibit the increase of cytosolic calcium ion concentration which in turn prevents calcium-induced potassium efflux. The disadvantage of this principle is obvious: These drugs will interfere with any physiologic process which involves calcium-release from internal stores.
3) Prevention from calcium-induced potassium outflux would be a highly desirable principle because it enables an interruption of dysregulation at an early stage.
4) Membrane depolarization can be inhibited by a number of drugs called membrane stabilizers. Again, difficulties arise from unspecificity since these drugs tend to act on physiologic regulations throughout the organism.
5) Membrane depolarization induces the opening of plasmalemma voltage dependent calcium channels and increases a leak of calcium directly through the lipid bilayer. Drugs inhibiting calcium entry through channels (calcium channel blockers) should act protective; however, they also act on physiologic regulations involving the voltage dependent calcium channel. Drugs which reduce the leak of calcium through the lipid bilayer are more specifically active under pathologic conditions since they prevent primarily calcium overload (calcium overload blockers) and do not affect physiologic activities of classic types of calcium channels.

References

1. Campbell, A.K. (1985). Intracellular calcium, its universal role as regulator. Wiley & Sons, Chichester.
2. Mutch, W.A. & Hansen, A.J. (1984). Extracellular pH changes during spreading depression and cerebral ischemia: Mechanisms of brain pH regulation. J. Cereb. Blood Flow Metab., 4: 17-27.
3. Jacobson, K. & Papahadjopoulos, D. (1975). Phase transitions and phase separations in phospholipid membranes induced by changes in temperature, pH, and concentration of bivalent cations. Biochemistry, 14: 152-161.

4. Lüllmann, H. & Peters, T. (1977). Plasmalemmal calcium in cardiac excitation-concentration coupling. Clin. Exp. Pharmacol. Physiol., 4: 49-57.
5. Peters, T. (1986). Calcium in physiological and pathological cell function. Eur. Neurol., suppl. 1, 25: 27-44.
6. Zwaal, R.F.A., Roelofsen, B. & Colley, C.M. (1973). Localization of red cell membrane constituents. Biochim. Biophys. Acta, 300: 159-182.
7. Fabiato, A. (1985). Use of aequorin for the appraisal of the hypothesis of the release of calcium from the sarcoplasmic reticulum induced by a change of pH in skinned cardiac cells. Cell calcium, 6: 95-108.
8. Astrup, J., Siesjö, B.K. & Symar, L. (1981). Thresholds in cerebral ischemia - the ischemic penumbra. Stroke, 12: 723-725.
9. Latorre, R., Coronado, R. & Vergara, C. (1984). K^+ channels gated by voltage and ions. Annu. Rev. Physiol., 46: 485-495.
10. Hansen, A.J. & Zeuthen, T. (1981). Extracellular ion concentration during spreading depression and ischemia in the rat brain cortex. Acta Physiol. Scand., 113: 437-445.
11. Siesjö, B.K. (1981). Cell damage in the brain: A speculative synthesis. J. CBF Metab., 1: 155-185.
12. Hansen, A.J. (1985). Effect of anoxia on ion distribution in the brain. Physiol. Rev., 65: 101-148.
13. Höller, M., Dierking, H., Dengler, K., Tegtmeier, F. & Peters, T. (1986). Effect of flunarizine on extracellular ion concentration in the rat brain under hypoxia and ischemia. In N. Battistine, P. Fiorani, R. Courbier, F. Plum & C. Fieschi (Eds.), Acute brain ischemia medical and surgical therapy. Raven Press, N.Y.
14. Akerman, K.E.O. & Heinonen, E. (1983). Qualitative measurements of cytosolic calcium ion concentration within isolated guinea-pig nerve endings entrapped arsenazo III. Biochim. Biophys. Acta, 732: 117-121.15.
15. Harris, R.J., Symon, L., Branston, N.M. & Bayhan, M. (1981). Changes in extracellular calcium activity in cerebral ischemia. J. CBF Metab., 1: 203-209.
16. Govoni, S., Trabucchi, M., Magnoni, M.S., Battaini, F. & Paoletti, R. (1985). Abnormal transmitter release and calcium entry blockers. In T. Godfraind, P.M. Vanhoutte, S. Gavoni & R. Paoletti (Eds.), Calcium entry blockers and tissue protection. Raven Press, N.Y.
17. Kuriyama, H. (1981). Excitation contraction coupling in various visceral smooth muscles. In E. Bülbring, A.F. Brading, A.W. Jones & T. Tomita (Eds.), Smooth muscle: An assessment of current knowledge. Edward Arnold Ltd, London.

Psychological Determinants of When Stressors Stress

J. Bruce Overmier

Last October 12, Holger - member of a local polar bear club - accidently swamped his canoe while tending his fishing nets 100 meters from shore. He swam to shore safely but had to be treated for shock and later developed mild hemorrhagic gastric erosions. Yet, just the preceding December 25, he and a number of his fellow polar-bear club members had chopped through ice so that they could swim in a 100 meter race; Holger had suffered no ill effects on that occasion. This vignette makes the issue clear: When do potential stressors in fact constitute a debilitating psychobiological challenge? They don't always do so as is clear from both anecdotes and the scientific study of humans and animals.

We have posed an important question but hardly a new one (1-5). Answering the question has at least three parts: (1) defining stress, (2) defining potential stressors, and (3) determining the conditions under which the putative stressors do and do not lead to the specific effect. The present paper is more a strategic proposal than a direct answer to the question.

I shall not undertake to define "stress." There are those who spent many years in defining this term, Selye (6), without satisfying all critics (7, 8). Moreover, I do not really want to follow Selye in this matter because for many psychologists the use of the term is more consistent with what Selye called "distress" and this is what laymen mean as well. (To accept Selye's definition is to have to argue to unions and others that "stress" is sometimes a good thing (eustress) and this makes a muddle of all the discussion - and negotiations - that follow. See also (9)). What we are interested in are the conditions that constitute sufficient psychobiological challenge with the potential to result in behavioral and/or physiological impairments and which, given the opportunity, the organism will defend against. When such defense or coping fails, the result is "distress." This "distress" - which I may sometimes simply call "stress" - and the conditions which permit defense are the current focus.

I shall not undertake to define the features of potential stressors that could cause distress. Nor shall I attempt an exhaustive list of the members of the class of potential stressors. None now exists, nor is one likely ever to be constructed. In the absence of such a complete list, one cannot be sure that one has an adequate definition. Moreover, such a definition or list is not really necessary to achieving the goals here, which is the consideration of *some* of the psychological context features which modulate - or more precisely, allow the organism to modulate - the impact of *some* (hopefully representative) potential or real stressors. I will finesse the issue even further in the pages that follow by attending only to physical events known to be aversive such as electric shocks, cold water immersions, and the like.

In determining the conditions under which the putative stressors cause distress, we are tackling a complex problem that includes not only the organism's past history with physical events but its psychological state, and this last may be a function of the former as well as of current contextual features (10). It is well known that the distress caused by a given physical experience is a function of the organism's prior physical experiences with that or other stressors (11-14).

Choice of a Strategy

In defining stressors, one strategy many have adopted is to define situations and events broadly in terms of both physical events and psychological factors *interfused* (15, 16). The argument is that the psychological state is integral to the definition of the stressor, that one must include not only the description of the physical event but also the "meaning" of that event (17-19). But the psychological factors have been multitudinous, nonsystematic, and sometimes inconsistent with one another. These have included things such as social supports, competitive challenges, perceptions, expectancies, attributions about the reasons for the stressor, attributions about the self and/or others, personality traits (e.g., "internality" vs. "externality"), imaginal style, "immersion" among many others. Worse, some of these "factors" may really be consequents of the stressor challenge rather than antecedents. These things are without doubt of importance, if one chooses this strategy.

Alternatively, I would suggest that for the present we treat the psychological meaning factors *not as components* of the stressor *per se* but rather as separable modulators of the stressfulness of the fundamental physical event(s). (For a similar approach see 20, 21). To be more concrete, consider a physical treatment like severe physical restraint for 4 hours. We can sensibly ask how does changing the illumination level modulate the stressfulness of the basic physical challenge? In the same way, we can ask what psychological contextual factors modulate (ameliorate or augment) the impact of the restraint. Does restraining the organism in the presence of a social group modulate the stressfulness of the physical challenge? And just as we need not define a new stressor for each possible brightness, we need not define a new stressor for each possible variant on a psychological contextual manipulation. The strategy here proposed then is to attempt in our analysis of stress to get a *separation* for analytic purposes between the physical event impacting upon the organism and the psychological context in which it occurs. This then lets us attribute specific properties to the psychological factors themselves!

Whether we ought to treat psychological contextual factors as primary (the first strategy above) or as moderator variables (the alternative strategy above) is an issue of continuing debate (22, 23). I have here argued for the latter as a matter of *productive strategy* rather than on a basis of received truth. Below, I extend this argument by reference to specific cases.

Psychologists tend to look at organism functioning in the world in their "normal, adaptive" ways and then, after studying this normal functioning, to study deviations from this normal functioning, seeking the causal variables responsible for these deviations. This is a specific view and approach to the analysis of biobehavioral phenomena and is exemplified by recent psychological research on two special phenomena of maladaptive behavior: Learned helplessness and learned irrelevance. We have neither the time nor the space to review these here (for reviews, see 24, 25). However, there are some strategic things to be learned by looking briefly at these problems.

Learned Helplessness and Learned Irrelevance

Learned helplessness is known to occur empirically in animals as a consequence of exposure to a severe sequence of uncontrollable (and unpredictable) aversive events. The phenomena involves subsequent motivational/behavioral failure to master new challenges, emotional changes, hormonal shifts, and biochemical depletion, among other features (24, 26, 27) . This phenomenon is a general one transcending species and environments (28). (It appears as an analog to the responses of people to disastrous events (29)). An animal showing learned helplessness is a clear instance of a distressed, noncoping organism.

Now what is the "cause" of this distress? We can approach the answer theoretically or operationally. There are merits in both. One theoretical account that has been given says that learned helplessness results from the cognition that behavioral responding in the face of aversive events is to no avail - a stable, general, cognition of "uncontrollability." One operational account that has been given is that it results from extensive exposure to uncontrollable aversive events. These two are similar but far from identical because the former invokes a hypothetical construct which is not tied in an absolute way to the inducing operations. Thus, in the theoretical approach one must find independent ways to assess the cognition and then determine the additional factors that modulate the cognition's establishment. This last is no small task because it involves understanding how organisms assess contingencies among events.

The study of how organisms (including humans) assess contingencies among events has been and is being studies rather extensively (30-33), and yet we still are unsure. Factors play a role besides the absolute operating dependencies (e.g., response frequency, Skinner; Wasserman) are differential weightings or biases among the four sets of dependencies that define a contingency.[1] Study of these differential weightings (i.e., strategies) is itself a subject meriting extensive analysis. Skinner (33) and Alloy and Tabachnik (32) have provided analyses of this difficult problem. This issue is further complicated by possible

1. The degree of contingency between two events, say a response and an outcome, is a function of the relative frequencies of 4 possible event-event occurences: (1) R and O, (2) R and not-O, (3) not-R and O, (4) not-R and not-O. These values may be subject to statistical decision treatment, signal detection treatment, or a variety of other treatments (Handbook of Mathematical Psychology) to yield an inference as to degree of contingency.

attributions that the organsism may make that may modulate all the other factors (34-36).

The point of the preceding is to illustrate that to the extent we are interested in proceeding to analyze the psychobiologic phenomenon rather than the cognitive one, we may be better advised for the nonce to focus upon operational features that we can directly assess and restrict our inferences to behavioral and psychological processes that we can more directly measure.

Similar arguments derive from the phenomenon of learned irrelevance (25). Learned irrelevance is known to occur empirically as a consequence of exposure to a long sequence of randomly related signals and aversive events (i.e., non-predicting signals and unpredictable aversive events - which by the way were also uncontrollable). The phenomenon involves subsequent interference with associative signals with, say, shocks when the latter are now predictable; moreover, we can presume that since these latter aversive events are effectively *not* "anticipated" the effects of these shocks as indexed by physiological measures will be greater that otherwise (37). This important phenomenon also seems to be a general one as is learned helplessness (38, 39).

The "cause" of learned irrelevance, too, may be identified theoretically (i.e., resulting from the cognition that events in the world are generally unrelated) or operationally (i.e., resulting from the exposure to the random events). And as before, if one chooses the former, one must first find ways to measure the cognition and then study extensively those things which may modulate the cognition (32, 40-43) - again taking us away, at least temporarily, from the psychobiological question we wish to address.

Another strategic issue has to do with one's reference condition. In learned helplessness, the effort is to study the deleterious effects of making controllable events or predictable events uncontrollable and unpredictable. In the present context, I suggest it is rather better to study the distress modulating effects of making known definable stressors controllable and/or predictable.

The shift in view here is subtle but important. Here I take the reference condition to be the psychobiological effects of the physical stressor events themselves unencumbered by any other organism-environment interactions.

Psychological context factors or "meaning" giving features are manipulated independently as *additions*.

To say that an event is a controllable one requires that the organism indeed exercises such control. If it does not, the *experimenter defined* controllability is without effect for the organism. Organism sensitivity to experimenter defined controllability and predictability are *measurable* - the former through observing the frequency of the defined controlling response and its sensitivity to shifts in demands (i.e., Thorndikian instrumental behavior), the latter through anticipatory responses during the predicting signal (i.e., Pavlovian conditional responses). And, on these empirical bases we can infer the presence of psychological sensitivity to the factors of controllability or predictability. But one cannot infer from lack of responses the opposite states - absence of responses does not insure a psychological state of uncontrollability. This logical asymmetry reinforces the strategy of "adding" psychologically meaningful variations in a form of reducing stress consequences rather than removing these psychological factors from the coping individual. The careful reader here will recognize that both procedures involve operationally the same groups but the new approach turns "learned helplessness" into a normal consequence of stressors rather than some special phenomenon of distorted behavioral processes. Hence, the reason I wish to use the response to "pure" physical event as the baseline for inferring whether psychological factors reduce the extent to which physical events are distressing - i.e., modulate when stressors stress.

This shift in focus for us psychologists that I have suggested has other simplifying advantages, as well, in terms of experimental design and interpretation. Demonstrations of learned helplessness typically utilize a special experimental design called the triadic design which compares a group that receives escapable shocks, a group that receives matched (yoked) inescapable shocks, and a group that receives no shocks. Klosterhalfen and Klosterhalfen (44) in a careful critique have noted that the "helplessness" interpretations depend upon obtaining a specific pattern of relations among all three groups. In contrast, the testing of whether adding control over aversive events alters the effects produced by uncontrollable events requires only a comparison of two groups. We do not care for the present purposes whether the obtained difference is attributable to learned helplessness or learned mastery or both. Similarly, demonstrations of learned irrelevance typically rely upon obtaining a particular pattern of results among three groups analogous to those of the triadic design (45) or among four groups (38, 46), depending upon the alternatives to be excluded, Here, too, testing of whether adding prediction of the aversive events alters the effects produced by unpredicted events requires only a comparison of two groups.[2] We do not care for the present purposes whether the obtained difference is attributable to associative interference or associative priming or both. In the present instance, I want merely to identify those conditions wherein the impact of the stressors are reduced by introducing some psychological contextual factor such as controllability and predictability.

Consequences of Stressors

In the above section, we have argued against assuming the primacy of psychological states as causes of stress and rather, argued for their treatment as modulators of stress. We now must turn to the consequences of exposure to stressors. These are many and might include personal reports of despair, frustration, impairment of memory, inability to coordinate movements, loss of appetite, anxiety, increased serum cortisol, depleted norepinephrine, gastric

2. In both cases, of course, one might well wish to include groups to insure that the observed differences are not attributable to the effects of responses per se, in former case, or to signals per se, in the latter case. However, to the extent that response production and/or novel signals themselves usually yield physiological arousal, then these potential contributors are directionally opposite of the ameliorating effects of control and prediction. Thus, absence of such treatment control groups most likely results in an underestimation of the ameliorating effects of control and prediction.

ulceration, and reduced resistance to disease (47-49). Some of these are classifiable as psychological manifestations, some as somatic.

Is one of these classes of response primary and the other secondary with the primary processes mediating the secondary ones? For example, do the psychological consequences beget the somatic ones as the term psychosomatic implies to so many? An example of the view would be that altered psychological functioning might be said to "cause" ulcers. Or, do the somatic consequences beget the psychological ones, as most reductionists would have it? On this view, for example, depletion of brain norepinephrine would "cause" the symptoms of learned helplessness. For either of these views to be accepted, considerable degrees of correlation between the biological and the psychological indices must exist - although such correlations still don't prove causality much less the direction of the "causal arrow." Moreover, either view is an invocation of mind-body dualism.

Considerable research has addressed in one way or another the degree of correlation between the psychological and the somatic indices. A number of researches are especially noteworthy in this regard (26, 49, 50-53), and some impressive degrees of covariation have been detected. But there also are extensive reports of desynchrony within and among and within biological, psychological, and behavioral measures as well (37, 54-56). Indeed, some have gone so far as to develop theories that assume substantial independence among classes of indices (57).

Thus, it seems to me, that the empirical uncertainty is such that for the purposes of research strategy we must treat the indices separately, allowing correlations among them to *emerge* from the database if they will. Such correlations may be found to operate only under some conditions, perhaps only when some psychological moderator is or is not present. But this is an issue best resolved empirically. Moreover, it is the desynchrony among measures that we will later wish to make use of to address important questions.

Application of the Strategy

It follows from the preceding that, given the demonstrated effects of a specific stressor, one manipulates as separate independent variables the basic physical stressor and those operational contingencies known to be psychologically important to organisms and one measures the changed physiological and/or psychological status of the organism relative to that seen to the stressor alone. Applications of this strategy requires that we attend to four issues:

1) specification of the basic stressor,
2) determination of its effects (relative to absence of the stressor),
3) identifying operational contingencies known to be psychologically important,
4) specifying one's dependent variable measure(s).

Let us comment on each in turn.There are such a wide variety of noxious events that one cannot help be struck by the fact that researchers have experimentally studied *so* few. Possibilities include electric shocks, pressure, cold, ischemia, loud noises, threats, endoscopic exams, dental drilling, even application of medication (e.g., injections or tropical iodine), to name a few.

How do we recognize a potential stressor event? One way is by observing marked physiologically important event-induced shifts in the organism *relative* to the resting state. Another is by observing impaired psychobiological functioning induced by the event relative to psychobiological functioning prior to the event. That there is a separate distinct status of distressed or "stressed" organisms equally implies a reference status of "not stressed" or "unstressed." Because we cannot *a priori* know whether any event is a stressor, we must choose as our initial reference the unstimulated resting organisms (58).

Because we here wish to examine the available data for patterns and because we wish to focus upon animal models, we must look to the one(s) most studied in animals: electric shocks. We need not assume that what is true for the electric shock stressors will necessarily be true for all others. (Indeed, for example, electric shock and cold exposure do differ in their effects over repeated exposures as indexed by shock induced brain norepinephrine depletion, (13).) The degree of congruence of the patterns of stress effects in various response systems and modulation of those effects by psychological factors is a matter of empirical determination. However, in the absence of data to the contrary, the best prediction is provided by the pattern experimentally obtained with another stressor. And, indeed it was the similarity of effects obtained across a wide variety of challenges that led Selye to posit "the general adaptation syndrome."

It is not necessary here for me to present a detailed review of the consequences of exposures to electric shocks as these have been discussed, from various viewpoints and with varying foci, elsewhere (2, 24, 37, 59-61,). The consequences of exposures are both acute and chronic or proactive, that is changes in the sensitivity of the organisms to reexposures to the initial challenge or to new challenges (62, 63), and are to be detected in both physiological and psychological measures (64, 65), from urine osmolarity (66) to perceptions of oneself (67). Because we have no certainty about which among these many possibilities are most central and these are not always perfectly correlated (11, 37), a variety must be considered to establish a "profile." Similarity between the profiles or patterns of any two *effects* (i.e., a strong correlation) may be taken to imply that the *possibility* of common causality or that one is a mediator of the other.

The identifying of operational contingencies that are psychologically important is a complex issue if we are to avoid circularity. That is, we dare not look at which such operations produce a change in the degree of distress that the organism reveals and then identify them as psychological factors. We need instead *independent* sets of observations that organisms are psychologically sensitive to the imposed operations. (See 68 for a similar argument.) For example? Well, learning seems a prototypic psychological process. What operational contingencies are factors in learning?

Establishing a signalling relationship between a neutral stimulus and a hedonically important event results in learning as was early demonstrated by

Pavlov and is called classical conditioning by some or sign learning by others. Indeed, Pavlov also showed that stimuli signalling the non-occurrence of such events also produced learning, albeit opposite in character to the former. We can *independently* confirm that signalling is psychologically important by allowing organisms to choose between two alternatives. The hedonic events presented in each alternative are the same but in one the hedonic events are signalled as to time of occurrence or magnitude while in the other these are not signalled. Under these circumstances animals reliably choose the signalled alternative (69); humans, it seems are somewhat less reliable and Miller (65) has related this to the hypothetical construct of coping style. Other confirming independent operations could be adduced here as well, however (70), but we need not belabor this point of independent observations as being necessary to break the chain of circularity.

Thus, we might identify signalling operation, or *predictability*[3] as one operational contingency of psychological importance to be explored for its moderator role with respect to stress.[4]

Establishing a dependency relation between the occurrence of a hedonically important event and some arbitrarily selected prior act by the organism results in a second kind of learning (71) as was early demonstrated by Thorndike and is called instrumental training by some or habit learning by others. Animals readily show increases in responding indicative of learning when occurrence of, say, food is made a consequence of the response, and they show a response decrease when the withdrawal of food is made a consequence. Similarily, animals readily show increases in responding indicative of learning when ommission or termination of a scheduled aversive event is made a consequence of the response, and they show a response decrease when the presentation of that noxious event is made the consequence. (See 72 for a survey of such research on giving animals control.) We can *independently* confirm that control over hedonic events is psychologically important by allowing organisms to choose between two alternatives. The hedonic events that occur in each alternative are the same but in one the occurrence of the events is under the organism's control while in the other they are not. Under these circumstances animals reliably choose the condition which affords control (73, 74). This preference for control is not quite so reliable in humans with up to 20% sometimes choosing "no-control" (75); Bandura (76) suggests this may be a result of perceived self inefficacy.

Thus, we might identify the dependency operation, or *controllability*, as another operational contingency of psychological importance to be explored for its moderator role with respect to stress.

There are other operations for which we can obtain independent evidence for the organism's psychological sensitivity in, say, learning paradigms. One example

3. Predictability is more complex a dimension than merely signalled vs. unsignalled (123).

4. To assert that something is psychological is not an assertion of independence from physiology, only that its physiology is not now understood. A reductionistic analysis of the mechanisms underlying the stress reducing properties is now underway and may involve reinstatable (conditioned) stress-induced analgesia mediated via endorphins (124, 125).

would be switching the hedonic value of the presented events (signalled or unsignalled, controlled or uncontrolled) between noxious and pleasurable or between pleasurable and neutral. Such "ambiguous" outcomes, which have been called "conflict" and "frustrating," respectively, result in "ambivalent" behaviors (77-79). However, because we do not undertake to review all psychological modulators of stress but rather an illustration of a strategy, the factors of predictability and controllability which we have developed will suffice. And, as they are perhaps the most systematically and certainly the most extensively studied, (see 80, for one recent review). They are probably best conceived of as evolution's "answer" to the unknowable future challenges to the organism's reproductive success (17, 81).

Our dependent variables for indexing any stress modulating effects, of course, would be those variables that were used to index stress in the first place. Note that the criterion comparison is between two groups. A difference on *one* or more of these index variables between groups exposed to the stressor event with and without the potential psychological factor present would reveal the importance of the *psychological* variable. It is *not* necessary that all or even most index variables change upon introduction of the psychological factor, although very powerful factors would be expected to modulate more of the index variables and possibly through greater range. The particular index (indices) which show change might well differ for different types of noxious events and this may interact with the choice of physical stressor event as well.

Towards a Periodic Table of Stress

To seek coherence, if there be any, we must organize our data on stressors, psychological factors, and psychobiological responses. And here we follow the usual practice of independent variables in one dimension and dependent variables in another. Table 1 is an implementation of this organizational scheme for a single stressor event; additional stressors would require replication of the table in the third dimension (see Table 1). The result is a set of cells into which we may enter empirical results. Each cell represents a specific kind of experimental procedure and a psychobiological measure.

Prediction of Onsets

Let us illustrate. For example, let us consider the effects of electric shock stressors as inducers of stress and how a psychological context variation alters the distress. Simple extended exposures to electric shocks are well known to contribute to gastric erosions (Basic Noxious Event's Effect in Table 1), and Caul, Buchanan, and Hays (82) reconfirmed this by simply presenting randomly distributed uncontrollable shocks to resting rats and comparing the effect to that seen in resting rats. They also showed in another group that if those shocks were merely signalled, the degree of ulceration was significantly reduced.[5] That providing prediction of uncontrollable shocks is stress reducing when stress is indexed by gastric erosion has been confirmed by Tsuda, Tanaka, Nishikawa, Hirai, and Pare (83) and by Guile and McCutcheon (84), despite earlier speculations by some (85, 86) that prediction of uncontrollable shocks might well increase the animal's level of distress.

Table 1. Periodic Table of Stress.

(BIOLOGICAL) ←---------- EFFECTS ---------→ (PSYCHOLOGICAL)

CAUSES AND MODULATORS	IMMUNO-LOGICAL	TARGET ORGAN	NEURO-CHEMICAL	HORMONAL (e.g.) CORTICOID ACTH	EMOTIONAL	MOTIVATIONAL	ASSOCIATIVE	COGNITIVE
NOXIOUS EVENT EFFECT								
PREDICTION: ONSET								
PREDICTION: SEVERITY								
PREDICTION: TERMINATION								
CONTROL: ONSET								
CONTROL: SEVERITY								
CONTROL: TERMINATION								
COMBINATIONS: CONTROL ON&OFF; PRED. ON								
COMBINATIONS: CONTROL ON&OFF; PRED. ON&OFF								

NOXIOUS EVENT: SHOCK, COLD, ...

In a similar fashion, Overmier (45) based upon more complete reporting of data obtained by Dess, Linwick, Patterson, Overmier, and Levine (62), presented data using cortisol as the index which suggest that providing prediction of onsets of uncontrollable shocks is stress reducing. While restrained dogs showed a 279% increase in serum cortisol, randomly shocked dogs showed a 437% increase; but dogs which were given a signal before each shock showed only a 352% increase. We may see the distress-reducing effects of signalling uncontrollable shocks in other indices, as well, including more psychological ones. Signalling uncontrollable shocks reduces the chronic fear measured by the conditioned emotional supression of baseline responsing (see 69 for a thorough

5. Of course, these groups are from a single experiment and the shocked groups were literally wired in series to insure identical physical stressor exposure. This use of a yoked "triplet" follows the classical initial use of this procedure by Weiss (97) and is similar to the "triadic" design of Seligman and Maier (94). In so far as possible, I will restrict my review to experiments using such designs.

review.) And, Overmier and Wielkiewicz (38) reported that signalling uncontrollable shocks reduced the interference with future associative learning that is produced by random shocks and signals.

We may present these findings in the table by inserting downward pointing arrows in the appropriate cells to characterize the "stress-reducing" effects of prediction of the occurrence of inescapable, unavoidþble noxious events. These arrows are shown inserted in Table 2.

Table 2. Periodic Table of Stress.

	(BIOLOGICAL) ←---------- EFFECTS							---------→ (PSYCHOLOGICAL)	
CAUSES AND MODULATORS	IMMUNO-LOGICAL	TARGET ORGAN C-V	TARGET ORGAN G-I	NEURO-CHEMICAL	HORMONAL (e.g.) CORTICOID ACTH	EMOTIONAL	MOTIVATIONAL	ASSOCIATIVE	COGNITIVE
NOXIOUS EVENT EFFECT	INCOM-PETENCE	HYPER-TENSION	ULCERS	DEPLETE	HYPER: SECRETE	FEAR	IMPAIRED	SLOWED LEARNING	HELPLESS HOPELESS
PREDICTION: ONSET	↑	?	↓		↓ [↑]	↓		↓	
PREDICTION: SEVERITY									
PREDICTION: TERMINATION			( )			( )			
CONTROL: ONSET			↑						
CONTROL: SEVERITY									
CONTROL: TERMINATION	↓	?	↓		↓	↓	↓	↓	
COMBINATIONS: CONTROL ON&OFF; PRED. ON	?	↓	↓	↓	↓	↓			
COMBINATIONS: CONTROL ON&OFF; PRED. ON&OFF									

Although I have painted a uniform picture, things may be more complicated, because Bassett, Cairncross, and King (87) reported finding that signalled shocks resulted in greater corticoid response than did unsignalled shocks; this was true both when they were inescapable and escapable. Thus, the pattern of data from the corticoid index is more mixed than and not perfectly congruent with that from, say, the ulcer index. In a similar vein, we may note that Friedman, Ader, and Glasgow (88) reported that signalled shocks, as compared to unsignalled shocks or no shocks, *decreased* resistance to viral (Coxsackie B) infection, that is, increased immunoincompetence, and we indicate this by an upward arrow in Table 2.

Control of Duration

So far, we have looked at the pattern of effects in one *row* of the table. Let us now look at the pattern in another row. We now look to see how a different psychologically important factor modulates the several indices of stress: The effects of control over the duration of unsignalled shocks - a simple escape task in which the animal can terminate the random shocks once they begin.

The number of relevant studies here is surprisingly few.[6] The problem is that the procedure most often used to provide control is a discriminative escape-avoidance procedure which confounds control of duration or termination (escape) with control of onset (avoidance) and moreover provides a signal to set the occasion for making the response. Although such experiments are of interest, and we shall consider some of them a bit later, they do not allow us to be certain about which aspect of control is important.

Returning to the few pure escape of signalled shocks, we note that Davis, Porter, Livingston, Herrman, McFadden, and Levine (89) have shown (in a non-yoked procedure) that control by rats over the termination of the shocks resulted in reduced corticoid response relative to that seen in the absence of control. Murison and Isaksen (90) confirmed this in yoked animals and also observed that while inescapable shocks sensitized rats to the ulcerogenic effects of restraint, escapable shocks did not. Additionally, Sklar and Anisman (91) have shown that the availability of the escape contingency reduces the high degree of susceptability to tumor growth (P 815) produced by exposure to equal inescapable shocks (92).[7]

Turning to more psychological indices, Mineka, Cook, and Miller (93) found that the fearfulness induced in rats by exposure to inescapable shocks was reduced in the group for which they were escapable. Finally, exposure to inescapable electric shocks impairs performance in subsequent shock escape/avoidance tasks (94) and in water-escape tasks (95) whereas exposure to the same amounts of escapable shocks does not. Finally, Jackson, Alexander and Maier (96) have shown that the interferences with choice learning that results from exposure to inescapable shocks is reduced when those same shocks are escapable and that this effect cannot be explained by non-associative factors.

These results too may be placed in the table as downward arrows. These results are also incorporated into Table 2.

It would be of interest to compare the above effects of control over termination to those of control over onsets of shocks that are unpredictable - a pure avoidance task. Here we find as set of classic - if disputed - studies by Brady and his associates commonly referred to as the "executive monkey" experiments (3). They compared monkeys (the executives or masters) that were allowed to control scheduled brief shocks by responding anticipatorily to prevent them with yoked monkeys that received the same shocks but over which they could exercise no control. They found that masters developed massive ulcers and died, whereas the yoked monkeys did not.

6. I make no claims to have been exhaustive in my searches in preparing this paper, but base this statement on the relative frequency of their appearance among hundred read.

7. The effects obtained with immunological indices must be viewed with caution for they may or may not be "direct" effects. Rather they may be mediated by one of our other indices (e.g., corticoids, ACTH); moreover, various sarcomas respond very differently. For an enlightening analysis see Newberry, Liebelt, and Boyle (126) but also Maier, Laudenslager, and Ryan (127).

This result has been, as we all know, criticized for a design flaw (97): The animals were not randomly selected but "self selected" into their roles by their performances on the initial days. Weiss (97) carried out a formally *similar* experiment with rats but obtained the opposite pattern of results. But we should note that Brady et al. used unsignalled shocks (so called, Sidman avoidance schedule) and used brief, avoidable-but-inescapable shocks, whereas Weiss (97) used signalled avoidance schedule and, after a few trials, escapable shocks - one of those "combinations" shown at the bottom of Tables 1 and 2. Therefore, as interesting as Weiss's data are in their own right, they neither disconfirm Brady et al. nor do they demonstrate that Brady et al.'s results were attributable to this experimental flaw. And, to my view, a later experiment which I detail below confirms Brady et al.'s initial observation. The point of this present discussion is to emphasize how very careful we must be in identifying the features of the experimental operation which we recognize. Brady's and Weiss' experiments both involved control, even avoidance, but Weiss' also included other features that we have already noted *also* act to reduce ulcers: prediction of onset and control of termination.

Returning to the Brady paradigm, Barbaree and Harding (98) compared rats randomly assigned to the unsignalled avoidable shock condition or the yoked uncontrollable shock condition. They too found that the "executives" showed more ulcerations than their yoked partners (but see 99). So we shall for the moment enter a sign of increasing "stress" in the "control of onset x target organ" cell of Table 2.

Combination and Confounding

By far, the bulk of the experimental research on the question of the effect(s) of predictability and controllability of events as psychological factors modulating the organism's response to the event have not used the "simple" single factor procedures of the type we have just reviewed above. Rather, they have used procedures which *explicitly* at least partially conflated these two factors and/or the various aspects of the events to which these operational factors are relevant, i.e., onset, severity, or termination. Why would researchers opt for experiments that combine factors about which we can have separate questions?

One partial account of this, is that some researchers held theoretical positions that *a priori* asserted an "equivalence" between prediction and control. For example, Averill (75) reduces the role of controllability to merely affording the organism prediction: If you can control the event, you know when it will occur and/or how severe it will be and/or how long it will last. Indeed, Mowrer and Viek (100) in their early classic paper, "An Experimental Analogue of Fear from a Sense of Helplessness," argued that the rat's fear of the inescapable shocks arose from uncertainty about how long they would last. In sharp contrast, Taylor (19), Perkins (101), and Lykken (102) reduce prediction to "control" in the form of allowing the organism to make anticipatory covert responses to modulate the impending event. (These two positions should be distinguished from those that argue that there is an interaction between prediction and control such that the latter is permissive of or modulates the expression of the former - e.g., that prediction is only arousal-reducing when the organism also has explicit control over the event, (80, 85, 103, 104)). Both are speculations.

A second partial account is the metatheoretical belief in learnig as a single unitary construct capturing the properties of a complex but single underlying mechanism. This metatheoretic view underlies many of the "grand" theories of lea ning (105-107). These have never really proved satisfactory (71, 108). But, one can readily see that if you believe that learning about signals for onsets of events is the same process as learning how to escape them, then when one asks questions about how learning may influence stress, one will be relatively insensitive to what learning contingencies are operating. While perhaps satisfactory for initial experiments, this attitude quickly begins to create ambiguities.

Another partial account of this conflation is that many of the experiments were generated in a theoretial context that did not make precise distinctions. For example, the theory of learned helplessness (109), which necessarily derived from the initial experimental observations (10, 94), argued that "uncontrollability" was critical without distinguishing among the possible things that might be controlled or not. An example of a relevant question that seems never to have been considered nor answered is "Would a long series of electric shocks that were controllable in terms of severity (e.g., succesive responses could reduce the intensity of the shocks) but were uncontrollable in terms of onset (unavoidable) and termination (inescapable) induce learned helplessness or not?"

Such a question is not just an attempt at a *tour de force;* rather it is central to some of the issues raised with respect to *possible* kinds of "cognitive" control that might be exercised by humans in the *absence of explicit operational control* over onsets or terminations (19, 63, 75, 104). These have been suggested to include such forms of "control" as attentional, beliefs, cognitive, decisional, illusional, imaginal, informational interpretive, retrospective, and vicarious. One might suggest that these hypothetical processes are, in one sense, a restatement of the fact that forms of prediction have an effect. When they do so and we then ask the person "Why?," they give us an "answer." But as Nisbett and Wilson (110) have so clearly argued and shown in their paper, "Telling more than we can know...," these answers, although providing interesting information about inferential processes, may have little validity as to the actual process of adjustment to the potential stressor.[8]

8. All this is not to discount non-operational factors because, I must agree, that one can demonstrate that such can play an important role. One clear case is "potential" control. In such an experiment the human subject is told that they can (or will be able to) "control" the aversive event but are asked not to; under these circumstances the control is potential and in that it is not exercised, yet the subjects with this "potential" control show less distress to the aversive event than those without control (128). Because these subjects with potential control have never exercised the response the effect must arise from some process other than an experienced operational contingency. This phenomenon contains within it a serious warning to those who wish to study the problems of stress and control or learned helplessness. This is because new U.S.A laws require that human subjects be informed that they may withdraw from the experiment at any time without penalty. Thus, in any experiment all human subjects have potential control which may eliminate the effect of your experimental treatment (129, 130).

The consequence of such operational and/or conceptual conflation, confounding, and confusion is that the causal variables of some important phenomena in stress research are ill understood. Take for example, the classic experiment by Coover, Ursin, and Levine (111) in which they illustrate "coping." In this experiment the experimental rats were trained in a discrete trial discriminated avoidance task in which the signalled shocks if not avoided were escapable. Over trials, as the animals learned to avoid to asymptote, the distress level of the rats declined dramatically as indexed by corticosterone-which they called "coping." Not only does this experiment not include controls receiving matched patterns of shocks and confuse the dependent variable with the hypothetical construct, but it does not enable one to disambiguate which of the operational features - prediction of onsets, control of onset, or control of termination - is critical. Of course, at first, it *is* important to know you *do have* a phenomenon. But follow-up experiments continue to be plaqued by the same problems (112, 113).

One beneficial result of trying to fit experiments into Table 2 has been to alert us to these problematic conflations that we should seek experimentally to prevent. But, to the extent, that control does provide a potential basis for prediction despite operationalized independence (62, 114), then we must find new, more powerful experimental designs (see 31 for discussion of details of one approach). But, until these are implemented, we must make do with the data at hand.

Combination Procedures

Because experiments have sometimes studied the effects of control-of-onsets of events in a confounded procedure that also afforded control-of-termination to the experimental group and signalling of onsets for both the experimental and the reference groups does not mean results obtained are of no value or interest. If the experimental subjects differ from the reference group we do know that the *some* aspect of the control afforded is important; we just don't know whether it is control-of-onset or termination. Indeed, Weiss has been using such procedures rather creatively in his "triplet" design for several years (13, 97, 115 etc.) and many have partially patterned their research after his (116).

Clearly, when enough such triplet experiments have been done, we shall have evidence as to how the simple effects *interact*, but still no *direct* evidence on the pure effects of the factors. I must admit that I think it is strategically better to study first the simple pure cases, then the simple compounds of one form of prediction and one form of control. It is true that this leaves unanswered questions such as "Are the effects of control-of-onset and control-of-offset synergistic and interactive with one or both forms of prediction?" But, then, the complex compounds alone cannot answer that either. They can only point towards the simple single factor effects one at a time.

But, let us briefly see what these compound experiments do suggest.

Data

Probably the most cited of experiments of this form are those by Weiss (97). Weiss was initially interested in the issue of control. Experimental animals were given discriminated (signalled) escape/avoidance training and compared to animals yoked to the experimental group in terms of signals and shocks, but the yoked animals could neither escape nor avoid the shocks. Weiss measured gastric lesions and body weights and showed fewer ulcers; indeed they were close to normal. In a related experiment (117), they found inescapable, unavoidable shocks induced depletion of brain norepinephrine that was fully alleviated in rats for which the shocks were fully controllable. Also Buchholz, et al. (116) found that affording similar control over shocks reduced the persistent hypertensive reactions seen in yoked animals receiving uncontrollable shocks. Dess, et al. (62) reported reduced serum cortisol levels in the escape/avoidance dogs relative to those yoked but without control.

Turning to less physiological measures, Starr and Mineka (118) trained animals in a signalled escape/avoidance task and had animals yoked to these, hence receiving the same patterns of signals and shocks but having no control. When compared in terms of their fear of the CS, those animals which could control the shocks showed much less fear (see also 119 for a similar result when control was via escape only). We can summarize all these findings on our Table 2 by entering downward arrows in the respective cells at the bottom.

At this point, I should like to end my illustrative overview of some typical experiments and data, not because the review is in any sense complete. Indeed by further search we could find many more relevant experiments with shock, and, of course we have not even considered other potential stressors the data for which would be entered in successive layers in the third dimension of Table 1. I stop here because my aim is merely to *illustrate* an analytic strategy that includes the data patterns we detect in applying the strategy. A key factor in the analysis is the desynchrony (often lamented) among the measures of distress and the different outcomes of the under the "learning treatments."

What does the Table Tell Us?

The effort expended to devise and to compile our table will have been waste if we are not informed more by the patterns to be found than we were by the individual experiments. However, our time has not been wasted. There is a great deal to see, use and be guided by.

First of all, there are lots of empty cells, and that is not all attributable to this reviewer's laziness. Researchers simply have not asked all the experimental questions implied by the empty cells in Tables 1 and 2. Oh, I am sure you can fill in a few more - but not all, and please note that under "combinations" I have listed but two of the possible experimental procedures. Consider groups 10 through 16 in Table 3. All the possible contrasts are shown in Table 3 for reference.

That there are many empty cells can imply the simplistic "There is always more research to be done," or it can be taken to imply that the field is flailing

Table 3. Design Testing for Psychological Factors.

Group[1]	Experimental signal			Group Treatment control			Contrast Group
	no	on	off	no	on	off	
1	x			x			0 (rest)
2	x				x		1 (0)
3	x					x	1 (0)
4		x		x			1 (0)
5			x	x			1 (0)
6		x			x		1 (2,4)
7		x				x	1 (3,4)
8			x		x		1 (5,2)
9			x			x	1 (5,3)
10		x	x	x			1 (4,5)
11	x				x	x	1 (2,3)
12		x			x	x	1 (6(2,4))
							1 (7(3,4))
							1 (11(2,3))
13			x		x	x	1 (8(5,2))
							1 (9(5,3))
							1 (11(2,3))
14		x	x		x		1 (8(5,2))
							1 (6(2,4))
							1 (10(4,5))
15		x	x			x	1 (9(5,3))
							1 (7(3,4))
							1 (10(4,5))
16		x	x		x	x	1 (14(8;5,2)(6;2,4)(10;4,5))
							1 (15(9;5,3)(7;3,4)(10;4,5))
							1 (12(6;2,4)(7;3,4)(11;2,3))
							1 (13(8;5,2)(9;5,3)(11;2,3))

1. In brackets are necessary subsidiary comparisons.

forward without a clearly predicated overall strategy. To be sure microstrategies are being persued in each laboratory to answer important but rather specific local questions. The strategy proposed here and captured in part in Table 2 is, I dare say, perhaps too broad for any one laboratory, but it does afford us some systematic approach to the answers to some old questions that have plagued us for a long time. So let's look at the patterns.

We have a fair number of entries in three rows and one column and they mostly are downward arrows. But not all are. Thus, we can compare patterns across rows and across columns, and if the data are from the same experiment we might even do quantitative comparisons *within* columns.

As one example of comparisons of rows to answer a question, consider the following: The combination row ("control-on, control-off; prediction-on") in which we explored the effects of control can be compared to the other two filled rows ("prediction-of-onset" and "control-of-termination"). Where comparisons cell to cell are possible, the combination procedure does not differ from either of the other rows. That is, *on the available data* presented we cannot decide whether the combination procedure is more like that of the prediction-of-onset procedure or that of the control-of-termination procedure both of which features it has. More data are needed and our Table 2 tells us exactly which data should address the issue. One relevant set would come from an experiment in which the immunological consequences of the combination procedure are explored: If the combination procedure resulted in increased susceptibility to disease, then we might infer greater similarity to the prediction-of-onset procedure. If the result were decreased susceptibility, then we might infer greater similarity to control-of-termination. *This* conclusion ought to be of special interest to those using the combination procedure who choose to think of the control they are providing the animal as one of control over onsets, i.e., avoidance. The simple entry in the control-of-onset row is directly at odds with the entry in the same column (Target Organ) for the combination procedure.

We agree (see footnote 7) that the immunological data are probably subject to vagaries that we have yet to appreciate, and so we might choose to let Table 2 direct us to another locus for analysis. Well, we have a result for the effects of the combination procedure on cardiovascular hypertension, but no information in our Table on this index in the other two rows. Experiments to determine these effects might be useful in guiding our inferential processes, certainly more so than one more experiment on emotion.

I do not seriously propose the above as genuine cases because the data I have included are too meagre. Yet the above illustrates my point that such a table can direct us to experimental comparisons which, when properly made *within* a single experiment, are most likely to yield discriminating data. Such discriminations would allow us to begin to answer the question about the absolute and relative importance of and the relationship among the several psychological features we have entered into the left margin of the table. And the reader recognizes, of course, that those entries are themselves not exhaustive and are only illustrative.

We might use Table 2 to address other questions. Earlier we noted that it is argued whether control achieves its effects through affording some form of prediction. To adress this question, we begin by asking "prediction of what." When an organism responds to terminate a shock, a sensory feedback from the completed response accompanies the end of the shock and signals a period of time free from shock. If the beneficial effects of the controlling response are attributable to such feedback prediction of the post-shock period, then we ought to be able to show that the prediction-at-termination procedure produces the same effects as control-of-termination.

In fact, this strategy has been recently applied comparing conditions in which one group could escape from shock and a yoked group that got the same shocks *plus* a brief signal at the end of shocks when the escape animal made its response (93). The finding was, using fear as the index, that the brief signal functioned for the yoked animals just as effectively as did the response for the escape animals to reduce fear relative to a reference group that had no control nor received the feedback signal. And, extending this, Overmier, Murison, and Skoglund (120) also found, using gastric erosions as the index, that safety signals functioned to mimic responses in reducing the ulcerogenic effects of prior shocks (90). These two findings do not prove that control-of-termination has as its stress-reducing mechanism the prediction of post-shock safety, but they are consistent with that hypothesis. This instance of using the table for guidance towards key experiments has been particularly enlightening for me because, having worked for a long time in the "learned helplessness" tradition, I had come to believe controlling responses held very special meaning for organisms. The value of a schemata becomes clear to one when it directs you to an experiment that you otherwise might not have done and when additionally the result is contrary to your expectations, as in this case.

Now, this finding and a look at Table 2 suggests that, since we know that the combination "control-on, control-off; predict-on" has stress reducing properties (whatever their source), we might find "control-on, control-off; predict-on, predict-off" might have even *greater* stress reducing effects. Recently, Cook, Mineka, and Trumble (manuscript) carried out an experiment that allows exactly this comparison over 50 and 200 trials of avoidance training. Their observation was that the extra feedback upon response resulted in faster avoidance learning again emphasizing the role of feedback. And Weiss (115) had earlier shown that such exteroceptive response feedback reduces the number of gastric ulcers that an animal shows after a prolonged unsignalled escape/avoidance behavior, relative to an animal that has the same escape/avoidance task but no feedback stimulus. In fact, the latter group showed almost as much pathology as a yoked group which had no control at all. This series of findings leads one to begin to question whether, in the phenomenon of coping, the response plays any unique role at all, and if so, is it a stress reducing one? The single relevant entry in the table suggests not (see control-of-onset only).

Before concluding, there are other potential uses to which we can put a "periodic table" if we add a substantial number of entries for shock *and* for other noxious challenges that constitute potential stressors. First, we can ask the degree of congruence among the successive "slices" for each new physical challenge. It is remotely possible that the psychological factors will modulate responses to each just as they do the effects of shocks. If so, a dramatic simplification could be achieved by ignoring the specific challenge event. More likely, this will not be the case, and we will be reduced to looking for similarities and differences of patterns across stressors. Those stressors that are modified in the same ways by the various psychological factors could be grouped together into "families" of stressors that are similar in terms of the psychological factors that the organism can use to adjust. Those psychological factors themselves that modulate the effects of the stressors in similar ways may be grouped together in "families" and their common features sought (as was illustrated above for control-of-termination and prediction-at-termination). Finally, we just might uncover the answer to the conundrum of the general arousal/

alarm reaction and the precision with which different organs suffer - symptom specificity. This could be the product of the three-way (at least) interaction of stressors x psychological factor the organism brings to bear x that factor's efficacy in reducing the activation of particular response systems arising from the fact that the psychological process of learning does not proceed equally well under all circumstances that are operationally equivalent (121, 122) but is dependent upon the specific features of each dimension we have included in our Table 1 above: The contingency, the stimuli, the response system.

To the extent then that there are teleological biological constraints on learning and that learning is one of the organism's most powerful "coping" mechanisms, then we should not be surprised to find just the systematicities I suggest if we organize our "Periodic Table of Stress" correctly. This paper has been an effort to get us to try to see the potential for such a systematic approach. In chemistry, Emile Beguyer de Chancourtois and John Alexander Reina Newlands were ridiculed for their attempts (which it turns out were reasonably close to the mark). Mendeleev finally convinced the world. I wait for our Mendeleev.

References

1. Selye, H. (1974). Stress without distress. Lippincott, Philadelphia.
2. Weiner, H. (1977). Psychobiology and human disease. Elsevier, N.Y.
3. Brady, J.V., Porter, R.W., Conrad, D.G. & Mason, J.W. (1958). Avoidance behavior and the development of gastroduodenal ulcers. J. Exp. Anal. Behav., 1: 69-72.
4. Mason, J.W. (1959). Psychological influences on the pituitary-adrenal cortical system. In G.Pincus (Ed.), Recent progress in hormone research, Vol. 15. Academic Press, N.Y.
5. Mason, J.W. (1975). A historical view of the stress field. J. Hum. Stress, 1: 6-12 and 22-36.
6. Selye, H. (1976). Stress of life (2nd ed.). McGraw-Hill, N.Y.
7. Hinkle, L.E. (1977). The concept of "stress" in the biological and social sciences. In Z.J. Lipowski, D.R. Lipsett & P.C. Whybrow (Eds.), Psychosomatic medicine: Current trends and clinical applications. Oxford Univ. Press, N.Y., p. 27-49.
8. Ursin, H. (1980). Personality, activation and somatic health: A new perspective. In S. Levine & H. Ursin (Eds.), Coping and health. Plenum Press, N.Y., p. 259-279.
9. Ursin, H. & Murison, R.C.C. (1984). Classification and description of stress. In G.M. Brown et al. (Eds.), Neuroendocrinology and psychiatric disorder. Raven Press, N.Y., p. 123-131.
10. Overmier, J.B. & Seligman, M.E.P. (1967). Effects of inescapable shock upon subsequent escape avoidance responding. J. Comp. Physiol. Psychol., 63: 28-33.
11. Murison, R., Overmier, J.B. & Skoglund, E.J. (in press). Serial stressors: Prior exposure to a stressor modulates its later effectiveness on gastric ulceration and corticosterone. Behav. Neural Biol.
12. Richter, C. (1957). On the phenomenon of sudden death in animal and man. Psychosom. Med., 19: 191-198.
13. Weiss, J.M., Glazer, H.I., Pohorecky, L.A., Brick, J. & Miller, N.E. (1975). Effects of chronic exposure to stressors on avoidance-escape behavior and on brain norepinephrine. Psychosom. Med., 37: 522-533.
14. Zigmond, M.J. & Harvey, J.A. (197Þ). Resistance to central norepinephrine depletion and decreased mortality in rats chronically exposed to electric foot shock. J. Neuro-Visc. Relat., 31: 373-381.
15. Lazarus, R.S. & Folkman, S. (1984). Stress, appraisal, and coping. Springer-Verlag, N.Y.
16. Lazarus, R.S., DeLongis, A., Folkman, S. & Gruen, R. (1985). Stress and adaptional outcomes. Am. Psychol., 40: 770-779.
17. Burchfield, S. (1979). The stress response: A new perspective. Psychosom. Med., 41: 661-672.
18. Mandler, G. (1979). Thought processes, consciousness, and stress. In V. Hamilton & D.M. Wartburton (Eds.), Human stress and cognition: An information processing approach. Wiley, London, p. 179-201.

19. Taylor, S.E. (1983). Adjustment to threatening events: A theory of cognitive adaptation. Am. Psychol., 38: 1161-1171.
20. Dohrenwend, B.S., Dohrenwend, B.P., Dodson, M. & Shrout, P.E. (1984). Symptoms, hassles, social supports, and life events: Problem of confounded measures. J. Abnorm. Psychol., 93: 222-230.
21. Dohrenwend, B.P. & Shrout, P.E. (1985). "Hassles" in the conceptualization and measurement of life stress variables. Am. Psychol., 40: 780-785.
22. Lazarus, R.S. (1984). On the primacy of cognition. Am. Psychol., 39: 124-129.
23. Zajonc, R.C. (1984). On the primacy of affect. Am. Psychol., 34: 117-123.
24. Maier, S.F. & Seligman, M.E.P. (1976). Learned helplessness: Theory and evidence. J. Exp. Psychol.: Gen., 105: 3-46.
25. Mackintosh, N.J. (1973). Stimulus selection: Learning to ignore stimuli that predict no change in reinforcement. In R.A. Hinde & J. Stevenson-Hinde (Eds.), Constraints on learning. Academic Press, London, p. 75-96.
26. Anisman, H. (1975). Time dependent variations in aversively motivated behaviors: Noassociative effects of cholinergic and catecholaminergic activity. Psychol. Rev., 82: 359-385.
27. Hellhammer, D.H., Rea, M.A., Bell, M., Belkien, L. & Ludwig, M. (1984). Learned helplessness: Effects on brain monoamines and the pituitary gonadal axis. Pharmacol. Biochem. Behav., 21: 481-485.
28. Overmier, J.B. (1986). Strategic lessons from learned helplessness. Rev. Latino. Am. Psicol., 18: 387-404.
29. Engle, G.L. & Schmale, A.H. (1972). Conservation-withdrawal: A primary regulatory process for organismic homeostasis. In CIBA, Physiology, emotions, and psychosomatic illness. Elsevier, Amsterdam.
30. Wasserman, E.A., Chatlosh, D.L. & Nuenaber, D.J. (1983). Perceptions of causal relations in humans: Factors affecting judgment. Learn. Motiv., 14: 406-432.
31. Hammond, L.J. (1985). An empirical legacy of two-process theory: Two-term versus three-term relations. In F.R. Brush & J.B. Overmier (Eds.), Conditioning, affect, and cognition: Essays on the determinants of behavior. Lawrence Erlbaum, Hillsdale.
32. Alloy, L.B. & Tabachnik, N. (1984). Assessment of covariation by humans and animals: The joint influence of prior expectations and current situational information. Psychol. Rev., 91: 112-148.
33. Skinner, E.A. (1985). Actions, control judgments, and the structure of control experience. Psychol. Rev., 92: 1-38.
34. Abramson, L.Y., Seligman, M.E.P. & Teasdale, J.D. (1978). Learned helplessness in humans: Critique and reformulation. J. Abnorm. Psychol., 87: 49-74.
35. Alloy, L.B. & Seligman, M.E.P. (1979). On the cognitive component in learned helplessness and depression. In G. Bower (Ed.), The psychology of learning and motivation, Vol 13. Academic Press, N.Y.
36. Miller, I.W. & Norman, W.H. (1979). Learned helplessness in humans: A review and attribution theory model. Psychol. Bull., 86: 93-118.
37. Abbott, B., Schoen, L.S. & Badia, P. (1984). Predictable and unpredictable shock: Behavioral measures of aversion and physiological measures of stress. Psychol. Bull., 96: 45-71.
38. Overmier, J.B. & Wielkiewicz, R.M. (1983). On unpredictability as a causal factor in "learned helplessness." Learn. Motiv., 14: 324-337.
39. Dess, N.K. & Overmier, J.B. (under review). Signals and shocks: Generalized proactive effects on Pavlovian conditioning in dogs.
40. Alloy, L.B., Abramson, L.Y. & Kossman, D.A. (1985). The judgment of predictability in depressed and non-depressed college students. In F.R. Brush & J.B. Overmier (Eds.), Affect, conditioning, and cognition. Hillsdale, N.J., L.E.A., p. 229-246.
41. Ajzen, I. (1977). Intuitive theories of events and the effects of base-rate information on prediction. J. Pers. Soc. Psychol., 35: 303-314.
42. Arkes, H.R. & Harkness, A.R. (1983). Estimates of contingency between two dichotomous variables. J. Exp. Psychol.: Gen., 112: 117-135.
43. Dickenson, A., Shanks, D. & Evenden, J. (1984). Judgment of act-outcome contingency: The role of selective attribution. Q. J. Exp. Psychol: A Hum. Exp. Psychol., 36: 29-50.
44. Klosterhalfen, W. & Klosterhalfen, S. (1983). A critical analysis of the animal experiments cited in support of learned helplessness. Psychol. Beitr., 25: 435-458.
45. Overmier, J.B. (1985). Toward a reanalysis of the causal structure of the learned helplessness syndrome. In F.R. Brush & J.B. Overmier (Eds.), Conditioning, affect, and cognition: Essays on the determinants of behavior. Lawrence Erlbaum, Hillsdale, p. 211-227.
46. Baker, A.G. (1976). Learned irrelevance and learned helplessness. J. Exp. Psychol.: Anim. Behav. Proc., 2: 130-142.

47. Natelson, B.H., Tapp, W.N., Adamus, J.E., Mittler, J.C. & Levin, B.E. (1981). Humoral indices of stress in rats. Physiol. Behav., 26: 1049-1054.
48. Stone, E.A. (1975). Stress and catecholamines. In A.J. Friedhoff (Ed.), Catecholamines and behavior, Vol. 2. Plenum Press, N.Y., p. 31-72.
49. Ursin, H., Baade, E. & Levine, S. (1978). Psychobiology of stress. Academic Press, N.Y.
50. Anisman, H. (1978). Neurochemical changes elicited by stress. In H. Anisman & G. Bignami (Eds.), Psychopharmacology of aversively motivated behavior. Plenum Press, N.Y., p. 119-171.
51. Levine, S., Madden, J., Conner, R.L., Moskal, J.R. & Anderson, D.C. (1973). Physiological and behavioral effects of prior aversive stimulation (preshock) in the rat. Physiol. Behav., 10: 467-471.
52. Weiss, J.M., Goodman, P.A., Losito, B.G., Corrigan, S., Charry, J.M. & Bailey, W.H. (1981). Behavioral depression produced by an uncontrollable stressor: Relationship to norepinephrine, dopamine, and serotonin levels in various regions of the rat brain. Brain Res. Rev., 3: 167-205.
53. Maier, S.F. & Jackson, R.L. (1979). Learned helplessness: All of us were right (and wrong): Inescapable shock has multiple effects. In G. Bower (Ed.), The psychology of learning and motivation, Vol. 13. Academic Press, N.Y.
54. Lang, P.J. (1968). Fear reduction and fear behavior: Problems in treating a construct. In J.M. Shlien (Ed.), Research in psychotherapy, Vol. III. American Psychological Assn., Washington, p. 90-103.
55. Mineka, S. & Gino, A. (1980). Dissociation between CER and extended avoidance performance. Learning and motivation, 11: 476-502.
56. Overmier, J.B., Patterson, J. & Wielkiewicz, R.M. (1980). Environmental contingencies as sources of stress in animals. In S. Levine & H. Ursin (Eds.), Coping and Health. Plenum Press, N.Y., p. 1-38.
57. Rachman, S. (1978). Fear and courage. Freeman, San Francisco.
58. Engle, G.L. (1953). Homeostasis, behavioral adjustment and the concept of health and disease. In R. Grinker (Ed.), Midcentury psychiatry. Charles C. Thomas, Springfield, Ill.
59. Mason, J.W. (1968). A review of psychoendocrine research on the pituitary-adrenal cortical system. Psychosom. Med., 30: 576.
60. Miller, N.E. & Weiss, J.M. (1969). Effects of the somatic or visceral responses to punishment. In B.A. Campbell & R.M. Church (Eds.), Punishment and aversive behavior. Appleton Century Crofts, N.Y., p. 343-374.
61. Barchas, J.D. & Freedman, D.X. (1963). Brain amines: Response to physiological stress. Biochem. Pharmacol., 12: 1232-1235.
62. Dess, N.K., Linwick, D., Patterson, J., Overmier, J.B. & Levine, S. (1983). Immediate and proactive effects of controllability and predictability on plasma cortisol responses to shocks in dogs. Behav. Neurosci., 97: 1005-1016.
63. Thompson, S.C. (1981). Will it hurt less if I can control it? A complex answer to a simple question. Psychol. Bull., 90: 89-101.
64. Cannon, W.B. (1953). Bodily changes in pain, hunger, fear and rage (2nd ed.). Branford, Boston.
65. Miller, N.E. (1980). A perspective on the effects of stress and coping on disease and health. In S.Levine & H. Ursin (Eds.), Coping and health. Plenum Press, N.Y., p. 323-353.
66. Corson, S.A. & Corson, E.O. (1980). Biopsychogenic stress. In H. Selye (Ed.), Selye's guide to stress research, Vol. 2. Van Nostrand Reinhold Co.
67. Gathel, R.J., Paulus, P.B. & Maples, C.W. (1975). Learned helplessness and self report affect. J. Abnorm. Psychol., 84: 732-734.
68. Meehl, P.E. (1950). On the circularity of the law of effect. Psychol. Bull., 47: 52-75.
69. Badia, P., Harsh, J. & Abbott, B. (1979). Choosing between predictable and unpredictable shock conditions: Data and theory. Psychol. Bull., 86: 1107-1131.
70. Hymowitz, N. (1979). Suppression of responding during signalled and unsignalled shock. Psychol. Bull., 86: 175-190.
71. Mowrer, O.H. (1947). On the dual natures of learning - A reinterpretation of "conditioning" and "problem-solving." Harv. Educ. Rev., 17: 102-148.
72. Bitterman, M.E., LoLordo, V.M., Overmier, J.B. & Rashotte, M.E. (1979). Animal learning: Survey and analysis. Plenum Press, N.Y.
73. Osborne, S.R. (1977). The free food (contra-free-loading) phenomenon: A review and analysis. Anim. Learn. Behav., 5: 221-235.
74. Knapp, R.K., Krause, R.H. & Perkins, C.C.Jr. (1959). Immediate vs. delayed shock in T-maze performance. J. Exp. Psychol., 58: 357-362.
75. Averill, J.R. (1973). Personal control over aversive stimuli and its relationship to stress.

Psychol. Bull., 80: 286-303.

76. Bandura, A. (1977). Self efficacy: Toward a unifying theory of behavioral change. Psychol. Rev., 84: 191-215.
77. Amsel, A. (1958). The role of frustrative nonreward in noncontinuous reward situations. Psychol. Bull., 55: 102-119.
78. Brown, J.S. (1948). Gradients of approach and avoidance responses and their relation to motivation. J. Comp. Physiol. Psychol., 41: 450-465.
79. Mineka, S. & Kihlstrom, J. (1978). Unpredictable and uncontrollable events: A new perspective on experimental neurosis. J. Abnorm. Psychol., 87: 256-271.
80. Mineka, S. & Henderson, R.W. (1985). Controllability and predictability in acquired motivation. Annu. Rev. Psychol., 36: 495-529.
81. Hollis, K.L. (1982). Pavlovian conditioning of signal-centered action patterns and autonomic behavior: A biological analysis of function. Adv. Study. Behav., Vol. 12: 1-64.
82. Caul, W.F., Buchanan, D.C. & Hays, R.C. (1972). Effects of unpredictability of shock on incidence of gastric lesions and heart rate in immobilized rats. Physiol. Behav., 8: 669-672.
83. Tsuda, A., Tanaka, M., Nishikawa, T., Hirai, H. & Pare, W.P. (1984). Effects of unpredictability versus loss of predictability of shock on gastric lesions in rats. Physiol. Psychol., 11: 287-290.
84. Guile, M.N. & McCutcheon, N.B. (1984). Effects of naltrexone and signalling inescapable electric shock on nocioception and gastric lesions in rats. Behav. Neurosci., 98: 695-702.
85. Weinberg, J. & Levine, S. (1980). Psychobiology of coping in animals: The effect of predictability. In S. Levine & H. Ursin (Eds.), Coping and health. Plenum, N.Y., p. 39-60.
86. Miller, S.M. (1980). When is a little information a dangerous thing? Coping with stressful events by monitoring versus coping. In S. Levine & H. Ursin (Eds.), Coping and health. Plenum Press, N.Y., p. 145-169.
87. Bassett, J.R., Cairncross, K.D. & King, M.G. (1973). Parameters of novelty, shock predictability and response contingency in corticosterone release in the rat. Physiol. Behav., 10: 901-907.
88. Friedman, S.B., Ader, R. & Glasgow, L.A. (1965). Effects of psychological stress in adult mice inoculated with coxsackie B viruses. Psychosom. Med., 27: 361.
89. Davis, H., Porter, J.W., Livingstone, J., Herrman, T., MacFadden, L. & Levine, S. (1977). Pituitary adrenal activity and lever-press shock escape behavior. Physiol. Psychol., 5: 280-284.
90. Murison, R.C.C. & Isaksen, E. (1982). Gastric ulceration and adrenocortical activity after inescapable and escapable preshock in rats. Scand. J. Psychol., Suppl. 1: 133-137.
91. Sklar, L.S. & Anisman, H. (1981). Stress and cancer. Psychol. Bull., 89: 369-406.
92. Visintainer, M.A., Volpicelli, J.R. & Seligman, M.E.P. (1982). Tumor rejection in rats after inescapable or escapable shock. Science, 216: 437-439.
93. Mineka, S., Cook, M. & Miller, S. (1984). Fear conditioned with escapable and inescapable shock: Effects of a feedback stimulus. J. Exp. Psychol: Anim. Behav. Proc., 10: 307-323.
94. Seligman, M.E.P. & Maier, S.F. (1967). Failure to escape traumatic shock. J. Exp. Psychol., 74: 1-9.
95. Caspy, T., Frommer, R., Weiner, I. & Lubow, R.E. (1979). Generality of US pre-exposure effects: Effect of shock or food pre-exposure on water escape. Bull. Psychon. Soc., 14: 15-18.
96. Jackson, R.L., Alexander, J.H. & Maier, S.F. (1980). Learned helplessness, inactivity, and associative deficits: Effects of inescapable shock on response choice escape learning. J. Exp. Psychol.: Anim. Behav. Proc., 6: 1-20.
97. Weiss, J.M. (1968). Effects of coping on stress. J. Comp. Physiol. Psychol., 65: 251-260.
98. Barbaree, H.E. & Harding, R.K. (1973). Free-operant avoidance behavior and gastric ulceration in rats. Physiol. Behav., 11: 269-271.
99. Tsuda, A. & Hirai, H. (1977). Effects of coping responses on chronic stress in rats. Jap. J. Psychosom. Med., 17: 121-129. (in Japanese, English abstract)
100. Mowrer, O.H. & Viek, P. (1948). An experimental analogue of fear from a sense of helplessness. J. Abnorm. Soc. Psychol, 43, 193-200.
101. Perkins, C.C. (1968). An analysis of the concept of reinforcement. Psychol. Rev., 75: 155-172.
102. Lykken, D.T. (1962). Perception in the rat: Autonomic response to shock as a function of the lenght of warning interval. Science, 137: 665-666.
103. Weiss, J.M. (1977). Psychological and behavioral influences on gastrointestinal lesions in animals. In J.D. Maser & M.E.P. Seligman (Eds.), Psychopathology: Experimental models. Freeman, San Francisco, p. 232-269.

104. Miller, S.M. (1979). Controllability and human stress: Method, evidence, and theory. Behav. Res. Ther., 17: 287-304.
105. Pavlov, I.P. (1928). Lectures on conditioned reflexes. (Edited and translated by W. Horsley Gantt.). International Publ., N.Y.
106. Guthrie, E.R. (1935). The psychology of learning. Harper & Row, N.Y.
107. Hull, C.L. (1943). Principles of behavior. Appleton Century Crofts, N.Y.
108. Tolman, E.C. (1949). There is more than one kind of learning. Psychol. Rev., 56: 144-155.
109. Maier, S.F., Seligman, M.E.P. & Solomon, R.L. (1969). Pavlovian fear conditioning and learned helplessness. In B. Campbell & R.M. Church (Eds.), Punishment and aversive behavior. Appleton Century Crofts, N.Y.
110. Nisbett, R.E. & Wilson, T.D. (1977). Telling more than we can know: Verbal reports on mental processes. Psychol. Rev., 84: 231-259.
111. Coover, G.D., Ursin, H. & Levine, S. (1973). Plasma corticosterone levels during active avoidance learning in rats. J. Comp. Physiol. Psychol., 82: 170-174.
112. Berger, D.F., Starzec, J.J. & Mason, E.B. (1981). The relationship between plasma corticosterone levels and lever press avoidance vs. escape behaviors in rats. Physiol. Psychol., 9: 81-86.7

Discussion:

Recent Approaches in Psychological Research

O. Berndt Scholz

I should like to start my discussion of the previous contributions to this section with a few reflections on the systematic prerequisites, stated quite explicitly by Dr. Overmier. He depicted a system that includes all relevant dimensions of contemporary stress research. His remarks have to be seen as a call for a rigorous turn away from positivistic or fashion-oriented research technologies. This call embraces the physical stimulation characteristics of stressors as well as the transformation of these occurrences into psychological terms - in accordance with Klix (1), one could speak of "significance-marking." His system furthermore explicates a class of organismic "coping-responses" as well as a level of stress effects. This system can therefore be seen as heuristic, in so far as it is preliminary and offers the researcher maxims for dealing with furthering or specifying studies. In this context, the question arises whether the dimensions and subdivisions implicit in the system can also be seen as representative for applied clinical - psychological research.

The problem connected with this can clearly be illustrated via one of our own studies: We concerned ourselves with the contingencies between stress-coping and life events in patients with ulcus ventriculae and duodeni (2). As expected, these patients reported significantly more distressful life events. It is however surprising, that these events practically happened overnight, or in other words, unpredictably for the person and still lingered on during the florid phase of the illness. Thus, even their effects are of an uncontrollable quality to the person and serve as daily hassles. In most cases, these stressors are concerned with the interpersonal relationships of the patients. With the help of this and comparable studies, preliminary statements can be made about the psychological characteristics of the stressors, the coping responses and the response classes. But our knowledge about onset, termination and other physical situational characteristics is very patchy. Neither an objective definition, nor the definition of the contents of stress research in man are yet prototypical. Therefore, the question arises over the extent to which those stress conditions known to be easily controlled in animal experiments can be realized in human experiments. Seeing these problems, Dr. Overmier has called for animal research rather than human experiments (3, 4). The extent to which results of such research can be transferred to the special needs of research in humans still remains uncertain.

As far as the paradigm of learned helplessness is concerned, it must be seen as Dr. Overmier's accomplishment to have shown us that the process of increasing helplessness is accompanied by endocrinological and neurochemical changes. Helplessness research seems to have been deeply rooted within a social sciences orientation. The consequence of nearly all research results of the group around Overmier and Henn, i.e., that learned helplessness is not a singular phenomenon, has to be seen as equally important as the somatic support for this concept. This gives rise to the question whether the paradigm of learned helplessness can be used as a general model of explanation for the multitude of so called psychosomatic illnesses and if it can be put side by side with the Selye's concept. The latter concept has after all recently enjoyed a kind of renaissance in neuropsychoimmunology (5).

When one is talking about learned helplessness, the studies of Dr. Henn certainly have to be taken into consideration. It would be stimulating to discuss the explications both on the basis of their comprehensive aspects of general research directions as well as with regard to their consequences for behavioral medicine. For lack of space, the discussion shall concentrate on the first of the two aspects.

Dr. Henn's team study the effects of learned helplessness at different biological levels. He and his co-workers have been able to show that rodents, made helpless in an experiment, were not only less active and slept less than controls. The animals in the experimental group also showed better responses to administration of thymoleptics than to sedatives, neuroleptics or tranquilizers. These findings thus support the concept of learned helplessness as a paradigm for clinically relevant depression. However, special attention has to be given to the experimentally found indications for the development of a genetic disposition for helplessness, if the ancestors learned to behave helplessly. The proof of a neuroanatomical representation of depressive behavior through findings of a higher ß-receptor density in the hippocampus has to be considered equally important.

Because of their methodological basis, the experiments mentioned offer the possibilities of cross-experiments. If it is possible to breed rats completely resistent to the development of a deficit in flight behavior in the fourth generation, one must also be able to breed rats that are especially prone to develop such flight behavior under the same conditions. Furthermore, if the results of Dr. Henn are replicable, one must have to be able to produce animals that lose their flight deficit when cross bred with genetically non-helpless animals. To be able to pinpoint hereditability as the source of variance, one would have to prevent all possibilities for learning in these rodents. This would clearly demonstrate the value of the genetic and stress components of the learned helplessness model.

Analogies to this can be made for a useful cross-breeding experiment with regard to the changes in the density of ß-receptors in the hippocampus. Their density should not only be used as an indicator for learned helplessness, but also as indicative of parameter renormalization due to behavior modification procedures.

Such research will be able to further validate and specify learned helplessness as an analogue for depressive symptoms. This will also make it necessary to discuss the question of specifity of this paradigm with regard to the various clinical depressive syndromes, which has been largely excluded so far. If this question proves relevant, one would have to consider its applicability.

The question of application orientation for biopsychological matters should be especially relevant with regard to the research of Dr. Peters. His initial question is the search for effective calcium antagonists that would, for instance, make it possible to treat cardiac arrhythmia. Among other reasons, such disturbances can be consequences of an increased cellular calcium influx coinciding with a dysfunction of the calcium pump. This results in an intra-cellular oxygen deficit, which in turn causes a decrease in peripheral blood supply. The oxygen-calcium imbalance thus results in a decrease of the speed of neuronal impulse conduction, respectively a decrease in the contractibility of the smooth muscles. Symptoms of this kind come into being with the influence of epinephrine, norepinephrine and cortisone. Psychologists like to call these substances stress hormones, which could be an indication of a link between cell biochemistry and psychological research.

The reality of the depicted situation is much more complicated. One should indeed take into account the immense difference between the behavioral and biochemical aspects of a cardiac arrhythmia. Both aspects are in a way opposite ending points on a common line. Does the question arise for the biochemist or the pharmacologist if and how one should consider stress as an experimental condition? If this is the aim to keep the intracellular calcium concentration as low as possible and taking the fact into consideration that calcium exerts an influence on the release of other neurotransmitters resulting in an interaction effect, then biopsychological stress research and those aspects of cell pathology studied by Dr. Peters are complementary areas of research. To what extent is the thesis justified that a high intracellular calcium concentration can be interpreted as an indicator of the failed mastering of a stressor? A stressor in this context is any stimulus the reaction to which requires the body to set free additional reserves to be able to continue functioning as a stable system.

Methodologically, the evaluation of the intracellular calcium concentration is too complicated to be useful as a routine parameter in stress research. Would it be possible to use the calcium concentration in serum for this purpose? Which functional interrelations are known between the intracellular and the serum cortisol level that would have to be taken into account? - Considerations of this kind can further the research, because the importance of magnesium for stress research is a well known fact. Magnesium is seen as a sensitive, methodologically reliable and at the same time easily obtainable stress parameter. Ising's group could for example determine interrelations between chronic noise pollution and increased secretion of catecholamines as well as changes in the concentration of electrolytes in blood. These effects are enhanced by a lack of magnesium. Stress and a magnesium deficit amplify each other and lead to an increased risk of cardiovascular disorders. Are these parallel processes increasing intracellular calcium and decreasing the magnesium concentration? Can these interrelations only be observed in the case of cardiovascular disorders or could they also be established for other stress related illnesses?

The contribution of Dr. Wallin is extraordinarily interesting not only because of its information content. Some of his research shows that the "psycho-physiological conditions" within the autonomic nervous system are far more complicated than the extent to which they are taken into consideration in experimental designs might lead us to think. One must therefore not be surprised if those conditions, when varied in laboratory research, do not show the wanted effects.

It is rather tempting to study phenomena such as sympathetic innervation of the skin, that can point out situational and interindividual variations at a high retest validity. This is certainly the case for expressional and emotional psychology which have recently come into fashion again. It will most probably still be a long way before the method developed by Dr. Wallin will be applied to the examination of emotionally tainted influences (e.g., anger) on the performing ability of patients with different pain syndromes, also taking into account measurement of skin resistance level, muscle activity and blood pressure. According to Funkenstein (6), the latter parameters can typify an anger-in-pattern characteristic for migraine patients. Dr. Wallin has repeatedly pointed out in the past (7) that sudomotorical, vasoconstrictive, baroreflectative, thermoregulatory and last but not least environmental influences add to the emotional characteristics resulting in a certain sympathetic skin and muscle innervation pattern, although emotional characteristics were the main research objective in this example.

This question is of very concrete significance: Scholz, Goepel, & Grothgar (8) compared their self reports, the expressional behavior and a few cardiovascular parameters in migraine patients, chronic patients and healthy subjects in laboratory situations with varying degrees of anger provocation. Compared to the other two experimental groups, the migraine patients showed a definite drop in diastolic blood pressure. How can this result which has previously been reported by Feuerstein (9) and Gerber (10) for comparable experimental conditions be interpreted meaningfully? Could it be, that the migraine patients initially show an increase in diastolic blood pressure, but that the sympathetic activity sinks reflectively under anger provocation conditions? The consequence of this, taking Wallin's findings into account, would have to be a redistribution of blood resources within the skeletal musculature, accompanied by a reduction of diastolic blood pressure. Since measurements in the study of Scholz, Goepel and Grothgar could not be taken analogously, only the reduced diastolic blood pressure in migraine patients under anger conditions could be observed. Or could these findings be more adequately explained through the involvement of vasoactive substances? Support for these results of Scholz, Goepel & Grothgar through the findings of Wallin is certainly not only of interest to the biologically or the behaviorally oriented psychologist. The inadequate dealing with anger is also attributed to many different syndromes by the representatives of psychodynamic schools. Possibly, different fields of research could concern themselves with problems of similar generality. The paradigm of learned helplessness, respectively the effects of stress on the physiology and biochemistry of man, can be seen as progressive research approaches, the personnel and financial support of which should be hoped for.

References

1. Klix, F. (1971). Information und Verhalten. Deutscher Verlag der Wissenschaften, Berlin/DDR.
2. Scholz, O.B., Kutschke, T. & Leonhardt, G. (in press). Coping behavior and stressful life events in peptic ulcer patients. Psychology and Health.

3. Overmier, J.B., Patterson, J. & Wielkiewicz, R. M. (1980). Environmental contingencies as sources of stress in animals. In S. Levine & H. Ursin (Eds.), Coping and health. Plenum Press, N.Y., p. 1-38.
4. Overmier, J.B. (1981). Interference with coping. Acad. Psychol. Bull., 3: 105-118.
5. Jemmott, J.B. & Locke, S.E. (1984). Psychosocial factors, immunologic mediation, and human susceptibility to infectiouns diseases: How much do we know? Psychol. Bull., 95: 78-108.
6. Funkenstein, D.H., King, S.H. & Drolette, M. (1954). The direction of anger during a laboratory stress inducing situation. Psychosom. Med., 16: 405-413.
7. Wallin, G. (1983). Intraneural recording and autonomic function in man. In R. Bannister (Ed.), Autonomic failure. Oxford University Press, London.
8. Scholz, O.B., Goepel, R. & Grothgar, B. (1984). On specific behavior of headache patients in an anger provoking situation. Paper read at 23. International Congress of Psychology, Acapulco.
9. Feuerstein, M., Bush, C. & Corbisieros, R. (1982). Stress and chronic headache: A psychophysiological analysis of mechanism. J. Psychosom. Res., 26: 167-182.
10. Gerber, W.D. (1982). Psychophysiologische Untersuchung. In W.D. Gerber & G. Haag (Eds.), Migräne: Diagnostik und Therapie für Ärzte und Psychologen. Springer-Verlag, Berlin.

5.

Central Control of the Pituitary-Adrenal Axis I

Limbic-Midbrain Mechanisms and Behavioral Physiology of Interactions with CRF, ACTH and Adrenal Hormones

Béla Bohus

The terms limbic system and emotion (1), emotion and disease (2), emotion, stress, adrenal and disease (3) have been linked for some decades. In the early fifties when it was recognized that emotional stimuli are among the strongest stressors that activate the adrenal cortex studies have been initiated to elucidate the role of limbic structures in the control of the pituitary adrenal axis. Porter (4) was the first to report that the eosinopenic response to noxious stimuli, that was used as the index of pituitary-adrenal activity is inhibited by electrical stimulation of the hippocampus in the monkey. Measurement of the plasma 17-hydroxycorticosteroid level as a more direct index of adrenal activity in stressed monkeys led Mason (5) to a similar conclusion. In a more extended study, we subsequently demonstrated that electrical stimulation of the dorsal hippocampus inhibits the response of the pituitary-adrenal system to both neural (painful electric footshock) and humoral (epinephrine, histamine) stimuli in several species (6). An inhibitory influence of the hippocampus on the pituitary-adrenal system in man was demonstrated by Rubin et al. (7) using low frequency stimulation of CA_2 and CA_1 layers of the hippocampus. Observations in animals bearing lesions in the hippocampus or in the afferent or efferent pathways of this structure (e.g., medial septum, anterior cingulate cortex, sub- and supra-collosal cortex) (8-10) also favored the hypothesis that the role of hippocampus in controlling ACTH release is primarily an inhibitory one. Subsequent studies then revealed the involvement of other limbic structures such as the amygdala, pyriform, enthorhinal and orbitofrontal cortex and of midbrain areas in the control of basal and stress-induced ACTH release (11).

These areas appeared to be of importance also in suprahypothalamic control of autonomic functions including that of the adrenal medulla (12). The endocrine and autonomic findings together presupposed a key function of the limbic-midbrain system in emotional behavior and accompanying physiological and endocrine processes. However, such a few seemed to be rather speculative because the different pieces of jigsaw puzzle failed to fit into a coherent picture. Reasons for incoherency could be related to the absence of integrated studies (behavior, physiology and endocrinology), the use of anesthetized animals in many studies, etc.

These studies were supported in part by the Saal van Zwanenberg Stichting, Stichting Farmacologisch Studiefonds, Utrecht and the Canadian Medical Research Council. The valuable contributions of Drs. J. Borrell, S. del Cerro, G.A. Cottrell, E.R. de Kloet & J. van der Meulen to different studies described here, are greatly acknowledged. The author thanks Mrs. Joke Poelstra-Hiddinga for her secretarial aid.

The results of the last one and a half decades primarily because of a substantial development of the knowledge on neuroendocrine communications allow now a view on the limbic system and its connection to the endocrine apparatus. First of all, it appears that the limbic-midbrain system possesses multiple neuroendocrine output channels. Beside the classically known outputs, namely the hypothalamus (Corticotropin Releasing Factor; CRF) - pituitary (Adrenocorticotrophin; ACTH) - adrenal cortical (corticosteroids) axis and the hypothalamus - autonomic nervous system (ANS) and the adrenal medulla (catecholamines) one should consider the function of CRF and opiomelanocortins (ß-endorphin, ACTH/α-MSH; γ-MSH) as independent messengers of limbic-midbrain activity. Emotional stressors may affect differentially the activity of the pituitary-adrenal, ANS-catecholamine axis and the release of peptides (CRF and opiomelanocortins) (see 13, Smelik in this volume).

Secondly, it appears that four neuroendocrine input channels of the CRF-opiomelanocortin-adrenal neuroendocrine system to the limbic-midbrain structures exist. The limbic structures, particularly the hippocampus, septum and amygdala contain neuronal receptor systems for corticosteroids (14-17). CRF- and opiomelanocortin-containing neuronal systems, originating from the hypothalamic paraventricular, respectively the arcuate nuclei reach a number of limbic-midbrain areas (17, 18). These peptides, in particular opiomelanocortins from the pituitary, may also reach the brain via hormonal routes (16). Finally, an increasing number of evidence suggest that circulating catecholamines, particularly epinephrine, probably through indirect mechanisms, play an important role in modulating limbic midbrain function and thereby the behavior (19, 20).

The present paper describes neurophysiological, behavioral and autonomic physiological experiments in rats that demonstrate the significance of CRF, ACTH, corticosteroids and catecholamines in limbic-midbrain functions. Accordingly, attention is focussed on the input channels. It has recently been recognized that the endocrine state of the brain as an important target organ of hormones plays a key factor in an integrated stress response (21). Therefore, in addition to describing the experimental findings in relation to physiology, an attempt is made to integrate these data into a view on the role of neuroendocrine states in psychosomatic diseases.

Limbic Kindling: Neurophysiology and Behavior

Kindling is an experimental model for limbic epilepsy (22). It entails the administration of one low amperage electrical stimulation per day, to a limbic structure such as the hippocampus or the amygdala. It is characterized by the gradual lengthening of the evoked after-discharge (AD) with the accompanying appearance of behavioral components such as immobility, head nodding, and chewing, and finally, a tonic-clonic convulsion. This is the ictal phase. This phase is followed by an immobility behavior defined as postictal depression or behavioral depression (BD). The animal is temporarily torpid or immobile and it displays drastically reduced responsiveness to environmental stimuli. Physiologically speaking, changes in the neurophysiological and behavioral consequences of kindling reflect alterations in the excitability of the kindled structure.

The first electrophysiological studies using the synthetic CRF suggested that the peptide induces spontaneous electrical seizures in limbic and cortical areas in the rat (23). It was therefore of interest to investigate its effect on the AD and BD of hippocampal-kindled rats (Cottrell and Bohus, unpublished). The peptide (porcine-CRF; Penninsula Labs. Inc.) was given into a lateral cerebral ventricle in rats with established seizures. The doses and the treatment-test interval (60 min) were selected on the basis of behavioral studies in a learning situation (Veldhuis, pers. comm.). Table 1 shows that although there was a tendency to decrease both the duration of AD and BD by low doses of CRF, the differences did not reach a statistically significant level. The highest dose- i.e., 30 ng i.c.v. - as used in this study, slightly increases AD, but decreases BD. However, these differences were also not significant.

Table 1. Intracerebroventricular administered corticotrophin releasing factor (CRF) and hippocampal kindling-induced after-discharge (AD) and behavioral depression (BD).

Treatment dose	0.03	0.3	2.0	30.0 ng
N =	11	9	8	7
AD	-0.20 ± 0.12	-0.19 ± 0.18	-0.20 ± 0.13	0.08 ± 0.09
BD	-0.65 ± 1.45	-0.25 ± 0.76	-0.11 ± 0.55	-1.91 ± 1.85

AD and BD: duration of AD (BD) expressed in min as studied 60 min after CRF administration minus the duration on the day before peptide treatment (i.e., following i.c.v. saline injection).
N = number of observations. Data from Cottrell and Bohus (unpublished).

These principally negative results were somewhat surprising in the light of the aforementioned seizure-inducing effect of CRG. Although one could list a number of factors that may explain negative findings in the ictal phase (e.g., the dose, the treatment-test interval, the site of kindling, etc.), it is obvious that CRF cannot be considered as a peptide that readily influences ictal and postictal processes in physiological or near physiological concentrations.

In contrast, melanocortins (ACTH/α-MSH and γ-MSH-like peptides) markedly affected the ictal processes and the postictal consequences of hippocampal kindling-induced seizures even with peripheral administration of these peptides (24). Table 2 summarizes the influence of various ACTH fragments and analogs on the duration of AD and BD in hippocampally kindled rats following subcutaneous administration in a dose range of 3 to 100 μg/kg. The only exception was an ACTH 4-16 analogue which was given in doses of 0.1 to 10 μg/kg. The duration of AD was reduced by a number of ACTH-related peptides such as ACTH 1-16, α-MSH, ACTH 7-16, 7-D-Phe-ACTH 7-16, ACTH 4-16 (4-Met-(0), 8-D-Lys, 9-Phe, 11-D-Lys-ACTH 4-16) and γ-MSH 1-12. The fragments ACTH 4-10, 7-D-Phe-ACTH 4-10 and γ-MSH 1-11 were ineffective.

Table 2. Melanocortins and hippocampal kindling-induced after-discharge and behavioral depression.

	1	2	3	4	5	6	7	8	9	10	11	12	13	14	15	16
ACTH 1-16	Ser-	Tyr-	Ser-	Met-	Glu-	His-	Phe-	Arg-	Tyr-	Gly-	Lys-	Pro-	Val-	Gly-	Lys-	Lys
γ-MSH 1-12	Tyr-	Val-	Met-	Gly-	His-	Phe-	Arg-	Try-	Asp-	Arg-	Phe-	Gly				

Peptide	After-discharge	Behavioral depression
ACTH 1-16	-	-
α-MSH (Ac-ACTH 1-13)	-	0
ACTH 4-10	0	0
7-D-Phe-ACTH 4-10	0	-
ACTH 7-16	-	0
7-D-Phe-ACTH 7-16	-	-
ACTH 4-16 analogue	-	-
γ-MSH 1-11	0	0
γ-MSH 1-12	-	-

- : reduction; 0 = no effect. Data from Cottrell et al. (24).

Immobility that is to say BD, was reduced by ACTH 1-16, ACTH 4-16 analogue, 7-D-Phe-ACTH 4-10 and 7-D-Phe-ACTH 7-16. All L fragments 4-10 and 7-16, and α-MSH appeared to be ineffective. γ-MSH 1-12 reduced the duration of BD but γ-MSH 1-11 was not active. The ACTH 4-16 analogue was the most potent to affect both the ictal and postictal events.

Recent studies suggest the involvement of endogenous opioid mechanisms in postictal events. Frenk et al. (25) reported that BD is eliminated or at least reduced by the opiate antagonist naloxone in amygdala-kindled rats. We have replicated this finding and additionally showed that naltrexone also reduces the duration of BD in hippocampally kindled rats (26). The doses of the antagonist that were minimally effective to reduce BD were almost 1000 times less than that required to block analgesic or catatonic action or morphine. This suggests the involvement of high-affinity mu-opiate receptor mediated processes. Interestingly, similarities exist in the structural requirements of melanocortins for reducing BD and for the partial agonist/antagonist properties on opiate receptors. Both the sequences 4-7 and 13-16 seem to be essential for an action on the BD. These two active sites seem to act in a cooperative way. Introduction of the D-enantiomer of 7-Phe in the molecule results in an appearance of activity in fragments that contain only one of the active sites. A similar phenomenon has been observed in reaction to the antianalgesic and grooming activities of melanocortins (27, 28). These similarities and the very potent action of opiate antagonist drugs (26) suggest that a functional antagonism of a subpopulation of mu-opiate receptors may underlie these peptide effects. That the functional mu-antagonist endogenous peptide γ-MSH 1-12 (29) that originates from the N-terminal portion of the proopiomelanocortin precursor molecule (30) share reducing properties with ACTH-related peptides also support a view on the involvement of opioid mechanisms. However, the differences in the structural requirements for the reduction of the duration of AD and BD may suggest that different opioid mechanisms are involved in the ictal and postictal events.

Adrenal cortical hormones also affect seizure-behavior in animals and people. Some corticosteroids increase an animal's susceptibility to seizures and lower convulsive threshold (31, 32). The hippocampus was implicated in this hormonal action (33-35). In order to specify the physiological role of the adrenal hormonal system in the excitability of the hippocampus the effect of adrenalectomy (ADX) and corticosterone (CS) replacement was studied on seizures induced by hippocampal kindling in rat (36). Corticosterone is the natural main secretory product of the rats' adrenal and the hippocampus contains a large number of receptor sites specific for CS (14, 15).

A complex series of changes occurred in AD and BD during the immediate hours after ADX, culminating at day 1 in markedly decreased AD and BD, which returned to normal over the next several days. These changes in the early stage (4 and 24 h) were normalized after replacement of the ADX rats with low doses of CS (Table 3). These results suggest that the expression and maintenance of hippocampal kindled seizures is under short-term control of corticosterone in the rat. The data indirectly imply that corticosterone receptors, probably in the hippocampus, are involved in the maintenance of kindled seizure, as the AD and BD are disrupted by removal of the source of endogenous corticosterone and reinstated by a physiological dose of the same steroid. However, it seems that the animal can adapt to a change in its hormonal milieu after ADX as kindled seizure related events return to baseline with time. It remains to be shown whether the reinstatement is due to an "escape" from adrenal cortical control or whether other neuroendocrine mechanisms of peptidergic nature compensate for the absence of corticosteroids.

Table 3. Adrenalectomy (ADX) and corticosterone (CS) replacement affects hippocampal kindling-induced after-discharge and behavioral depression.

	After-discharge						Behavioral depression					
Groups/ADX-test interval	1h	4h	8h	24h	48h	72h	1h	4h	8h	24h	48h	72h
Sham-op	-	0	0	0	0	0	-	0	0	0	0	0
ADX	-	-	-	-	0	0	-	+	-	-	-	0
ADX + CS	nd	0	nd	0	0	0	nd	0	nd	0	0	0

- : a reduction; + : an enhancement; 0 = no difference to pre-operative level; nd: not determined.
Data from Cottrell et al. (36).

The 1 h effect is probably a generalized stress effect as evoked by the surgical procedure. Oliverio et al. (37) also found a reduction in electroconvulsive shock-induced seizures following immobilization stress.

Taken together, experiments in rats with kindled seizures suggest that neurophysiological and behavioral consequences of brain seizures are under a complex control of the CRF-opiomelanocortin-adrenal cortex neuroendocrine system. ACTH-related peptides reduce the consequence of epileptiform seizures. Adrenal cortical hormones, at least on a short run, maintain such activity. Accordingly, this neuroendocrine system bears a potential to ameliorate or to potentiate the syndromes of seizure behavior affecting limbic excitability.

The question of the role of stress in seizure behavior is not clear yet. The present data suggest that it ameliorates the severity of both the ictal and postictal components. This is, however, a short-term effect because the measured parameters return to prestress level 24 h later. It remains to be determined whether "classical" stress-hormones (e.g., catecholamines) or pituitary and/or brain born peptides are involved.

Hormones and Emotional Behavior

The term emotional behavior is rather ill defined but it may be a useful expression if one discusses issues such as emotional stress, the limbic system and hormones and emotional stress, the limbic system and behavior and physiology. The term would then cover all kinds of behavioral alterations that are related to fear, anxiety, frustration, disappointment, pleasure, etc. In relation to the issue of stress and behavior it has recently been proposed (21) that behavioral stress responses are organized at the limbic-midbrain system- i.e., at the first level of organization of stress responses in general, and they may be of specific and non-specific nature. Learning, retention (memory) and extinction can be considered as specific behavioral stress responses. The specifity lies on the assumption that learning of one particular behavioral response means adaptation to a given environment. Even minor changes in the environment may require new strategies in which older learned behavioral patterns may be incorporated, but the old patterns may also disturb the acquisition of new patterns. The non-specific behavioral stress responses may occur in different environments with or without interfering with specific reactions. Exploration, displacement behaviors, analgesia and reflex immobility are considered to belong to this group of adaptive responses. These responses occur as unconditioned species specific behaviors in novel environment.

Clinical observations in the fifties already suggested that ACTH and corticosteroids affect emotionality in man. Subsequent studies in animals then demonstrated a dissociation within the pituitary-adrenal system: ACTH and corticosteroids have differential behavioral effects (38, 39). The validity of this notion has been shown for man as well (40). The present state of art suggests more dissociations in the actions of hypothalamus-pituitary-adrenal hormones in relation to specific and non-specific behavioral stress response.

The first dissociation is in the action of CRF and the rest of the hormones, particularly in relation to non-specific behavioral stress responses. It is suggested that intracerebroventricular administration of CRF in the rat elicits changes in exploratory and grooming behavior that occur under the influence of "stressors" (41, 42). This interpretation is certainly vague and needs further elaboration.

The second and third dissociation are (1) between ACTH and the rest of the hormones and (2) within the peptide system. As far as (1) is concerned, it is well established that ACTH-related peptides and corticosteroids affect specific behavioral stress responses (learning, memory and extinction) often in an opposite way (40). The effects of ACTH and adrenal catecholamines, however, may be similar. ACTH and related peptides and epinephrine share a dose-related effect on retention when given as a post-learning treatment in intact and ADX rats (43-45). The dissociation within the ACTH-related peptides is related to the issue of their putative receptor mechanisms in the brain. Subsequent to the recognition that fragments of the ACTH are behaviorally in extinction more active than the parent molecule (38) and ACTH and α-MSH share a number of behavioral actions (46), it was suggested that the "message" for the avoidance extinction behavior is carried by the 4-7 sequence of ACTH/α-MSH (47). A second active site may be embedded in the 7-9 sequence but it does not become expressed unless there is a C-terminal elongation. The discovery of endorphins and that endorphins and ACTH/α-MSH originate from the common precursor proopiomelanocortin molecule (48) has changed our view on the behavioral action of ACTH-related peptides. According to pharmacological studies ACTH and related fragments have some affinity for opiate receptors (partial agonist/antagonist property) and the peptide diminishes the analgesic action of morphine. However, the structural requirements for these pharmacological actions appeared to be different from those described for extinction behavior (28, 49). In addition, a functional opiate antagonist sequence, "namely γ-MSH," has been identified within the opiomelanocortin molecule (29). Extensive studies of the possible physiological function of the multiple opiomelanocortin fragments in the regulation of behavioral stress responses also showed that the actions of ACTH on learning, retention and extinction should be related to the complex effects of the whole opiomelanocortin molecule on these processes (50). ACTH or its fragments sometimes mimics the action of ß-endorphin, the agonist of the opiomelanocortin system, sometimes that of the antagonist γ-MSH. Therefore, ACTH/α-MSH may be regarded as functional partial agonist/antagonist of endorphins. This view is also valid for non-specific stress responses such as grooming, analgesia, etc.

The differential behavioral effects may be related to the opioid receptor or to putative opiomelanocortin receptor mediated processes (50). However, a "non-opioid" receptor system may exist also for ACTH/α-MSH-related peptides (51-53), Thus, the opioid or opiomelanocortin-like vs. the non-opioid effects of ACTH/α-MSH represent also a dissociation within the peptide system. It is not clear yet whether the "opioid" and "non-opioid" mechanisms represent different compartments of origin, i.e., multiple origin such as the anterior and intermediate pituitary and the brain, or the differentiation is embedded in the receptor specifity in the brain.

Although many indirect evidences suggest the interactions of ACTH-related peptides with limbic-midbrain mechanisms few direct data are available on the exact localization of action. Studies on extinction behavior of the rats bearing limbic-midbrain lesions suggest that destruction of the amygdala, septum, thalamic parafascicular area and lesion in the dorsal hippocampus prevents the action of α-MSH or ACTH 4-10 (54). As far as non-specific stress-related behavior is concerned, ACTH-induced excessive grooming is attenuated by total hippocampectomy (55) but the primary actions are most probably localized in the substantia nigra (56).

The next dissociation concerns the differential role of adrenal cortical and medullary hormones. The way of controlling a stressful situation determines whether adrenal medullary or cortical hormones are indispensible for a proactive effect on the expression of behavior. This conclusion is suggested by the following studies. A one-trial learning inhibitory avoidance training allows two kinds of tests of what has been learned from an aversive experience (light painful footshock) a day earlier. The rat can be tested for inhibitory avoidance as learned behavior. In this case, the rat actively controls the environment by deciding to re-enter or not to enter a compartment where it received the aversive experience. However, if the animal is placed directly to this compartment from where no escape is possible the rat displays immobility. This immobility reflects no active control or loss of control about the environment.

Short-term ADX impairs behavioral performance both in the avoidance and immobility situation (43, Bohus & del Cerro, to be published). Peripheral administration of epinephrine immediately after learning in ADX rats in physiological doses normalizes the avoidance behavior. Corticosterone is unable to correct for this deficit in the avoidance situation. In contrast, the behavior of the rats in a situation that they cannot control actively is under the influence of corticosterone. Short-term ADX rats receiving corticosterone immediately after learning show immobility behavior in contrast to their ADX controls. The findings of an experiment in which the rat received corticosterone after learning and then tested for immobility and subsequently for avoidance are summarized in Table 4.

Table 4. Adrenalectomy (ADX), adrenomedullectomy (ADMX), corticosterone (CS) or dexamethasone (DEX), replacement, immobility, and subsequent avoidance in the rat.

Surgery/Treatment	Immobility	Avoidance
Sham-ADX	+	+
ADX	-	-
ADXM	+	-
ADX + CS	+	-
ADX + DEX	-	-

Data from Bohus and Del Cerro (in preparation).

The dissociation in the function of medullary and cortical systems is also supported by the findings in adrenomedullectomized rats. Removal of the source of circulating epinephrine does not affect significantly immobility behavior but impairs avoidance behavior. The differential effect of corticosterone and dexamethasone will be dealt with below.

These experiments suggest that optimal hormonal states provided by the two adrenal hormone systems are essential but for different mechanisms that serve behavior in actively controllable and uncontrollable situations. These mechanisms are embedded in the same individual and the proper one may be selected according to the environmental requirements. However, one cannot exclude the possibility that individual differentiation in behavioral and neuroendocrine adaptation means a preferable use of the one above the other mechanism. Such a differentiation has been proposed by Henry (57) in mice - i.e., fight/flight vs. depression or conservation-withdrawal - and corroborated by Fokkema (58) in rats and Koolhaas et al. (59) in rats and mice, respectively. According to Henry (57) the fight-flight type of behavior is probably organized by amygdala-related mechanisms and reflected in high sympathetic and/or adrenal medullary system activities. The conservation-withdrawal mechanisms are according to Henry (57) hippocampus-septum related and reflected in high pituitary-adrenal activity.

The last dissociation is in the receptor systems that are involved in the action of corticosterone in various forms of emotional behavior. Extinction of a fear-motivated behavior using a so-called forced extinction procedure in the rat is attenuated by short-term ADX and restored by corticosterone but not by dexamethasone, progesterone, or deoxycorticosterone (60). The observations on immobility behavior as described above also show a selective action of corticosterone vs. the potent glucocorticoid dexamethasone.

Recent observations by de Kloet and his associates (17) suggest that the rat brain contains at least two kinds of receptors for corticosteroids: corticosterone receptor (CR) and glucocorticoid receptors (GR). CR receptors are primarily localized in the hippocampal neurons, have much higher affinity for corticosterone than for dexamethasone, and most receptor sites are occupied by endogenous corticosterone under basal conditions. This function may be described as a tonic (permissive) one. The GR receptors are primarily localized in the lateral septum, central and cortical amygdala and the hypothalamus, have higher affinity for glucocorticoids such as dexamethasone than for corticosterone, and most receptor sites are unoccupied under basal conditions. The function of these neuronal and glial receptors may be described as a phasic one and probably mediate a feedback action of corticosteroids on stress-activated brain processes. Since the majority of the receptor sites with specifity for corticosterone is localized in the hippocampus it is therefore reasonable to suggest that this area is the major target of corticosterone-specific behavioral changes such as forced extinction and immobility behavior and CR receptors are involved. Behavioral effects of all glucocorticosteroids as described in intact rats (39, 61) are probably mediated by GR receptors. The localization of these actions is rather widespread in the limbic system (39, 61) and corresponds to the distribution of the GR receptors (62).

However, not every kind of immobility behavior is specifically affected by corticosterone. Jefferys et al. (63) found that the retention acquired immobility during forced swimming is impaired by adrenalectomy. Administration of corticosterone or dexamethasone before the acquisition normalizes the retention of acquired immobility. Recently, Veldhuis et al. (64) reported that GR receptors are involved in the steroid action on this immobility behavior. The differential involvement of CR- and GR-mediated processes in various forms of immobility behavior suggests that the significance of the dissociation between the function of CR and GR receptors in behavioral adaptation may lie in the emotional rather than the motor component of the behavior.

Emotional Behavior, Physiology and Hormones

Abundant evidence suggests that the limbic system, particularly amygdaloid and septal structures profoundly influences cardiovascular, respiratory and gastrointestinal functions (65-68). Within the amygdala complex the central nucleus is indicated as a major controller of autonomic functions in relation to emotional behavior (69). From a behavioral point of view the medial nucleus of the amygdala may also be of importance. Lesioning these nuclei bilaterally either electrolytically or with the aid of neurotoxins impairs emotional behavior in social (aggressive) situations (70-72). In addition, studies by McGaugh and his associates (20) suggest intimate relation between the amygdala and the adrenal medulla in behavioral modulation. These amygdaloid areas are also rich in various neuropeptides. Among others, CRF containing perikarya and fibers have been localized in the central amygdala (73) and opiomelanocortin-containing neurons also project to the amygdala complex (16). Additionally, corticosterone reception is suggested by a distinct uptake of corticosteroid in neuronal cell nuclei of the various subcomponents of the amygdala complex (74).

Neuroanatomical observations suggest that the control of the autonomic nervous system and thereby cardiovascular, respiratory and gastrointestinal functions may be exerted through two different pathways. One pathway is represented by the numerous direct projections from the amygdala complex to brainstem areas such as the parabrachial nuclei, the nuclei of the solitary tract, the dorsal motor nucleus of the vagus nerve and the central grey (72, 73). The other pathway is the innervation of the autonomic hypothalamus and its subsequent connection to the brainstem or to the spinal cord (75, 76).

Indirect evidence suggests that the CRF-opiomelanocortin-adrenal neuroendocrine system affect autonomic physiology in relation to emotional behavior. Peripheral administration of ACTH 4-10, which is a behaviorally active fragment of ACTH (77), causes tachycardia and a facilitation of emotional behavior in an inhibitory avoidance situation. The control rats display a relative bradycardiac response in this situation as determined by radiotelemetric recording of the electrocardiogram of the free-moving animal (78, 79). The increased heart rate of ACTH 4-10 treated rats is probably the consequence of an increased sympathetic influence on the heart rhythm. That neonatal chemical sympathectomy prevents the occurrence of the tachycardia response of the peptide-treated rats (80) supports this view. Sympathetic influences on the heart are generally evoked by intense stressor and/or when the organism is actively engaged in the preparation or execution or somato-motor activities (81). The somatic pattern of the rats' behavior during inhibitory avoidance is not affected by ACTH 4-10. Therefore, tachycardia in ACTH 4-10 treated rats may occur because the peptide signals intense stress to the appropriate brain centers and causes a facilitated arousal state. This signalization then causes a shift in the autonomic control of the heart from a moderate vagal control to a more pronounced sympathetic influence. The arousal hypothesis is valid for man too. ACTH 4-10 increases heart rate and the magnitude of tendon reflexes in young healthy volunteers during a binary choice reaction test (82). Improved task performance, increased forearm blood flow and tachycardia is caused by ACTH 4-10 in extrovert subjects during a battery of tests that produces psychological stress. The performance and the autonomic reaction of introverted subjects are suppressed by ACTH 4-10 (83). These latter behavioral and physiological reactions may be due to an overarousal.

The function of opioid peptide ß-endorphin in autonomic physiology in relation to emotional behavior is not clear yet. Although ß-endorphin profoundly affects cardiovascular functions (84) the opiate antagonist naltrexone fails to modify a bradycardiac response to an emotional stressor of uncontrollable behavioral situations. Remarkably, naltrexone abolishes the hyperthermic stress response to the same stimulus (85). Since the temperature response as determined from the anal temperature may be related to circulatory changes, further studies using cardiovascular measures other than the heart rate are necessary. It should be mentioned that combined behavioral and physiological studies concerning CRF are also missing. Beside the arousing behavioral actions, the peptide seems to cause a sympathetic activation when given intracerebrally in somewhat large amounts. This is suggested by an increased blood pressure, heart rate and plasma catecholamine level (86-88).

Table 5. Adrenalectomy (ADX) diminishes behavioral hypertension and bradycardia in the rat in an inhibitory avoidance situation under avoidance and immobility conditions.

	Blood pressure		Heart rate	
	Control	ADX	Control	ADX
Before aversive stimulation	115.5 ± 3.3	116.6 ± 2.0	123.3 ± 3.0	126.6 ± 2.9
After stimulation				
Avoidance	127.4 ± 7.5[1]	115.3 ± 4.3	128.2 ± 4.7[1]	131.5 ± 2.0[1]
Immobility	132.4 ± 7.2[1]	108.4 ± 3.7*	125.0 ± 2.61	30.2 ± 2.6[1]

Mean blood pressure in mmHg. Mean interbeat interval in msec. All values are given as means ± S.E.M. of 6-6 rats.
Significance: * $p<0.05$ (two-tailed t-test, control vs. ADX); 1 $p<0.05$ (paired t-test for values before and after aversive stimulation). Data from van der Meulen and Bohus (89).

Recent findings in our laboratory suggest that adrenal hormones play an important role in behavioral hypertension (89). These experiments were carried out in the inhibitory avoidance situation in rats equipped with a catheter implanted in the descending aorta for direct blood pressure measurements. The rats were tested for avoidance or immobility alternatively every other day up to 8 days after the aversive stimulus or footshock (0.6 mA, 2 sec). Table 5 shows that short-term adrenalectomy (4 days prior to the aversive stimulation) prevents the blood pressure response to emotional stressor in both the avoidance and immobility situation. The animals served as their own controls compairing their blood pressure (and heart rate) before and various times after the aversive stimulation. Short-term ADX fails to affect pre-stress blood pressure (and heart rate).

The overall bradycardiac response as given in Table 5 is not pronounced and adrenalectomy has less influence on this measure. It should be mentioned that the cardiac response in both the controllable and uncontrollable situation is rather complex (85). During avoidance a more or less continuous relative bradycardia (so-called tonic response) and short phases of further heart rate decrease occur (phasic response). The phasic response accompanies conflict behavior - i.e., approaching-withdrawing of the compartment of former aversive stimulation. During immobility behavior in the latter compartment an early marked bradycardiac response is shifting to slight tachycardia within a 5 min observation period. More detailed analysis of the heart rate data (which is in progress) may give a better picture of the adrenal involvement in this measure. The avoidance and immobility behavior of the adrenalectomized rats is impaired. Accordingly, behavioral deficits are accompanied by the absence of one physiological response - i.e., the hypertension. It remains to be shown whether the behavioral impairment is of primary importance or the behavioral and physiological responses are organized parallely but separately. That the bradycardiac stress response is less affected by short-term ADX favors a separate organization.

Taken together, these observations suggest that ACTH-related peptides and adrenal hormones affect certain physiological functions in relation to emotional behavior. The parallelism between behavioral and physiological actions presuppose a neuroendocrine input to brain mechanisms which are involved in the control of both emotional behavior and physiology. This input may be related to a direct action of the neuroendocrine principles on limbic structures such as the amygdala. The presence of cell bodies and/or terminals of peptidergic neurons in this area, as discussed in the introduction of this section, supports this view. However, reciprocal connections exist between limbic and brainstem structures, and both terminals and cell bodies of CRF and opiomelanocortins have been described in brainstem autonomic areas such as in the central grey, parabrachial nuclei, nuclei of the tractus solitary, etc. (16, 73). Accordingly, changes in emotionality through limbic influences may alter peptidergic autonomic regulatory mechanisms at the level of the brainstem.

The observations in adrenalectomized rats suggest the involvement of adrenal hormones. It remains to be shown whether adrenal catecholamines or corticosteroids play an essential role in behavioral hypertension or like in the case of behavior their function depends upon the controllability of the situation. As far as adrenal cortical hormones are concerned their site of action may be both of limbic or brainstem level as suggested by autoradiographic studies of nuclear corticoid uptake (74, 90). It is, however, maintained that peripherally circulating catecholamines cannot pass the blood-brain barrier. Circumventricular organs that lie outside this barrier (91) in the vicinity of the limbic system (e.g., organum vasculosum laminae terminalis, subfornical organ) or the brainstem (e.g., area postrema) and communicate with neighboring brain structures may be of the site(s) of behavioral and physiological actions of epinephrine and/or norepinephrine.

Closing Comments

Neurophysiological, behavioral and physiological evidences as reviewed here suggest complex interactions between limbic-midbrain mechanisms and the CRF-opiomelanocortin-adrenal neuroendocrine system. Each component of the system produces a different neuroendocrine state in the brain. The diversity is partially embedded in the hierarchy of the level of control. CRF may act independently as neuroendocrine messenger through the pituitary or as a neural messenger through peptidergic transmission/neuromodulation. Opiomelanocortin release of pituitary origin depends upon the neuroendocrine function of CRF. Adrenal cortical and medullary hormonal systems are in multiple ways d pendent on the CRF-opiocortin system. Accordingly, the dependence of a neuroendocrine state in the brain on the activity of the other components of the system is increasing with the level of hierarchy. However, each component of the system can convey different messages to the same limbic-midbrain structure.

While discussing the interactions between limbic-midbrain mechanisms and CRF-opiocortin and adrenal neuroendocrine system the emphasis has been placed on the anterior pituitary as the source of opiocortins, in particular of ACTH, ß-LPH. The release of these peptides without doubt is controlled by CRF. However, in the rat, the intermediate lobe of the pituitary is also the source of opiomelanocortins such as α-MSH, CLIP and ß-endorphins. The release of the intermediate lobe peptides is controlled by the circulating catecholamines (92). Thus, the complexity of the organization of a certain neuroendocrine state is further extended. In addition, the existence of a opiomelanocortinergic neuronal system in the brain, originating from the arcuate nuclei of the hypothalamus and terminating among others in limbic-midbrain areas (16, 17) questions whether the hormonal or the neural systems are of primary importance to determine this peptidergic neuroendocrine state of the brain. Some behavioral and physiological findings (50) suggest that the pituitary source serves adaptive functions in relation to stress. Furthermore, it has been suggested recently that vasopressin rather than CRF is the releaser of ß-endorphin from neuronal pools in the brain (93).

The complexity of a neuroendocrine mechanism that serves stress and adaptation may assure the maintenance of behavioral and physiological functions within extreme stressful conditions. However, such complexity also includes the possibility that dysfunction of one or more components of the neuroendocrine system contribute to the disintegration of adaptive brain mechanisms. In these ways neuroendocrine imbalance - either hyper- or hypoactivity in interaction with environmental factors may serve both as etiological factor or modulator of the outcome of mental and psychosomatic disease. The psychosomatic aspect of this hypothesis (94, 95) is primarily based upon observations on cardiac responses to emotional stressors. Recent observations on behavioral hypertension and on the kindling model of epilepsy provide additional support of a neuroendocrine view of psychosomatic diseases.

The arrhythmogenic potential of the central nervous system in both coronary and non-coronary types of sudden cardiac death syndromes (SCDS) has been well recognized (96, 97). A dysbalance of the autonomic or hormonal control of cardiac rhythm can be viewed as a predisposing factor to SCDS. Sympathetic overactivity in the early phase of myocardial infarction is a classic severe danger for ventricular fibrillation. An imbalance in favor of the parasympathetic control may lead to syncope or ectopic electrical activity of the heart. The impact of the central nervous system on the autonomic and hormonal system as a component of the stress reaction implies that emotional factors may be important precursors of psychosomatic events leading to SCDS. Observations in infra-human species (98-100) suggest that the relation between emotional stress and SCDS is a general biological phenomenon. The acute cardiovascular (heart rhythm and blood pressure) response to emotional stressors in the rat and its relation to the behavioral component of the stress response, as presented in this paper, may thus serve as a model of psychosomatic disturbances. An extrapolation from animal experiments to man in real life situations is obviously risky, but models that use semi-natural situations (e.g., social interaction in rodents) make it possible to integrate available information to recognize the failures and to suggest further research.

A neuroendocrine hypothesis of mind-body relationships is somewhat different from former psychosomatic views. For example, Alexander (2) postulated that particular emotional states determine the diversity of bodily responses. Such strong specifity has been denied by later proposals (101) but - although sometimes in indirect ways - emotionality remained an important factor in psychosomatic theories. Recently, Ursin (102) emphasized the role of neuroendocrine factors in psychosomatic pathology. It is suggested that sustained activation causes disease. The specifity of psychosomatic pathology depends on personality traits and their related dominating endocrine system.

A generalized activational hypothesis cannot explain the development of various organ pathologies as a consequence of psychosocial stressors. Interactions between "personality factors" (e.g., fight-flight vs. depression strategies; 57), active or passive characteristics (59), environmental properties (e.g., controllability and predictability; 103-105), the properties of stressor, stress reactions and the behavioral and physiological systems involved (106) determine ultimately the quality and quantity of stress-related pathology.

The proposed neuroendocrine model for psychosomatic disease consists of five elements. The first element is a brain state which is induced by the biotic or non-biotic environment. The brain state (activation, non-specific arousal) activates (or inhibits) physiological and neuroendocrine systems and certain non-specific behavioral responses. The second element is to establish a certain "neuroendocrine state." The neuroendocrine state is determined by the availability of stress hormones and the functional properties of their receptors both in the periphery and the brain. The third element is that the neuroendocrine state by modulating the original brain state results in an "integrated brain state." The integrated brain state also depends on recent experiences of the environment (controllability, predictability) and on exper-iences acquired in the past (e.g., ontogeny) and on genetical factors. The fourth element is the organization of an "integrated" physiological response and also of more specific behavior. Although a peripheral interaction between peptides and steroid hormones and organs of the cardiovascular system, gastrointestinal tract, etc. cannot be excluded, the present hypothesis considers the brain as the major target. The last element is the development and outcome of the psychosomatic (eventually mental) disease. Since the integrated brain state is highly dependent on the neuroendocrine state, neuroendocrine imbalance in the brain may be followed by behavioral and somatic imbalance and different degrees of disease. If this neuroendocrine view of the mind-body interaction is correct the reinstallation of neuroendocrine imbalance by peptides and/or other hormone treatment or by specific hormone antagonists may be curative in psychosomatic diseases.

References

1. Papez, J.W. (1937). A proposed mechanism of emotion. Arch. Neurol. Psychiat., 38: 726-744.
2. Alexander, F. (1950). Psychosomatic Medicine. Norton, N.Y.
3. Selye, H. (1950). Stress. The physiology and pathology of exposure to stress. Acta Medica Publ., Montreal.
4. Porter, R.W. (1954). The central nervous system and stess-induced eosinophenia. Recent Progr. in Horm. Res., 10: 1-27.
5. Mason, J.W. (1957). The central nervous regulation of ACTH secretion. In H.H. Jasper, L.D. Proctor, R.S. Knighton, W.C. Noshay & R.T. Costello (Eds.), Reticular formation of the brain. Little, Brown, Boston, p. 645-670.
6. Endröczi, E., Lissák, K., Bohus, B. & Kovács, S. (1959). The inhibitory influence of archicortical structures on pituitary-adrenal function. Acta Physiol. Acad. Sci. Hung., 16: 17-22.
7. Rubin, R.T., Mandell, A.J. & Crandall, P.H. (1966). Cortiosteroid responses to limbic stimulation in man: Localization of stimulus sites. Science, 153: 767-768.
8. Endröczi, E. & Lissák, K. (1960). The role of the mesencephalon, diencephalon and archicortex in the activation and inhibition of the pituitary-adrenocortical system. Acta Physiol. Acad. Sci. Hung., 17: 39-55.
9. Bohus, B. (1961). The effect of central nervous lesions on pituitary-adrenocortical function in the rat. Acta Physiol. Acad. Sci. Hung., 20: 373-377.
10. Knigge, K.M. (1961). Adrenocortical response to immobilization in rats with lesion in hippocampus and amygdala. Ped. Proc., 20: 185.
11. Lissák, K. & Endröczi, E. (1960). Die neuroendokrine Steuerung der Adaptionstätigkeit. Akademischer Verlag, Budapest, p. 172.
12. Kaada, B.R. (1972). Stimulation and regional ablation of the amygdaloid complex with reference to functional representations. In B.E. Eleftheriou (Ed.), The neurobiology of the amygdala. Plenum Press, N.Y., p. 205-281.
13. Henry, J.P. & Stephens, P.M. (1977). Stress, health, and the social environment. A sociobiologic approach to medicine. Springer-Verlag, N.Y.
14. McEwen, B.S. (1982). Glucocorticoids and hippocampus: Receptors in search of a function. In D. Ganten & D. Pfaff (Eds.), Current topics in neuroendocrinology, Vol. 2. Adrenal actions on the brain. Springer-Verlag, Berlin, p. 1-22.
15. Bohus, B., de Kloet, E.R. & Veldhuis, H.D. (1982). Adrenal steroids and behavioral adaptation: Relationships to brain corticoid receptors. In D. Ganten, D. Pfaff (Eds.), Adrenal actions to brain. Springer-Verlag, Berlin, p. 108-140.
16. De Kloet, E.R., Palkovits, M. & Mezey, E. (1986). Opioid peptides: Localization, source and avenues of transport. In D. de Wied, W.H. Gispen & Tj.B. van Wimersma Greidanus (Eds.), Neuropeptides and behavior, Vol. 1. Pergamon Press, Oxford, p. 1-41.
17. De Kloet, E.R., Reul, J.M.H.M., de Ronde, F.S.W. & Veldhuis, H.D. (1986). Brain corticosteroid receptor systems: Heterogeneity, function and plasticity. In D. de Wied & W. Ferrari (Eds.), Central actions of ACTH and related peptides. Symposia in neuroscience, Vol. 4. Liviana Press, Springer-Verlag, p. 115-129.

18. Olschowka, J.A., O'Donohue, T.L., Mueller, G.P. & Jacobowitz, D.M. (1982). The distribution of corticotropin releasing factor-like immunoreactive neurons in rat brain. Peptides, 3: 995-1015.
19. Borrell, J., de Kloet, E.R. & Bohus, B. (1984). Corticosterone decreases the efficacy of adrenaline to affect passive avoidance retention of adrenalectomized rats. Life Sci., 34: 99-105.
20. McGaugh, J.L. (1985). Peripheral and central adrenergic influences on brain systems involved in the modulation of memory storage. Ann. N.Y. Acad. Sci., 444: 150-161.
21. Bohus, B. (1984). Neuroendocrine interactions with brain and behavior: A model for psychoneuroimmunology? In R.E. Ballieux (Ed.), Breakdown in human adaptation to stress. Towards a multidisciplinary approach. Martinus Nijhoff Publ., The Hague, p. 638-652.
22. Goddard, G.V., McIntyre, D.C. & Leech, C.L. (1969). A permanent change in brain functions resulting from daily electrical stimulation. Exp. Neurol., 25: 295-330.
23. Ehlers, C.L., Hendriksen, S.J., Wang, J., Rivier, J., Vale, W. & Bloom, F.E. (1983). Corticotropin-releasing factor produces increases in brain excitability and convulsive seizures in rats. Brain Res., 278: 332-336.
24. Cottrell, G.A., Nyakas, C., Bohus, B. & de Wied, D. (1983). ACTH and MSH reduce the after-discharge and behavioural depression following kindling. In E. Endröczi, D. de Wied, L. Angelucci & U. Scapagnini (Eds.), Integrative neurohumoral mechanisms. Developments in neuroscience, Vol. 16. Elsevier, Amsterdam, p. 91-97.
25. Frenk, H., Engel, J.Jr., Ackerman, R.F., Shavit, Y. & Liebeskind, J.C. (1979). Endogenous opioids may mediate post-ictal behavioural depression in amygdala kindled rats. Brain Res., 167: 435-440.
26. Cottrell, G.A., Nyakas, C. & Bohus, B. (1984). The behavioural depression of hippocampal kindled rats is attenuated by subcutaneous and intracerebroventricular naltrexone. Prog. Neuro- Psychopharmacol. Biol. Psychiat., 8: 673-676.
27. Gispen, W.H., Wiegant, V.M., Greven, H.M. & de Wied, D. (1975). The induction of excessive grooming in the rat by intraventricular application of peptides derived from ACTH: Structure activity studies. Life Sci., 17: 645-652.
28. Gispen, W.H., Buitelaar, J., Wiegant, V.M., Terenius, L. & de Wied, D. (1976). Interaction between ACTH fragments, brain opiate receptors and morphine-induced analgesia. Eur. J. Pharmacol., 39: 393-397.
29. Van Ree, J.M., Bohus, B., Csonton, K., Gispen, W.H., Greven, H.M., Nijkamp, F.P., Opmeer, F.A., de Rotte, G.A., van Wimersma Greidanus, Tj.B., Witter, A. & de Wied, D. (1981). Behavioral profile of gamma-MSH: Relationship with ACTH and ß-endorphin action. Life Sci., 28: 2879-2888.
30. Nakanishi, S., Inoue, A., Kita, T., Nakamura, M., Chang, A.C.Y., Cohen, S.N. & Numa, S. (1979). Nucleotide sequence of cloned cDNA for bovine corticotropin-ß-lipotropin precursor. Nature, 278: 423-427.
31. Heuser, G. & Eidelberg, E. (1961). Steroid-induced convulsions in experimental animals. Endocrinology, 69: 915.
32. Woodbury, D.M. (1958). Relation between the adrenal cortex and the central nervous system. Pharmacol. Rev., 10: 275-345.
33. Endröczi, E. (1969). Brain stem and hypothalamic substrate of motivated behaviour. In K. Lissák (Ed.), Results in neurophysiology, neuroendocrinology, neuropharmacology and behaviour. Recent developments of neurobiology in Hungary, Vol. 2. Akadémiai Kiadó, Budapest, p. 27-46.
34. Feldman, S. (1973). The interaction of neural and endocrine factors regulating hypothalamic activity. In A. Brodish & E.S. Redgate (Eds.), Brain-pituitary-adrenal interrelationships. Karger, Basel, p. 224-238.
35. Halmy, L., Bohus, B., Frey, Z. & Endröczi, E. (1970). Direct metyrapone effect on central nervous system. Endocrinology, 57: 139-141.
36. Cottrell, G.A., Nyakas, C., de Kloet, E.R. & Bohus, B. (1984). Hippocampal kindling: Corticosterone modulation of induced seizures. Brain Res., 309: 377-381.
37. Oliverio, E., Castellano, C. & Puglisi-Allegra, S. (1983). Anticonvulsant effects of stress: Role of endogenous oipoids. Brain Res., 271: 193-195.
38. De Wied, D. (1969). Effects of peptide hormones on behavior. In W.F. Gangon & L. Martini (Eds.), Frontiers in neuroendocrinology. Oxford University Press, N.Y., p. 97-140.
39. Bohus, B. (1970). Central nervous structures and the effect of ACTH and corticosteroids on avoidance behaviour: A study with intracerebral implantation of corticosteroids in the rat. In D. de Wied & J.A.W.M. Weijnen (Eds.), Pituitary, adrenal and the brain. Progress in Brain Research, Vol. 32. Elsevier, Amsterdam, p. 171-184.
40. Bohus, B. & de Wied, D. (1980). Pituitary-adrenal system hormones and adaptive behaviour.

In I. Chester-Jones & I.W. Henderson (Eds.), General, comparative and clinical endocrinology of the andrenal cortex, Vol. 3. Academic Press, London, p. 256-347.

41. Sutton, R.E., Koob, G.F., Le Moal, M., Rivier, J. & Vale, W. (1982). Corticotropin releasing factor produces behavioral activation in rats. Nature, 297: 331-333.
42. Britton, D.R., Koob, G.F., Rivier, J. & Vale, W. (1982). Intraventricular corticotropin-releasing factor enhances behavioral effects of novelty. Life Sci., 31: 363-367.
43. Borrell, J., de Kloet, E.R., Versteeg, D.H.G. & Bohus, B. (1983). Inhibitory avoidance deficit following short-term adrenalectomy in the rat: The role of adrenal catecholamines. Behav. Neural Biol., 39: 241-258.
44. Borrell, J., de Kloet, E.R., Versteeg, D.H.G., Bohus, B. & de Wied, D. (1984). Neuropeptides and memory: Interactions with peripheral catecholamines. In E. Usdin, R. Kvetnansky & J. Axelrod (Eds.), Stress. The role of catecholamines and other transmitters. Gordon and Breach, N.Y., p. 391-402.
45. McGaugh, J.L. (1983). Hormonal influences on memory. Ann. Rev. Psychol., 34: 297-323.
46. Kastin, A.J., Miller, L.M., Nockton, R., Sandman, C.A., Schally, A.V. & Stratton, L.O. (1973). Behavioral aspects of melanocyte-stimulating hormone (MHS). In E. Zimmerman, W.H. Gispen, B.H. Marks & D. de Wied (Eds.), Drug effects on neuroendocrine regulation. Progress in Brain Research, Vol. 39. Elsevier, Amsterdam, p. 461-470.
47. De Wied, D., Witter, A. & Greven, H.M. (1975). Behaviourally active ACTH analogues. Biochem. Pharmacol., 24: 1463-1468.
48. Chrétien, M., Benjannet, S., Gossard, F., Gianoulakis, C., Crine, P., Lis, M. & Seidah, N.G. (1979). From ß-lipotropin to ß-endorphin and "pro-opiomelanocortin." Canad. J. Biochem., 57: 1111-1121.
49. Terenius, L., Gispen, W.H. & de Wied, D. (1975). ACTH-like peptides and opiate receptors in the rat brain: Structure-activity studies. Eur. J. Pharmacol., 33: 395-399.
50. Bohus, B. (1984). Opiomelanocortins and behavioral adaptation. Pharmac. Ther., 26: 417-451.
51. Gispen, W.H., Van Ree, J.M. & de Wied, D. (1977). Lipotropin and the central nervous system. Intern. Rev. Neurobiol., 20: 209-250.
52. Jacquet, Y.G. (1978). Opiate effects after adrenocorticotropin or ß-endorphin injection in the periaqueductal gray matter of rats. Science, 201: 1032-1034.
53. Kastin, A.J., Olson, R.D., Schally, A.V. & Coy, D.H. (1979). CNS effects of peripherally administered brain peptides. Life Sci. 25: 401-414.
54. Van Wimersma Greidanus, Tj.B., Bohus, B., Kovács, G.L., Versteeg, D.H.G., Burbach, J.P.H. & de Wied, D. (1983). Sites of behavioral and biochemical action of ACTH-like peptides and of neurohypophyseal hormones. Neurosci. Biobehav. Rev., 7: 453-463.
55. Colbern, D., Isaacson, R.L., Bohus, B. & Gispen, W.H. (1977). Limbic-midbrain lesions and ACTH-induced excessive grooming. Life Sci., 21: 383-402.
56. Gispen, W.H. & Isaacson, R.L. (1981). ACTH-induced exsessive grooming in the rat. Pharmacol. Ther., 12: 209-246.
57. Henry, J.P. (1980). Present concept of stress theory. In E. Usdin, R. Kvetnansky & I.J. Kopin (Eds.), Catecholamines and stress: Recent advances. Elsevier North Holland Inc. Amsterdam, p. 557-571.
58. Fokkema, D.S. (1985). Social behavior and blood pressure: A study of rats. Ph.D. Thesis, Groningen, Netherlands.
59. Koolhaas, J.M., Fokkema, D.S., Bohus, B. & van Oortmerssen, G.A. (1986). Individual differentiation in blood pressure reactivity and behaviour of male rats. In T.M. Dembroski, T.H. Schmidt & G. Blümchen (Eds.), Biobehavioral factors in coronary heart disease. Springer-Verlag, p. 517-526.
60. Bohus, B. & de Kloet, E.R. (1981). Adrenal steroids and extinction behavior: Antagonism by progesterone, deoxycorticosterone, and dexamethasone of a specific effect of corticosterone. Life Sci., 28: 433-440.
61. Bohus, B. (1973). Pituitary-adrenal influences on avoidance and approach behavior of the rat. In E. Zimmerman, W.H. Gispen, B.H. Marks & D. de Wied (Eds.), Drug effects on neuroendocrine regulation. Progress in Brain Research, Vol. 39. Elsevier, Amsterdam, p. 407-420.
62. Reul, J.M.H.M. & de Kloet, E.R. (1986). Anatomical resolution of two types of corticosterone and receptor sites in rat brain with in vitro autoradiography and computerized image analysis. J. steroid Biochem., 24: 269-272.
63. Jefferys, D., Copolov, D., Irby, D. & Funder, J.W. (1983). Behavioural effect of adrenalectomy: Reversal by glucocorticoids or (D-ala^2-met^5) enkephalinamide. Eur. J. Pharmacol., 92: 99-103.
64. Veldhuis, H.D., de Korte, C.C.M.M. & de Kloet, E.R. (1985). Glucocorticiods facilitate the retention of acquired immobility during forced swimming. Eur. J. Pharmacol., 115: 211-217.

65. Hilton, S.M. & Zbrozyna, A.W. (1963). Amygdaloid region for defense reactions and its efferent pathway to the brain stem. J. Physiol., 165: 160-173.
66. Henke, P.G. (1979). The hypothalamus-amygdala axis and experimental gastric ulcers. Neurosci. Biobehav. Rev., 3: 75-82.
67. Kapp, B.R., Frysinger, R.C., Gallagher, M. & Haselton, J.R. (1979). Amygdala central nucleus lesions: Effect on heart rate conditioning in the rabbit. Physiol. Behav., 23: 1109-1117.
68. Harper, R.M., Frysinger, R.C., Trelease, R.B. & Marks, J.D. (1984). State-dependent alteration of respiratory cycle timing by stimulation of the central nucleus of the amygdala. Brain Res., 306: 1-8.
69. Smith, O.A. & DeVito, J.L. (1984). Central neural integration for the control of autonomic responses associated with emotion. Ann. Rev. Neurosci., 7: 43-65.
70. Bolhuis, J.J., FitzGerald, R.E., Dijk, D.J. & Koolhaas, J.M. (1984). The corticomedial amygdala and learning in an agonistic situation in the rat. Physiol. Behav., 32: 575-579.
71. Bohus, B. & Koolhaas, J.M. (1985). Neuropeptides, neurotransmitters and memory: Socio-sexual aspects. In J. McGaugh (Ed.), Contemporary psychology: Biological processes and theoretical issues. Elsevier, Amsterdam, p. 3-16.
72. Luiten, P.G.M., Koolhaas, J.M., de Boer, S. & Koopmans, S.J. (1985). The cortico-medial amygdala in the central nervous system organization of agonistic behavior. Brain Res., 332: 283-297.
73. Veening, J.G., Swanson, L.W. & Sawchenko, P.E. (1984). The organization of projections from the central nucleus of the amygdala to brainstem sites involved in central autonomic regulation: A combined retrograde transport-immunohistochemical study. Brain Res., 303: 337-357.
74. Stumpf, W.E. & Sar, M. (1975). Anatomical distribution of corticosterone-concentration neurons in rat brain. In W.E. Stupf & L.D. Grant (Eds.), Anatomical neuroendocriology. Karger, Basel, p. 254-261.
75. Swanson, L.W. & Sawchenko, P.E. (1983). Hypothalamic integration: Organization of the paraventricular and supraoptic nuclei. Ann. Rev. Neurosci., 6: 269-324.
76. Luiten, P.G.M., ter Horst, G.J. & Steffens, A.B. (1987). The hypothalamus, intrinsic connections and outflow pathways to the endocrine system in relation to the control of feeding and metabolism. Progr. Neurobiol., 28: 1-54.
77. Bohus, B. (1979). Effects of ACTH-like neuropeptides on animal behavior and man. Pharmacology, 18: 113-122.
78. Bohus, B. (1974). Telemetered heart rate responses of the rat during free and learned behavior. Biotelemetry, 1: 193-201.
79. Bohus, B. (1977). Pituitary neuropeptides, emotional behavoir and cardiac responses. In W. de Jong, A.P. Provoost & A.P. Shapiro (Eds.), Hypertension and brain mechanisms. Progress in Brain Research, Vol. 47. Elsevier, Amsterdam, p. 277-288.
80. Bohus, B., de Jong, W., Provoost, A.P. & de Wied, D. (1976). Emotionales Verhalten und Reaktionen des Kreislaufs und Endokriniums bei Ratten. In A.W. von Eiff (Ed.), Seelische und körperliche Störungen durch Stress. Gustav Fischer Verlag, Stuttgart, p. 140-157.
81. Obrist, P.A. (1981). Cardiovascular psychophysiology. A perspective. Plenum Press, N.Y., London, p. 141-231.
82. Brunia, C.H.M. & Van Boxtel, A. (1978). Alpha-MSH/ACTH 4-10 and task induced increase in tendon reflexes and heart rate. Pharmacol. Biochem. Behav., 9: 615-618.
83. Breier, C., Kain, H. & Konzett, H. (1979). Personality dependent effects of the ACTH 4-10 fragments on test performance and on concomitant autonomic reactions. Psychopharmacol., 65: 239-245.
84. Holaday, J.W. (1983). Cardiovascular effects of endogenous opiate systems. Ann. Rev. Pharmacol. Toxicol., 23: 541-594.
85. Bohus, B. (1985). Acute cardiac responses to emotional stressors in the rat: The involvement of neuroendocrine mechanisms. In J.F. Orlebeke, G. Mulder & L.J.P. Van Doornen (Eds.), Psychophysiology of cardiovascular control. Models, methods and data. Plenum Press, N.Y., p. 131-150.
86. Brown, M.R., Fisher, L.A., Rivier, J., Spiess, J., Rivier, C. & Vale, W. (1982). Corticotropin-releasing factor: Effects on the sympathetic nervous system and oxygen consumption. Life Sci., 30: 207-210.
87. Brown, M.R., Fisher, L.A., Spiess, J., Rivier, C., Rivier, J. & Vale, W. (1982). Corticotropin-releasing factor actions on the sympathetic nervous system and metabolism. Endocrinology, 111: 928-931.
88. Fisher, L.A., Rivier, J., Rivier, C, Spiess, J., Vale, W. & Brown, M.R. (1982). Corticotropin-releasing factor (CRF). Central effects on mean arterial pressure and heart rate in rats. Endocrinology, 110: 2222-2224.

89. Van der Meulen, J. & Bohus, B. (1984). Adrenalectomy prevents behaviourally induced hypersensive reponses in the rat. Neurosci. Lett. Supl., 18: 442.
90. Stumpf, W.E. & Sar, M. (1979). Glucocorticosteriod and mineralcorticosteroid hormone target sites in the brain: Autoradiographic studies with corticosterone, aldosterone and dexamethasone. In M.J. Jones, B. Gillham, M.F. Dallman & S. Chattopadhyay (Eds.), Interaction within the brain-pituitary-adrenocortical system. Academic Press, London, N.Y., Toronto, Sydney, San Francisco, p. 137-147.
91. Weil-Malharbe, H., Axelrod, J. & Tomchick, R. (1959). Blood-brain barrier for adrenaline. Science, 129: 1226-1227.
92. Berkenbosch, F., Vermes, I., Binnekade, R. & Tilders, F.J.H. (1981). ß-adrenergic stimulation induces an increase of the plasma levels of immunoreactive alpha-MSH, ß-endorphin, ACTH and of corticosterone. Life Sci., 29: 2249-2254.
93. Barna, I., Wiegant, V.M., Veldhuis, H.D. & de Wied, D. (1986). Vasopressin is a potent releaser of ß-endorphin from stores in the central nervous system. Proc. 27th Dutch Federation Meeting, Abstr. No 15.
94. Bohus, B. (1980). Effects of neuropeptides on adaptive autonomic processes. In D. de Wied & P.A. Van Keep (Eds.), Hormones and the brain. MPT Press Ltd., Lancaster, p. 129-139.
95. Bohus, B. (1984). Endocrine influence on disease outcome: Experimental findings and implications. J. Psychosom. Res., 28: 429-438.
96. Crampton, R.S. & Schwartz, P.J. (1978). Some aspects of sudden cardiac death. In P.J. Schwartz, A.M. Brown, A. Malliani & A. Zanchetti (Eds.), Neural mechanisms of cardiac arrhythmias. Raven Press, N.Y., p. 1-6.
97. Elliot, R.S. & Buell, J.C. (1983). Role of central nervous system in sudden cardiac death. In T.M. Dembroski, S. Petersburg, T.H. Schmidt & G. Blümchen (Eds.), Biobehavioral bases of coronary heart disease. Karger, Basel, p. 257-269.
98. Richter, C.P. (1957). On the phenomenon of sudden death in animals and man. Psychosom. Med., 19: 191-197.
99. Hughes, C.W. & Lynch, J.J. (1978). A reconsideration of psychological precursors of sudden death in infrahuman animals. Am. Psychol., 33: 419-429.
100. Lown, B. & Verrier, R.L. (1978). Neural factors and sudden death. In P.J. Schwartz, A.M. Brown, A. Malliani & A. Zanchetti (Eds.), Neural mechanisms of cardiac arrhythmias. Raven Press, N.Y., p. 87-98.
101. Ladder, M. (1972). Psychophysiological research and psychosomatic medicine. In CIBA Found. Symp. 8 (new series), Physiology, emotion and psychosomatic illness. Elsevier, Amsterdam, p. 297-311.
102. Ursin, H. (1980). Personality, activation and somatic health. A new psychosomatic theory. In S. Levine & H. Ursin (Eds.), Coping and health. Plenum Press, N. Y., p. 259-279.
103. Weiss, J.M. (1970). Somatic effects of predictable and unpredictable shock. Psychosom. Med., 32: 397-408.
104. Bassett, J.R. & Cairncross, K.D. (1976). Myocardial sensitivity to catecholamines following exposures of rats to irregular, signalled footshock. Pharmac. Biochem. Behav., 4: 27-37.
105. Sklar, L.S. & Anisman, H. (1979). Stress and coping factors influence tumor growth. Science, 205: 513-515.
106. Bohus, B., Benus, R.F., Fokkema, D.S., Koolhaas, J.M., Nyakas, C., Van Oortmerssen, G.A., Prins, A.J.A., de Ruiter, A.J.H., Scheurink, A.J.W. & Steffens, A.B. (in press). Neuroendocrine states and behavioral and physiological stress responses. In E.R. de Kloet (Ed.), Neuropeptides and brain functions. Progress in Brain Research. Elsevier, Amsterdam.

Differential Control of ACTH-Related Peptides and the Importance of the Behavioral Situation

Peter G. Smelik

Experimental stress research in the past has focussed mainly on the pituitary-adrenocortical response to acute aversive or damaging stimuli. A wealth of data has been collected on a wide variety of stressful agents and situations, inducing a prompt and standardized adrenal response. The mechanisms by which the adrenocortical reaction is controlled (hypothalamic factors, corticosteroid feedback) have been amply studied and analyzed.

Considerably less attention has been paid to the question whether cognitive and emotional factors may contribute to the intensity or pattern of the stress response. It is conceivable that the behavioral and physiological response to stressful situations can only be modified by conditions such as past experience, perception of the stimulus, expectancy, and coping capability. Psychological variables, such as these, can only be studied in individual animals, using adequate behavioral methods. This is in contrast with the classical endocrinological approach in which results are obtained by comparing experimental and control groups, and by presenting the mean values of a group. It becomes increasingly clear now that the most interesting cases may be those which are deviating from the statistical mean.

Stress research taking into account individual variables in experiencing and handling of a stressful situation has been conducted mainly by psychologists, following Mason's adagium that "the stress concept should not be regarded primarily as a physiological concept but rather as a behavioral concept" (1).

Another interesting shift in stress research is that from the acute damaging stimulus to a chronic situation. Originally, the main focus was on stimuli like pain, surgical interventions or toxic agents. In view of the psychological factors modifying the stress response, it became pertinent to study types of stress in which the emotional component was more significant than the somatic component. Situational stress, particularly when involving social interactions, seems to be a condition which reflects more accurately human stress conditions. Consequently, the psychosocial aspects of demanding, threatening or aversive situations have gained considerable research interest.

A third, more recent development is the acknowledgment that the neuroendocrine response to stress is not restricted to adrenocortical activation but involves a number of physiological systems. This notion is not new, however. Long before Selye's theories on the adaptation syndrome became popular, Cannon had proposed that the sympatho-adrenomedullary system is activated by noxious or threatening stimuli, and that this system readily mobilizes a number of physiological defense mechanisms. The overwhelming impact of Selye's concept, together with the methodological difficulties in finding reliable and accurate parameters for adrenomedullary activity, have obscured for a long period the significance of Cannon's findings.

Apart from this, the development of radio-immuno assays for peptide hormones made it possible in recent years to study more directly the response of pituitary hormones to stress. From such studies it appeared that the pituitary secretes more stress-labile hormones than ACTH. The question arises what the functional significance of such hormones may be in stress conditions.

These hormones include: Corticosteroids, catecholamines, testosterone, ACTH, endorphins and prolactin.

In our own studies we came across a possible differential response to stress, depending on the type of stress involved as well as on the individual situation of the animal. This idea resulted from an analysis of the control mechanism for intermediate lobe peptides in the rat. Studies on the control of αMSH secretion from melanotroph cells revealed that the main controlling system is an inhibitory dopaminergic innervation (2). In further studies it was found that peripheral ß-adrenergic stimulation results in release of αMSH and other intermediate lobe peptides such as ß-endorphins (3). Interestingly, it appeared more recently that emotional but not somatic stress stimuli induce a release of these peptides from melanotrophs mediated by a ß-adrenergic mechanism (5, 6). We have now some indications that in the rat, stimuli inducing a high level of anxiety (without concomitant motor behavior) provokes an adrenomedullary discharge of adrenaline which is sufficient to turn on intermediate lobe peptide secretion. This suggests that, apart from the classical CRF- ACTH- corticosteroid axis, a sympathetic-adrenaline-intermediate lobe axis may also operate in response o fear-providing stimuli (Figure 1).

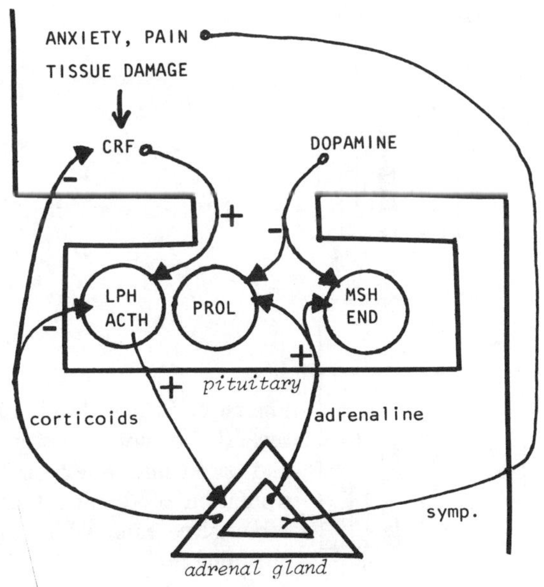

Figure 1. Control mechanisms for anterior lobe and intermediate lobe peptide hormones responsive to stress stimuli.

It has been shown by several groups that fear reduction can be obtained by adequate coping behavior (for reviews see 7, 8). A chronic anxiety state can be induced when any behavioral response to aversive stimulation is prevented ("learned helplessness"). Conversely, if defense or escape mechanisms can be used successfully, the physiological stress response is extinguished. In this connection, it would be interesting to know whether the presence of adequate coping behavior would modify the endocrine response to threatening stimuli.

Recently, we have started experimental work on hormonal responses in social encounters between rats living in a colony (H. Dijkstra, to be published). It is well known that within a group of males a hierarchy is developed. The hierarchical position of an animal can range from dominant or subdominant to subordinate or submissive. Dominant animals possess adequate coping behavior: They are aggressive, competitive and regular winners in confrontations. Submissive rats are avoiding, apprehensive and apathetic. It can be anticipated that the behavioral response of a dominant male towards the appearance of an unknown, new male will be quite different from the response of a submissive rat. The question was whether this difference in position, experience, emotional status and defensive behavior also would be reflected in a different pattern of hormonal response.

Accordingly, blood levels of several stress-labile hormones were measured in dominant or submissive rats after confrontation with intruding males. Among these hormones were the steroids corticosterone and testosterone, and the pituitary hormones ACTH, ß-endorphin, αMSH and prolactin. The results (Figure 2) show that indeed substantial differences in hormonal reactivity exists.

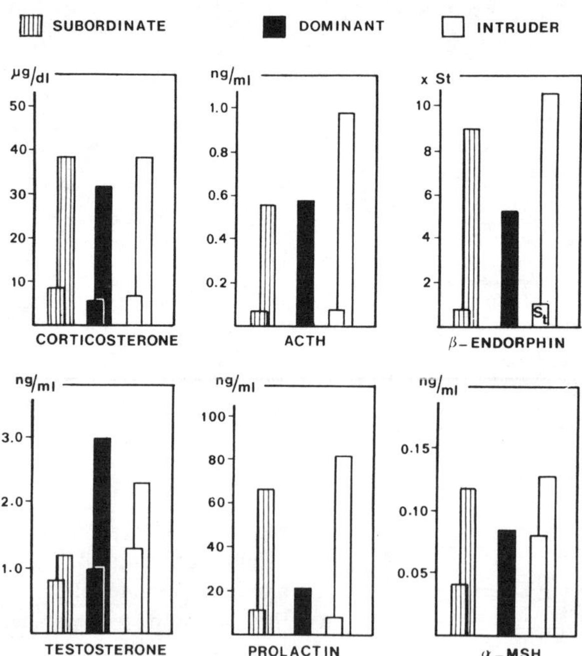

Figure 2. Plasma levels of several hormones before and x 20 min after confrontation of dominant or submissive rats with an intruding male rat.

The testosterone response is remarkably low in submissive and high in dominant animals. This in accordance with the results from studies in man and animals that testosterone levels correspond with aggressive behavior, self-confidence and performance.

Another striking difference is that notably the prolactin, but also the endorphin and MSH response is lower in dominants compared to submissive or intruding rats. It may not be a coincidence that these hormones are the only ones with an inhibitory dopaminergic control. Anyway, this suggests that these three hormones may be more involved in defense, fear and uncertainty.

Although the adrenocortical response reflects a considerable level of stress in all groups, they nevertheless do show differences in hormonal pattern, which seem to be related to individual situations, cognitions and emotions.

This conclusion may have some bearing on human stress research. It is feasible that also in humans correlations can be found between blood levels of certain pituitary hormones and particular emotional stress or coping strategies. Unfortunately, very little work has been done on peptide hormone levels during stressful episodes in man. In the past, the main drawback has been the tedious assay procedure for peptides, but recent developments render it possible to measure such substances routinely. It could be anticipated that pituitary hormones can be used as early biological markers for coping capability.

References

1. Mason, J. (1971). A re-evaluation of the concept of "non-specifity" in stress theory. J. Psychiat. Res., 8: 323-333.
2. Tilders, F.J.H., Mulder, A.H. & Smelik, P.G. (1975). On the presence of a MSH-release inhibiting system in the rat neurointermediate lobe. Neuroendocrinology, 18: 125-130.
3. Berkenbosch, F., Vermes, I., Binnekade, R. & Tilders, F.J.H. (1981). ß-Adrenergic stimulation induces an increase of the plasma levels of immunoreactive alpha-MSH, ß-endorphin, ACTH and corticosterone. Life Sci., 29: 2249-2256.
4. Tilders, F.J.H., Berkenbosch, F. & Smelik, P.G. (1982). Adrenergic mechanisms involved in the control of pituitary-adrenal activity in the rat: A ß-adrenergic stimulatory mechanism. Endocrinology, 110: 114-120.
5. Berkenbosch, F., Tilders, F.J.H. & Vermes, I. (1983). ß-Adrenoceptor activation mediates stress induced secretion of ß-endorphin related peptides from intermediate but not anterior pituitary. Nature (London), 305: 237-239.
6. Berkenbosch, F., Vermes, I. & Tilders, F.J.H. (1984). The ß-adrenoceptor blocking drug propanolol prevents secretion of immunoreactive ß-endorphin and alpha-melanocyte stimulating hormone in response to certain stress stimuli. Endocrinology, 115: 1051-1059.
7. Levine, S., Weinberg, J. & Ursin, H. (1978). Definition of the coping process and statement of the problem. In H. Ursin, E. Baade, & S. Levine (Eds.), Psychobiology of stress. A study of coping men. Academic Press, N.Y., p. 3.
8. Ursin, H. (1985). The instrumental effects of emotional behavior. In P.P.G. Bateson & P.H. Klopfer (Eds.), Perspectives in ethology. Plenum Publ. Corp., 6: 45-62.

Permissive Effects of Prolactin on Cellular Immunity in Vivo: Implications Relating Behavioral Stress and Host Defenses[1]

Edward W. Bernton, Monte S. Meltzer and John W. Holaday

Over the past several decades, in vitro analysis has permitted great advances in our understanding of the physiology and pathophysiology of immune responses. One weakness of such approaches is that these *in vitro* observations can lead to a reductionist oversimplification of mechanisms that regulate host defenses in the intact animal. *In vitro* immunological studies eliminate and thus obscure the influence of factors such as the innervation of immune organs and the effects of the endocrine environment, both of which may serve to integrate immune function into the *milieu internal.*

There is evidence that personality structure, life events, behavioral stressors, and mechanisms of adaptation to stress alters the course of autoimmune, infectious and neoplastic disease (1). Lymphocytes from individuals exposed to psychosocial stressors such as bereavement have an altered proliferate capacity in response to *in vitro* stimulation (2). Recent research also suggests that interactions among the central nervous system (CNS), the neuroendocrine axis, and the immune system provide additional mechanisms for mutual interregulation (3). These mechanisms include but are not limited to the pituitary-adrenocortical axis. Although increases in ACTH and corticosteroids occur with both infectious and psychosocial stressors, and in some cases corticosteroids markedly inhibit immune function, a variety of data clearly suggest that mediators other than corticosteroids play a role in the CNS modulation of immune function. For example, suppression of lymphocyte proliferative responses in rats following repeated footshock is not abolished by adrenalectomy (4).

Histologic studies show immune tissues to be extensively and intimately innervated by autonomic fibers, many of which contain and release neuropeptides as well as classical neurotransmitters (5). Immune tissues such as the spleen also include cells with chromogranin, a marker for cells of the "diffuse endocrine system" (6), i.e., cells capable of secreting a variety of neuroactive amines and peptides. Recent evidence shows that various immune cell functions are modulated *in vitro* by a remarkable variety of neuropeptides and hormones: i.e., prolactin (7), ACTH (8, 9), endogenous opioids (10, 11), thyroid stimulating hormone (12), somatostatin (13), somatomedin-C (14), and

Research was conducted in compliance with the Animal Welfare Act, and other Federal statutes and regulations relating to animals and experiments involving animals and adheres to principles stated in the Guide for the Care and the Use of Laboratory Animals, NIH publication 85-23. The views of the authors do not purport to reflect the position of the Department of the Army or the Department of Defense, (para 4-3), AR 360-5.

vasoactive intestinal peptide (15). Furthermore, brain lesions in areas closely involved in the regulation of pituitary hormone secretions dramatically affect immune responses. For example, lesions of the anterior basal hypothalamus (but not ventral or posterior lesions) prevent *in vivo* development of delayed hypersensitivity in immunized guinea pigs (16). Similarly, lesions of the tuberoinfundibular region of the hypothalamus in mice permanently abrogate "natural killer cell" activity (17). Taken together, this evidence suggests that immune cells are capable of secreting peptides which may act on the CNS or on endocrine target organs. Conversely, physiologic and anatomic substrates must exist to allow the brain to regulate immune host defenses via CNS actions upon the neuroendocrine axis or the autonomic nervous system. Thus, there is a reciprocal relationship between the immune system and the CNS. The actual physiologic significance of these potential interactions largely remains to be elucidated, particularly in the context of clinically relevant models of infectious challenge of host-defenses or pathophysiologic manifestations of autoimmune diseases.

Stress, Prolactin, and Immune Function

Although the neuroendocrine literature concentrates on hormonal responses and regulation following a single acute stress, most stressors involved in life require adaptation and tend to be repetitive and chronic. Environmental stressors clinically associated with changes in host defense mechanisms are also chronic in nature. The well known effects of chronic stress on adrenocorticotropic hormone (ACTH) and corticosteroid responses are basically a continuation of their sustained secretion provoked by a single acute stress.

We are particularly interested in the role of prolactin in immune responses. Prolactin is in fact a "stress hormone" since acute physical or behavioral stressors induce a rapid and significant increase in prolactin levels in mammals. Unlike ACTH and corticosteroids, prolactin secretion follows a strikingly biphasic pattern. Acute stress evokes a rapid increase in prolactin release; this is followed by decreased prolactin secretion and then refractoriness to further stimulation with repetition of the acute stress (18-20). Since the release of prolactin is under the inhibitory control of dopamine, the effects of stress may be mediated by alterations in dopaminergic tone in neurons descending to the pituitary via the tuberoinfundibular pathway.

During prolonged restraint stress in rats, not only does plasma prolactin fall towards basal levels, but also morphine is no longer capable of evoking prolactin secretion. At the level of the pituitary, however, prolactin release following administration of the dopamine receptor antagonist haloperidol remains unaffected by chronic stress (21). These observations suggest that inhibition of the prolactin response to repeated stress may be mediated at the supra-pituitary level, perhaps through opioidergic neurons in the hypothalamus. Opioids such as morphine reduce activity of tuberoinfundibular dopaminergic neurons, thus diminishing the tonic dopaminergic inhibition of prolactin release (22).

Corticosteroids also decrease prolactin release: Attenuation of prolactin release with chronic or repeated stress temporally coincides with the increase in circulating corticosteroids. Indeed, the decrease in prolactin release in response to repeated footshock in rats is abolished by adrenalectomy, and restored by doses of corticosterone that mimic levels present in intact rats following repetitive footshocks (23). To summarize, the prolactin response to an acute stress is rapidly attenuated with continued stress. The adaptation seems to be mediated at least in part by the elevation of circulating corticosteroids sustained during continued stress. Thus, the adaptation of prolactin release following sustained stress may be mediated by corticosteroid actions at the suprapituitary level which activate tuberoinfundibular dopamine release and thus decrease the secretion of prolactin.

The target organ of stress-induced prolactin release in males and non-lactating females is unknown. Several lines of evidence suggest that prolactin may play a role directly and/or indirectly in the modulation of cellular immune responses. Prolactin levels change markedly in pregnancy, coincident with marked alterations in cellular immunity (24). The marked inhibition of immune responses following hypophysectomy can be reversed by treatment with prolactin; and bromocryptine treatment, which inhibits prolactin release, likewise abrogates these immune responses (25). Several other lines of evidence further support the role of prolactin in altering immune responses. For example, lymphocytes express receptors for prolactin; prolactin induces ornithine decarboxylase, an enzyme required for cell proliferation in lymphoid tissues; and cyclosporine, a potent immunosuppressant drug, competitively inhibits prolactin binding to lymphocytes (26).

These observations led us to hypothesize that prolactin secretion in response to either environmental stimuli, reproductive events or pharmacological manipulation could affect cellular immunity. It was our objective to demonstrate a trophic or permissive action of prolactin using an *in vivo* model of T-cell dependent immunity, and to elucidate prolactin's mechanism(s) of action in that system. A correlary of this hypothesis would be that immunosuppression associated with chronic stress could be mediated by adaptive responses causing an impaired or refractory secretion of prolactin, and reversible with the exogenous administration of this hormone.

Secretory Events Associated with Immune Recognition

Immune responses involve a network of both cell-to-cell physical interactions and the potent actions of their respective groups of autocrine (and in some cases endocrine) secretory proteins, the monokines from macrophages and the lymphokines from lymphocytes. The immune response to antigen first involves processing of the foreign antigenic protein to macrophages. These phagocytic cells then present processed fragments of this protein to T-lymphocytes. Lymphocytes are unable to respond to antigenic determinants on foreign proteins until they have been processed and presented in concert with histocompatibility markers (markers for "self" recognition) expressed on the macrophage membrane. Accompanying antigen processing, macrophages lymphocytes to produce interleukin-2 (IL-2), a T-cell growth factor produced by appropriately triggered T-cells. Under the proliferative effects of IL-2, a great expansion of the clone of T-cells that respond to antigen occurs. The macrophages can also turn off this proliferation of T-cells since macrophages have the capacity to secrete prostaglandin E_2 (PGE_2). PGE_2 increases induction of suppressor T-lymphocytes, which then inhibit this T-cell proliferative response.

Antigen-activated T-cells also become directly cytotoxic effector cells after interaction with antigen; T-cells stimulate B-lymphocytes to secrete antibodies that specifically bind the antigen and T-cells also secrete lymphokines such as γ-interferon. γ-interferon in turn has several stimulant effects on immune cells including the activation of "natural killer" cells to become nonspecifically cytotoxic, the activation of macrophages to result in augmented phagocytosis, enhanced intracellular killing of organisms and increased cytotoxicity to tumor cells, and greater efficiency of macrophage presentation of antigen due to increased histocompatibility protein expression.

Secretory products of macrophages, such as IL-1, PGE_2, and tumor necrosis factor (or cachectin) have endocrine and paracrine effects on many tissues besides immune cells. IL-1 is essentially hormonal in its ability to alter trace metal metabolism, induce fever, alter the composition of liver-secreted serum proteins, and increase the production of prostaglandins by the blood vessel endothelium (27, 28). In addition, IL-1 and other macrophage products may also exert potent effects on the neuroendocrine axis.

We (see below) and others have found a suppression of prolactin and elevation of luteinizing hormone (LH) levels in mice following a variety of antigenic stimuli (29). Recombinant-derived IL-1, at picomolar concentrations, stimulates ACTH and LH secretion and inhibits prolactin secretion from cultured rat pituitary cell monolayers (30). Consistent with this result is the report that endotoxin, a potent stimulus for macrophage IL-1 secretion, suppresses serum prolactin levels in lactating pigs (31). Others have reported both IL-1 and the monokine hepatic-stimulating factor directly stimulate ACTH release by ATT-20 pituitary adenoma cells (32).

Collectively, the data reviewed above suggest that IL-1 and other monokines and lymphokines signal the neuroendocrine apparatus in response to antigenic stimuli and immune events. This signal results in changes in pituitary hormone secretion which, in turn, either enhance or regulate immunologic as well as metabolic responses to infection or antigenic challenge.

Assessment of in vivo Activation of Macrophages Following Infectious Challenge: Effects of Prolactin Suppression with Dopamine Agonists

In order to assess the role of prolactin in immune responses, we used a mouse model of T-cell immunity to infection. As reviewed above, tumoricidal activation of macrophages occurs following *in vivo* or *in vitro* exposure to lymphokines secreted by T-lymphocytes. Importantly, resident or irritant (starch)-elicited peritoneal macrophages do not kill tumor cells unless activated by lymphokines. In our model of infection, killed *Propriobacterium acnes (P. acnes)* were injected intraperitoneally in mice to evoke an inflammatory response which, over time, results in: (1) the formation of a peritoneal exudate rich in macrophages and (2) a T-lymphocyte response that includes secretion of lymphokines such as γ-interferon. Interferon, in turn, activates peritoneal macrophages to acquire both tumoricidal and microbiocidal capacities. Eight to ten days following *P. acnes* injection, the macrophage "peritoneal exudate cells" (PEC) were harvested by sterile peritoneal lavage, purified by adherence to plastic wells, and their tumoricidal activation measured by incubation with radio-labelled tumor cells. During the ten day period leading to activation of macrophages following *P. acnes* injection, the mice can either be exposed to various stressors or to drugs and hormones to manipulate their neuroendocrine responses. Hormone levels were also measured over time before and after injection of *P. acnes* or other antigens.

We examined the effects of bromocryptine and pergolide (two dopamine type 2 (DA_2) agonists that inhibit pituitary prolactin release (33)) treatment on the *in vivo* activation of macrophages following intraperitoneal (i.p.) injection of 0.2 mg of killed *P. acnes.* Male C3H/HEN mice (6/group) were injected daily i.p. with 0.2 mg bromocryptine, 0.1 mg pergolide, or an equal volume of vehicle for 5 days beginning 1 day prior to the injection of *P. acnes.* All experiments were completely replicated on at least 2 separate occasions. Tumoricidal activity of macrophages was estimated by measuring radiolabel released into culture fluids at 48 h and expressed as a percentage of total counts of tumor-cell label. It is important to note that in the following tables, absolute % cytotoxicity is not comparable among experiments due to interassay variabilities.

Table 1. The effect of bromocryptine and pergolide treatment on induction of tumoricidal macrophages in *P. acnes*-treated mice[1].

Mice treated with:	Macrophages/well: 4×10^5	2×10^5	1×10^5
saline	10%*	10%*	10%
P. acnes + saline	85%	65%	20%
P. acnes + bromocryptine	20%*	20%*	10%
P. acnes + pergolide	15%*	10%*	10%

1. Tumor cytotoxicity is expressed as a % of total tumor cell label.
* $p<0.05$ when compared to "P. acnes + saline" control group, demonstrating a significant reduction of tumoricidal activity in the DA_2 agonist-treated mice.

Both bromocryptine and pergolide treatments diminished tumoricidal activity to levels comparable to resident macrophage controls (Table 1). Thus, *P. acnes*-treated mice which received either of these two DA_2 agonists failed to develop tumoricidal macrophages, possibly as a result of DA_2 inhibitory effects on prolactin release.

Since six to ten days is required for *P. acnes* to induce activated, tumoricidal peritoneal macrophages, we were interested in assessing which stage of this process is most responsive to DA_2 agonist treatment. The effects of pergolide treatment on the induction of tumoricidal macrophages during days 1-5 following *P. acnes* injection were compared to the effects of pergolide treatment on days 1-2 only versus days 4-7 only (Table 2). Whereas continued pergolide treatment (0.1 mg/day) on days 1-5 blocked tumoricidal activation, treatment on days 1-2 or 4-7 was not sufficient to inhibit macrophage activation by *P. acnes*. Thus, an early step in macrophage activation may be blocked by DA_2 agonists, but several days of sustained drug treatment is required. These findings also argue against a direct toxic effect of pergolide on macrophages since treatment on days 4-7 allows less time for PEC macrophages themselves to recover from drug exposure before their harvest by lavage.

Table 2. Treatment time requirements for inhibition of macrophage activation by pergolide.

Mice treated with:	Tumor cytotoxicity[1]
saline	25%*
P. acnes + saline	45%
P. acnes + pergolide on:	
days 1-5	25%*
days 1-2	50%
days 4-7	50%

1. Tumor cytotoxicity is expressed as a % of total tumor cell label.
* $p<0.05$ when compared to "P. acnes + saline" control group, demonstrating that pergolide treatment on days 1-5, but not 1-2 or 4-7 is required to reduce tumoricidal activity.

Having demonstrated the effects of DA_2 agonists on tumoricidal activation of macrophages *in vivo*, it was important to elucidate whether they altered tumoricidal effector mechanisms, acted directly upon macrophages to impair their activation, or acted indirectly via other immune cells. Pergolide or prolactin were tested for their possible direct effects on tumoricidal effector mechanisms as well as on the *in vitro* activation of starch-elicited (unactivated) macrophages incubated with lymphokines. Pergolide, even at concentrations exceeding those achieved *in vivo*, did not inhibit *in vitro* activation of macrophages by added lymphokines, nor did prolactin potentiate activation. In other experiments, prolactin could not substitute for lymphokines to activate macrophages, nor did pergolide added *in vitro* inhibit tumor-killing by macrophages activated *in vivo* by *P. acnes*. Significantly, non-tumoricidal macrophages from DA_2 agonist-treated mice could acquire tumoricidal activity when incubated with lymphokines *in vitro*.

The data above suggest that DA_2 agonists such as pergolide and bromocryptine inhibit macrophage activation *in vivo* but not *in vitro*. From this evidence, it is apparent that an earlier step in immune cell function is involved, probably by a mechanism which decreases the production of lymphokines by T-cells. This mechanism may not necessarily involve the action of DA_2 agonists on pituitary prolactin release. Therefore, we determined if treatment with exogenous prolactin could reverse the effects of bromocryptine treatment.

Table 3. Simultaneous administration of ovine prolactin prevents inhibition of macrophage tumoricidal activation of bromocryptine injection on day 1-5 following *P. acnes*.

Mice treated with:	Tumor Cytotoxicity
saline	5%
P. acnes and:	
saline	45%
bromocryptine	20%
Bromocryptine + prolactin	40%

Mice received i.p. injections of vehicle, bromocryptine (0.2 mg), or bromocryptine and ovine prolactin (100 μg) daily for the same 5-day treatment regime used in prior experiments with *P. acnes*. Simultaneous prolactin treatment prevented the inhibition of macrophage tumoricidal activity seen in bromocryptine-treated mice (Table 3). While the inhibition of tumoricidal activation of bromocryptine and its restoration by prolactin could involve unrelated mechanisms, this experiment strongly suggests that the effects of bromocryptine depend on its ability to inhibit prolactin release.

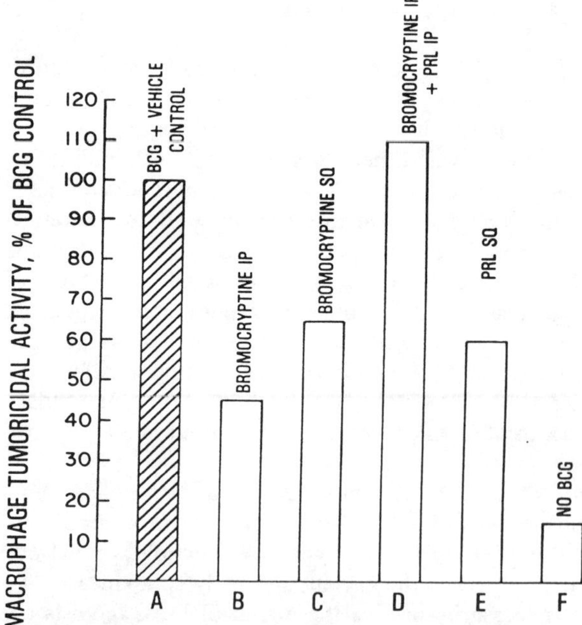

Figure 1. All groups except group F received an i.p. injection of fresh frozen BCG on day 2, and were treated with the drugs shown, 200 μg/mouse daily on days 1 through 5. On day 10 peritoneal macro-phages were assessed for tumoricidal activity against radiolabelled TU-5 target cells. Percent of target radiolabel released into supernatant was measured in replicate wells and normalized against activity of macrophages from BCG- and vehicle treated controls. These are the average results calculated from duplicate experiments which closely replicated. 4 male C3H/Hen mice were used per group.

These experiments described above involved the use of killed *P. acnes* as the antigenic stimulus for immune responses. It was important to determine whether similar responses following drugs and prolactin challenge could be reproduced in a live organism model of infection. In these experiments, mice were injected with BCG, a live, replicating mycobacterial pathogen that causes intracellular infection of macrophages and T-cell dependent macrophage activation. The effects of bromocryptine and prolactin described above, following *P. acnes* administration were completely replicated in this live organism infectious model (Figure 1). Additionally, it was found in this and subsequent studies, that while interperitoneal injection of prolactin reversed the effects of bromocryptine, the same dose of prolactin administered subcutaneously was ineffectual, and if anything tended to independently inhibit macrophage activation.

Serum Prolactin Response to Antigenic Challenges

We examined prolactin levels 4 and 20 hours following injection of killed *P. acnes* or saline in mice treated 2 hours earlier with 0.2 mg of bromocryptine or saline vehicle (Table 4). A significant decrease in serum prolactin also occurred after injection of *P. acnes* in mice *not* pre-treated both bromocryptine. Injection of another antigen, sheep red blood cells, caused similar decreases in prolactin levels. We found that injection of 25 units of purified IL-1 also caused a significant and rapid (2 hours) depression in prolactin levels, suggesting that this lymphokine may mediate the *in vivo* responses described above. This hypothesis is further supported by our recent evidence that rat pituitary cell prolactin release is suppressed by the addition of picomolar concentrations of IL-1 to monolayer pituitary cultures (30). Thus, the antigens or infectious agents themselves suppress prolactin release, possibly by the release of IL-1.

Table 4. Changes in serum prolactin (ng/ml ± SEM) at 4 and 20 h following bromocryptine treatment or injection with *P. acnes*.

	Time following bromocryptine treatment:	
Mice treated with:	4 hours	20 hours
saline/saline	22.0 ± 6.0	17.0 ± 3.0
saline/bromocryptine	0.3 ± 0.1*	0.2 ± 0.1*
P. acnes/saline	7.0 ± 3.0*	11.0 ± 4.0
P. acnes/bromocryptine	0.2 ± 0.1*	0.3 ± 0.1*

* $p < 0.05$ when compared to respective saline/saline controls.

Discussion

Our results demonstrate that treatment with DA_2 agonists severely inhibits the *in vivo* tumoricidal activation of peritoneal macrophages following administration of *P. acnes* or BCG, two well-characterized inducers of activated macrophages. Several lines of evidence indicate that impaired production of macrophage-activating factors by T-cells following antigenic stimulation is responsible for the effects of these drug treatments. These data include: (1) the treatment time requirements of this effect, (2) the reversibility *in vitro* by lymphokines, and (3) the lack of direct inhibition by DA_2 agonists of macrophage activation or tumoricidal effector mechanisms *in vitro*.

Although our data indicate that the *in vivo* restitution of prolactin levels by i.p. injections following endogenous suppression by DA_2 agonists reverses the immunosuppressive effects of DA_2 agonists, the direct involvement of prolactin remains unclear. For example, we have been unable to demonstrate a direct augmentation of lymphocyte proliferation or lymphokine production by addition of prolactin to lymphocytes *in vitro*. Paradoxically, additions of low concentrations of prolactin appear to suppress both lymphocyte proliferation and lymphokine production *in vitro* (unpublished data). This could mean that a secondary mediator is involved since spleen cells removed from bromocryptine and prolactin-treated mice do produce more lymphokines than cells from mice treated with bromocryptine alone (unpublished data). Research is presently underway to clarify these paradoxical findings and to identify possible "immunopermissive" mediators of prolactin's *in vivo* effects. The observation that intraperitoneal but not subcutaneously administered prolactin is able to reverse suppression by bromocryptine, invites the speculation that perhaps the liver is the source of such mediators. This organ contains the largest mass of PRL receptors in the body and PRL administered i.p. would be largely delivered, via the entero-hepatic circulation, to the liver. Our current studies are addressing this issue.

The *in vivo* effects of prolactin or prolactin-induced mediators on T-cell production of macrophage activating factors (such as the lymphokine γ-interferon) could be due to several factors. These substances could effect maturation of mature helper T-cells possessing Thy 1.2 surface markers, a process viewed as thymus-dependent. They could effect the production or response to IL-2, a T-cell growth factor allowing expansion of the responding clones of T-helper cells. Alternately they could effect the secretion of γ-interferon or other macrophage-activating factors by the expanded clone of T-helper cells. Future work to explain the phenomena presented above will need to address these questions.

Several other lines of evidence further support our observations regarding the importance of prolactin as an immunostimulant. For example, nude (athymic, T-cell deficient) mice have been shown to have very low levels of prolactin. Transplantation of a normal thymus into such mice not only restores cellular immunity but normalizes prolactin levels (34). Treatment of nude mice with antisera against crude anterior pituitary extract (absorbed against thymus and lymphocytes to remove any antibodies binding to immune tissues) prior to transplantation of a thymus into these mice prevents reconstitution of thymic-dependent (cellular) immunity even though the thymus appears histologically normal (34). Thus, from the point of view of ontogeny, thymic factors may be necessary for development of normal pituitary function and certain anterior pituitary hormones may be necessary for development of normal thymic-dependent immunity.

Such ontologic interrelationships between pituitary and thymic tissues remain poorly understood. As far as functional inter-relationships, our data lead us to speculate that IL-1 may lower prolactin levels and increase LH and ACTH as part of a neuroendocrine feedback loop to limit or down-regulate certain T-cell dependent immune responses. The actions of DA_2 agonists in our experiments could be viewed as pharmacologic mimicry of the physiologic effects of IL-1 on pituitary hormone release.

We hypothesize that chronic stress acts to suppress cellular immunity via the pituitary axis, not only by increasing ACTH secretion and consequently adrenocortical steroids, but also by inhibiting prolactin release. Such stress may inhibit either the basal level of this hormone or possibly inhibit increases in response to *antigenic* stimuli and release of unidentified immune secretory messengers evoked by such stimuli.

These observations, in concert, raise new possibilities regarding the physiologic control of cellular immunity by neuroendocrine hormones which are themselves affected by the CNS response to behavioral stressors, as well as by sexual and reproductive influences. The predominant inci ence of certain autoimmune diseases, such as lupus erythematous and rheumatoid arthritis in females, (diseases which tend to remit during pregnancy and to flare post-partum), may represent a reflection of the sexual dimorphism of male and female pituitary and hypothalamic function. The availability of human recombinant monokines and lymphokines should make it possible to further explore the endocrine effects of these substances in primates, and the role of such effects in the regulation of immune responses. The possibility that chronic stress affects cellular immunity via neuroendocrine mechanisms should now be specifically examined with appropriate experimental models. Such efforts will require close collaboration among practitioners of behavioral science, endocrinology, pharmacology, and immunology.

References

1. Schindler, B.A. (1985). Stress, affective disorders and immune function. Med. Clin. North Am., 69: 585-597.
2. Schleifer, S.J., Keller, S.E., Camerino, M., Thornton, J.C. & Stein, M. (1983). Suppression of lymphocyte stimulation following bereavement. JAMA, 250: 374-377.
3. Blalock, J.E. (1984). The immune system as a sensory organ. J. Immunol., 132: 1067.1069.
4. Keller, S.E., Weiss, J.M., Schleifer, S.J., Miller, N. & Stein, M. (1983). Stress-induced suppression of immunity in adrenalectomized rats. Science, 221: 1301-1302.
5. Felten, D.L., Felten, S.Y., Carlson, S.L., Olschowka, J.A. & Livnat, S. (1985). Noradrenergic and peptidergic innervation of lymphoid tissue. J. Immunol., 135: 755s-765s.
6. Angeletti, R.H. & Hickey, W.F. (1985). A neuroendocrine marker in tissues of the immune system. Science, 230: 89-90.
7. Russell, D.H., Matrisian, L., Kibler, R., Larson, D.F., Poulos, B. & Magun, B.E. (1984). Prolactin receptors on human lymphocytes and their modulation by cyclosporine. BBRCU 121: 899-906.
8. Johnson, H.M., Smith, E.M. & Torres, B.A. (1982). Neuroendocrine hormone regulation of in vitro antibody production. Proc. Natl. Acad. Sci. USA, 79: 4171-4173.
9. Johnson, H.M., Torres, B.A., Smith, E.M., Dion, L.D. & Blalock, J.E. (1984). Regulation of lymphokine (gamma-IF) production by corticotropin. J. Immunol., 132: 246-250.

10. Kay, N., Allen, J. & Morley, J.E. (1984). Endorphins stimulate normal human peripheral blood lymphocyte natural killer activity. Life Sci., 35: 39-59.
11. Smith, E.M., Harbour-McMenamin, D. & Blalock, J.E. (1985). Lymphocyte production of endorphins and endorphin-mediated immunoregulatory activity. J. Immunol., 135: 779s-782s.
12. Blalock, J.E., Johnson, H.M., Smith, E.M. & Torres, B.A. (1984). Enhancement of the in vitro antibody response by thyrotropin. BBRC, 30: 30-32.
13. Payan, D.G. & Goetzl, E.J. (1985). Modulation of lymphocyte function by sensory neuropeptides. J. Immunol., 135: 783s-786s.
14. Schimpff, R.M., Repellin, A.M., Salvatoni, A., Thieriot-Prevost, G. & Chatelain, P. (1983). Effect of purified somatomedins on thymidine incorporation into lectin-activated human lymphocytes. Acta Endocrinol., 102: 21-26.
15. O'Dorisio, M.S., Wood, C.L. & O'Dorisio, T.M. (1985). Vasoactive intestinal peptide and neuropeptide modulation of immune response. J. Immunol., 135: 792s-801s.
16. Macris, N.T., Schiavi, R.C., Camerino, M.S. & Stein, M. (1970). Effects of hypothalamic lesions on immune processes in the guinea pig. Am. J. Physiol., 219: 1205-1209.
17. Forni, G., Bindoni, M., Santoni, A., Belluardo, N., Marchese, A. & Giovarelli, M. (1983). Radiofrequency destruction of the turboinfundibular region of the hypothalamus permanently abrogates NK cell activity in mice. Nature, 306: 181-184.
18. Taché, Y., Du Ruisseau, P., Taché, J., Selye, H. & Collu, R. (1976). Shift in adenohypophyseal activity during chronic intermittent immobilization of rats. Neuroendocrinology, 22: 325-336.
19. Taché, Y., Du Ruisseau, P., Ducharme, J.R. & Collu, R. (1978). Pattern of adenohypophyseal hormone changes in male rats following chronic stress. Neuroendocrinology, 26: 208-219.
20. Euker, J.S., Meites, J. & Riegle, G.D. (1975). Effects of acute stress on serum LH and prolactin in intact, castrate and dexamethasone-treated male rats. Endocrinology, 96: 85-92.
21. Fekete, M.I.K., Kanyicska, B., Szentendrei, T., Simonyi, A. & Stark, E. (1984). Decrease of morphine-induced prolactin release by a procedure causing prolonged stress. J. Endocrinol., 101: 169-172.
22. Moore, K.E. & Johnson, C.A. (1982). The median eminence aminergic control mechanisms. In E.E. Muller & R.M. Macleod (Eds.), Neuroendocrine perspectives, Vol. 1, Elsevier Press, N.Y., p. 23.
23. Yelvington, D.B., Weiss, G.K. & Ratner, A. (1984). Effects of corticosterone on the prolactin response in psychological and physical stress in rats. Life Sci., 35: 1705-1711.
24. Brabom, B.J. (1985). Epidemiology of infection in pregnancy. Rev. Infect. Dis., 7: 579-597.
25. Nagy, E., Berczi, I., Wren, G.E., Asa, S.L. & Kovacs, K. (1983). Immunomodulation by bromocryptine. Immunopharmacol., 6: 231-243.
26. Russell, D.H., Larson, D.F., Cardon, S.B. & Copeland, J.G. (1984). Cyclosporine inhibits prolactin induction of ornithine decarboxylase in rat tissues. Mol. Cell. Endocrinol., 35: 159-166.
27. Oppenheim, J.J. & Gery, I. (1982). Interleukin^{-1} is more than an interleukin. Immunol. Today, 3: 113.
28. Albrightson, C.R., Baenziger, N.L. & Needleman, P. (1985). Exaggerated human vascular cell prostaglandin synthesis mediated by monocytes: Role of monokines and interleukin^{-1}. J. Immunol., 135: 1872-1877.
29. Pierpaoli, W. & Maestroni, G. (1977). Pharmacological control of the immune response by blockade of the early hormonal changes following antigen injection. Cell. Immunol., 31: 355-363.
30. Beach, J.E., Bernton, E.W., Holaday, J.W., Smallridge, R.C. & Fein, H.G. (in press). Interleukin^{-1} modulates secretion by rat pituitary cell in monolayer culture. (Abstract), Neuroendocrinology. Beach, J. & Fein, H. (submitted).
31. Smith, B.B. & Wagener, W.C. (1984). Suppression of prolactin in pigs by Escherichia coli endotoxin. Science, 224: 605-607.
32. Woloski, B.M.R., Smith, E.M., Meyer, W.J., Fuller, G.M. & Blalock, J.E. (1985). Corticotropin-releasing activity of monokines. Science, 230: 1035-1037.
33. Rao, M.R., Bartke, A., Parkening, T.A. & Collins, T.J. (1984). Effect of treatment with different doses of bromocryptine on plasma profiles of gonadotropins, prolactin, and testosterone in mature male rats and mice. Int. J. Androl., 7: 258-268.
34. Pierpaoli, W., Kopp, H.G. & Bianchi, E. (1976). Interdependence of thymic and neuroendocrine functions in ontogeny. Clin. Exp. Immunol., 24: 501-506.

Stress and the Immune Response

Rudy E. Ballieux and Cobi J. Heijnen

The nervous system and the immune system show a certain degree of congruence. Their main function is to provide contact between the individual and the often hostile and threatening "Umwelt." The immune response has several characteristics in common with the response evoked in the nervous system. Just to mention three: Communication at a distance (which in the immune system is based on cell traffic), the capability to develop memory (which in the immune system is stored in long living lymphocytes) and the use of chemical messengers (monokines and lymphokines) to transfer messages between the cells. This has led a number of investigators to assume that the two systems are functionally connected and consequently that environmental conditions of psychosocial or of physical nature may influence the body's defense. And indeed, we now begin to see a functional interdependence of the mind and the immune system. As a consequence studies of interdisciplinary nature in this field, which is often referred to as psychoimmunology, neuroimmunology, psychoneuroimmunology, behavioral immunology or neuroimmunomodulation, have been intensified in the last few years. The results of these investigations are no longer to be found in papers exclusively published in journals related to behavioral sciences. Even journals like the *Journal of Immunology, New England Journal of Medicine, The Lancet, Science* and *Nature* carry articles and editorials on emotions and immunity, conditioning of the immune response and stress and the immune system. In this (mini) review a few aspects in relation to the issue "stress and immune function" will be discussed.

Stress-Induced Immunomodulation: Fancy or Fact?

The first item to be considered is the question whether the reports on modulation of the immune response by stress are still to be considered as "anecdotal," lacking solid experimental support. In our opinion we have passed this stage. There are several well designed studies, even of prospective nature, which show that stress can alter immune reactivity. In general, a suppressive effect has been noted, both in animal models and in studies analyzing the immune response in man.

One of the first (now almost classical) studies in humans, is that of Bartrop and co-workers reported in 1977 in *The Lancet* (1). These investigators analyzed the proliferative response of blood lymphocytes to mitogens in subjects whose

This review includes data from research carried out in the authors' laboratories. Part of these investigations have been supported by grants from the Dutch Asthma Foundation (grant no. 84.21) and from Organon International, Oss, The Netherlands.

spouses had died 6 weeks earlier. They found a small but significant decrease in the response of T lymphocytes. In blood samples taken 1-3 weeks and 6 weeks after bereavement the mean serum levels of classical stress hormones such as cortisol and prolactin were not different from control persons; unfortunately data on hormone profiles immediately after the stressful life event were not available. As will be discussed later (*vide infra*), measurement of hormone levels at the onset of severe stress may be essential for a better understanding of the mechanisms involved in stress-induced immunoregulation. Nevertheless, Bartrop's findings mark the first time that severe psychological stress has been shown to produce a measurable change in immune function. These studies have been followed by other investigations, in particular by the group of Stein (2), which confirm and extend the results obtained by Bartrop.

Long-Term or Short-Term Stress

The studies in human on the effect on the immune response of bereavement, of abortion, of unemployment or of severe mental depression all concern long-term stress. The question arises whether short-term stress can also induce changes in immune reactivity. The answer is yes. In animal models as well as in human beings immune parameters are altered in this condition. Thus, Ursin and colleagues (3) found that an acute type of occupational stress induced a change in IgM plasma levels. Several other groups have studied the effect of academic examinations on plasma levels of immunoglobulin, on antibody responses of B lymphocytes or on NK cell function (4, 5). In almost all instances a decline in the parameters measured was noted. This is also true in animal models. However, in these animal experiments, the stressors applied are often of physical nature, such as electric footshocks, being subjected to rotation, being placed on a hot plate and so on. Furthermore, in some instances the stressors are applied repeatedly. This implies that the stressful condition cannot be considered to be of short-term nature.

Psychological Stress in Animals

Only few studies have been carried out in animals using stress stimuli of psychological nature. Dantzer et al. (6) used the resident-intruder paradigm to analyze cellular immune functions in rats of different social status. In these experiments a reduced cellular immunocompetence was found in the subordinate animals. The stressful situation induced by the difference in social status of the dominant and subordinate animals in the resident-intruder dyads can be considered to be of long-term nature since it lasted 11 days. We have investigated the effects of an acute form of emotional stress in rats as provoked by the one-trial passive avoidance test, originally developed by Ader and colleagues (7). As a correlate of immune reactivity, the proliferative response of spleen lymphocytes *in vitro* upon stimulation with a T cell mitogen as well as a B cell mitogen were investigated. Control animals were subjected to the same experimental procedure but the short-term, mild electric footshock was omitted during the learning trial. In the majority of experiments the mitotic activity of T as well as B cells of the experimental animals was found to be decreased when tested already 15 minutes after the stressful experience produced by the retention test in the passive avoidance procedure. It was noted that the animals in the control group had higher lymphocyte stimulation values than home-cage control animals. Preliminary results of ongoing studies suggest that the arousal, caused by the experimental "control situation," results in an increased lymphocyte activity. The emotional stress induced by the retention session seems to "neutralize" this effect. These observations could be of basic interest since we observed that in a short-term immobilization-paradigm the lymphocytes of the experimental animals also had an increased mitotic response compared to home cage controls. Thus it seems that arousal stimulates immune reactivity whereas anxiety has a suppressive effect.

Our investigations using the one-trial passive avoidance paradigm were more recently complemented by analyzing the effect of this particular form of short-term emotional stress on the antibody response *in vivo*. To that end the rats were immunized with sheep red blood cells (SRBC) immediately after the retention trial. Thus the animal was exposed to the antigen very shortly after the stressful event. The antibody response was measured 5 days later. It was found that the stressed rats had a less efficient production of anti SRBC antibody by spleen plasmacells. This finding establishes that the encounter of an antigen (e.g., a virus) during a stress-period may lead to a reduced immune response at a later stage. The clinical significance of this observation is as yet unknown. It is important, however, to consider the possibility that a short stressful experience may have an effect on bodily function well separated in time.

Coping, Control and Opiates

These findings mentioned above touch upon an important second aspect: Why is it that some individuals are vulnerable to the effect of stress and show impaired immune reactions, and others do not? The answer to this challenging question still is incomplete. However, there is strong evidence that individual characteristics or personality type may determine the outcome. These properties may be reflected in the behavior of the individual and in his or her ability to cope with the stressful situation. Thus Stein and his co-workers (8) reported recently that severe depression is associated with subnormal mitotic responses of blood lymphocytes. Locke et al. (9) have presented evidence that poor coping capacity, more than the stressful event per se, may determine the modulation of the immune response. A second element seems important in determining the effect of stress on immune function. It has been observed in various studies that the possibility to control the stressful event may counterbalance the suppression induced by stress. This is clearly shown in experiments by

Laudenslager et al. (10) on the effect of control of stressors on tumor growth. Rats were given mild electric shocks to the tail. In the controllable-stressor group the rats could turn off the shock whenever it occurred by turning a wheel. The animals in the uncontrollable-stressor group were in the same experimental condition with the exception that the shocks were controlled by the behavior of the rats in the first group. It was found that transplanted tumors grew more rapidly and were less often rejected in the rats exposed to the shocks in the uncontrollable situation. This correlates very well with a diminished T cell activity and NK cell function in this group of animals. An important finding is that in the uncontrollable situation the effect on the immune system involves opiates. Pharmacological drugs that antagonize opiate activity seem to keep uncontrollable stressors from promoting tumor growth, most probably because the immune system is no longer suppressed. Essentially identical results were obtained by Shavit et al. (11) using two different inescapable footshock stress paradigms. In this respect the findings by Heijnen et al. (12) on the effect of endorphins on immune responses in the human are interesting. She stimulated human B lymphocytes in cell cultures with the antigen ovalbumin (OA). This resulted in the production of anti-OA antibodies of the IgM-class. The cellular processes taking place in this experimental *in vitro* system are considered to reflect a genuine immune response as it occurs in lymphoid tissues in the body. It was found that α-endorphin, when added to the cell cultures, blocks anti-OA production. Most probably this effect is mediated via opiate-receptors, since des-tyr-α-endorphin does not have any effect. The addition of ß-endorphin does not result in suppression of the antibody response, in spite of the fact that the N-terminal aminoacid sequence (which binds to the opiate receptor) of the first 16 aminoacids of α- and ß-endorphin is identical (unpublished results). Since endogenous opioids, released by stress, seem to interfere with immune reactivity, more detailed analyses are needed to understand the molecular events involved in stress-related immuno-modulation. This brings us to the question of mechanisms which is really a complicated one. We will merely comment briefly on this question and will, furthermore, not discuss the complicated methodological aspects of studies on stress-induced changes in immune reactivity.

Regarding mechanisms involved in neuroimmunomodulation one could state that two main pathways exist. One is of humoral nature and involves pituitary and adrenal hormones and peptides. Among these are the enkephalins and endorphins (*vide supra*), ACTH, vasopressine and oxytocine. It should be emphasized that stress-induced reduction of lymphocyte functions is not necessarily corticosteroid dependent; Keller and Stein (13) have documented that in adrenalectomized rats stress can induce suppression of mitotic response of spleen lymphocytes.

The second pathway is represented by the nervous innervation of lymphoid tissues such as thymus, spleen, lymph nodes and even bone marrow (14, 15). In this circuit neurotransmitters may locally modulate immune reactivity; receptors for substanc s like VIP and catecholamines have been identified on lymphocytes.

Before bringing this paper to an end we would like to mention briefly two interesting issues.

Conditioning of the Immune Response

Research in this area of behavioral immunology was initiated some 10 years ago by Ader using the taste-aversion paradigm. Ader and Cohen (16) produced in rats (and later on also in mice) conditioned immunosuppression by pairing the conditioned stimulus (saccharin flavored drinking water) with the injection of the immunosuppressive drug cyclophosphamide, which represents the unconditioned stimulus. Conditioned animals that were exposed to the conditioned stimulus at a larger stage, showed a significant decrease in immune reactivity.

These experiments have been confirmed and extended by Gorczynski, using tumor growth (17) and graft rejection (18) as immunological read-out system and by the Klosterhalfens (19) in an adjuvant arthritis model in rats. Very recently, Gorczynski (17) reported that conditioning is a T cell dependent process and that conditioned immune suppression in mice could be reversed by cimetidine. This strongly suggests that histamine-receptor carrying T suppressor cells are involved in conditioned immune suppression. If this can be confirmed, it represents the first link of immunopharmacology with behavioral pharmacology.

Feedback: Is there a Lymphoid-Brain Axis?

Besedovsky et al. (20) have shown, already a number of years ago, that an ongoing immune response induces changes in neurotransmitter levels in the spleen of the animal and increases the firing rate of neurons. This means that not only the brain influences the immune system, but that the immune system may reciprocally effect the central nervous system. This notion has been strongly supported by the studies of Blalock and co-workers. They found that murine lymphocytes, after proper activation produce molecules which apparently are identical to pituitary hormones of the neuroendocrine circuit (21). Thus mouse T lymphocytes produce ACTH and endorphine-like material. Using a monoclonal antibody specific for the first four N-terminal aminoacids of endorphins and enkephalins, Cobi Heijnen could demonstrate that human mononuclear blood cells produce molecules which carry this opioid receptor specific sequence (unpublished results). Studies are underway now at the level of DNA and RNA to establish the molecular relationship between the brain-derived and lymphocyte-derived hormones. It is obvious that lymphocytic "neurotransmitters" may very well influence behavior. This again will bring the behavior-scientist, the neuropharmacologist and the immunologist together in a joint effort to elucidate the effect of the interaction between the central nervous system and the immune system.

References

1. Bartrop, R.W., Lazarus, L., Luckhurst, E., Kiloh, L.B. & Penny, R. (1977). Depressed lymphocyte function after bereavement. The Lancet, i: 834-836.
2. Schleifer, S.J., Keller, S.E., Camerino, M., Thornton, J.C. & Stein, M. (1983). Suppression of lymphocyte stimulation following bereavement. J. Am. Med. Assoc., 250: 374-377.

3. Ursin, H., Mykletun, R., Tonder, O., Vaernes, R., Relling, G., Isaksen, E. & Murison, R. (1984). Psychological stress-factors and concentrations of immunoglobins and complement components in human. Scand. J. Psychol, 25: 340-347.
4. Dorian, B., Garfinkel, P., Brown, G., Shore, A., Gladman, D. & Keystone, E. (1982). Aberrations in lymphocyte subpopulations and functioning during psychological stress. Clin. Exp. Immunol., 50: 132-138.
5. Kiecolt-Glaser, J.K., Garner, W., Speicher, C., Penn, G.M., Holliday, J. & Glaser, R. (1984). Psychosocial modifiers of immunocompetence in medical students. Psychosom. Med., 46: 7-14.
6. Raab, A., Dantzer, R., Michaud, B., Mormede, P., Taghzouti, K., Simon, H. & Le Moal, M. (1985). Behavioral, physiological and immunological consequences of social status and aggression in chronically coexisting resident-intruder dyads of male rats. Physiol. Behav., 36: 223-228.
7. Ader, R., Weijnen, J.A.W.M. & Moleman, P. (1972). Retention of a passive avoidance response as a function of the intensity and duration of electric shock. Psychon. Sci.; Sect. Anim. Physiol. Psychol., 26: 125-128.
8. Schleifer, S.J., Keller, S.E., Siris, S.G., Davis, K.L. & Stein, M. (1985). Lymphocyte function in ambulatory depressed patients, hospitalised schizophrenic patients, and patients hospitalised for herniorrhaphy. Arch. Gen. Psychiatry, 42: 129-133.
9. Locke, S.E., Kraus, L., Leserman, J., Hurst, M.W., Heisel, J.S. & Williams, R.M. (1984). Life change stress, psychiatric symptoms, and natural killer cell activity. Psychosom. Med., 46: 441-453.
10. Laudenslager, M.L., Ryan, S.M., Drugan, R.C., Hyson, R.A. & Maier, S.F. (1983). Coping and immunosuppression: Inescapable but not escapable shock suppresses lymphocyte proliferation. Science, 221: 568-570.
11. Shavit, Y., Lewis, J.W., Terman, G.W., Gale, R.P. & Liebeskind, J.C. (1984). Opioid peptides mediate the suppressive effect of stress on natural killer cell cytotoxicity. Science, 223: 188-190.
12. Heijnen, C.J., Bevers, C., Kavelaars, A. & Ballieux, R.E. (1986). Effects of alpha-endorphin on the antigen-induced primary antibody response of human blo d B cells in vitro. J. Immunol., 136: 213-216.
13. Keller, S.E., Weiss, J.M., Schleifer, S.J., Miller, N.E. & Stein, M. (1983). Stress-induced suppression of immunity in adrenalectomized rats. Science, 221: 1301-1304.
14. Bulloch, K. & Pomerantz, W. (1984). Autonomic nervous system innervation in wild-type and nude mice. J. Comp. Neurol., 228: 57-63.
15. Felten, D.L., Felten, S.Y., Carlson, S.L., Olschowka, J.A. & Livnat, S. (1985). Noradrenergic and peptidergic innervation of lymphoid tissue. J. Immunol., 135: 755s-765s.
16. Ader, R. & Cohen, N. (1975). Behaviorally conditioned immunosuppression. Psychosom. Med., 37: 333-340.
17. Gorczynski, R.M., Kennedy, M. & Ciampi, A. (1985). Cimetidine reverses tumor growth enhancement of plasmacytoma tumors in mice demonstrating conditioned immuno-suppression. J. Immunol., 134: 4261-4266.
18. Gorczynski, R.M., Macrae, S. & Kennedy, S. (1982). Conditioned immune response associated with allogeneic skin grafts in mice. J. Immunol., 129: 704-709.
19. Klosterhalfen, W. & Klosterhalfen, S. (1983). Pavlovian conditioning of immunosuppression modifies adjuvant arthritis in rats. Behav. Neurosci., 97: 663-666.
20. Besedovsky, H.O., del Rey, A.E. & Sorkin, E. (1985). Immune-neuroendocrine interactions. J. Immunol., 135: 750s-754s.
21. Blalock, J.E. (1984). The immune system as a sensory organ. J. Immunol., 132: 1067-1070.

Discussion:

Central Control of the Pituitary-Adrenal Axis I

Karl Heinz Voigt

Research in the regulation of the hypothalamus-pituitary-adrenal (HPA) axis represents a prominent example of a successful cooperation of such different scientific disciplines as endocrinology, psychology and immunology. Thus, the presentations of this session cover important parts of neuroendocrinology, psychoendocrinology, and psychoneuroimmunology. The most common connection between the very different contributions might be described as the adrenal mediated stress response by the three major integrative systems of the body: CNS, endocrine and immune systems. In this respect the chimeric term "stress" was not defined but used very flexibly for any defense situation.

Before discussing some of the interesting issues of the papers, new information on the HPA axis which may be relevant for their understanding should be summarized.

1) The adrenocorticotropic hormone (ACTH) is synthesized by the pituitary corticotroph as part of the much larger precursor molecule pro-opiomelanocortin (POMC). Its bioactive portions like the opioid ß-endorphin, ACTH and γ-MSH were secreted concomitantly under all circumstances (1).

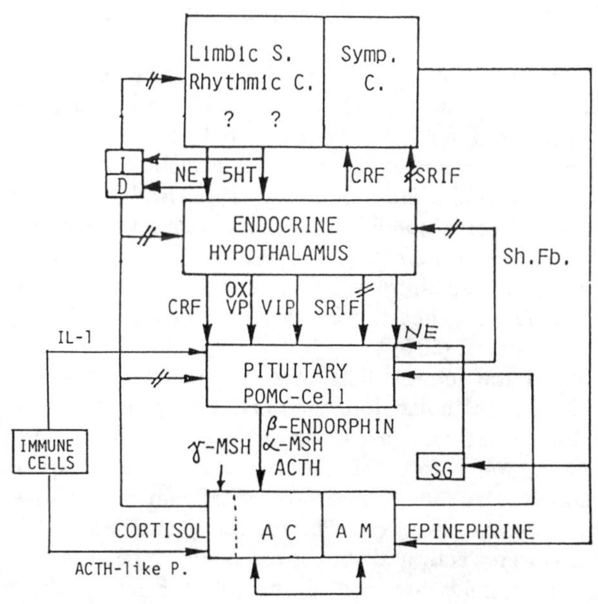

Figure 1. The regulatory systems for the hypothalamo-pituitary-adrenal axis: (a) Differential and integral negative feedback control by cortisol, (b) Modulation of cortisol secretion by neurotransmitters, neuropeptides and by pituitary POMC-peptides, (c) Influence of adrenergic substances and (d) Stimulation of ACTH by Interleukin-1 and production of ACTH-like peptides by immune cells.

2) A number of neuropeptides including not only CRF, but also vasopressin, oxytocin, VIP, somatostatin as well as adrenergic neurotransmitter substances are supposed to be direct regulators of pituitary ACTH and ß-endorphin (2).
3) Some of these "corticotropin" releasing substances influence the sympathetic centers of the hypothalamus and in turn the sympathetic outflow of the adrenal medulla and the spinal ganglia. Thus, a circuit of plasma adrenalin and noradrenalin together with cortisol from the adrenal cortex is established as a new regulatory principle of HPA activity (3, 4).
4) In addition to the anterior pituitary, ACTH is produced also by adrenal medullary cells in close contact to cortisol-producing adrenocortical cells (and in other peripheral organs as well). Furthermore, lymphocytes are able to synthesize and release ACTH-like substances (5). These and other unknown mechanisms are probably responsible for the phenomenon of ACTH unrelated cortisol secretion (6).
5) Recently, three different types of receptors for adrenocorticosteroids have been found in rat brains. Of particular interest is the specific corticosterone receptor, preferentially localized in hippocampal structures, which are involved in the regulation of cognitive processes, emotional state and termination of stress-induced activation of the HPA axis (7).

In particular these latter aspects of the behavioral physiology of hypothalamic CRF, pituitary ACTH and adrenal steroids are described by Bohus.

In summarizing more than a decade of an intensive study in his laboratory, Bohus introduced a new model for psychosomatic disease. It is based on neuroendocrine-brain interactions during stress, various types of extinction of learned avoidance behavior, and more recently experiments with limbic kindling, and the endocrine control of vegetative functions. His hypothesis is very stimulating, especially with respect to the interactions of hormones from the adrenal cortex with catecholamines from the medulla. Also, the observations of differential effects of adrenocorticosteroids due to binding at specific receptors give new insights into the modulation of emotional behavior in rats. However, recently the occurrence of different receptors for corticosterone and for pure glucocorticoids has not been demonstrated in humans. Circulating catecholamines and peptides obviously do not enter the brain. Steroids freely cross the blood brain barrier (8). Thus, interpretation of corresponding experiments should take this into consideration. Since the CNS neurons are able to produce all the regulatory peptides including ACTH, MSH and ß-endorphin, which are also synthesized in peripheral organs (endocrine glands, gut, heart, skin) (9), the brain peptides act synaptically as transmitters and regulators (10).

The secretion of hormones of the intermediate lobe of the rat pituitary is under inhibitory control by tuberoinfundibular dopamine (11) thus representing a powerful model for brain-endocrine interactions. However, a functional role for the intermediate lobe was not known before the experiments by the group of Smelik. They found, that emotional but not somatic stress influences a release of intermediate lobe hormones (γ-MSH, ß-LPH). The release is mediated by ß-adrenergic mechanisms, which were activated by stress with "high level of anxiety." Since circulating glucocorticoids are not suppressive for intermediate lobe hormones (in contrast to those from the anterior pituitary) and, on the other hand, stress induced catecholamines stimulate their secretion, the resulting relative amounts of pituitary stress hormones (e.g., γ-MSH vs. ACTH/ß-endorphin) in plasma may be a valuable marker for certain types of "emotional" stress in rats. In humans, the pituitary intermediate lobe appears only for a short period in fetal life. In adult humans, the secretory patterns of pituitary prolactin during stress are probably as specific as those of rat intermediate lobe hormones, because both cell types are tonically inhibited by hypothalamic dopamine (12).

The presentation by Bernton, Meltzer and Holaday has contributed much to the knowledge of a new physiological role for prolactin as an immune modulator during stress. The influence of prolactin on T-cell mediated immune response is most probably in balance with the well known immunomodulatory action of glucocorticoids (13) induced by different types of stress. In addition, many other neuropeptides are able to modulate immune cell functions. On the other hand, interleukin-[1], a product of macrophages and monocytes is a powerful stimulating factor for ACTH (14) and abolishes prolactin secretion. Thus prolactin, considered in the past as a hormone "in search of a mission" now becomes a member of the immune modulating humoral factors. Recently, prolactin was found to predict cardiac allograft rejection in patients under immunosuppressive medication (15). Research on prolactin secretion during acute and chronic stress and its relation to immune cell function seems to be a promising approach for a better understanding of the communication between the CNS and the immune system, mediated by two kinds of circulating chemical factors: Hormones and products of immune cells (monokines and lymphokines).

The intriguing observation by Blalock and coworkers (16) of synthesis and release of ACTH related hormones by activated lymphocytes is the most evident example for an interdependence of the immune and the neuroendocrine systems. Ballieux and Heijnen have critically reviewed the relevance of immune modulation induced by different types of stress and in particular the involvement of endogenous opioids in this process. The opioid peptides preferentially block immune responses in animal models (17). Ballieux and Heijnen presented evidence for suppression of antibody production by human B-lymphocytes, when incubated with ß-endorphin. The effect was obviously not mediated by known opioid receptors. In an animal model for emotional stress they observed different proliferative responses of spleen lymphocytes due to arousal compared with anxiety situations. This is in accordance with the distinct neuroendocrine reactions induced by different kinds of stress described by Bohus and by Smelik.

One would predict that simultaneous measurements during identical stress experiments of both the parameters used by the neuroendocrinologists (e.g., Bohus and Smelik) and the immunological markers reported by Ballieux and also by Bernton should considerably enhance our understanding of some stress-induced disturbances in the endocrine and immune systems.

References

1. Herbert, E., Roberts, J., Phillips, M., Allen, R., Hinman, M., Budarf, M., Policastro, P. & Rosa, P. (1980). Biosynthesis, processing and release of corticotropin, ß-endorphin, and melanocyte-stimulating hormone in pituitary cell cultures. Front. Neuroendocrinol., 6: 67-101.
2. Axelrod, J. & Reisine, D. (1984). Stress hormones: Their interaction and regulation. Science 224: 452-459.
3. Brown, M.R. & Fisher, L.A. (1984). Brain peptides as intracellular messengers. JAMA, 251: 1310-1315.
4. Borell, J., de Kloet, E.R., Versteeg, D.H.G. & Bohus, B. (1983). Inhibitory avoidance deficit short-term adrenalectomy in the rat: The role of adrenal catecholamines. Behav. Neural. Biol., 39: 241-258.
5. Smith, E.M., Morrill, A.C., Mayer III., W.J. & Blalock, J.E. (1986). Corticotropin releasing factor induction of leukocyte-derived immunoreactive ACTH and endorphins. Nature, 321: 881-882.
6. Fehm, H.L., Voigt, K.H. & Born, J.: This volume.
7. De Kloet, E.R., Reul, J.M.H.M., de Ronde, F.S.W. & Veldhuis, H.D. (1986). Brain corticosteroid receptor systems: Heterogeneity, function and plasticity. In D. De Wied & W. Ferrari (Eds.), Central actions of ACTH and related peptides. Liviana Press, Padova, p.115-129.
8. Pardridge, W.M. (1983). Neuropeptides and the blood-brain barrier. Ann. Rev. Physiol. 45: 73-82.
9. Krieger, D.T. (1984). Brain peptides. Vitam. Horm., 41: 1-50.
10. Schmitt, F.O. (1984). Molecular regulators of brain function: A new view. Neuroscience, 13: 991-1001.
11. Stoll, G., Martin, R. & Voigt, K.H. (1984). Control of peptide release from cells of the intermediate lobe of the rat pituitary. Cell Tissue Res., 236: 561-566.
12. Ben-Jonathan, N. (1985). Dopamine: A prolactin-inhibiting hormone. Endocr. Rev., 6: 564-589.
13. Munk, A., Guyre, P.M. & Holbrock, N.J. (1984). Physiological functions of glucocorticoids in stress and their relation to pharmacological actions. Endocr. Rev., 5: 25-44.
14. Besedovsky, H.O., Del Rey, A.E., Sorkin, E. & Dinarello, C.A. (1986). Immunoregulatory feedback between interleukin-1 and glucocorticoid hormones. Science, 233: 652-654.
15. Larson, D.F., Copeland, J.G. & Russell, D.H. (1985). Prolactin predicts cardiac allograft rejection in cyclosporin immunosuppressed patients. Lancet, 6: 53.
16. Smith, E.M., Harbour-McMenamin, D. & Blalock, J.E. (1985). Lymphocyte production of endorphins and endorphin-mediated immunoregulatory activity. J. Immunology, 135: 779s-782s.
17. Teschemacher, H. & Schweigerer, L. (1985). Opioid peptides: Do they have immunological significance? Trends Pharmacol. Sci., 7: 368-370.

6.

Central Control of the Pituitary-Adrenal Axis II

Expectancy and Activation:
An Attempt to Systematize Stress Theory

Holger Ursin

This paper represents an attempt to formalize a set of observations in man and animals on the relationship between external events (stimuli - "stressors"), overt behavior (response - coping attempts) and the internal physiological state of the individual (stress response).

Two major assumptions will be made, one relating to Activation, and one to Expectancy. *Activation* is defined as the process in the central nervous system (CNS) which increases the activity in the brain from a lower level to a higher level, and maintains this high level. *Expectancy* is simply the ability of the brain to store relationships between stimuli, and responses and stimuli, in the form that one precedes the other.

The First Assumption: When Does Activation Occur?

Activation occurs in all situations where "novel" stimuli occur, in situations where there is a homeostatic imbalance (if the proper incentives are available), and during emotions, in particular in situations where there is a threat to the organism. The *first assumption* is that all these situations have common logical features to them, and that activation occurs according to a very simple principle from general control theory (1, 2). I assume that the brain is a self-regulating logical net which functions according to general cybernetic principles. For each variable controlled by the brain there exists a "set value" (SV) which is the value on which the brain is "set" on for that particular variable at that particular time. The brain compares this SV with the actual value (AV) of that variable:

(1) SV = AV ?

If there is a discrepancy, the brain is wired in such a way that this produces the non-specific activation response:

(2a) (SV ≠ AV) = > Activation and
(2b) (SV = AV) = > No activation.

The *(2a)* statement is to be read: When the set values differs from the actual value this implies (= >) activation. The only part of this definition which differs from ordinary control theory is that for this particular system, a generalized alarm system called activation is activated by discrepancies between set values and actual values.

Activation affects the brain, the vegetative processes, the skeletomuscular system, all endocrine systems (3, 4), and probably the immune system (5). No characteristic of the somatic "stress" response, as described by Selye or in the stress-literature, differs from activation, except for the assumption that there is a relation to disease. In this paper, therefore, the stress response is identical to the activation response.

Since activation is assumed to be essentially a biological mechanism, the response must be assumed to be "adaptive." The biological significance of the response is its effect on behavior. The essence in this thinking may be expressed as follows: Activation will sustain itself until activation affects mechanisms that serve to solve the underlying discrepancy, by changing the actual values, or the set values, or shifting to other motivational systems (see below). Eventually activation turns off activation:

(3) $S \Rightarrow$ Activation $\Rightarrow$ Somatic and/or psychological processes $\Rightarrow$ $R \Rightarrow \overline{S}$,

where $\overline{S}$ symbolizes abolished stimulation by responses (R). This statement is to be read: A stimulus which implies activation implies somatic and/or psychological responses which imply responses which abolish that stimulus. Or, stated in easier language: Stimuli that elicit activation also elicit responses which abolish that particular stimulus. The essence of this formulation is that it is the responses that abolish the stimulation, which gave the activation. The same meaning may be written this way: Since *(2):*

(4) $(SV - AV \neq 0) \Rightarrow$ Activation $\rightarrow ((SV - AV) \rightarrow 0)$,

which is to be read: When the set value differs from the actual value this implies activation which, in turn, leads to this difference being reduced or abolished. The relationship to pathology, inherent in the "stress" concepts, must be assumed to have something to do with situations where these mechanisms do not work properly. To elaborate on these aspects the second term is required.

The Second Assumption: What is Expectancy?

The second assumption to be made is that brains are able to learn that certain stimuli or responses precede other stimuli. This is an essential property of brains. To perform complex acts like catching a prey the predator must direct its movements to where the prey is expected to be in the next time interval. Learning theory used to deal with simpler stimulus situations, but we now find an increasing degree of references to complex stimuli and processes of active information sampling like attention and preparation (6-9). When the brain has established that something precedes something, the brain "expects" the second stimulus when the first stimulus has been presented, or the response has been performed. *Expectancy* then, is a particular brain function of registering, storing and using the particular information that one stimulus precedes a second stimulus, or one response precedes ("brings") a particular outcome.

When one stimulus (S1) predicts the occurrence of another event (S2) (S1 = > S2) this is referred to as *stimulus expectancy* (10). When performance of a response (R1) brings a certain S2 (R1 = > S2) this is referred to as *response outcome expectancy* (10). When an animal learns an instrumental response for food, it typically first learns that certain cues predict food, and then learns that certain responses produce food. In an avoidance situation it first learns the stimulus contingencies predicting shock, and then learns how to avoid them (see 10 for definitions and review). This is, essentially, a two process learning theory. Several formulations exist (11-13), the common elements being that there are two stages in any learning situation. Stimulus-stimulus learning may be regarded as classical conditioning, response learning as instrumental conditioning. In Pavlovian and Konorskian literature the corresponding terms are Type 1 and Type 2 conditioning (14).

Stimulus Expectancies

There is substantial agreement (9) that in classical conditioning the subject learns that the previously neutral stimulus (CS) precedes or predicts the shock or the food (UCS) (10, 11, 15, 16). The conditioned response, therefore, is no "reflex" but a response to an acquired "expectancy" (E). When the subject has learned that S1 (CS) precedes (predicts) S2 (UCS), a stimulus expectancy has been established. The formal definition of a stimulus expectancy is then:

(5) ${}_{S1}E_{S2} = (S1 => S2)$

which should be read: The S1 (CS) expectancy of S2 (UCS) means that S1 (CS) implies S2 (UCS).

Stimulus expectancy, then, is stored information on the relationship between stimuli, or on a "new order of things in the environment" (10). The event S2 may be any event, for instance the UCS in the classical conditioning paradigm. The essential requirement is the time course of events (time contiguity). The concept is overlapping with, but not identical to "associative bonds" between S1 and S2 (or CS and UCS), as it is used by learning theorists (7).

Response Outcome Expectancies

Brains do not only register relationships between stimuli. They are, of course, also able to register relationships between their responses and the environment. Tolman referred to this as "knowledge." In this paper this dimension will be referred to as response outcome expectancies (Bolles (10), Irwin (17): Act outcome expectancy). Response outcome expectancy will be referred to formally as:

(6) ${}_{R1}E_{S2}$,

where R1 is a response, and S2 the outcome of that response. This concept is essential for the discussion of coping, helplessness and hopelessness. These terms are, again, necessary in order to be able to discuss the internal states that may be elicited by different types of expectancy.

Bolles (10) has argued that while the stimulus expectancy corresponds rather accurately with the true stimulus outcome contingencies, the response outcome contingency may be a much "less faithful representation" of the contingencies. An essential element in the present paper is that it is the perceived relationship that counts, not the objectively true contingencies. Bolles has discussed this in detail, and this was an essential part of his 1972 argumentation, and in the discussion that followed that paper. This position is one of the most important reasons for the usefulness of these concepts, as opposed to ordinary learning theory. It also marks a point of departure from most applications of statistical decision theory and optimal foraging theory, where there is little or no allowance for variance and differences between true and perceived probabilities (18, 19).

Quantification of Expectancies

From a theoretical point of view it seems necessary to quantify expectancies along several dimensions. In the following it will be assumed that these dimensions are independent (orthogonal), but this is not a necessary assumption. Future multivariate research is required to determine how many scales really are required and what the interrelations really are.

Bolles (10) operated with two dimensions, the "strength" of the expectancy, and the perceived probability of the outcome. He also discussed the "value" of that outcome. In human motivation theory, there is frequent reference to the incentive value of the expected outcome (17, 20). Coover (21) concentrated on the value aspect of the expectancy, referring to positive and negative expectancies. All three dimensions will be used in this paper, *acquisition strength, perceived probability, affective value*. All three dimensions will be assumed to be quantifiable, and will be given numeric values.

The "expectancy" comprises all three dimensions. This is a learned function. The $_{S1}(E)_{S2}$ is an individual characteristic. For one particular subject S1 implies S2, after a learning stage. Therefore, E has an *acquisition strength*, which depends on properties of the S1 and S2, the contiguity in the presentation, the number of presentations, and the predictive value of S1. The acquisition of this dimension follows the general principles of learning theory. In this paper the acquisition strength will be referred to as H ("habit value"), which will be assumed to have values between 0 (minimum) and 1 (maximum). Formally, the strength of S1 = > S2 is expressed by $H(_{S1}E_{S2})$ and has values between 0 and 1:

(7a) $H(_{S1}E_{S2}) \in (0,1)$.

Or, in more detail:

(7b) $\forall_{S1}E_{S2}, \exists \quad H(_{S1}E_{S2}) \in (0,1)\{0\}$.

This statement is to be read: For all ${}_{S1}E_{S2}$ there is a H-value between 0 and 1. If the H-value approaches zero, there is no expectancy ($\{0\}$). In the following only the simple version of *(7)* will be used, and this will also be the principle for other formalizations. The same is true for ${}_{R1}E_{S2}$:

(8) $H({}_{R1}E_{S2}) \in (0,1)$.

Expectancy also implies that the brain allocates a certain probability to the possibility that S1 implies R1, or that R1 implies S2. This subjective evaluation of the probability will be referred to as *perceived probability* (PP). PP is not necessarily equal to the true or objective probability since PP represents a subjective evaluation. It may be a true picture of the outside world, but there may also be variance in this concept as referred to previously. For the stimulus expectancies *predictability* has been used, for response outcome expectancy the subjective evaluation of the probability may be referred to as *control*. These terms require further comments, and they are not necessarily overlapping or identical terms.

The time contiguity between S1 and S2 or a response R1 and S2 is important for learning to occur. In objective terms this relationship may be referred to as "probability" (P), and is usually assigned values from 0 to 1. Formally:

(9) $P(S1 => S2) \in (0,1)$.

The subjective predictability and control which is referred to as "perceived probability" (PP) will also be attributed values between 0 (very low perceived probability) and 1 (very high perceived probability). Formally, for stimulus expectancies:

(10) $PP({}_{S1}E_{S2}) \in (0,1)$.

For response expectancies:

(11) $PP({}_{R1}E_{S2}) \quad (0,1)$.

The difference between perceived probability and the true probability may be particulary pronounced in some situations, as, for instance, when we evaluate risks. There are situations where it is quite improbable that S1 or R1 will lead to S2, the true probability is very low, but the perceived probability may be high.

Expectancies may also be quantified beyond acquisition strength and perceived probability. The value of the expected event is important (10, 21). The reinforcing or attractive/aversive value of the expected outcome or stimulus event will be referred to as the *affective value* (A):

(12) $A(_{S1}E_{S2})$,

and will be allocated values from -1 (highly unattractive) to +1 (highly attractive). Formally:

(13) $A(_{S1}E_{S2})$ (-1, +1), and $A(_{R1}E_{S2})$ (-1, +1).

The affective value of an expectancy depends on (is a function (f) of the expected event (S2). Therefore:

(14) $A(_{S1}E_{S2}) = f(A(S2))$ and $A(_{R1}E_{S2}) = f(A(S2))$.

The affective value corresponds in part to the concept of "intensity" of the US (22). In a simple one-stimulus learning situation with one reinforcer or UCS, the Hullian concept of intensity may be sufficient. For many complex situations involving more than one motivational system, and comparisons between them, intensity alone cannot be used for comparative judgments. This makes an A scale necessary. The dimension is also useful for a proper understanding of a relative reinforcement concept. S2-type of events are not just either neutral or reinforcing, but should be represented on a continuous value scale (23, 24).

As already mentioned, no exact knowledge is available at the present time about the angle between these three dimensions in a multivariate space, or, more simply, to what extent the scales are independent. However, it is still an important aspect of the theory that the PP scale and the H scale may be independent in some cases. It is possible to have a high H-value and very low PP-value, for instance, when a subject has learned that a response does not work, or a stimulus does not bring another, specific stimulus ("inhibitory" conditioning). Rather than assuming a decrement in some association bond it is postulated that the brain simply stores information that the response or class of responses does not bring the desired outcome.

Set Values and Expectancies

The set value referred to in Statement *(2)* may be acquired, as mentioned before, including the "template" referred to in the Sokolov theory of orienting behavior. Other types of acquired set values are goals, ambitions, social expectancies, and attitudes. All such "values" may be regarded as the S2 in the expectancy statements, occurring in specific stimulus situations or contexts (S1). For instance, in the habituation situation, after a number of trials the general stimulus situation (stimulus background, context) signals the appearance, or probability of appearance, of S2. Activation is produced if the S2 does not occur, or occurs in a different context. It is possible to argue that dis-habituation is partly a change of context, therefore producing a response to S2. For the activation that occurs when an expected stimulus does not appear, or when a response expectancy is not met, for instance in early extinction trials (25, 26):

(15a) for stimulus expectancies:
If $H({}_{S1}E_{S2}) \Rightarrow 1$, $PP({}_{S1}E_{S2}) \Rightarrow 1$, and $S1 \neq> S2$
then activation,
since *(2)*: $(SV = (S1 => S2)$ and $AV = (S1 \neq> S2))$.

(15b) same statement for response expectancies.

Within this framework the "novelty" of the stimulus in the orienting response design shrinks to a special, reversed case of *(15)*, where the expectancy (SV) is $S1 \neq> \overline{S2}$, S2 is not expected in this particular stimulus situation (S1), and activation will occur.

Expectancies and Activation

Activation is not a linear function of deprivation unless there are cues or incentives present signalling that there is some probability that the actual value of that particular variable may be corrected (27). From a biological point of view it would be inadequate if, for instance, the food or water-deprived animal kept running around in its cage when food or water is not available. When the individual has established that no food or water is available by any strategy, the best strategy is to conserve energy or water, sit still and hope for better times. The theory developed from Statement *(2)* must also consider the simple fact that there is more to life than food or water. The brain has more than one set value. Some attention or selection mechanism must be operating. Detailed and complex models for such shifts have been introduced both in ethology (28) and in human motivation theory (29). The selection mechanisms must also be assumed to have consequences for the activation system.

Deprived animals follow the sensible strategy mentioned earlier. They are quiet until some cue signals that the deprivation period may be over. When such cues are presented, activity increases (30, 31). Activation measured by hormones follow the same principle. There is a rise in plasma norepinephrine levels 15 minutes before feeding in pigs maintained on a fixed schedule (32). There is a considerable set of data on "circadian rhythms" in rats which seem to confirm these findings, but they have been interpreted differently by the authors reporting them, possibly because of a lack of the expectancy concept.

The corticosterone levels in plasma of rats fed once daily are no longer dominated by the light-dark cycle, but by the feeding schedule. There is a general agreement that there is a peak in corticosterone levels at feeding time, but this peak occurs before feeding, regardless of the light schedule, and also in blinded rats (33). It disappears after prolonged starvation. The light-dark related changes in corticosterone in non-deprived rats also show the same phenomenon, there is an increase related to darkness, but it starts before lights are turned off. The food-regulated rhythm is interpreted as an "entrained" rhythm. It takes about 10 days to establish. But what does "entrained" mean? Kato, Saito and Suda suggested that the regulation was due to "some endogenous mechanism," and similar hypotheses are generally found in this literature. In this case it seems as if the train not only arrives at the station before the locomotive, it also moves before the locomotive has started. Unless one assumes that the feeding is run by the steroids, the steroids are either run by the same clock that runs the experimenters and their laboratories, or by a hypothetical clock in the brain.

This raises the interesting question about the relationship between circadian rhythms and the expectancy functions. Why does the rat increase his activity before the lights are turned off? Are internal clocks always faster than real time, or is the rat simply using the available cues in the laboratory and animal quarter environment? The most parsimonious explanation seems to be that these rhythms are probably not entrained: they are simply trained.

The clearest relationships and the best control over the stimulus situation seem to be in the work by Coover and his associates (34) (see Figure 1). In my opinion, their use of expectancy concepts with inherent, but not explicit use of the three subscales (H, A, and PP), have clarified these relationships.

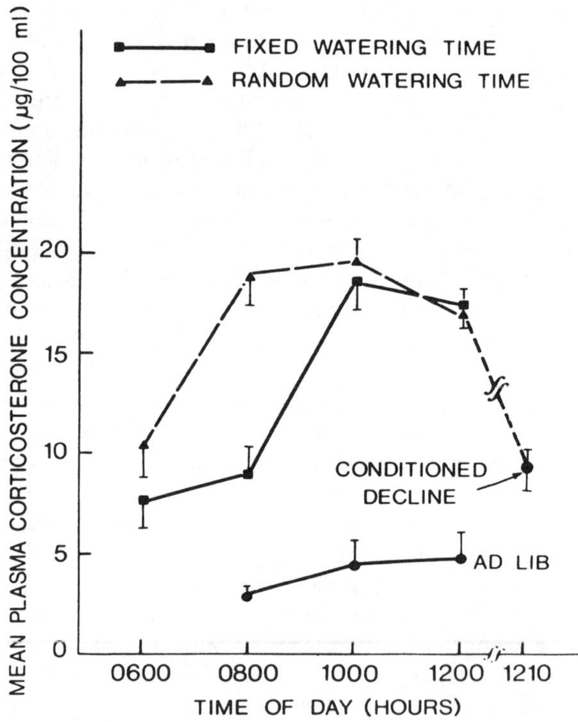

Figure 1. Prewatering plasma corticosterone levels in rats maintained for 8 weeks on three different schedules for watering: Ad Lib (free access to water); Fixed Watering Time (water available for 20 min at pr. 1.00 hours); and Random Watering Time (water available for 20 min sometime between 8.00 and 12.00). Conditioned Decline shows the effect of strong cues signalling that water was imminent for the Random Watering Group (34).

Deprived rats have a higher basal value than ad lib watered rats, but the initial levels measured are low, well within what is regarded as "basal values" from other laboratories. The striking differences between groups occur later in the day, when cues accumulate that water may be coming for the group that was given water at random, between 8.00 and 12.00 hours. Particularly striking is the delay in the prewatering rise in the group given water at 12.00 each day. Coover's data have been replicated also for feeding (35). There was basically a curvilinearity in the plasma corticosterone level in the hungry rat, high levels when there was uncertainty about whether food was coming or not, and low levels when there was a very high or very low probability that food was coming.

The perceived probability of success, therefore, has a decisive influence on the activation level, and statement *(2)* must be modified taking this complex "probability of success" variable into account. Set values that have at least a certain perceived probability (PP) of being resolved $(SV - AV = 0)$ should have access to the activation system, while for set values where there is a low or no perceived probability that the set value and the actual value will be equal, there is a low access to the activation system. Formally, for one particular motivational system with a set value SV_1 and actual value AV_1, and where there is a low perceived probability that the difference between the set value and the actual value is eliminated, the following assumption may be made:

(16) If $SV_1 \neq AV_1$, and if $PP((SV_1 - AV_1) \rightarrow 0) \rightarrow 0$
then activation is low.

This is what is assumed to explain the low values observed before cues are given (see Figure 2).

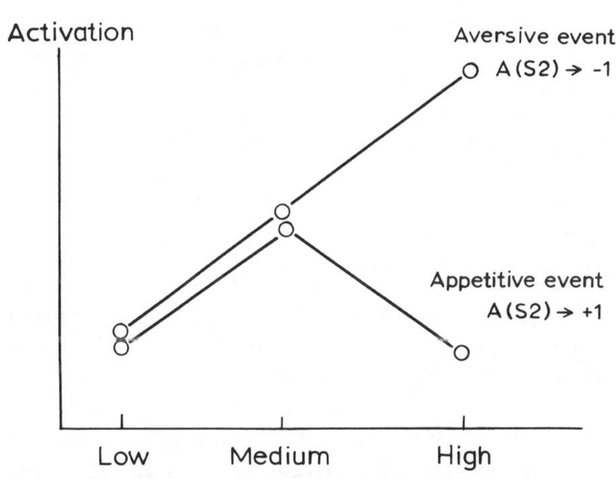

Figure 2. Relationship between the perceived probability of an event (the PP dimension of expectancy) and activation.

The apparent bidirectionality in the corticosterone response for appetitive events seen in Figure 2 suggests a particular mechanism turning off activation. Bidirectionality in the response was first described by Goldman, Coover and Levine (36). Rats were trained to barpress for water on continuous reinforcement (CRF) or a variable interval (VI) schedule. When the VI trained rats were suddenly exposed to the CRF schedule, their corticosterone level decreased during the session. This did not take place in the CRF trained rats, and shifts to extinction produced the expected rise in corticosterone (Statement *15b*). The corticosterone decline may be conditioned to neutral cues (37, 38), in other words, the strong expectancy of the positive event produced the fall (21). Formally:

(17) If $SV_1 \neq AV_1$, and if $PP((SV_1 - AV_1) \rightarrow 0) \rightarrow 1$, then activation is low.

This statement is in apparent contradiction with the fact that increasing the magnitude of reinforcement often increases the speed of running (39, 40). Increased magnitude of reward is an important element in previous reward expectancy formulations of learning theory (41), and presumably also for the low corticosterone values. Coover suggests that sufficiently large rewards are necessary to observe a corticosterone decline during an instrumental conditioning session (21). But the lack of correlation between increased running speed and decreased activation is another example of the fact that the activation level cannot be evaluated by the external, overt behavior. The Crespi phenomenon may perhaps be explained as an increase in "arousal" (42) and phasic activation (see below). Another attractive hypothesis is that the running speed increases when there is less uncertainty, and less concern with alternative, competing strategies (see 43, for similar argument for the relationship between emotion (activation) and performance).

The bidirectionality in the response may be due to an active deactivating mechanism, possibly serotonergic, possibly related to post-reinforcement synchronization and drowsiness (44). The decline produced by food cues depends on the ventromedial hypothalamic nucleus (45), but may be effectuated via reduced or inhibited activity in the general activation system.

Set Values and Motivational Systems

The selection mechanism that must determine which SV is to be considered for its corresponding AV at any given point in time has been given more attention by ethologists than by psychologists, probably because experimental control has been such an essential part of the psychological tradition. The shift from one "motivational system" to another has been left to the experimenter, not to the subject itself. In ethology, the lack of stimulus control has helped in the realization of the complexity and interaction of motivational systems. It seems reasonable to assume that the gating of the access to the activation system (Statements *16, 17*) may have implications also for the necessary ranking and shifting between motivational systems. Traditional motivation theories (28) require a system for weighing the different set values. In this paper this is taken care of by the A dimension (A(SV)), since set values have the properties of expectancies. In addition to this principle it is possible that an expectancy function orders the hierarchy according to the probability of success for the available responses:

(18) If $SV_1-AV_1 \neq 0$ and $SV_2-AV_2 \neq 0$ and if
$PP(R_1 => (SV_1-AV_1) -> 0) > PP(R_2 => (SV_2-AV_2) -> 0)$
and if $A(SV_1) \sim A(SV_2)$ then
$P(R_1) > P(R_2)$,

where R_1 is the response or behavior involved in the solution to the first problem, and R_2 the response for the second problem, and P is the true probability for R_1 or R_2 to be executed. Probability of success also influences how hard a human subject will work (29).

According to the Utility theory for decision-making (46), humans make rational decisions based on the highest expected utility. This is a response outcome expectancy system, and the highest gain is cho en. Deviations from this rational behavior may be explained by a modification called Prospect theory (47). Values (corresponding to the A-scale) are associated with the outcomes, and "decision rate" is associated with the probability (corresponding to the PP-scale in the present system). Individual differences in how probabilities are perceived depends on previous experience, personality factors, the motivational situation and on individual differences in how abilities are perceived (48-50).

Predictability and Probability

The curvilinear relationship between probability of appetitive events and activation (Figure 2) (Statements *16*, *17*) may be reduced to a linear relationship if we insert a new term, *predictability* (see Figure 3). A highly probable as well as a highly improbable event are both predictable. This is the optimum of predictability. Low predictability is when there is an even chance of an event occurring or not occurring ($P(S2) = P(\overline{S2}) = 0.5$). The maximum of unpredictability exists when S1 and S2, or CS and UCS, occur randomly with respect to one another (51).

This occurs when

(19) $P(S1 => S2) = P(\overline{S1} => S2)$,

which is to be read: The probability of S2 (or UCS) occurring after S1 (CS) equals the probability of S2 occurring given no S1 (CS). A similar statement is valid for the relationship between responses and the expected event. There is empirical support for animals and humans preferring predictable to unpredictable aversive events (52-54) and, in general, the somatic consequences of signalled shocks are less severe than those resulting from unsignalled shocks. However, predictability in itself is not enough to predict the internal state, or the behavioral consequences. Supporting this theoretical position are findings of seemingly paradoxical deleterious effects of predictable events (55, 56).

In situations where the affective value of the expected event is close to -1, that is highly unattractive, high perceived probability leads to high activation rather than low. Since occurrence of an unattractive event is very much against

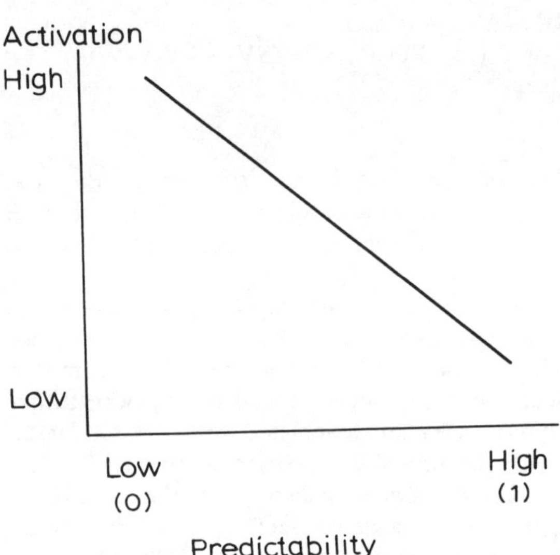

Figure 3. The function underlying Figure 2 (appetitive events) transferred to a monotonous function of predictability (or uncertainty), for appetitive events (A –> +1). For expected aversive events (A –> -1), the function is inverse.

the set values of an organism, this follows directly from *(2)*. This is a reasonable definition of *fear*. If the perception is of a chance probability that an unattractive event might occur, that is, the perceived probability is close to 0.5, the activation is still high. Only when the perceived probability of the unattractive event is low, the activation is low. This occurs under *coping* (see below). *Anxiety* may be characterized by a perceived chance level of an expected, unattractive event, or with a generalized fear without clear S2-expectancies. In this case, the acquisition value may be high, but the perceived probability is vague or ill defined, perhaps best expressed by 0.5. If the probability contingencies became clarified, anxiety may be transferred to fear. Both fear and anxiety may be reduced by learning about the true probability levels. Many fear reducing strategies, therefore, are not extinction of conditioned reflexes in the classical sense, but learning of a more exact or true expectancy.

Defense

Information about the true stimulus contingencies often works as an anxiety and fear reducing factor, but also depends on personality factors like defense (57), or "blunting" (58). Humans may defend themselves against threatening stimuli by distorting them or denying them. This particular "perceptual" type of defense has only been demonstrated in humans, and consists of cognitive strategies redefining the threat (57).

Defense, therefore, is related to stimulus expectancies as defined in this paper, and acts by restructuring the expectancies by distorting or redefining the signals about the true nature of the S2 contingencies. This makes defense a strategy which may be rather dangerous to use, in particular when the S2 really is signalling physical danger. Support for this assumption is found in repeated demonstrations of defense, measured by perceptual methods (59), predicting inadequate behavior in many different types of dangerous tasks (60). In previous theories of stress, defense mechanisms have sometimes been regarded as an essential part of the total coping resources (61, 62). However, in the present paper defense is regarded as a separate phenomenon related to *stimulus expectancies*, rather than to response expectancies.

Coping

The adequate way of reducing activation to a threat is to reduce or eliminate the threat itself by action, which changes the threat. If the subject has a response available, which will abolish the S2, and the individual learns that this is the case, a *positive response outcome expectancy* may be developed. This is *coping*.

When an organism has learned that a certain event S1 implies a dangerous or unattractive event S2, the activation level in that organism becomes high *(2)*. This drives the organism to a particular instrumental behavior, which, once established reduces the activation level *(3)*. There is direct empirical evidence for this in a series of rat experiments by Coover and collaborators (63). Rats trained in an avoidance situation show a high level of activation when they are given the shocks the first time, and also when they have learned the signal value of the warning signal. When they acquire the initial escape and avoidance responses, activation is still high. However, when the avoidance response has been overtrained, there is a clearcut reduction in the corticosterone level indicating that the animals have learned not only a correct response, but also that this response eliminates the shocks. Coping has been used as the term for this type of learning, which goes beyond the performance of the animals. A formal definition of c ping is:

(20) $H({}_{R1}E_{\overline{S2}}) \rightarrow 1$, $PP\ ({}_{R1}E_{\overline{S2}}) \rightarrow 1$, $A(S2) \rightarrow -1$.
Since $A(S2) \rightarrow -1$, R1 is abolishing a negative event,
therefore $A({}_{R1}E_{\overline{S2}}) \rightarrow +1$.

It follows from the general statement *(17)* that the activation level is expected to be low. In short, coping is a positive response outcome expectancy. It also follows from *(20)* that the discussions on whether avoidance behavior is maintained by "safety" or "residual fear" is a sham problem. Since *-(-1)* = *+1* there is no logical reason to prefer one of the two expressions, it is really the same whether one deals with the negative affect of S2, or the positive affect of $\overline{S2}$.

This is an essential part of many formulations of two factor theory of avoidance learning, where the initial part of the learning consists of stimulus expectancy learning (or classical conditioning), which then is followed by response expectancy learning. The additional postulate in the present theory is that this should lead to a reduced activation level, since the set value in this case is to abolish the unattractive stimulus. Empirical support for this has been provided in rats, dogs, and primates (55, 56, 63-65) and from humans (4), and this activation fall has even been used as a criterion for coping having taken place (66).

The term coping has also been used for all efforts to obtain this state (62, 67), even defense, as mentioned above. Haan (57) uses coping for the strategies used, but only for the strategies that are associated with accepting the true nature of the situation. In other words, she uses the term coping only for strategies that do not involve defensive distortions of reality. In this paper the term coping does not refer to the coping attempts, but the result of successful coping attempts.

Since coping is regarded as a "state," there have to be signals present to elicit it, a stimulus expectancy eliciting the particular response expectancy. Once this state occurs, the positive response outcome expectancy seems to have a particular tendency to generalize to other situations, and to other responses. The self-efficacy concept of Bandura (68) seems closely related to this more general coping concept, and Rotter's (69) internal locus of control scale measures to what extent an individual believes that reinforcements in his life are under his control. The general coping concept also relates to the "mastery" concept of Pearlin, Lieberman, Menaghan, and Mullen (70), the "instinct of mastery" of Hendrick (71), and the effectance concept of White (72).

A necessary condition for coping to occur is that there is information about the relationship between responses and their results. This is referred to as "feedback" and is an important element in prevention of stomach ulcerations in animals (73). Low feedback, for instance shifting from fixed ratio of reinforcement to variable ratio, results in higher levels of corticosterone in rats (36) and more stomach ulcerations (74). The term "control" is also partly used for this dimension. Lack of control over the stimulus environment produces "emotional behavior" (75), more rapid tumor growth (76), and greater changes in brain catecholamines (64). The term "control," however, does not show a totally consistent relationship to the internal state, as pointed out by Folkman (77), in a recent review. However, if the PP-scale and the A-scale is used for response outcome expectancies, it seems possible to avoid these inconsistencies.

Helplessness

What happens when coping is impossible? This may occur in experimental situations with uncontrollable and unsignalled negative events, or in humans subjected to unpleasant life events beyond their control. However, in animals there is a surprising degree of coping even in situations that appear to be without solution (78). Response and stimulus expectancies are subjective dimensions, and many set values may be redefined. Most people subjected to bereavement and dramatic life events survive and show no trace of somatic or psychic illness (79). However, these capabilities may be overtaxed.

The classical experimental situation is the experimental neurosis situation of Pavlov (80) and Masserman (81). In a review of this literature (82), Mineka and Kihlstrom concluded that the common thread running through this literature is that disturbances occur when important life events become unpredictable or uncontrollable, or both.

Mowrer and Viek (83) pointed out that the effects of aversive events were less disruptive for an approach task if escape was possible. They used the term "sense of helplessness" for the condition arising from the non-escape situation. Overmier and Seligman (84) found that "helplessness" may generalize to situations where control is possible. Dogs with previous experience with inescapable shocks do not learn avoidance tasks. The particular situation producing this phenomenon is when:

(21) $P(R1 => \overline{S2}) = P(\overline{R1} => \overline{S2})$.

In words: The probability of avoiding the aversive stimulus with a response is the same as for no response. The response is without any consequence for the occurrence of the aversive event. The organism has no control (51). In the present terminology, the essential feature of the response outcome expectancy is that "nothing helps." This has consequences for the PP, perhaps it appears even close to zero.

Formally, therefore, helplessness exists when:

(22) $H({}_{R1}E_{\overline{S2}}) \to 1,\ PP({}_{R1}E_{\overline{S2}}) \to 0,\ A(S2) \to -1,$
$PP({}_{R1}E_{\overline{S2}}) \sim PP({}_{\overline{R1}}E_{\overline{S2}})$.

From formulations *(16)* and *(17)* it might be expected that the activation value could be low, but these statements have only been tested when A(S2) is positive. Since, in this case, the A value is negative, it is also a situation eliciting fear and, therefore, high activation. The predictions for activation, therefore, is problematic. It is possible that the so-called helplessness may be an instrumental response in some situations, at least when the helplessness is shown by freezing. The "freezing" type of fear behavior may be an effective and useful strategy (44). If so, lack of movements in an avoidance box may not be "helplessness" at all, as defined by Statement *(22)*, even if shocks might occur.

An essential feature of the helplessness concept is that this response expectancy also tends to generalize. However, there are data that suggest that generalization is easier to establish to stimulus expectancy than to response expectancy. Dess et al. (56) found that while plasma cortisol was higher in dogs with no control as compared with dogs with control over the pretreatment shocks, the important variable in later tests was predictable vs non-predictable shocks.

Seligman has suggested that helplessness might be related to depression, and to changes in brain biochemistry. This is only relevant for the type of helplessness where the response is not instrumental and the activation level is high. Lewinsohn's (85) view of depression as being due to low rate of response contingent positive reinforcement seems also covered by a hypothesis of a relation between statement *(22)* and depression. There is at least substantial evidence for severe behavior disturbances in learning experiments that follow the pre-shock treatment which produced helplessness in the original work by Overmier and Seligman (84, see also (16) for review). Similar findings have been made for problem solving in humans (86).

Hopelessness

Depressive patients are perhaps better described as having no hope than having no control. It is not only that responses and outcome is unrelated *(22)*: It is worse than that. There is an element of guilt and despair which is stronger than what helplessness *(22)* covers. Several authors stress hopelessness as a crucial aspect of depression (87, 88). This is also an important element in Beck's negative cognitive set and negative self esteem (89). The essential element in hopelessness is that whatever the subject is doing, punishment will occur. This is more truly the opposite of coping, everything the individual does will be punished. For hopelessness:

$$(23)\quad H({}_{R1}E_{S2}) \rightarrow 1,\ PP({}_{R1}E_{\overline{S2}}) \rightarrow 1,\ A(S2) \rightarrow -1.$$

This should produce high activation levels. In his review of the depression literature Blaney (90) concluded that even if the behavioral elements referred to in statements *(22)* and *(23)* are important in depression, none were proven to be necessary antecedents of depression. However, the findings of biochemical CNS changes due to prolonged or strong activation (64, 91) suggest that these response expectancies may well be causal.

On the other hand, even if all responses are punished, activation may not be sustained indefinitely. This particular state and expectancy may elicit specific strategies in others, that, in turn, may be instrumental and activation-reducing. Forrest and Hokanson (92) hypothesized that the self-demeaning displays of depressives controlled the aversiveness and threats from other individuals, and found that positive reward for self-punitive responses gave faster autonomic arousal reduction in depressed than in non-depressed control subjects. Similarly, Coyne (93) has pointed out that the soliciting of support from depressives tends to inhibit direct expressions of annoyance and hostility from others.

Sustained Activation and Psychosomatic Illness

In a healthy organism a short lasting tonic or general activation has no proven ill effects. When coping has been established, there is still a short lasting phasic activation ("arousal": (42); (94)) when individuals cope with potentially dangerous tasks. In humans this activation seems to be limited to epinephrine (not norepinephrine) (95), pulse rate increase (96-98), and a modest testosterone rise (99), again without any known pathogenic effect. This activation pattern, therefore may have training effects, but, to the best of our knowledge, no straining effects (94, 100). The response seems to be characterized as an anabolic response of benefit to elderly patients (101), and probably for the rest of us, too.

However, the non-coping individual may show a sustained tonic activation pattern when facing an unsolved problem *(3)*. This activation pattern is the general activation response, which affects all systems. If shortlasting, there is probably no ill effects in the healthy organism. However, if this general activation is sustained several systems may be challenged beyond their capacity, and straining effects may result. Particular interest is focused on the sustained high levels of norepinephrine, cortisol, vagal discharges, and thyroxin and the related changes in the gastrointestinal system, the cardiovascular system, the immunological system, and biochemical changes in the brain itself (102). Such situations are ifficult to reproduce under strict experimental control in humans for simple ethical reasons. There is, however, animal data with a high degree of consistency. Rats develop gastric ulcerations when food deprived and then immobilized or presented with inescapable shocks. Pre-shock treatment of rats increases their adrenocortical response to mild stress (open field) one week later (103, 104, Murison, this volume). These sensitized animals also show greater susceptibility to gastric ulceration under immobilization stress (104) as long as their previous experience was with inescapable shock. Pretreatment with inescapable shock, on the other hand, reduces below non-shock control levels the susceptibility to ulceration under later immobilization stress (104). In the food deprived stomach, with intact vagal innervation, a sustained activation will eventually lead to ulceration, probably due to a breakdown in the mucous barrier which defends the stomach wall against self digestion (105). The cardiovascular system also breaks down upon sustained activation (106). The media part of the wall in the arteries become irreversibly damaged in mice subjected to psychosocial situations which are difficult to control (107). These mice develop hypertension, and heart infarctions have also been produced in this and other species in similar situations. The psychological situation seems characterized by several common variables, either a highly threatening situation with poor means of control, or at least poor feedback as in the celebrated "executive" monkey study by Brady, Porter, Conrad and Mason (108), combined with a high response demand (73, 105). Lack of sleep and rest may also be important factors (109).

The CNS itself shows biochemical changes in rats that are unable to control their situation (64). These changes occur in the monoamine systems which probably are involved in depression and in schizophrenia (91). Even the immune systems show changes in situations with poor coping possibilities (76, Ballieux this volume), which in turn, affects the resistance to infections and tumor growth (110, 111). This may also take place in humans (112).

Weiss has made the most detailed model for the animal studies, in his case for the ulceration model. According to him ulcerations occur when rats have poor response feedback, and high task demands (see Figure 4). This model shows a remarkable correspondence to similar models from epidemiological psychosocial research in humans (113, 114), covering a large number of occupations.

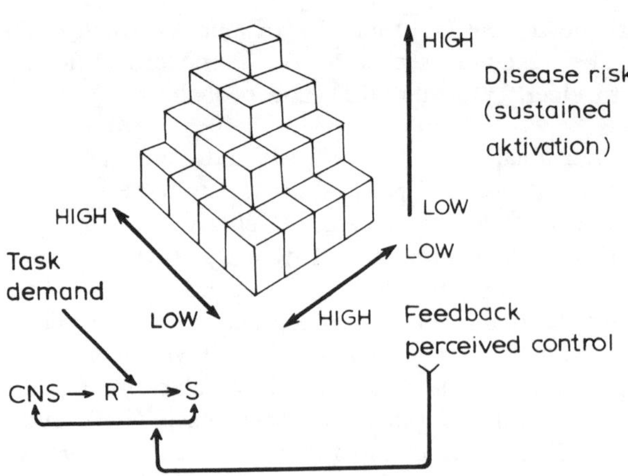

Figure 4. Disease risk, task demand and feedback of information (control) in animals and men.

Figure 4 suggest that the dimensions involved are orthogonal (independent) factors, but this is not a necessary assumption. The important thing is that there are two axes, which we will refer to as task-demand and control. In situations where $SV - AV \neq 0$, and with high numeric A-value for the variables or motivational systems involved, sustained activation may occur if *SV and/or AV* are incorrigible. If the individual then is unable to uncouple this motivational system, sustained activation may be the result, with its possible relation to pathology. Finally, sustained activation may be produced by poor response feedback (73), as for instance in the Sidman avoidance situation. In this situation the animal that formally has control over the situation develops psychosomatic symptoms.

"Sustained activation," therefore, is an acceptable pathophysiological mechanism for psychosomatic disease. There is a brain substrate, and reasonably well known peripheral mechanisms to explain the psychosomatic contribution to somatic disease. There is no organ specificity in this model, and the contribution from the brain mechanisms must be assumed to be additive or interacting with other pathophysiological mechanisms. This model, therefore, is compatible with contemporary views of disease as a multi-causal event.

Conclusion

For the relationship between the external world and the internal state of an individual these "soft" terms seem to be useful, in my opinion even necessary for the understanding of the processes underlying psychsomatic complaints and psychosomatic disease. But the use of such terms is treacherous if they are not strictly defined. The definitions offered in this paper may not be the best, and they are definitely not the only possible or proper definitions. However, they are at least defined in a way which should make it possible for readers to decide what the definitions are, and whether or not it agrees with the readers' preferences.

References

1. Wiener, N. (1961). Cybernetics. Wiley, N.Y.
2. Toates, F. (1975). Control theory in biology and experimental psychology. Hutchinson Educational Ltd., London.
3. Mason, J.W. (1971). A re-evaluation of the concept of "non-specificity" in stress theory. J. Psychiat. Res., 8: 323-335.
4. Ursin, H., Baade, E. & Levine, S. (Eds.) (1978). Psychobiology of stress: A study of coping men. Academic Press, N.Y.
5. Locke, S.E. & Hornig-Rohan, M. (1983). Mind and immunity. Institute for the Advancement of Health, N.Y.
6. Kamin, L.J. (1969). Predictability, surprise, attention and conditioning. In B.A. Campbell & R.M. Church (Eds.), Punishment and aversive behavior. Appleton-Century-Crofts, N.Y., p. 279-296.
7. Rescorla, R.A. & Wagner, A.R. (1972). A theory of Pavlovian conditioning: Variations in the effectiveness of reinforcement and nonreinforcement. In A.H. Black & W.F. Prokasy (Eds.), Classical conditioning II: Current research and theory. Appleton-Century-Crofts, N.Y., p. 64-99.
8. Mackintosh, N.J. (1974). The psychology of animal learning. Academic Press, London.
9. Dickinson, A. (1980). Contemporary animal learning theory. Cambridge University Press, Cambridge.
10. Bolles, R.C. (1972). Reinforcement, expectancy and learning. Psychol. Rev., 79: 394-409.
11. Rescorla, R.A. & Solomon, R.L. (1967). Two-process learning theory: Relationships between Pavlovian conditioning and instrumental learning. Psychol. Rev., 74: 151-182.
12. Mowrer, O.H. (1960). Learning theory and behavior. Wiley, N.Y.
13. Gray, J.A. (1975). Elements of a two-process theory of learning. Academic Press, London.
14. Konorski, J. (1967). Integrative activity of the brain. University of Chicago Press, Chicago.
15. Seligman, M.E.P. (1975). Helplessness: On depression, development and death. Freeman, San Francisco.
16. Overmier, J.B., Patterson, J. & Wielkiewicz, R.M. (1980). Environmental contingencies as sources of stress in animals. In S. Levine & H. Ursin (Eds.), Coping and health. Plenum Press, N.Y., p. 1-38.
17. Irwin, F.W. (1971). Intentional behavior and motivation. J.B. Lippincott, Philadelphia.
18. McNamara, J.M. & Houston, A.I. (1980). The application of statistical decision theory to animal behaviour. J. Theor. Biol., 85: 673-690.
19. McFarland, D.J. (Ed.) (1982). Functional ontogeny. Pitman, London.
20. Vollmer, F. (1978). Motivational and physiological arousal. In H. Ursin, E. Baade & S. Levine (Eds.), Psychobiology of stress: A study of coping men. Academic Press, N.Y.
21. Coover, G.D. (1983). Positive and negative expectancies: The rat's reward environment and pituitary-adrenal activity. In H. Ursin & R. Murison (Eds.), Biological and psychological basis of psychosomatic disease. Pergamon Press, Oxford, p. 45-60.
22. Hull, C.L. (1943). Principles of behavior. Appleton-Century-Crofts, N.Y.
23. Premack, D. (1959). Toward empirical behavior laws: I. Positive reinforcement. Psychol. Rev., 66. 219-233.
24. Malone, J.C. (1975). The „paradigms" of learning. Psychol. Record, 25: 479-489.
25. Amsel, A. (1958). The role of frustrative nonreward in non-continous reward situations. Psychol. Bull., 55: 102-119.
26. Coover, G.D., Goldman, L. & Levine, S. (1971). Plasma corticosterone increases produced by extinction of operant behavior in rats. Physiol. Behav., 6: 261-263.
27. Malmo, R.B. (1966). Studies of anxiety: Some clinical origins of the activation concept. In C.D. Spielberger (Ed.), Anxiety and behavior. Academic Press, N.Y., p. 157-177.
28. McFarland, D.J. (1975). Motivational control systems analysis. Academic Press, N.Y.
29. Atkinson, J.W. & Feather, N.T. (1966). A theory of achievement motivation. Wiley, N.Y.
30. Amsel, A. & Work, M.S. (1961). The role of learned factors in "spontaneous" activity. J. Comp. Physiol. Psychol., 54: 527-532.
31. Sheffield, F.D. & Campbell, B.A. (1954). The role of experience in the "spontaneous" activity of hungry rats. J. Comp. Physiol. Psychol., 47: 97-100.
32. Ingram, D.L., Dauncey, M.J., Barrand, M.A. & Callingham, B.A. (1980). Variations in plasma catecholamines in the young pig in response to extremes of ambient temperature compared with exercise and feeding. In E. Usdin, R. Kvetnansky & I.J. Kopin (Eds.),

Catecholamines and stress: Recent advances. Elsevier, N.Y.
33. Kato, H., Saito, M. & Suda, M. (1980). Effect of starvation on the circadian adrenocortical rhythm in rats. Endocrinology, 106: 918-921.
34. Coover, G.D., Heybach, J.P., Lenz, J. & Miller, J.F. (1979).Corticosterone "basal levels" and response to ether anesthesia in rats on a water deprivation regimen. Physiol. Behav., 22: 653-656.
35. Coover, G.D., Murison, R., Sundberg, H., Jellestad, F. & Ursin, H. (1984). Plasma corticosterone and meal expectancy in rats: Effects of low probability cues. Physiol. Behav., 33: 179-184.
36. Goldman, L., Coover, G.D. & Levine, S. (1973). Bidirectional effects of reinforcement shifts on pituitary-adrenal activity. Physiol. Behav., 10: 209-214.
37. Coover, G.D., Sutton, B.R. & Heybach, J.P. (1977). Conditioning decreases in plasma corticosterone levels in rats by pairing stimuli with daily feedings. J. Comp. Physiol. Psychol., 91: 716-726.
38. Levine, S. & Coover, G.D. (1976). Environmental control of suppression of the pituitary-adrenal system. Physiol. Behav., 17: 35-37.
39. Crespi, L.P. (1942). Quantitative variations of incentive and performance in the white rat. Am. J. Psychol., 55: 467-517.
40. Shanab, M.E. & Cavallaro, G. (1975). Positive contrast obtained in rats following a shift in schedule, delay, and magnitude of reward. Bull. Psychosom. Soc., 5: 109-112.
41. McHose, J.H. & Moore, J.N. (1976). Expectancy, salience and habit: A noncontextual interpretation of the effects of changes in the conditions of reinforcement on simple instrumental responses. Psychol. Rev., 83: 292-307.
42. Pribram, K.H. & McGuinness, D. (1975). Arousal, activation and effort in the control of attention. Psychol. Rev., 82: 116-149.
43. Spence, J.T. & Spence, K.W. (1966). The motivational components of manifest anxiety: Drive and drive stimuli. In C.D. Spielberger (Ed.), Anxiety and behavior. Academic Press, N.Y., p. 291-326.
44. Ursin, R. (1980). Deactivation, sleep and serotonergic functions. In M. Koukkou, D. Lehmann & J. Angst (Eds.), Functional states of the brain: Their determinants. Elsevier, Amsterdam.
45. Coover, G.D., Welle, S. & Hart, R.P. (1980). Effects of eating, meal cues, and ventromedial hypothalamic lesions on serum corticosterone, glucose and free fatty acid concentration. Physiol. Behav., 25: 641-651.
46. Fishburn, P. (1970). Utility theory for decisionmaking. Wiley, N.Y..
47. Tversky, A. & Kahneman, D. (1981). The framing of decisions and the psychology of choice. Science, 211: 453-458.
48. Kukla, A. (1972). Foundations of an attributional theory of performance. Psychol. Rev., 79: 454-470.
49. Feather, N.T. & Simon, J.G. (1973). Fear of success and causal attribution for outcome. J. Pers., 41: 525-542.
50. Meyer, W.U. (1973). Leistungsmotiv und Ursachenerklärung von Erfolg und Misserfolg. Klett, Stuttgart.
51. Seligman, M.E.P., Maier, S.F. & Solomon, R.L. (1971). Unpredictable and uncontrollable aversive events. In F.R. Brush (Ed.), Aversive conditioning and learning. Academic Press, N.Y., p. 347-400.
52. Badia, P., Harsh, J. & Abbott, B. (1979). Choosing between predictable and unpredictable shock conditions: Data and theory. Psychol. Bull., 86: 1107-1131.
53. Monat, A., Averill, J.R. & Lazarus, R.S. (1972). Anticipatory stress and coping reactions under various conditions of uncertainty. J. Pers. Soc. Psychol., 24: 237-253.
54. Pervin, L.A. (1963). The need to predict and control under conditions of threat. J. Exp. Psychol., 31: 570-585.
55. Weinberg, J. & Levine, S. (1980). Psychobiology of coping in animals. The effects of predictability. In S. Levine & H. Ursin (Eds.), Coping and health. Plenum Press, N.Y.
56. Dess, N.K., Linwick, D., Patterson, J., Overmier, J.B. & Levine, S. (1983). Immediate and proactive effects of controllability and predictability on plasma cortisol responses to shocks in dogs. Behav. Neurosci., 97: 1005-1016.
57. Haan, N. (1978). Coping and defending. Academic Press, N.Y.
58. Miller, S.M. (1980). When is a little information a dangerous thing? Coping with stressful events by monitoring versus blunting. In S. Levine & H. Ursin (Eds.), Coping and health. Plenum Press, N.Y., p. 145-169.
59. Kragh, U. (1960). The defense mechanism test: A new method for diagnosis and personnel selection. J. Appl. Psychol., 44: 303-309.

60. Vaernes, R.J. (1982). The defense mechanism test predicts inadequate performance under stress. Scand. J. Psychol., 23: 37-43.
61. Lazarus, R.S. (1966). Psychological stress and the coping process. McGraw-Hill, N.Y.
62. Moos, R.H. & Billings, A.G. (1982). Conceptualizing and measuring coping rescources and processes. In L. Goldberger & S. Breznitz (Eds.), Handbook of stress. Theoretical and clinical aspects. Free Press, N.Y., p. 212-230.
63. Coover, G.D., Ursin, H. & Levine, S. (1973). Plasma-corticosterone levels during active-avoidance learning in rats. J. Comp. Physiol. Psychol., 82: 170-174.
64. Anisman, H. (1978). Neurochemical changes elicted by stress. Behavioral correlates. In H. Anisman & G. Bignami (Eds.), Psychopharmacology of aversively motivated behavior. Plenum Press, N.Y.
65. Levine, S. (1980). A coping model of mother-infant relationships. In S. Levine & H. Ursin (Eds.), Coping and health. Plenum Press, N.Y., p. 87-99.
66. Levine, S., Weinberg, J. & Ursin, H. (1978). Definition of the coping process and statement of the problem. In H. Ursin, E. Baade & S. Levine (Eds.), Psychobiology of stress: A study of coping men. Academic Press, N.Y.
67. Folkman, S. & Lazarus, R.W. (1980). An analysis of coping in a middle-age community sample. J. Health Soc. Behav., 21: 219-239.
68. Bandura, A. (1982). Self-efficacy mechanisms in human agency. Am. Psychol., 37: 122-147.
69. Rotter, J.B. (1966). Generalized expectancies for internal control of reinforcement. Psychol. Monogr., 80: 609.
70. Pearlin, L.I., Lieberman, M.A., Menaghan, E.G. & Mullen, J.T. (1981). The stress process. J. Health Soc. Behav., 22: 337-356.
71. Hendrick, I. (1943). The discussion of the "instinct to master." Psychoanal. Q., 12: 561-565.
72. White, R.W. (1959). Motivation reconsidered: The concept of competence. Psychol. Rev., 66: 297-333.
73. Weiss, J.M. (1972). Influence of psychiological variables on stress-induced pathology. In R. Porter & J. Knight (Eds.), Physiology. Emotion and psychosomatic illness. CIBA Foundation Symposium 8. Elsevier, Amsterdam.
74. Tsuda, A., Tanaka, M., Nishikawa, T. & Hirai, H. (1983). Effects of coping behavior on gastric lesions in rats as a function of the complexity of coping tasks. Physiol. Behav., 30: 805-808.
75. Hunt, H.F. & Brady, J.V. (1955). Some effects of punishment and intercurrent "anxiety" on a simple operant. J. Comp. Physiol. Psychol., 48: 305-310.
76. Sklar, L.S. & Anisman, H. (1980). Social stress influences tumor growth. Psychosom. Med., 42: 347-365.
77. Folkman, S. (1984). Personal control and stress and coping processes: A theoretical analysis. J. Pers. Soc. Psychol., 46: 838-852.
78. Murison, R.C.C. (1983). Time course of plasma corticosterone under immobilisation stress in rats. IRCS Med. Sci., 11: 20-21.
79. Rabkin, J.G. & Struening, E.L. (1976). Life events, stress and illness. Science, 194: 1013-1020.
80. Pavlov, I.P. (1926). Conditioned reflexes. Oxford, reprinted: Dover (1960), N.Y.
81. Masserman, J.H. (1943). Behavior and neurosis. University of Chicago, Chicago.
82. Mineka, S. & Kihlstrom, J.F. (1978). Unpredictable and uncontrollable events: A new perspective on experimental neurosis. J. Abnorm. Psychol., 87: 256-271.
83. Mowrer, O.H. & Viek, P. (1948). An experimental analogue of fear from a sense of helplessness. J. Abnorm. Psychol., 43: 193-200.
84. Overmier J.B. & Seligman, M.E.P. (1967). Effects of inescapable shock upon subsequent escape and avoidance responding. J. Comp. Physiol. Psychol., 63: 28-33.
85. Lewinsohn, P.M. (1974). Clinical and theoretical aspects of depression. In K.S. Calhoun, H.E. Adams & K.M. Mitchell (Eds), Innovative treatment methods in psychopathology. Wiley , N.Y.
86. Hiroto, D.S. & Seligman, M.E.P. (1975). Generality of learned helplessness in man. J. Pers. Soc. Psychol., 31: 311-327.
87. Erickson, R.C., Post, R.D. & Paige, A.B. (1975). Hope as a psychiatric variable. J. Clin. Psychol., 31: 324-330.
88. Prociuk, T.J., Breen, L.J. & Lussier, R.J. (1976). Hopelessness, internal-external locus of control and depression. J. Clin. Psychol., 32: 299-300.
89. Beck, A.T. (1967). Depression: Clinical, experimental and theoretical aspects. Hoeber, N.Y.
90. Blaney, P.H. (1977). Contemporary theories of depression: Critique and comparison. J. Abnorm. Psychol., 86: 203-223.
91. Coover, G.D., Ursin, H. & Murison, R. (1983). Sustained activation and psychiatric illness.

In H. Ursin & R. Murison (Eds.), Biological and psychological basis of psychosomatic diesease. Pergamon Press, Oxford.
92. Forrest, M.S. & Hokanson, J.E. (1975). Depression and autonomic arousal reduction accompanying self-punitive behavior. J. Abnorm. Psychol., 84: 346-357.
93. Coyne, J.C. (1976). Toward an interactional description of depression. Psychiatry, 39: 28-40.
94. Ursin, H. (1980). Personality, activation and somatic health: A new psychosomatic theory. In S. Levine and H. Ursin (Eds.), Coping and health. Plenum Press, N.Y., p. 259-279.
95. Hansen, J.R., Stoa, K.F., Blix, A.S. & Ursin, H. (1978). Urinary levels of epinephrine and norepinephrine in parachutist trainees. In H. Ursin, E. Baade, & S. Levine (Eds.), Coping men - A study in human psychobiology. Academic Press, San Franscio, p. 63-74.
96. Blix, A.S., Stromme, S.B. & Ursin, H. (1974). Additional heart rate - an indicator of psychological activation. Aerosp. Med., 45: 1219-1222.
97. Stromme, S., Wikeby, P., Blix, A.S. & Ursin, H. (1978). Additonal heart rate. In H. Ursin, E. Baade & S. Levine (Eds.), Psychobiology of stress. A study of coping men. Academic Press, N.Y.
98. Ursin, H., Grahnstedt, S., Walther, B., Opstad, P., Myhre, K. & Andersen, H. (1983). Attention, performance and sustained activation in air traffic controllers. AGARD Conference Proceedings No. 338, 22.1-22.10.
99. Davidson, J.M., Smith, E.R. & Levine, S. (1978). Testosterone. In H. Ursin, E. Baade & S. Levine (Eds.), Psychobiology of stress. A study of coping men. Academic Press, N.Y., p. 57-61.
100. Ursin, H. (1978). Activation, coping and psychosomatics. In H. Ursin, E. Baade & S. Levine (Eds.), Psychobiology of stress. A study of coping men. Academic Press, N.Y., p. 201-228.
101. Arnetz, B. (1984). The potential role of Þsychosocial stress on levels of hemoglobin Alc(HbA1C) and fasting plasma glucose in eldery people. J. Geront., 39: 424-429.
102. Ursin, H. & Murison, R. (Eds.) (1983). Biological and psychological basis of psychosomatic disease. Pergamon, Oxford.
103. Levine, S., Madden, J., Conner, R.L., Moskal, J.R. & Anderson, D.C. (1973). Physiological and behavioral effects of prior aversive stimulation (preshock) in the rat. Physiol. Behav., 10: 467-471.
104. Murison, R.C.C. & Isaksen, E. (1982). Gastric ucleration and adrenocortical activity after inescapable and escapable pre-shock in rats. Scand. J. Psychol., Suppl. 1: 133-137.
105. Murison, R. & Isaksen, E. (1983). Biological and psychological bases of gastric ulceration. In H. Ursin & R. Murison (Eds.), Biological and psychological basis of psychosomatic disease. Pergamon Press, Oxford, p. 239-248.
106. Ursin, H. & Knardahl, S. (1985). Personality factors, neuroendocrine response patterns, and cardiovascular pathology. In G. Mulder & J.F. van Doornen (Eds.), Psychophysiology of cardiovascular control. Models. Plenum Press, N.Y.
107. Henry, J.P. & Stephens, P.M. (1977). Stress, health and the social environment. A sociobiologic approach to medicine. Springer, N.Y.
108. Brady, J.V., Porter, R.W., Conrad, D.G. & Mason, J.W. (1958). Avoidance behavior and the development of gastroduodenal ulcers. J. Exp. Anal. Behav., 1: 69-72.
109. Murison, R., Ursin, R., Coover, G.D., Lien, W. & Ursin, H. (1982). Sleep deprivation procedure produces stomach lesions in rats. Physiol. Behav., 29: 693-694.
110. Riley, V. (1981). Psychoneuroendocrine infuences on immuncompetence and neoplasia. Science, 212: 1100-1109.
111. Ader, R. (Ed.) (1981). Psychoneuroimmunology. Academic Press, N.Y.
112. Ursin, H., Mykletun, R., Isaksen, E., Murison, R., Vaernes, R. & Tonder, O. (1983). Immunoglobulins as a stress marker? In R.E. Ballieux, I.F. Fielding & A. L'Abbate (Eds.), Breakdown in human adaptation to "stress." Towards a multidisciplinary approach. Nijhoff, Boston, p. 681-690.
113. Gardell, B. (1977). Psychological and social problems of industrial work in affluent societies. Int. J. Psychol., 12: 125-134.
114. Karasek, R.A.Jr. (1979). Job demands, job decision latitude and mental strain: Implications for job redesign. Adm. Sci. Quart., 24: 285-308.

Adrenocortical Activity and Disease, with References to Gastric Pathology in Animals

Robert Murison and J. Bruce Overmier

Since the work of Selye and Mason, adrenocortical activity has been accepted as one of the major indices of the stress response. Activation of the hypothalamo-pituitary-adrenocortical axis is observed whenever the organism is subjected to a new unexpected stimulus situation, in response to certain expectancy cues (1), or in response to fear-inducing stimuli such as shock. Ursin (this volume) defines stress in terms of central activation, and, since adrenocortical output is controlled by central mechanisms, corticosterone levels should be a good index of the animal's stress response. To recapitulate Ursin, stress becomes pathological when it is sustained.

Another index of the stress response according to Selye is gastrointestinal bleeding (gastric mucosal erosions) which has similarities to but is not necessarily identical to peptic ulcer in man, one of the so-called classical psychosomatic disorders (2). Whether the phenomenon of gastric erosions in animals is identical to the ulcer phenomenon in man is a question we shall not dwell on here. Glavin (this volume) has already mentioned the desired criteria for stress ulcer models.

It has often been suggested or assumed that elevated levels of circulating corticosterone might cause gastric bleeding, and that these two stress indices are in some way causally linked. Review of some of the evidence for such a uniform stress model is now given, examining which behavioral situations yield either one of these stress responses, how they might relate to each other, and the evidence that high adrenocortical activity in itself might be pathological.

The most striking evidence for a close relationship between the excretion of endogenous corticosteroids and the development of gastric erosions followed a series of experiments by Weiss (3-5). Briefly, Weiss (3) demonstrated that the severity of shock-induced gastric lesions was modulated by the ability of the animal to do something about the aversive shock, either by escaping or avoiding the shock stimulus. Those animals who were able to perform a *simple* coping response developed less severe gastric erosions than animals unable to control the shock delivery, although the amount of shock (duration and intensity) received by the two groups was identical. Addition of a discrete warning signal reduced the severity of erosions in rats both with and without the availability

The work reported in this paper was supported by the Norwegian Research Council for Science and the Humanities. J.B. Overmier's participation was supported in part by a fellowship from the J.E. Fogarty Center for Advanced Study in the Health Sciences (FO-TW00976) and awards from the James McKeen Cattell Foundation and the Bush Foundation.

of an avoidance/escape response. Moreover, in both conditions the severity of gastric erosions was positively correlated to plasma corticosterone levels at the end of the 48-hour test session (5). Complementary to this, animals learning an avoidance task exhibit a reduction of plasma corticosterone levels after learning (6, 7), a phenomenon sometimes referred to as "coping." In addition, Weiss (4) reported that rats subjected to predictable uncontrollable shock for five or ten hours exhibited less severe gastric erosions and lower plasma corticosterone levels than rats subjected to similar amounts of unpredictable shock.

Complementary to these correlational data, Murphy et al. (8) demonstrated that rats with lesions of the hippócampus, a structure rich in corticosterone receptors, developed more severe gastric erosions and higher levels of plasma corticosterone than unlesioned control animals during a five hour simple restraint stress, or restraint combined with intermittent shock. Furthermore, the severity of the gastric erosions correlated with circulating levels of corticosterone.

Other ulcerogenic stress situations are also associated with high adrenocortical output, including restraint (9), 24-hour sleep deprivation using the classical flower-pot technique (10), immersion stress (11) and treatment of animals with corticosterone at high doses over long periods can result in gastric erosions (12, but see also 13). Brodie and Hanson (14) however reported increases in restraint-induced gastric erosions severity after adrenalectomy (but not hypophysectomy), suggesting that at least some adrenal output is protective in the face of challenge.

The kind of study referred to above has employed relatively long (5-72-hours) stress sessions, with corticosterone being measured at the end of the session at the same time as the ulcers are assessed, that is *after* the ulcerative process has been activated for some time. This type of model seems to be inappropriate in that such long-lasting severe stress is an uncommon phenomenon in real life. Rather, life is a stream of events, some of which m^a^ght be perceived by the organism as stressful, and others not, some giving rise to high adrenocortical secretion, and others not. What is interesting is how these cycles of precursor events and the stressfulness of them may have proactive effects on the response to later stressful experiences, both in terms of adrenocortical activation and gastrointestinal pathology.

Proactive Effects of Stressors on Adrenocortical Secretion and Gastric Erosions

Levine et al. (15) demonstrated that animals subjected to a single uncontrollable 3-minute shock each day for 5 days increased the animals' adrenocortical response to the mild stressor of exposure to an open field several days after the last shock experience. Murison and Isaksen (14, exp. 1) later demonstrated that, using exactly the same "preshock" procedures as Levine et al., rats could be made more susceptible to the development of gastric erosions under a 20-hour restraint stress ten days after the last of 5 pre-shock experiences. It thus appeared that animals known to respond with a higher than normal adrenocortical output in response to a mild stressor (open field exposure) were more likely to develop more severe gastric pathology disease under exposure to a strong stressor (restraint). In these data, there were no correlations or between group differences which could indicate any relationship between erosion severity and corticosterone levels at the end of the 20-hour restraint stress session.

Given the demonstrated importance of behavioral control in modulating the immediate ulcerogenic and adrenocortical consequences of shock, Murison and Isaksen in a second experiment in that series (16) exposed animals to a series of either 20 escapable or 20 inescapable (yoked) shocks for five days prior to the application of the 20-hour restraint stress. The animals which had earlier been able to escape shock, developed less severe and fewer gastric erosions under the restraint stress than did (1) the animals exposed to inescapable shock *and* (2) less severe and fewer erosions than animals which had not been pre-exposed to shock at all. In this experiment, the post-stress corticosterone levels mirrored the ulceration data; the previously escaping animals showed lower corticosterone levels at the end of the restraint period than non-escaping (yoked) animals or unshocked animals. The last-mentioned study, together with the original Weiss data, suggested importantly that providing animals with the experience of a coping response has not only immediate alleviating effects on both gastric erosions and corticosterone secretion but also proactive effects.

Within the psychological literature, there has been some discussion as to whether the beneficial effects of control over an aversive stimulus arise from control per se, or from the feedback (safety-signals) afforded by the termination of the stimulus (17, 18). In a conceptually similar study to the above, we therefore examined the effects of Pavlovian backward conditioning on the later response to restraint stress. Backward conditioning means that the animal is presented with a series of shock-signal pairings, with the signal being presented at the end of each shock period, much like an escape response signals the end of the shock period. Such a procedure results in lower corticosterone secretion than does similar inescapable shocks without the backward signal (19), presumably because the animal learns that the signal provides information about a safe period after every shock.

Following five daily sessions of 20 backward conditioning trials, our animals were subjected to the 20-hour restraint stress one week later. During conditioning, we used shock latencies, durations and inter-shock intervals generated by the escaping animals in the Murison and Isaksen (16) experiment. As expected, previous experience in the backward conditioning procedure led to less severe gastric erosions after 20 hours of restraint than was the case for animals previously subjected to either no shock or random presentations of shocks and signals. To our surprise however, and contrary to the results from the escape experiment, the group which showed the least gastric erosions post stress (the backward conditioning group), also exhibited the highest corticosterone levels at the end of the restraint period, although the overall correlation over groups between corticosterone and erosions was essentially zero. These data suggest that while coping behaviors might have a general positive proactive transfer effect, safety signals may result in more limited effects, in this case ameliorating ulceration severity, but in fact increasing the adrenocortical response to the later restraint stress. These results on *proactive* effects of backward conditioning procedures are therefore opposite to those of Hennessy et al. (19), looking at *immediate* effects on corticosterone.

These last experiments focused on the effects of prior exposure to one stressor on the ulcerogenic and adrenocortical responses to a new stressor. In a further study on proactive phenomena, we were interested in how repeated exposure to the *same* stressor - in this case partial immersion in water (19° C) combined with restraint (immersion stress) - might affect responses to a final similar stressor session. Earlier studies have indicated that the mortality of wild rats in the face of a cold-swim stressor is dependent on previous experience with that particular stressor (20), and Zigmond and Harvey (21) have reported modulation of neurochemical effects and mortality of rats under lethal shock exposure by previous experience with the same stressor. We exposed animals to either one or four, long (2 hours) or short (30 minutes) pre-exposures to an immersion stress prior to a final immersion stress session (75 minutes) after which the animals were killed. The corticosterone and ulceration data showed different effects of these treatments on the two indices of the stress response.

For gastric erosions, one prior exposure, but not four, yielded some protection against erosions under the final stress session. For corticosterone on the other hand, those animals receiving four but not one prior exposure exhibited lower corticosterone levels when compared to animals given no pre-exposure. This would seem to indicate that corticosterone response levels can develop "tolerance" after five sessions of water-restraint, but that the ulcerogenic response becomes sensitized. Since the outcomes of our manipulations were opposite for these two indices of stress, we ran a correlation between them, yielding a significant negative correlation, $r_s = -0.55$, $p < 0.05$. These data imply a more complex interaction between these stress indices than hitherto has been considered.

The Post-Stressor "Rest" Phenomenon

So far we have outlined some experiments in which proactive effects of one stressor were examined on corticosterone and erosions after a final stressor. A number of workers have shown that allowing the animals a period in their home cage ("rest" or "recovery" period) after the removal from the stressful situation prior to the assessment of gastric pathology significantly augments the ulcerogenic effects of the stressor, be the stressor shock (22), restraint (23), or water immersion (24).

It had been argued that the post-stress phenomenon is related to changes in the balance between the sympathetic and parasympathetic components of autonomic nervous activity. That is to say, the animal's response to restraint stress is primarily sympathetically dominated, associated with reduced gastric secretions and sympathetically induced vasoconstriction. After removal from the stressful immobilization experience, it is argued that there follows a period where the parasympathetic system dominates, associated with an increase in gastric secretions which may injure an already weakened mucosa (see 25 for discussion). Corroborative evidence is supported by the finding that treatment with rats during the post-stress period scopolamine significantly reduces severity of supine-restraint induced erosions (26).

In two recent experiments, Murison and Overmier undertook to explore how the two factors, previous experience with stress and post-stress rest, might interact with respect to their effects on adrenocortical activity and gastric pathology. In the first experiment, presenting animals during a post-immersion stress period with a signal (CS) previously associated with fear (shock) should increase the influence of the sympathetic system on the stomach, and should therefore modulate the *putative* parasympathetic rebound. Animals were therefore subjected to a conditioning procedure in which a series of 80 explicit tone-shock pairings were presented, two days before exposure to a short (2 hours) immersion stress. During a 2 hour post-stress period, some of the animals were again presented repeatedly with the stimulus previously associated with shock. Other animals were allowed to recover from the immersion stress without presentation of the previously aversive stimulus, while a third group of animals did not receive the initial preconditioning procedure but were presented with the, for them, neutral signal during recovery.

The ulceration data were contrary to our initial expectation, in that animals re-exposed to the danger cues after removal from the immersion stress developed *more*, not less, severe gastric erosions than the other animals. Of interest in the present context was the finding that that group of animals which were re-exposed to the danger signal and developed the *most* severe erosions *also* exhibited the *lowest* levels of adrenocortical activity during the post-immersion stress phase. In the three groups of animals described above, the overall correlation between plasma corticosterone levels and severity of gastric erosions was computed to be -0.65, $p<0.05$, suggesting that the extent of ulceration was *not* positively related to sustained corticosterone levels, but the opposite. The direction of the correlation within each of these three groups was also negative. While these data do not support the parasympathetic rebound hypothesis, they do again indicate a complex relationship between adrenocortical activity and gastric pathology.

At the risk of overstating the point, the data presented above strongly argue against a simple relationship between corticosterone and gastric erosions. Not only is there not always the type of positive correlation which would be expected from the earlier literature, thereby negating any simple causal relationship, there are under some circumstances negative correlations, which do not imply independence of the two measures, but an inverse relationship.

A Role for Corticosterone in Gastric Erosions - For and Against

The data described above were collected primarily to cast light on those psychological factors which might influence severity of stress-induced gastric erosions, but the data also cast some unusual and unexpected light on the relationship between adrenocortical activity and gastric pathology. Logically, we can conceive of three possible relations between corticosterone levels and severity of gastric erosions. First, that there is no direct relationship between these two dependent variables; second, that there is *always* a negative relationship, inferring either an inhibitory relationship, or consecutive control mechanisms for both; third, that there is *always* a positive relationship, inferring either a causal relationship, or at least control mechanisms which function together.

The bulk of the physiological/pharmacological literature supports an exacerbatory role for corticosterone in erosions. Apart from the ulcerogenic effects of treatment with corticosterone referred to above (12), corticoids have been reported to impair the healing of surgically induced ulcers (27). In addition, corticosterone has been seen to act as a permissive factor in the sympathetically-induced vasoconstriction associated with the stress response (28), which is also thought to play a role in the initial stages of ulcerogenesis (25). Furthermore, corticosterone is believed to inhibit the production and secretion of prostaglandins, which have been used to alleviate gastric pathology, possibly by strengthening the mucosal barrier or improving secretion of hydrocarbonate ions (29). The present state of our knowledge about prostaglandins seems inadequate, but it would appear reasonable to argue that these substances act to protect the organism from the damaging effects of stress exposure, but their release and effectiveness may be inhibited by high adrenocortical secretions.

The release of corticosterone from the adrenal cortex is permitted by release of ACTH from the pituitary gland, which in turn is controlled by the release of CRF (corticotropin releasing factor). Apart from its action on the anterior pituitary, CRF is also reported to bring about increased sympathetic activation when administered i.c.v. In addition CRF (i.c.v.) results in an inhibition of gastric secretion (30), which might be an important permissive factor in the development of immersion-induced gastric pathology. The effects of CRF on gastric secretion appear to be dependent on an intact adrenal gland, but not dependent on either an intact vagus or pituitary-adrenal system. This infers an important role in gastric secretion inhibition for the sympathetic innervation of the adrenal gland.

Pain, Conditioning, Opiates and Erosions

The physiological and pharmacological data point to either an exacerbatory or modulatory role for corticosterone in ulceration, while the data from psychological manipulations seem to indicate that the role might be excitatory under one set of circumstances (5, 8) and inhibitory under another (see above), allowing a fourth hypothesis: That corticosterone and severity of gastric erosions are not independent, but that the relationship between these two variables may not be fixed. A possible explanation for this puzzling phenomenon might be found in the heretofore unconnected field of stress-induced analgesia.

Under particular circumstances, exposure of animals to uncontrollable electric shock provides the animal with an analgesia which is reinstated when the animal is re-exposed to the shock 24 hours later. Those particular circumstances required are that the animal must be exposed to a certain number of shocks over a certain time period (31). This stress-induced analgesia (SIA) is reversed by treatment with naloxone and is therefore of an opiod nature (32), and can also be activated by a 30 minute restraint stress (33). To manifest SIA, it is unnecessary to re-expose the animal to the original aversive stimulus per se. It may also be reinstated by presenting the animal with a stimulus previously paired with the inducing stimulus (32, 34), that is, the effect is subject to learning in the form of classical conditioning.

Hypophysectomy abolishes the manifestation of SIA, as does treatment with dexamethasone, indicating a role for the pituitary-adrenal axis (35). Adrenalectomy also abolishes the manifestation of the SIA, whereas adrenalectomy plus corticosterone treatment can reinstate the effect, underlining a specific role for the adrenal cortex and corticosterone rather than any pituitary endorphin system. It has been suggested that the system functions such that uncontrollable shock or restraint stress leads to increases in corticosterone, which is an important factor in the rate limiting step in the production of serotonin, which in turn activates release of opioid material from the spinal cord and possibly other areas (35). It should also be remembered that endorphins are concurrently released with the secretion from the pituitary gland of ACTH.

The possible significance of this for ulceration becomes clearer when it is shown that erosions in 5-hour restrained rats may be ameliorated by morphine treatment (36), and exacerbated by treatment with the opiate antagonist naloxone. A similar picture also emerges when rats are subjected to cold supine restraint (37).

In our experiments, we have employed stress procedures which could potentially elicit some form of SIA, promoting the release of opioids and thus effecting the rate and amount of gastric secretion and gastric erosions. It should be noted that the largest concentration of opiod receptors outside the brain and central nervous system lies in the gastrointestinal tract (38).

In the experiment in which animals were pre-exposed to differing degrees of immersion stress prior to a final stressor session using the same immersion stress, a negative correlation was found between erosions and corticosterone. The highest negative correlations were found in those groups subjected to many long pre-exposures, closely followed by those subjected to many short pre-exposures. One might in speculate that the opioid releasing mechanism might in some way have become conditioned or at least sensitized during these pre-exposures so that the increased corticoid release during the final exposure would result in an elevated opioid release, reduced gastric secretions, and so lower gastric ulceration severity.

In a conditioning experiment, animals were first exposed to shock-tone pairings using similar parameters employed by others to establish SIA. After a later immersion stress, the CS was again delivered, and this procedure resulted in increased erosions, but erosions was negatively related to corticosterone. Again, a possible explanation might be found in the conditioning of SIA, reinstated by CS presentation, so that within that group the correlation should have been expected to be large and negative, which it was (-0.64) while the correlation for the animals who were not re-exposed to the CS was not significant, as was also the case for animals not subjected to the conditioning procedure at all.

Summering the data suggests that subjecting animals to prior stress procedures prior to a similar final stressor session somehow activates a mechanism whereby later stress-induced activation of the pituitary-adrenal axis has an inhibitory effect on gastric erosions induced by immersion stress, possibly via an opiod-mediated inhibition of gastric secretion. This hypothesis may be tested by manipulation of the opiod system, the serotonergic system, or the adrenocortical system. In contrast, where animals are not subjected to prior stress conditioning, generally one saw either no relationship between corticosterone and pathology, or a positive relationship. Given that the opioid hypothesis has any merit, it will still remain to explain the mechanisms by which corticosterone might have these different relationships to pathology. One might postulate here an explanation in terms of either changes in receptor sensitivity or in terms of possible dual control mechanisms for adrenocortical secretion (Fehm, this volume).

In conclusion, the original findings from Weiss should be reconsidered in the light of the present discussion. The Weiss data on the relationship between these two indices of stress are widely quoted, and together with the effects of long-term high dose treatments of corticosterone, have led many to assume a simple positive relationship, an assumption that for many has become fact. The evidence is unclear as to the exact relationship, but it is complex, and possibly open to modification by psychological manipulations.

References

1. Coover, G.D., Murison, R., Sundberg, H., Jellestad, F. & Ursin, H. (1984). Plasma corticosterone and meal expectancy in rats: Effects of low probability cues. Physiol. Behav., 33: 179-184.
2. Christie, M.J. (1981). Foundations of psychosomatics. In M.J. Christie & P.G. Mellett (Eds.), Foundations of psychosomatics. Wiley, London, pp.3-14.
3. Weiss, J.M. (1968). Effects of coping responses on stress. J. Comp. Physiol. Psychol., 65: 251-260.
4. Weiss, J.M. (1970). Somatic effects of predictable and unpredictable shock. Psychosom. Med., 32: 397-408.
5. Weiss, J.M. (1971). Effects of coping behavior in different warning signal conditions on stress pathology in rats. J. Comp. Physiol. Psychol., 77: 1-13.
6. Coover, G.D., Ursin, H. & Levine, S. (1973). Plasma corticosterone levels during active avoidance learning in rats. J. Comp. Physiol. Psychol., 82: 170-174.
7. Berger, D.F., Starzec, J.J. & Mason, E.B. (1981). The relationship between plasma corticosterone levels and lever-press avoidance vs. escape behaviors in rats. Physiol. Psychol., 9: 81-86.
8. Murphy, H.M., Wideman, C.H. & Brown, T.S. (1979). Plasma corticosterone levels and ulcer formation in rats with hippocampal lesions. Neuroendocrinology, 28: 123-130.
9. Murison, R. (1983). Time course of plasma corticosterone under immobilization stress in rats. IRCS Med. Sci., 11: 20-21.
10. Murison, R., Ursin, R., Coover, G.D., Lien, W. & Ursin, H. (1982). Sleep deprivation procedure produces stomach lesions in rats. Physiol. Behav., 29: 693-694.
11. Murison, R. & Overmier, J.B. (1986). Interactions amongst factors which influence severity of gastric ulceration in rats. Physiol. Behav., 36: 1093-1097.
12. Robert, A. & Nezamis, J.E. (1964). Histopathology of steroid-induced ulcers: An experimental study in the rat. Arch. Pathol., 77: 407-423.
13. Conn, H.O. & Blitzer, B.L. (1976). Non-association of adreno-corticosteroid therapy and peptic ulcer. New Engl. J. Med., 294: 473-479.

14. Brodie, D.A. & Hanson, H.M. (1960). A study of the factors involved in the production of gastric ulcers by the restraint technique. Gastroenterology, 38: 353-360.
15. Levine, S., Madden, J., Conner, R.L. & Anderson, D.C. (1973). Physiological and behavioral effects prior aversive stimulation (preshock) in the rat. Physiol. Behav., 10: 467-471.
16. Murison, R. & Isaksen, E. (1982). Gastric ulceration and adrenocortical activity after inescapable and escapable preshock in rats. Scand. J. Psychol., suppl. 1: 133-137.
17. Starr, M.D. & Mineka, S. (1977). Determinations of fear over the course of avoidance learning. Learn. Motiv., 4: 332-350.
18. Volpicelli, J.R., Ulm, R.R. & Altenfor, A. (1984). Feedback during exposure to inescapable shocks and subsequent shock-escape performance. Learn. Motiv., 15: 279-286.
19. Hennessy, J.W., King, M.G., McClure, T.A. & Levine, S. (1977). Uncertainty, as defined by the contingency between environmental events, and the adrenocortical response of the rat to electric shock. J. Comp. Physiol. Psychol., 91: 1447-1460.
20. Richter, C.P. (1957). On the phenomenon of sudden death in animals and man. Psychosom. Med., 19: 191-198.
21. Zigmond, M.J. & Harvey, J.A. (1970). Resistance to central NE depletion and decreased mortality in rats chronically exposed to electric footshock. J. Neuro. Visc. Relat., 31: 373-381.
22. Desiderato, O., MacKinnon, J.R. & Hissom, H. (1974). Development of gastric ulcers following stress termination. J. Comp. Physiol. Psychol., 87: 208-214.
23. Vincent, G.P. & Pare, W.P. (1982). Post-stress development and healing of supine-restraint induced gastric lesions in the rat. Physiol. Behav., 29: 721-725.
24. Overmier, J.B., Murison, R. & Ursin, H. (1986). The ulcerogenic effect of a rest period after exposure to water-restraint stress. Behav. Neural Biology, 46: 372-382.
25. Murison, R. & Isaksen, E. (1983). Biological and psychological basis of gastric ulceration. In H. Ursin & R. Murison (Eds.), Biological and psychological basis of psychosomatic disease. Pergamon Press, Oxford.
26. Glavin, G.B. (1980). Restraint ulcer: History, current research and future implications. In M.I. Grossman & D. Novin (Eds.), Experimental ulcer produced by behavioral factors. Brain Res. Bull., suppl. 1: 51-58.
27. Myhre, E. (1963). The effect of corticotropin and cortisone on the healing of gastric ulcer. In S.C. Skornya (Ed), Pathophysiology of peptic ulcer. McGill University, Montreal.
28. Zweifach, B.W., Shorr, E. & Black, M.M. (1953). The influence of the adrenal cortex on behavior of the terminal vascular bed. Ann. N.Y. Acad. Sci., 57: 626-633.
29. Allen, A. & Garner, A. (1980). Mucus and bicarbonate secretion in the stomach and their possible role in mucosal protection. Gut, 21: 249-262.
30. Taché, Y., Goto, Y., Gunion, M.W., Vale, W., River, J. & Brown, M. (1983). Inhibition of gastric acid secretion in rats by intercerebral injection of corticotropin releasing factor. Science, 222: 935-937.
31. Jackson, R.L., Maier, S.F. & Coon, D.J. (1979). Long-term analgesic effects of inescapable shock and learned helplessness. Science, 206: 91-93.
32. Maier, S.F., Sherman, J.E., Lewis, J.W., Terman, G.W. & Liebeskind, J.C. (1983). The opioid/nonopioid nature of stress-induced analgesia and learned helplessness. J. Exp. Psychol.: Animal Behavior Processes, 9: 80-90.
33. Amir, S. & Amit, Z. (1979). The pituitary gland mediates acute and chronic pain responsiveness in stressed and nonstressed rats. Life Sci., 42: 439-448.
34. Fanselow, M.S. & Bolles, R.C. (1979). Triggering of the endorphin analgesic reaction by CS previously associated with shock: Reversal with naloxone. Bull. Psychon. Soc., 14: 88-90.
35. MacLennan, A.J., Drugan, R.C., Hyson, R.L., Maier, S.F., Madden, J. & Barchas, J.D. (1982). Corticosterone: A critical factor in an opioid form of stress-induced analgesia. Science, 215: 1530-1532.
36. Arrigo-Reina, R. & Ferri, S. (1980). Evidence of an involvement of the opioid peptidergic system in the reaction to stressful conditions. Eur. J. Pharmacol., 64: 85-88.
37. Glavin, G.B. (1985). Effects of morphine and naloxone on restraint-stress ulcers in rats. Pharmacology, 31: 57-60
38. Smyth, D.G. (1984). Biosynthesis and targeting of ß-endorphin. Paper presented at the First Annual International Symposium Neuronal Control of Bodily Function - Basic and Clinical Aspects, Indianapolis.

Extrapituitary Mechanisms in the Regulation of Cortisol Secretion in Man

Horst-Lorenz Fehm, Karl Heinz Voigt and Jan Born

Figure 1 schematically depicts the complicated system controlling cortisol secretion, including its multiple- and multi-stage feedback loops. It is evident from this scheme that the brain and especially the hypothalamus plays a dominant role within this system. Despite its complexity, it represents an oversimplification in many respects. Obviously, it will be impossible to discuss all the different aspects here. Instead this section will focus on three topics only:

1) The corticosteroid feedback regulation of pituitary ACTH secretion with special reference to the importance of hypothalamic and extra-hypothalamic sites.
2) The significance of ACTH unrelated mechanisms in the regulation of cortisol secretion in man. This kind of influence has been ignored in the current conceptualization of the relationship between ACTH and cortisol.
3) The relationship between the sleep electroencephalogram and cortisol secretory bursts during sleep. This approach might help to define brain events triggering cortisol secretory bursts.

The Corticosteroid Feedback Regulation of Pituitary ACTH Secretion; Importance of Hypothalamic and Extra-Hypothalamic Sites

That adrenal corticosteroids can suppress pituitary ACTH secretion by a negative feedback was postulated already in 1947 by Sayers and Sayers (1). Since then, many experiments have tested this hypothesis. Later on, the existence of a dual corticosteroid feedback mechanism was demonstrated in the rat (2): After the administration of corticosteroids there were two periods of inhibition of stress-induced ACTH-release. The first one was brief and occurred immediately after the administration of the steroid; it was characterized by rate sensitivity and saturability. The second period of inhibition of ACTH release was much longer, did not occur until an hour after the steroid administration and was prolonged with increased dosages. These findings led us to study the kinetics of suppression of ACTH levels by corticosteroid administration in patients with ACTH hypersecretion secondary to adrenal insufficiency (Addison's disease) (3). Cortisol was administered according to different protocols which were chosen to provide extreme variations in the input signal. By this means, again two phases of suppression of ACTH levels could be differentiated. A first decrease occurred immediately whenever, and as long as, plasma cortisol levels were rising.

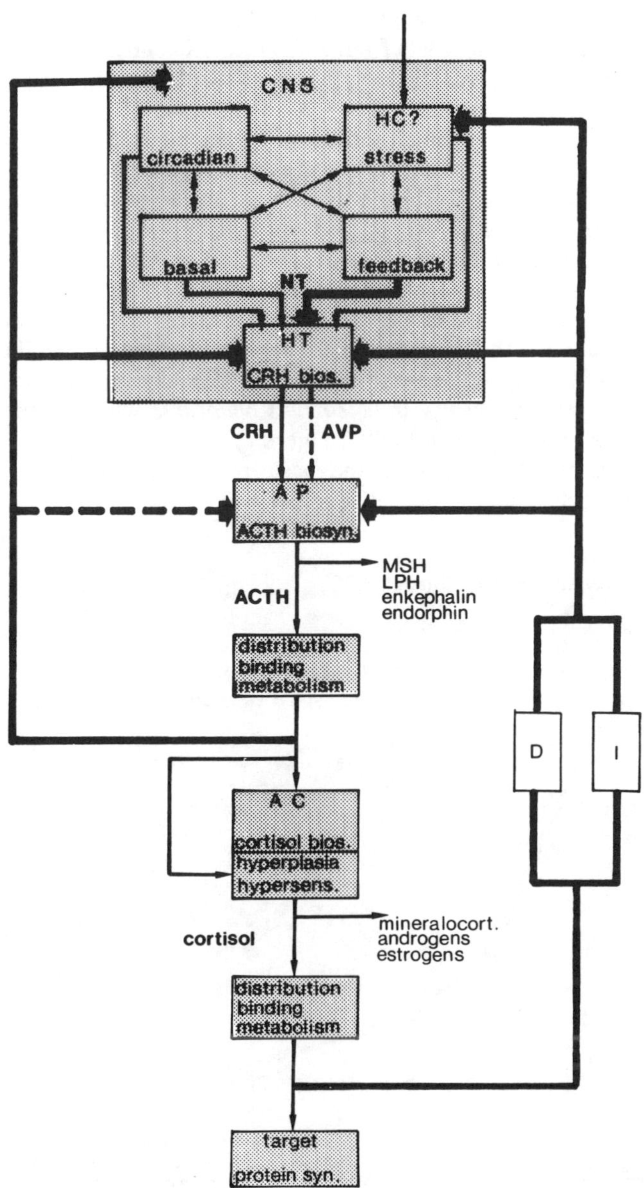

Figure 1. Schematic representation of the influences exerted by the brain on ACTH and cortisol secretion. The feedback loops are indicated by the thick lines.

The degree of suppression during this phase was correlated only to the rate in increase in cortisol, and not to absolute plasma concentrations. Therefore this mechanism was designated the differential or rate-sensitive mechanism. A second decrease in ACTH levels began after a silent period of about 30 min. In this case the degree of inhibition of ACTH levels was proportional to the cortisol dose administered (integral or dose sensitive mechanism). In sum, these findings are in accordance with the earlier data from animal experiments.

The next step was to analyze the function of this dual feedback mechanism in Cushing's disease, a disease characterized by a disturbance in feedback regulation. The failure to respond to small doses of dexamethasone with a complete suppression of endogenous cortisol secretion is still regarded as one of the most reliable means of identifying Cushing's disease. In order to define the nature of this disturbance in more detail, we studied the dynamic aspects of the ACTH response to corticosteroid administration in patients with Cushing's disease, who had been treated by total adrenalectomy. Previously we had observed that cortisol infusions in these patients induced a transient paradoxical rise in ACTH levels (4). The results of the more detailed analyses indicated that in Cushing's disease the differential, rate-sensitive feedback-mechanism is converted into a positive one (which results in a *circulus vitiosus*), whereas the integral, dose-sensitive mechanism is undisturbed (5; Figure 2).

This raises the question of what might be the basis for the conversion of the rate-sensitive feedback mechanism from negative to positive.

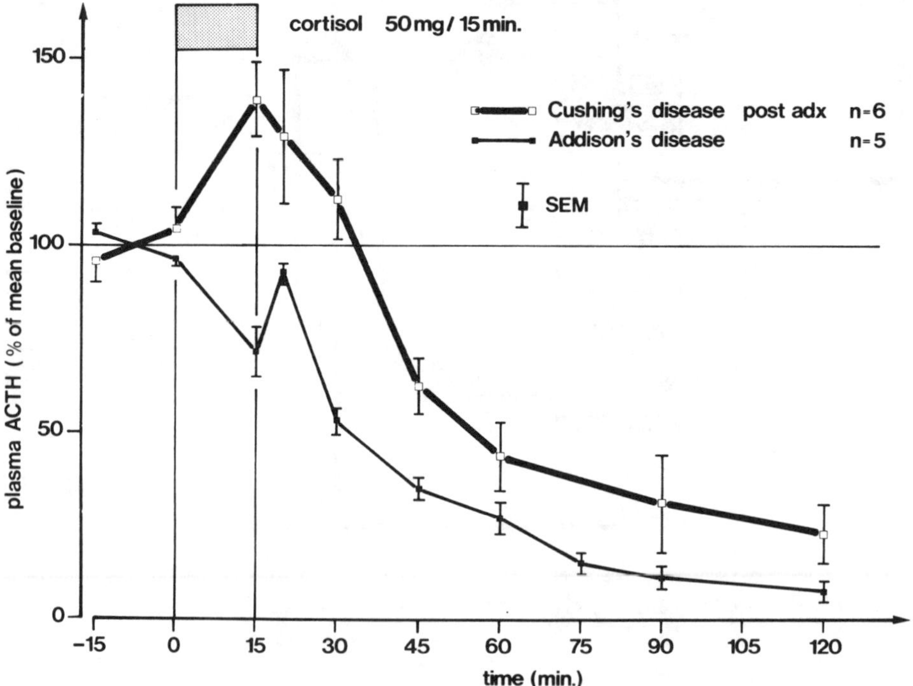

Figure 2. Time-course of plasma ACTH levels in response to an infusion of 50 mg cortisol during 15 min in patients with Cushing's disease after total adrenalectomy and in Addison's disease. During the phase of differential feedback inhibition in the addisonian patients, there was a paradoxical stimulation of ACTH secretion in the Cushing patients.

Here we have to consider briefly the results of Kaneko and Hiroshige (6) from animal experiments.

These authors demonstrated that norepinephrine neurons are involved in the differential feedback circuit and likewise serotonergic neurons in the integral feedback mechanism: In rats whose brain norepinephrine had been depleted by intraventricular injections of 6-hydroxy-dopamine, the rate-sensitive mechanism was eliminated while the delayed component was left intact. Conversely, after depletion of serotonin by administration of p-chlorphenylalanine the delayed component was abolished with an intact rate-sensitive mechanism. These results imply that the site of action of the rate-sensitive feedback is located in the central nervous system, probably in close association with catecholaminergic neurons.

On the basis of these considerations we studied the influence of neuroactive drugs on feedback affects in Addisonian patients (7). We used desipramine, a tricyclic compound, which is known to block preferentially norepinephrine re-uptake in central neurons, thus increasing norepinephrine receptor activity. Desipramine did not influence basal ACTH levels. However, when the rate-sensitive feedback elements were activated by infusions of cortisol, a paradoxical stimulation of ACTH secretion occurred. Obviously, under desipramine the negative differential feedback mechanism was converted into a positive one. The kind of disturbance in steroid feedback regulation produced by desipramine thus closely resembled the one occurring spontaneously in patients with Cushing's disease.

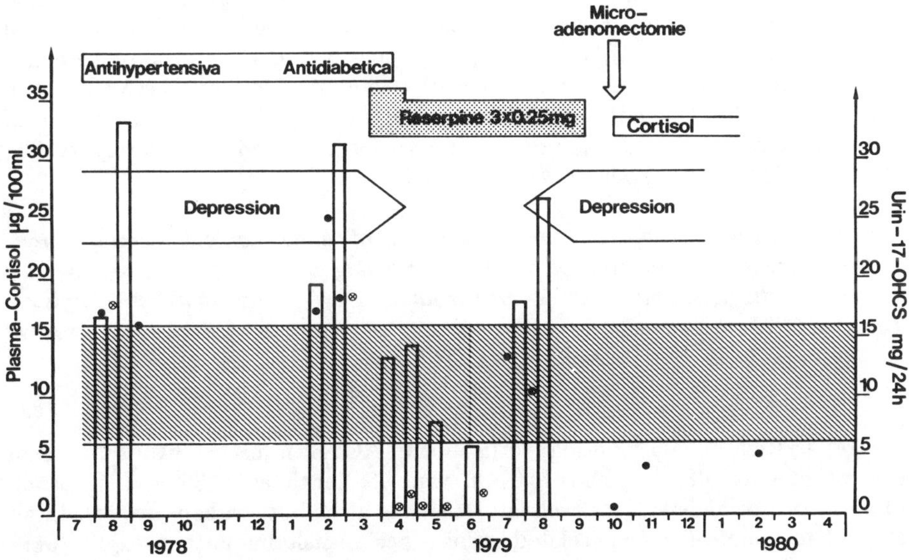

Figure 3. Reserpine-induced remission of Cushing's disease in a 56-year-old female patient.

On the other hand, the pre-existing disturbance of the differential feedback in patients with Cushing's disease could be abolished by depletion of norepinephrine granules by means of reserpine. Thus, also in man catecholaminergic neurons seem to be involved in the differential feedback mechanism and disturbances of this mechanism can be influenced by neuroactive drugs.

These considerations encouraged us to treat patients with Cushing's disease with reserpine. In Figure 3 the results of such a treatment in a 56-year-old female patient are shown. Already 2 weeks after initiation of reserpine treatment, urinary 17-hydroxycorticosteroids were normalized and plasma cortisol was completely suppressible in the 2 mg-overnight dexamethasone test. Surprisingly, symptoms of mental depression disappeared in parallel although reserpine is known to induce depression in some patients. After about 6 months there was relapse despite on-going reserpine treatment. Microsurgical pituitary exploration was performed, during which an ACTH-producing microadenoma could be removed.

Additional experience indicated that reserpine will induce remissions only in a small percentage of patients with Cushing's disease, and these remissions may be transient. In this respect, reserpine does not differ from other neuroactive drugs like cyproheptadine or bromocryptin, which have also been tried in Cushing's disease.

ACTH Unrelated Mechanism in the Regulation of Cortisol Secretion

The studies discussed up to this point were done in patients lacking endogenous cortisol. Thus, the question remains to be answered: Is negative feedback also important in the acute physiological regulation of ACTH secretion in normal subjects. To put it briefly, we failed -- as many before -- to observe feedback effects when plasma cortisol and the corresponding ACTH levels were studied in normal subjects. Instead, from these studies it appeared that a variety of well-known stimuli of cortisol secretion are not mediated by pituitary ACTH alone. The following hypothesis was generated:

Pituitary ACTH is necessary for biosynthesis of adrenocortical steroids. Physiological phenomena of cortisol secretion (morning peak, midday surge, exercise induced cortisol secretion etc.) are mediated by extrapituitary mechanisms. These ACTH independent mechanisms are at least as sensitive to negative feedback by adrenal corticosteroids as ACTH secretion.

Figure 4. Right panel: Plasma cortisol and ACTH levels in five subjects at bedrest between 08.00 h and 13.00 h, who ate lunch at 11.30 h. Left panel: Plasma cortisol and ACTH levels in 4 subjects at bedrest without a meal. In an attempt to imitate the meal-related cortisol peak, small amounts of ACTH were infused at 11.00 h. To prevent spontaneous cortisol peaks, 1 mg dexamethasone had been administered at 08.00 h.

See opposite

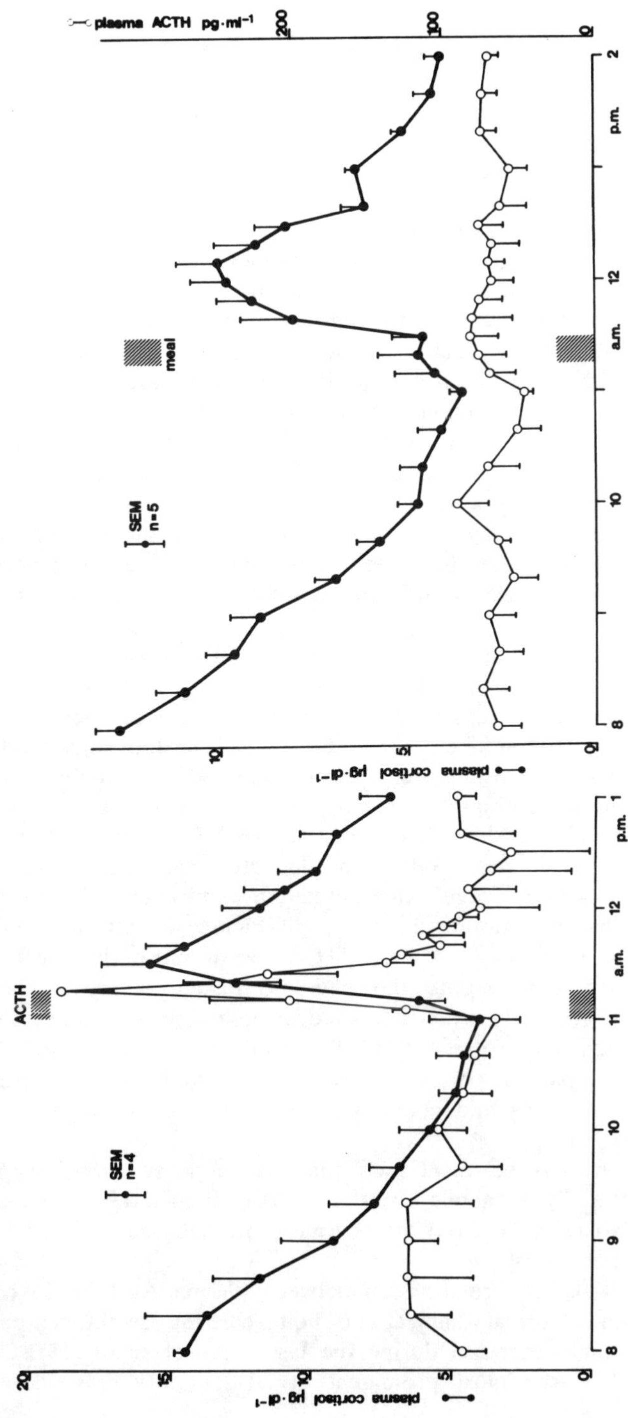
plasma ACTH pg·ml⁻¹
plasma cortisol μg·dl⁻¹
SEM n=5
meal
ACTH
SEM n=4
a.m.
p.m.

In the following, the data from which this hypothesis was derived, will be discussed in more detail.

First we tried to imitate a "physiological" cortisol secretory episode by infusing small amounts of exogenous ACTH (8). 0.01 U porcine ACTH per kg body weight, administered over 15 min by constant rate infusion, induced an increase in cortisol levels, which, considering the magnitude and duration of the increase, can be called physiological. The plasma ACTH levels necessary to induce such a cortisol peak were unexpectedly high (400 pg/ml). In our experience, ACTH levels in this range never occur under physiological conditions.

Of course, the adrenocortical activity of exogenous ACTH may differ from those of endogenous ACTH. ACTH is derived from a high molecular weight glyco-protein (proopiomelanocortin), the enzymatic processing of which yields ACTH and other proteins such as the lipotropins, the 164 fragment, p-endorphin, and γ_3-MSH. Several authors have demonstrated that the adrenocortical response to ACTH is potentiated by a part of the N-terminal region of proopiomelanocortin (9). To exclude this possibility we studied a situation where a cortisol peak is induced by endogenous ACTH. A well-documented example for this is the insulin induced hypoglycemia (insulin tolerance test). Again, maximal ACTH levels of about 400 pg/ml were observed to precede the increase in cortisol levels and clearcut elevated levels were demonstrable for a period of about 90 min. Thus, these results compare well with those of the cortisol peak induced by exogenous ACTH.

On the basis of these results we studied the ACTH/cortisol interrelationship during the so-called "mid-day surge" in plasma cortisol (10). The phenomenon of a large cortisol peak related apparently to the noon meal in subjects at rest has been described by Brandenberger and Follénius (11) and corroborated by Quigley and Yen (12). Our results are given in Figure 4: In recumbent subjects there was a continuous decrease in cortisol levels from 08.00 h to 11.00 h without any secretory episodes. The meal induced a large cortisol peak: However, this peak was not preceded by an adequate increase in ACTH levels. For comparison, a "mid-day surge" was imitated by infusing small amounts of ACTH in dexamethasone suppressed subjects (Figure 4, left side). ACTH infusions resulted in maximal plasma ACTH levels of more than 300 pg/ml. Dexamethasone did not accelerate the decrease in cortisol levels between 08.00 h and 11.00 h; obviously, even without dexamethasone, the adrenal cortex was completely inactive during this period. We conclude from these results that the mid-day surge in plasma cortisol cannot be mediated by immunoreactive ACTH alone. Similar results and conclusions have been published recently by Brandenberger et al. (13).

Furthermore, it should be mentioned that the mid-day surge in plasma cortisol is not induced by metabolic events related to food intake: An identical surge could be provoked at mid-day also by mere presentation of a meal or by mental stress instead of a meal (14).

Next we studied the interrelationship between plasma ACTH and cortisol levels during sleep. Normal subjects exhibit cortisol secretory patterns characterized by a sharp increase during the last hours of sleep (15). Usually this "morning peak" is the most prominent of all secretory episodes of the

24-hour cycle. In the subjects studied by us a main morning peak could usually be identified (16). Mean cortisol and ACTH levels were calculated time-locked to the onset of this main cortisol peak. By this procedure the individual main morning peaks occurring at different times were synchronized for statistical analysis. It appeared that again there was no increase in mean ACTH levels preceding the increase in cortisol. Thus, we have to conclude that the cortisol morning peak, too, is not mediated by pituitary ACTH. This assumption would implicate that a cortisol morning peak can also occur in ACTH deficient patients. Obviously, this is not the case. Therefore, we assumed that sub-threshold amounts of ACTH must be present so that the postulated extra-pituitary mechanisms can come into action. To test this hypothesis we studied cortisol patterns in 4 ACTH-deficient patients during long-term infusions of small amounts of ACTH. After priming with larger amounts of ACTH for 2 days (to restore functional atrophy of the adrenal cortex), ACTH infusions were slowed down to a rate of 0.05 U/h. With these minute amounts, cortisol levels fell to 4 to 5 μg/ml. Under these conditions, there were marked oscillations of cortisol values; in most patients an increase occurred during the morning hours, comparable to the physiological morning peak in healthy subjects. Plasma ACTH levels were always below detection limit with these minute amounts of ACTH.

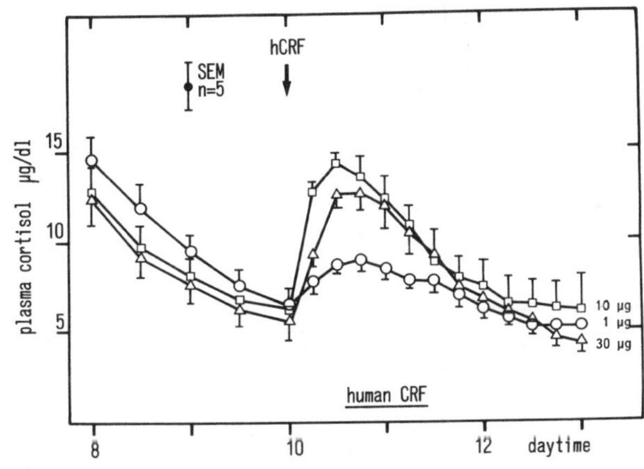

Figure 5. Plasma cortisol responses to different doses of human CRF, administered intravenously at 10.00 h in recumbent subjects.

The most recent advance in the field of pituitary-adrenal regulation is the isolation and synthesis of the corticotropin releasing factor CRF, which is now available for clinical use (17). There is preliminary evidence that even in CRF-induced cortisol secretion, extrapituitary mechanisms are involved. In Figure 5 the cortisol responses to different doses of human CRF are presented. The corresponding increase in ACTH levels to the largest CRF dose (30 μg i.v.) (Figure 6) was small and would not be considered adequate when compared with the ACTH levels during insulin tolerance test or following ACTH administration. Furthermore, we could demonstrate that CRF can induce cortisol secretory bursts in some ACTH deficient patients after priming with long-acting ACTH.

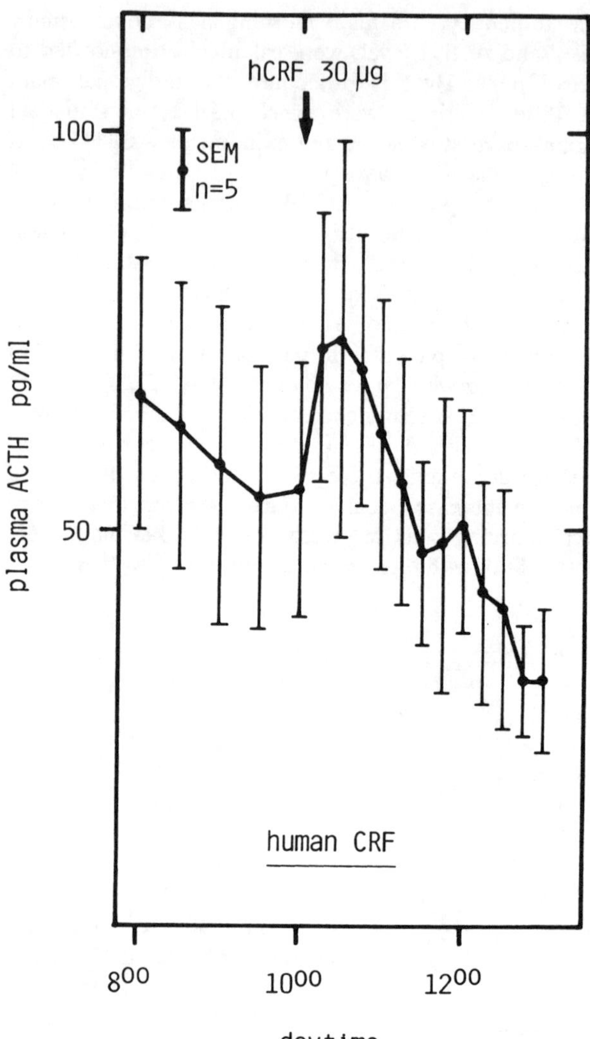

Figure 6. Plasma ACTH response to 30 µg human CRF in recumbent subjects. The corresponding cortisol values are given in Figure 5.

Taken together, we conclude from our results that ACTH induced cortisol bursts must be rather rare events. They do occur, for example, during insulin induced hypoglycemia or during surgical stress. In most physiological situations, however, cortisol release is brought about by ACTH unrelated mechanisms, for which the permissive effects of small amounts of ACTH are sufficient. The nature of these extrapituitary mechanisms remains obscure; several possibilities have to be considered:

1) Hypothalamic nuclei of the autonomic nervous system may influence the adrenal cortex directly via its autonomic innervation. Innervation of the adrenal cortex by postganglionic sympathetic fibers has been described by

Kiss (18) and at the ultrastructural levels by Unsicker (19). According to Ottenweller and Meier (20) adrenal innervation may be an extrapituitary mechanism able to regulate adrenocortical rhythmicity in rats.

2) The responsiveness of the adrenal cortex to ACTH may change in such a way that normal ACTH levels will stimulate cortisol secretion. The existence of ACTH-independent rhythms in adrenal responsiveness has been reported several times. In our experience, however, physiological amounts of ACTH produced identical increments in cortisol in the morning and in the evening.
3) Increases in cortisol secretion may be induced by metabolic events occurring in the periphery. Thus, changes in adrenal blood flow, changes in cortisol metabolism and distribution, changes in ion fluxes, particularly potassium fluxes, and many other possibilities could all account for increases in cortisol secretion.
4) More recently, it has been demonstrated that in humans the adrenal medulla is able to synthesize not only proenkephalin, but also proopiomelanocortin-related peptides including small amounts of ACTH (21). Thus, the possibility has to be considered that the adrenal medulla may influence the adrenal cortex by paracrine secretion of ACTH or ACTH-related peptides. Such an assumption would explain why stimulation of the adrenal medulla is usually accompanied by secretion of adrenal cortex hormones.

Relationship Between the Sleep EEG and Cortisol Secretory Bursts During Sleep

It is evident from the previous discussion that the term "stress" is inadequate at least for some stimuli of cortisol secretion. This holds true especially for the morning peak in plasma cortisol, which occurs during the late hours of nocturnal sleep. There is general agreement that the rhythms of cortisol release are driven by central nervous system mechanisms. From this, cortisol secretion during sleep - although not necessarily related to the regulation of sleep - can be expected to depend on sleep stages as defined by records of EEG activity. Results from studies correlating sleep stages with different measures of cortisol secretion were inconclusive. Weitzman et al. (22) observed no relationship between the occurrence of specific sleep stages and cortisol release in men, which were subjected to a prolonged 3-hour sleep-wake cycle. By contrast, Alford et al. (23) reported a positive relation between episodes of REM sleep or wakefulness and cortisol peaks. A recent report from Weitzman et al. (24) attempted to relate cortisol secretion and slow wave sleep.

Since from these results no one-to-one relation between any of the sleep stages and plasma cortisol could be expected, we hoped that the study of a single subject over a large number of nights (17) would reveal a more discrete pattern of interrelationships (25). In Figure 7 sleep EEG profiles and plasma cortisol patterns of three representative nights are shown. During the second part of the nights, beginning with a sudden and pronounced increase, plasma cortisol levels were elevated and REM stages prolonged. It is evident that REM sleep stages fell mainly into epochs of decreasing cortisol levels, suggesting that the adrenal cortex is less active during REM sleep.

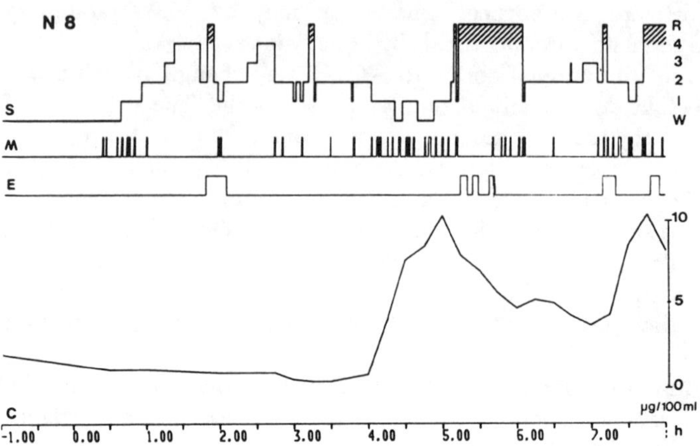

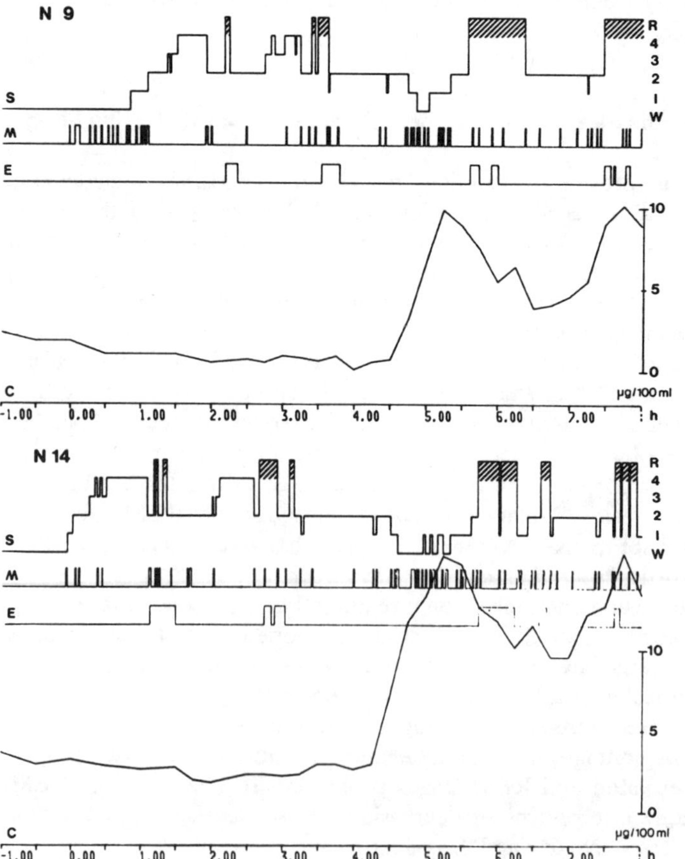

Figure 7. Sleep EEG profiles and plasma cortisol patterns during three nights in a healthy male volunteer, aged 26. Parameters measured were: S, sleep stages, 1, 2, 3, 4, W = wakefulness; REM = rapid eye movement; M, movements; C, plasma cortisol (μg/dl).

On the other hand wakefulness or stage I sleep occurred regularly during the period of rapid increase of cortisol.

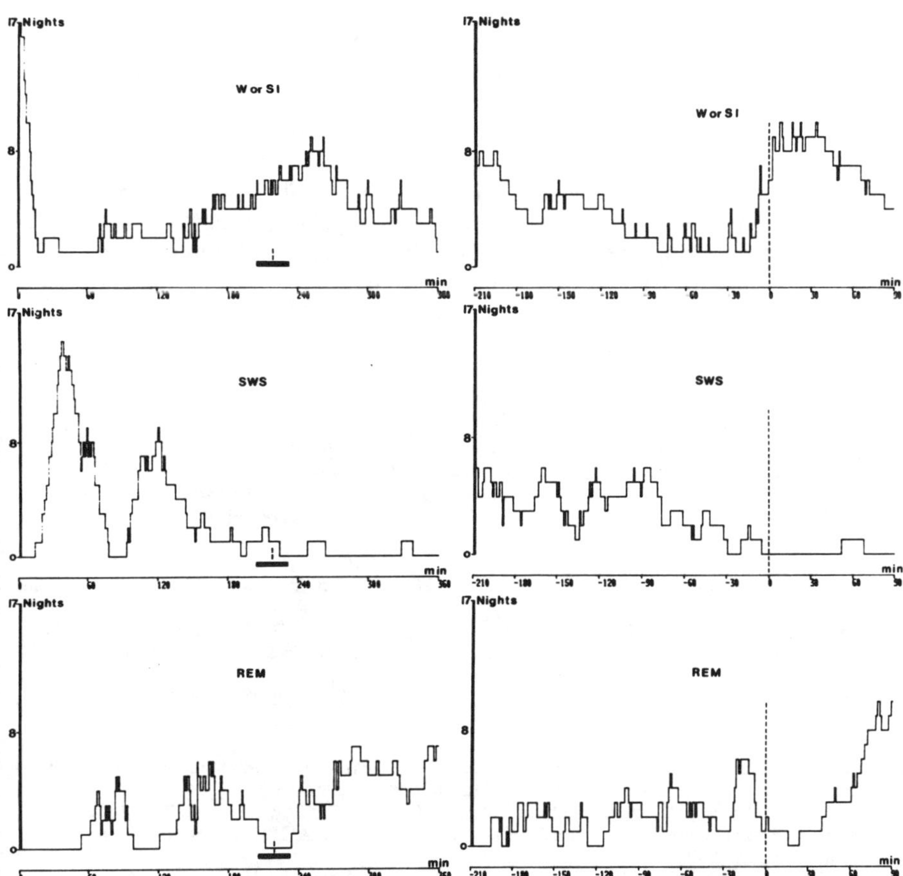

Figure 8. The frequency of occurrences of wakefulness or stage I sleep (upper panels), of slow wave sleep (SWS, middle panels), and of REM sleep (lower panels) in 17 experimental nights of a single subject. In the left panels, instances of the respective sleep stages were added up time-locked to the sleep onsets of the nights. The black bars on the bottom of each panel indicate the standard error of the mean latency of the onset of the morning cortisol peak. In the right panels, sleep pattern were synchronized with respect to the onsets of the first plasma cortisol peaks. The marked periodicity, which could be observed in the left panels, was replaced by flattened curves in the right panels, suggesting no specific temporal relation between the onset of the morning cortisol peak and SWS or REM sleep.

In order to see whether a certain sleep stage triggered the first cortisol peak during the night the appearance of each sleep stage was summed across all 17 nights, time-locked to the onset of the first cortisol peaks (Figure 8, right panel). These curves were contrasted with those obtained by summing instances of a particular sleep stage, time-locked to the sleep onsets (Figure 8, left panel). The marked periodicity, which could be observed for slow wave sleep and REM sleep in the left panels, were replaced by flattened curves in the right panels, suggesting no specific temporal relation between the onset of the morning cortisol peak and sleep patterns. On the other hand, wakefulness or stage I sleep were frequently observed just after the onset of the morning cortisol peak. Most of these findings could be replicated in a second study over 16 nights, each with a different experimental subject. Thus we have to conclude that there is no evidence for a specific sleep stage triggering the first rise of plasma cortisol during the night. It remains a matter of future research to define the characteristics of the brain events preceding cortisol secretory bursts.

References

1. Sayers, G. & Sayers, M.A. (1947). Regulation of pituitary adenocortitrophic activity during the response of the rat to acute stress. Endocrinology, 40: 265-273.
2. Dallman, M.F. & Yates, F.E. (1969). Dynamic asymmetries in the corticosteroid feedback path and distribution - metabolism - binding elements of the adrenocortical system. Ann. N. Y. Acad. Sci., 156: 696-721.
3. Fehm, H.L., Voigt, K.H., Kummer, G.W., Lang, R. & Pfeiffer, E.F. (1979). Differential and integral corticosteroid feedback effects on ACTH secretion in hypoadrenocorticism. J. Clin. Invest., 63: 247-253.
4. Fehm, H.L., Voigt, K.H., Lang, R.E., Deinert, K.E., Kummer, G.W. & Pfeiffer, E.F. (1977). Paradoxical ACTH response to glucocorticoids in Cushing's disease. New Eng. J. Med., 297: 904-907.
5. Fehm, H.L., Voigt, K.H., Kummer, G.W. & Pfeiffer, E.F. (1979). Positive rate sensitive corticosteroid feedback mechanism of ACTH secretion in Cushing's disease. J. Clin. Invest., 64: 102-108.
6. Kaneko, M. & Hiroshige, T. (1978). Site of fast, rate-sensitive feedback inhibition of ad enocorticotropin secretion during stress. Am. J. Physiol., 234: R46-R51.
7. Fehm, H.L., Steck, R., Hohnloser, J., Voigt, K.H. & Pfeiffer, E.F. (1983). Influence of neuroactive drugs on corticosteroid feedback regulation of ACTH secretion in man. Horm. Metab. Res., 15: 29-32.
8. Fehm, H.L., Holl, R., Steiner, K., Klein, E. & Voigt, K.H. (1984). Evidence for ACTH-unrelated mechanisms in the regulation of cortisol secretion in man. Klin. Wochenschr., 62: 19-24.
9. Pederson, R.C. & Drownie, A.C. (1980). Adrenocortical response to corticotropin is potentiated by part of the amino-terminal region of pro-corticotropin/endorphin. Proc. Natl. Acad. Sci. USA, 77: 2239-2243.
10. Fehm, H.L., Holl, R., Klein, E. & Voigt, K.H. (1983). The meal related peak in plasma cortisol is not mediated by radioimmunoassayable ACTH. Clin. Physiol. Biochem., 1: 329-333.
11. Brandenberger, G. & Follénius, M. (1973). Variations diurnes de la cortisolémie, de la glycémie et du cortisol libre urinaire chez l'homme au repos. J. Physiol. Paris, 66: 271-282.
12. Quigley, M.E. & Yen, S.S.C. (1979). A mid-day surge in cortisol levels. J. Clin. Endocrinol. Metab., 49: 945-947.
13. Brandenberger, G., Follénius, M. & Muzet, A. (1984). Interactions between spontaneous and provoked cortisol secretory epidodes in man. J. Clin. Endocrinol. Metab., 59: 406-411.
14. Holl, R., Fehm, H.L., Voigt, K.H. & Teller, W. (1984). The "midday surge" in plasma cortisol induced by mental stress. Horm. Metab. Res., 16: 158-159.

15. Weitzman, E.D., Fukushima, D., Nogeire, C., Roffwarg, H., Gallagher, T.F. & Hellman, L. (1971). Twenty-four hour pattern of the episodic secretion of cortisol in normal subjects. J. Clin. Endocrinol., 33: 14-22.
16. Fehm, H.L., Klein, E., Holl, R. & Voigt, K.H. (1984). Evidence for extrapituitary mechanisms mediating the morning peak of plasma cortisol in man. J. Clin. Endocrinol. Metab., 58: 410-414.
17. Vale, W., Spiess, J., Rivier, C. & Rivier, J. (1981). Characterization of a 41-residue bovine hypothalamic peptide that stimulates secretion of corticotropin and ß-endorphin. Science, 213: 1394-1397.
18. Kiss, R. (1951). Experimentell-morphologische Analyse der Nebenniereninnervation. Acta Anat. (Basal), 13: 81-89.
19. Unsicker, K. (1971). On the innervation of the rat and pig adrenal cortex. Z. Zellforsch., 116: 151-156.
20. Ottenweller, J.E. & Maier, A.H. (1982). Adrenal innervation may be an extrapituitary mechanism able to regulate adrenocortical rhythmicity in rats. Endocrinol., 111: 1334-1338.
21. Evans, C.J., Erdelyi, E., Weber, E. & Barchas, J.D. (1983). Identification of proopio-melanocortin derived peptides in the human adrenal medulla. Science, 221: 957-960.
22. Weitzman, E.D., Nogeire, C., Perlow, M., Fukushima, D., Sassin, J., McGregor, P., Gallagher, T.F. & Hellman, L. (1974). Effects of a prolonged 3-hour sleep-wake cycle on sleep stages, plasma cortisol, growth hormone and body temperature in man. J. Clin. Endocrinol. Metab., 38: 1018-1030.
23. Alford, F.P., Baker, H.W., Burger, H.G., de Kretzer, D.M., Hudson, B., Johns, M.W., Masterton, Y.P., Patel, G.C. & Rennie, G.C. (1973). Temporal patterns of integrated plasma hormone levels during sleep and wakefulness. J. Clin. Endocrinol. Metab., 37: 841-847.
24. Weitzman, E.D., Zimmerman, J.C., Czeisler, C.A. & Ronda, J. (1983). Cortisol secretion is inhibited during sleep in normal man, J. Clin. Endocrinol. Metab., 56: 352-358.
25. Fehm, H.L., Bieber, K., Benkowitsch, R., Fehm-Wolfsdorf, G., Voigt, K.H. & Born, J. (in press). Relationship between sleep stages and plasma cortisol: A single case study. Acta Endocrinol.

Adrenal Corticosteroids in the Endogenous Regulation of Blood-Brain Barrier Permeability: Functional Implications

Joseph B. Long and John W. Holaday

The blood-brain barrier regulates to a large degree the extracellular environment of the brain and protects the central nervous system from the changing milieu of the circulation (1, 2). While the entry into the central nervous system (CNS) of metabolic substrates and hormones required by CNS tissues is governed by carrier or transport mechanisms (3), the passage of most water soluble molecules from blood into the brain interstitium is restricted by several morphological characteristics unique to the microvasculature of the CNS. Tight injunctions or zonulae occludentes form belts around endothelial cells and prevent intercellular diffusion. Additionally, in contrast to the vasculature of the periphery, the virtual absence of fenestrations and pinocytotic vesicles prohibits solute permeation through endothelial cells of the cerebral vasculature. As a consequence, those substrates not transported by specific carrier mechanisms gain access to the CNS primarily on the basis of their lipid solubility and resultant ability to diffuse through the endothelial membranes (1, 2).

While these basic characteristics limiting permeability are well accepted, an understanding of the blood-brain barrier has evolved over the last several years so that it is no longer regarded as a static barrier sealing the brain off from the periphery, but may instead be appreciated as a dynamic interface. The dynamic aspects of this barrier function are reflected in the uniquely high concentrations of endothelial mitochondria and in the assortment of enzymes, carrier systems, receptors, and intracellular regulators that are specifically associated with the cerebral endothelium (1-4). Furthermore, it is increasingly apparent that the permeability and blood flow characteristics of the brain microvasculature are responsive to both neural and humoral influences. Following their initial observation of close anatomical associations between cerebral microvessels and adrenergic nerve terminals arising from the locus ceruleus (5, 6), Raichle and coworkers demonstrated that electrical and pharmacological stimulation of this population of neurons elicited a pronounced, rapid increase in the permeability of cerebral capillaries to water (7, 8). From these observations, it was concluded that central adrenergic neurons may serve to maintain a relatively constant cerebral volume through regulation of the cerebral microcirculation despite fluctuations in systemic arterial pressure and

---

This research was conducted in compliance with the Animal Welfare Act, and other Federal statutes and regulations relating to animals and experiments involving animals and adheres to principles stated in the Guide for the Care and Use of Laboratory Animals, NIH publication 85-23. The views of the authors do not purport to reflect the position of the Department of the Army or the Department of Defense, (para 4-3), AR 360-5.

osmolarity. Similar homeostatic mechanisms have been proposed for other regulatory substances such as acetylcholine (9), vasopressin (10), histamine (11), and the melanotrophic peptides *ACTH* and *MSH* (12, 13), based on the effects of these substances on the permeability of the brain to water or relatively impermeable water soluble substrates. Furthermore, the list of putative neurotransmitters and neuroregulators identified in perivascular nerve fibers making direct contact with cerebral blood vessels has grown to include acetylcholine, serotonin, substance P, neuropeptide Y, vasopressin, vasoactive intestinal polypeptide, calcitonin gene-related peptide, and cholecystokinin-8 (14, 15). In light of these abilities of these vasoactive substances to constrict and dilate blood vessels, these anatomical observations have furthered speculation over the involvement of putative chemical neuro-regulators in the coupling of blood flow to neuronal activity. Roles in the modulation of cerebrovascular permeability have similarly been proposed for CCK, vasopressin, and serotonin following historical observations that fibers containing these substances impinge on capillaries in the brain (14, 16-20).

From pharmacological observations, it appears that the cerebrovasculature may also be responsive to adrenal corticosteroids. Dexamethasone and other synthetic glucocorticoids have been widely used for the treatment of brain edema resulting from trauma and cerebral ischemia, with suggestions that therapeutic benefits result from restoration of vascular integrity and reductions in abnormal cerebrovascular permeability (21, 22). Dexamethasone has also been demonstrated to reduce the blood-brain barrier disruption produced by drug-induced hypertension (23), repeated convulsive seizure activity (24), or hyperosmotic perfusion of the brain (25). Furthermore, following dexamethasone administration and withdrawal in rats, brain water permeability and content decrease and increase, respectively, in the absence of any measurable changes in cerebral blood flow (2).

On the basis of these reports, we speculated that the normal, undisrupted brain microvasculature may be responsive to circulating glucocorticoids, and that the pituitary-adrenal axis may be involved in the endogenous regulation of the permeability characteristics of the brain microvasculature. As a result, alterations of circulating glucocorticoids by adrenal extirpation or stress may modify the access of macromolecules to the brain. To investigate this possibility, we recently examined the effects of adrenalectomy, adrenal demedullation, and corticosterone replacement on the permeability of the blood-brain barrier to the radiolabeled macromolecule ^{125}l-bovine serum albumin (^{125}l-BSA; 69,000 molecular weight) in rats (27).

Experimental observations

Bilaterally adrenalectomized, bilaterally adrenal demedullated, and sham-operated male Sprague Dawley rats (200-250 g; Zivic Miller, Allison Park, PA) were given laboratory chow ad libitum, and were provided with access to both a 0.9% saline drinking solution and tab water. At least two weeks following surgery, mean arterial pressures were recorded from catheterized tail arteries, and a 1.0 ml venous blood sample was withdrawn from each rat through external jugular catheters for plasma corticosterone and electrolyte determinations. Freshly prepared ^{125}I-BSA (10-20 μCi in 200 μl) was then administered through the external jugular catheder, and following a fixed circulation time, a 0.5 ml venous blood sample was removed. Immediately following removal of this blood reference sample, rats were anesthetized with pentobarbital (25 mg/kg, i.v.) and perfused in situ with approximately 160 ml of 0.9% saline. Brains were then removed and dissected into five regions, including the cerebellum (CER), brainstem (BS), rostral forebrain (RFB), ventral forebrain (VFB), and dorsal forebrain (DFB).

Cerebrovascular permeability of ^{125}I-BSA was calculated as the percentage of radioactivity in brain vs. blood ((cpm x mg brain $^{-1}$/cpm x mg blood $^{-1}$) x 100).

This measure of cerebrovascular permeability increased linearly in the brain areas through at least 80 minutes following injection of ^{125}I-BSA (Figure 1).

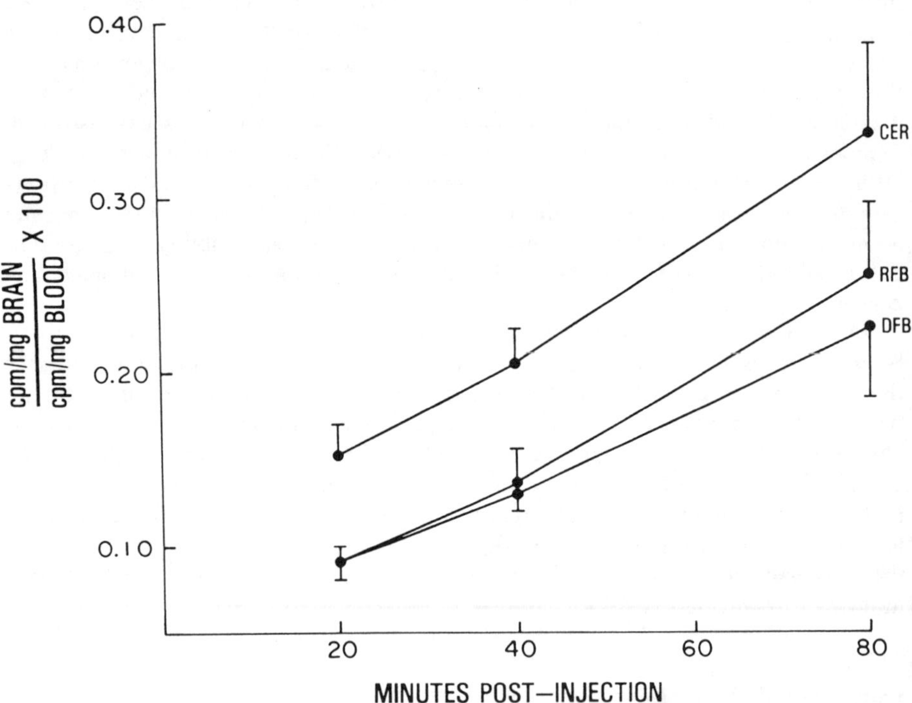

Figure 1. Time-dependent accumulation of radioactivity in rat brain following intravenous injection of ^{125}I-BSA. Radioactivity was measured in perfused, dissected brain samples obtained 20, 40 and 80 minutes following injection of 10 μCi of ^{125}I-BSA through external jugular catheders. Abbreviations: CER, cerebellum; BS, brainstem; RFB, rostral forebrain; and DFB, dorsal forebrain.

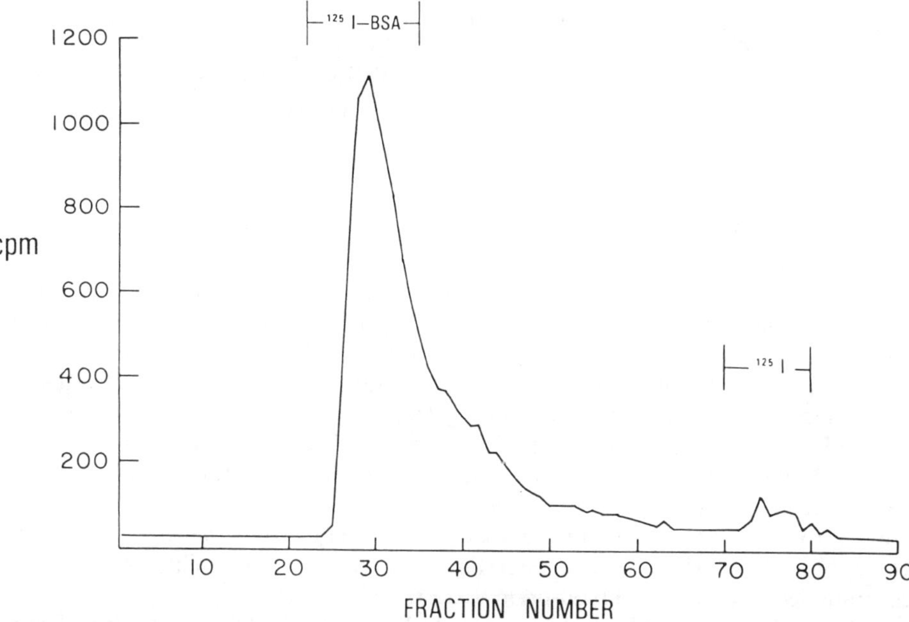

Figure 2. Gel filtration chromotography of radioactivity in rat brains following intravenous injection of ^{125}I-BSA. Perfused rat brains were homogenized in 0.1 M sodium phosphate buffer, pH 7.5 and centrifuged at 48,000 x g for 20 minutes. Supernatants were concentrated and passed over a column of Sephadex G-75 (1.5 cm by 45 cm, Pharmacia). Samples were eluted with 0.1 M sodium phosphate buffer, pH 7.5, and 1 ml fractions were collected and counted in a gamma counter. The elution profile of radioactivity extracted from brain tissue was identical to that seen following chromotography of freshly-prepared ^{125}I-BSA. Furthermore, elution profiles of radioactivity from brains of adrenalectomized rats did not differ from those obtained from sham-operated animals.

For subsequent experiments, a 20-minute circulation period was employed to minimize potential complications arising from longer circulation times, such as efflux from the brain of accumulated ^{125}I-BSA. Additionally, we anticipated that radioactivity measured in brain samples after a 20-minute circulation time period would principally represent the intact ^{125}I-BSA molecule, rather than free ^{125}I or ^{125}I-BSA fragments resulting from proteolytic activity in the periphery. Indeed, after perfusion of rats injected with ^{125}I-BSA 20 minutes earlier, homogenization of the brain and subsequent gel filtration chromatography of the supernatant verified that radioactivity in the brain was associated with a single peak of ^{125}I-BSA which co-migrated with freshly iodinated BSA (Figure 2). For this procedure to provide a valid estimate of cerebrovascular permeability to ^{125}I-BSA, it is essential that perfusion with saline completely removes intraluminal ^{125}I-BSA. To verify that perfusions adequately cleared the vasculature of residual ^{125}I-BSA and to evaluate the possibility of apparent differences in permeability resulting from actual differences in the removal by perfusion of intraluminal ^{125}I-BSA, rats were administered freshly prepared ^{51}Cr-labeled erythrocytes in addition to ^{125}I-BSA. Unlike ^{125}I-BSA, ^{51}Cr-labeled erythrocytes remain within the vascular lumen. Consequently, measurement of ^{51}Cr in brain tissue samples provides a direct index of the clearance of the vascular lumen of perfusion. In all instances, after perfusion ^{51}Cr in brain tissue samples was negligible (less than 1.5 times blank), indicating that our perfusion technique consistently cleared the vascular lumen of residual radioactivity in these experiments.

In consideration of the possibility that radioactivity measured in brain samples following perfusion was associated with ^{125}I-BSA adsorbed to the walls of the vascular lumen, rats were perfused with 1% BSA in saline to displace any adsorbed ^{125}I-BSA. This amount of unlabeled BSA administered in the perfusate is at least six orders of magnitude greater than the amount of ^{125}I-BSA injected as a bolus. Radioactivity in rat brains following perfusion with this BSA solution did not differ from radioactivity levels in brains perfused with saline alone, suggesting that adsorption of ^{125}I-BSA did not significantly contribute to measures of cerebrovascular permeability. Thus, we concluded that these procedures yield reasonable estimations of the permeability of the BSA macromolecule across the blood-brain barrier.

Adrenalectomy significantly increased the permeability of the blood-brain barrier to ^{125}I-BSA, with the magnitude of the increases ranging from 27 to 49% in the BS and DFB, respectively (Figure 3a). Adrenalectomy-induced increases in ^{125}I measurements were not accompanied by changes in ^{51}Cr measurements in brain tissue following perfusion of animals administered ^{51}Cr-labeled erythrocytes. Thus the apparent permeability differences were not the result of artefactual differences in perfusions of brains from two groups.

Additionally, concentrations of radioactivity in the blood were not changed by adrenalectomy, indicating that changes in this index of permeability were due to increases in ^{125}I-BSA accumulation in brain. In confirmation of the

Figure 3. Effects of (a) bilateral adrenalectomy, (b) bilateral adrenal demedullation, and (c) bilateral adrenalectomy with corticosterone replacement on the passage of intravenously injected ^{125}I-BSA into brains of rats. In corticosterone replacement experiments, approximately ten days following adrenalectomy or sham-surgery, rats were administered corticosterone (0.5 mg/kg, s.c. in 5% ethanol) or vehicle twice daily for four days. On the following day, rats were given a final injection of corticosterone (0.5 mg/kg, s.c.) or vehicle one hour prior to injection of ^{125}I-BSA. Blood radioactivity concentrations did not significantly differ among treatment groups within an experiment. Data were analyzed by two-way analysis of variance with repeated measures (Figures 3a and 3b) or one way analysis of variance (Figure 3c). Significant differences between means ($p < 0.05$) were determined by use of the Newman-Keuls test. Each bar represents mean + SEM; populations for experimental groups are defined in Table 1.

See opposite

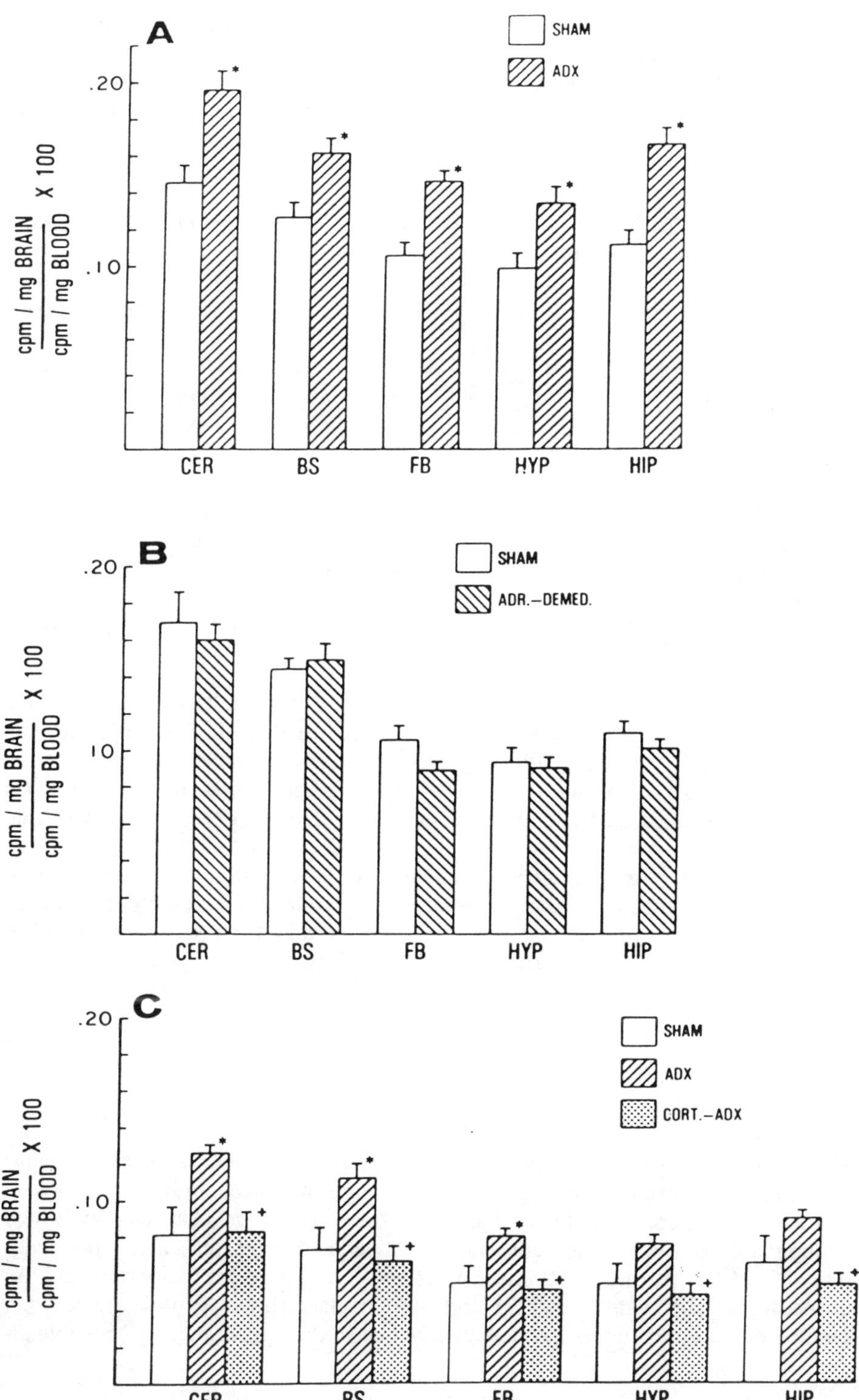
A
SHAM
ADX
.20
.10
cpm / mg BRAIN / cpm / mg BLOOD X 100
CER
BS
FB
HYP
HIP
B
SHAM
ADR.–DEMED.
.20
.10
cpm / mg BRAIN / cpm / mg BLOOD X 100
CER
BS
FB
HYP
HIP
C
SHAM
ADX
CORT.–ADX
.20
.10
cpm / mg BRAIN / cpm / mg BLOOD X 100
CER
BS
FB
HYP
HIP

completeness of adrenal extirpation, it was shown that adrenalectomized rats had significant reductions in MAP, and plasma corticosterone levels were reduced to the limits of detectability (Table 1). Possibly owing to the access of saline drinking solutions, plasma electrolyte levels in adrenalectomized rats did not differ from those of sham-operated animals.

Table 1. Mean arterial pressure (MAP) and plasma corticosterone values associated with rats having undergone (a) adrenalectomy, (b) adrenal demedullation and (c) adrenalectomy with corticosterone replacement (as described in Figure 3).

Treatment	n	MAP (mmHg)	Plasma Corticosterone (μg/dl)
(a) Sham-adrenalectomy	12	99.5 ± 2.3	13.9 ± 1.4
Adrenalectomy	12	73.4 ± 2.2*	0.5 ± 0.1*
(b) Sham-demedullation	16	109.5 ± 2.0	9.2 ± 1.7
Adrenal demedullation	16	108.5 ± 1.4	6.4 ± 1.1
(c) Sham-adrenalectomy	8	98.5 ± 3.0	10.9 ± 1.0
Adrenalectomy	7	75.0 ± 3.9*	0.6 ± 0.2*
Adrenalectomy and Corticosterone	7	91.4 ± 2.9	13.3 ± 1.5

* $p<0.05$, student's t-test.

In contrast to adrenalectomy, selective adrenal demedullation did not alter blood-brain barrier permeability to ^{125}I-BSA (Figure 3b). Plasma corticosterone, electrolytes, and MAPs also did not differ between sham-operated and adrenal demedullated rats (Table 1), indicating that normal adrenal cortical function was essentially preserved in these animals following removal of the adrenal medulla. Thus it appears that the absence of factor(s) associated with the adrenal cortex, and not with the adrenal medulla, were responsible for blood-brain barrier alterations associated with total adrenalectomy. Accordingly, physiological doses of corticosterone (0.5 mg/kg, s.c. twice daily for 4 days) reversed the adrenalectomy-induced increases in ^{125}I-BSA passage into the brain (Figure 3c). The decreased MAP associated with adrenalectomy was also reversed by corticosterone (Table 1).

Discussion

These data demonstrate that the pituitary-adrenal axis influences macromolecular permeability into the brain, and specifically implicate adrenal glucocorticoids as mediators in these alterations. However, the sites or mechanisms by which manipulation of the pituitary-adrenal axis influence blood-brain barrier permeability of ^{125}I-BSA are not clearly established by these experiments. As intracisternal injections of ACTH and other melanotrophic peptides have been reported to produce dose-dependent increases in the appearance of ^{125}I-albumin in the CSF of rabbits (12), the elevated levels of ACTH resulting from loss of adrenal glucocorticoid feedback in adrenalectomized rats may have contributed to the increased ^{125}I-BSA permeability. Alternatively, changes in permeability might have arisen from the sustained reductions in systemic arterial pressure associated with adrenalectomy (Table 1). While little is known about the cerebrovascular consequences of sustained hypotension such as occurs in adrenalectomized animals, two pieces of evidence argue against this hypothesis: (1) brain perfusion is autoregulated between 60 and 140 mmHg (28), and (2) we were unable to detect significant correlations between arterial pressures and cerebrovascular permeabilities within treatment groups. Thus, it appears unlikely that adrenal effects on blood-brain barrier permeability are due to arterial pressure differences.

In interpreting these results, consideration must be given to the effects of adrenalectomy on other adrenal cortical and medullary hormones, such as the loss of aldosterone and epinephrine. Blood-brain barrier changes do not appear to result from compromised adrenal mineralcortocoid function, since, with access to 0.9% saline drinking solutions, adrenalectomized rats maintained normal plasma electrolyte levels. Additionally, although pharmacological administration of adrenergic agonists has been reported (29, 30) to increase the extravasation of ^{125}I-BSA into the brain (apparently as a result of drastic acute increases in arterial pressure), the loss of circulating epinephrine due to adrenalectomy or adrenal demedullation did not significantly affect cerebrovascular permeability to ^{125}I-BSA (Figure 3). Thus, in contrast to catecholamines of central origin, catecholamines arising from the adrenal medulla appear not to appreciably influence the blood-brain barrier.

Passage of ^{125}I-BSA from the plasma into the brain may occur at the choroid plexus, the circumventricular organs, or the brain microvessels forming the blood-brain barrier. In measuring radioactivity associated with brain dissections, we can only speculate over the mechanisms and sites of entry underlying increased ^{125}I-BSA accumulation in the brains of adrenalectomized rats. Nevertheless, as the surface area of the capillaries comprising the blood-brain barrier is at least 5000 times greater than the surface area of the capillaries of the choroid plexus and circumventricular organs (31), it would appear likely that the quantitatively important site of ^{125}I-BSA entry into the brain resides at the blood-brain barrier.

Extravasation of macromolecules into the brain may involve transendothelial transport through pinocytotic vesicles or extracellular diffusion through endothelial tight junctions. Increased blood-brain barrier permeability of macromolecules has been associated with a number of experimental and clinical conditions such as hyperosmotic perfusions (32), acute hypertension (29, 30), hypoxia or ischemia (33), compression injury (34), seizures (35, 36, 37), or injections of vasoactive substances such as histamine (11) and cyclic nucleotides (38, 39), As these conditions are also accompanied by increased numbers of pinocytotic vesicles in the endothelium, transendothelial vesicular transport (pinocytosis) has been favored by a number of investigators as the important mechanism by which macromolecules enter into the CNS during blood-brain barrier dysfunction (4, 11, 33, 37-41).

Activation of brain endothelial pinocytotic activity by pathological and experimental circumstances suggests that rather than simply not existing, vesicular movement of macromolecules may be inactive or suppressed in the cerebral vasculature under normal conditions (40). Pharmacologically, glucocorticoids may reduce macromolecule entry into the CNS by suppressing the increased vesicular transport associated with these disruptive conditions. In turn, it is conceivable that endogenous circulating glucocorticoids may directly or indirectly participate in the cellular mechanisms by which vesicular transport is normally and uniquely suppressed in the cerebral vasculature. Consequently, under conditions of reduced glucocorticoids availability, such as adrenalectomy, increased vesicle-mediated ^{125}I-BSA entry into the brain may occur. Obviously, these proposals are highly speculative, as even the role of vesicles in blood-brain barrier transport are not uniformly agreed upon. Future examination of endothelial vesicle formation following adrenalectomy would adress not only the mechanisms underlying the increased permeability associated with adrenalectomy, but may also provide insights into the relevance of vesicles to macromolecule transport.

Recently, Tosaki et al. observed that Actinomycin D abolished dexamethasone-induced reductions in albumin leakage into the brain following global cerebral ischemia, prompting the suggestion that de novo protein synthesis is involved in the cerebroprotective effects of dexamethasone (42). Based upon observations of glucocoticoid actions in non-neural tissues (43), the phospholipase A_2 inhibitor macrocortin has been proposed as a likely secondary mediator for these steroid actions (42). Alternatively, a number of vasoactive regulators and experimental conditions which increase cerebrovascular permeability and pinocytotic vesicle formation have been shown to significantly increase adenylate cyclase activity in isolated cerebral capillaries (4). Furthermore, injections of the lipid soluble dibutyryl analogs of cyclic AMP and cGMP increase both macromolecule permeability and endothelial pinocytosis (4, 38, 39). Thus, cyclic nucleotides have been implicated as mediators involved in the regulation of cerebrovascular permeability, and effects of glucocorticoids on blood-brain permeability may involve cyclic nucleotides. Clearly, further study is necessary to define the mechanisms regulating permeability and specifically how glucocorticoids influence this process.

Implications

These results indicate that alterations of pituitary-adrenal function may modulate the entry of macromolecules into the CNS and thereby indirectly alter the central actions of hydrophilic drugs and humoral substances (Table 2). Such a possibility, which may extend to other hormones as well, has tremendous biological implications, particularly for research areas such as psychology, neuroendocrinology and psychoimmunology. For example, burgeoning research in these areas is revealing interactions and intercommunications among nervous, immune, and endocrine systems which were never previously considered due to the confinement of these systems to distinct central and peripheral compartments (see Bernton and Holaday chapter, this book). Neural and humoral influences on the cerebrovascular interface between these compartments may facilitate or inhibit intercommunications between systems and contribute to the overall integrated responses to various psychological and physiological conditions. Responses to environmental and psychological stressors, for example, include widespread neural, endocrine, and immune alterations. One means by which the nervous system can modulate responses in these other systems is through direct or indirect feedback mechanisms. Conceivably, under conditions in which appropriate hormones or transmitters are released, ensuing alterations in the blood-brain barrier may allow targets within the brain to be exposed to substances normally confined to the periphery, completing a feedback loop of sorts. In addition to integration of neural-endocrine-immunological regulatory axes, such exposures may also partly account for psychic responses to conditions such as stress and disease.

Much research interest in the blood-brain barrier stems from clinical consideration of how this barrier may be breached to deliver drugs to the CNS for treatment of a variety of conditions, such as neurologic disorders, infections, and malignant lesions within the CNS. While some success has been reported using hyperosmotic perfusions to reversibly disrupt blood-brain barrier integrity (44), the clinical usefulness of most of these manipulations has been limited by ineffectiveness, irreversibity, or neurotoxity. The research outlined above provides further evidence for the dynamic nature of the blood-brain barrier and specifically implicates altered glucocorticoid levels in the regulation of macromolecular access in the brain. While speculative, hormonal manipulation may serve as a viable means to enhance central drug delivery. Alternatively, the wisdom of high dose glucocorticoid therapy for the treatment of CNS malignancies or infections may be complicated by the effects of glucocorticoids in limiting the access of therapeutic drugs to the brain.

Table 2. Summary of Results and Implications.

Surgical procedure	Plasma epinephrine	Plasma corticosterone	Effect on blood-brain barrier
Sham adrenalectomy or demedullation	normal	normal	normal
Adrenalectomy	undetectable*	undetectable*	increased permeability
Adrenal demedullation	undetectable	normal	normal
Adrenalectomy plus corticosterone	undetectable	normal	normal
Stress ??	elevated	elevated	normal or decreased permeability

* "undetectable" indicates that values were below reliable limits of assay sensitivity.

References

1. Rapoport, S.I. (1976). Blood-brain barrier in physiology and medicine. Raven Press, N.Y.
2. Bradbury, M.W.B. (1979). The concept of a blood-brain barrier. Wiley, Chichester.
3. Pardridge, W.M. (1981). Transport of nutrients and hormones through the blood-brain barrier. Diabetolgia, 20:246-254.
4. Joo, F. (1985). The blood-brain barrier in vitro: Ten years of research on microvessels isolated from the brain. Neurochm. Int., 7: 1-25.
5. Hartman, B. (1973). The innervation of cerebral blood vessels by central noradrenergic neurons. In E. Usdin & S. Snyder (Eds.), Frontiers of catecholamine research. Pergamon Press, N.Y., p. 91-96.
6. Swanson, L., Connelly, M. & Hartman, B. (1977). Ultrastructural evidence for central monoaminergic innervation of blood vessels in the paraventricular nucleus of the hypothalamus. Brain Res., 136: 166-173.
7. Raichle, M., Eichling, J., Grubb, R. & Hartman, B. (1976). Central noradrenergic regulation of brain microcirculation. In H. Pappius & W. Feindel (Eds.), Dynamics of brain edema. Springer-Verlag, N.Y., p. 11-17.
8. Raichle, M., Hartman, B., Eichling, J. & Sharpe, L. (1975). Central noradrenergic regulation of cerebral blood flow and vascular permeability. Proc. Natl. Acad. Sci. USA, 72: 3726-3730.
9. Estrada, C., Hamel, E. & Krause, D.N. (1983). Biochemical evidence for cholinergic innervation of intracerebral blood vessels. Brain Res., 266: 261-270.
10. Raichle, M.E. & Grubb, R.L. (1978). Regulation of brain water permeability by centrally released vasopressin. Brain Res., 143: 191-194.
11. Gross, P.M., Teasdale, G.M., Angerson, W.J. & Harper, A.M. (1981). H_2 receptors mediate increases in permeability of the blood-brain barrier during arterial histamine infusion. Brain Res., 210: 396-400.
12. Rudman, D. & Kutner, M.H. (1978). Melanotropic peptides increase permeability of plasma/cerebrospinal fluid barrier. Am. J. Physiol., 234: E327-E332.
13. Goldman, H. & Murphy, S. (1980). An anlog of $ACTH/MSH_{4-9}$, ORG-2766, reduces permeability of the blood-brain barrier. Pharmacol. Biochem. Behav., 14: 845-848.
14. McCulloch, J. (1984). Perivascular nerve fibers and the cerebral circulation. TINS, 7: 135-138.
15. Edvinsson, L. (1985). Functional role of perivascular peptides in the control of cerebral circulation. TINS, 8: 126-131.
16. McCulloch, J. (1983). Peptides and the microregulation of blood flow in the brain. Nature, 304: 120.
17. Hendry, S.H.C., Jones, E.G. & Beinfeld, M.C. (1983). Cholecystokinin-immunoreactive neurons in rat and monkey cerebral cortex make symmetric synapses and have intimate associations with blood vessels. Proc. Natl. Acad. Sci. USA, 80: 2400-2404.
18. Jojart, I., Joo, F., Siklos, L. & Laszlo, F.A. (1984). Immunoelectronhistochemical evidence for innervation of brain microvessels by vasopressin-immunoreactive neurons in the rat. Neurosci. Lett., 51: 259-264.
19. Edvinsson, L., Degueurce, A., Daverger, D., MacKenzie, E.T. & Scatton, B. (1983). Central serotonergic nerves project to the pial vessels of the brain. Nature, 306: 55-57.
20. Griffith, S.G. & Burnstock, G. (1983). Immunohistochemical demonstration of serotonin nerves supplying human cerebral and mesenteric blood vessels. Lancet i: 561-562.
21. Pappius, H.M. & McCann, W.P. (1969). Effect of steroids on cerebral edema in cats. Arch. Neurol., 20: 207-216.
22. Fishman, R.A. (1982). Steroids in the treatment of brain edema. N. Engl. J. Med., 306: 359-360.
23. Johansson, B.B. (1978). Effect of dexamethasone on protein extravasation in the brain in acute hypertension induced by amphetamine. Acta Neurol. Scand., 57: 180-185.
24. Eisenberg, H.M., Barlow, C.F. & Lorenzo, A.V. (1970). Effect of dexamethasone on altered brain vascular permeability. Arch. Neurol., 23: 18-22.
25. Neuwelt, E.A., Barnett, P.A., Bigner, D.D. & Frenkel, E.P. (1982). Effects of adrenal cortical steroids and osmotic blood-brain barrier opening on methotrexate delivery to gliomas in the rodent: The factor of the blood-brain barrier. Proc. Natl. Acad. Sci. USA, 79: 4420-4423.
26. Reid, A.C., Teasdale, G.M. & McCulloch, J. (1982). The effects of dexamethasone administration and withdrawal on water permeability across the blood-brain barrier. Ann. Neurol., 13: 28-31.

27. Long, J.B. & Holaday, J.W. (1985). Blood-brain barrier: Endogenous modulation by adrenal-cortical function. Science, 227: 1580-1583.
28. Tyson, G.W. & Jane, J.A. (1982). Pathophysiology of head injury. In R.A. Cowley & B.F. Trump (Eds.), Pathophysiology and shock, anoxia, and ischemia. Williams and Wilkins, Baltimore, p. 570-600.
29. Johansson, B.B. & Martinsson, L. (1979). Blood-brain barrrier to albumin in awake rats in acute hypertension induced by adrenaline, noradrenaline and angiotensin. Acta Neurol. Scand., 60: 193-197.
30. Domer, F.R., Sankar, R., Cole, S. & Wellmeyer, D. (1980). Dose-dependent, amphetamine-induced changes in the permeability of the blood-brain barrier of normotensive and spontaneously hypertensive rats. Exp. Neurol., 70: 576-585.
31. Crone, C. (1971). The blood-brain barrier - Facts and questions. In B.K. Siesjo & S.C. Sorenson (Eds.), Ion homeostasis of the brain. Munksgaard, Copenhagen, p. 52-62.
32. Chiueh, C.C., Sun, C.L., Kopin, I.L., Fredericks, W.R. & Rapoport, S.I. (1978). Entry of (^{3}H)norepinephrine, (^{125}I)albumin and evans blue from blood into brain following unilateral osmotic opening of the blood-brain barrier. Brain Res., 145: 291-301.
33. Dux, E., Temesvari, P., Joo, F., Adam, G., Clementi, F., Dux, L., Hideg, J. & Hossman, K.A. (1984). The blood-brain barrier in hypoxia: Ultrastructural aspects and adenylate cyclase activity of brain capillaries. Neuroscience, 12: 951-958.
34. Beggs, J.L. & Waggener, J.D. (1976). Transendothelial vesicular transport of protein following compression injury to the spinal cord. Lab. Invest., 34: 428-439.
35. Lorenzo, A.V., Hedley-Whyte, T., Eisenberg, H.M. & Hsu, D.W. (1975). Increased penetration of horseradish peroxidase across the blood-brain barrier induced by metrazol seizures. Brain Res., 88: 136-140.
36. Pepito, C.K., Schaefer, J.A. & Plum, F. (1977). Ultrastructural characteristics of the brain and blood brain barrier in experimental seizures. Brain Res., 127: 251-267.
37. Westergaard, E., Hertz, M.M. & Bolwig, T.G. (1978). Increased permeability to horseradish peroxidase across cerebral vessels, evoked by electrically induced seizures. Acta Neuropath. (Berlin), 41: 73-80.
38. VanDeurs, B. (1980). Structural aspects of brain barriers, with special reference to the permeability to the cerebral endothelium and choroidal epithelium. Int. Rev. Cytol., 65: 117-191.
39. Joo, F., Rakonczay, Z. & Wolleman, H. (1975). cAMP-mediated regulation of the permeability in the brain capillaries. Experientia, 31: 582-583.
40. Joo, F., Temesvari, P. & Dux, E. (1983). Regulation of the macromolecular transport in the brain microvessels: The role of cyclic GMP. Brain Res., 278: 165-174.
41. VanDeurs, B. & Amtorp, O. (1978). Blood-brain barrier in rats to the hemepeptide microperoxidase. Neuroscience, 3: 737-748.
42. Tosaki, A., Koltai, M., Joo, F., Adam, G., Szerdahelyi, P., Lepran, I., Takats, I. & Szekeres, L. (1985). Actinomycin D suppresses the protective effect of dexamethasone in rats affected by global cerebral ischemia. Stroke, 16: 501-505.
43. Flower, R.J. & Blackwell, G.J. (1979). Anti-inflammatory steroids induce biosynthesis of a phospholipase A_2 inhibitor which prevents prostaglandin generation. Nature, 278: 456-459.
44. Neuwelt, E.A. & Rapoport, S.I. (1984). Modification of the blood-brain barrier in the chemotherapy of malignant brain tumors. Fed. Proc., 43: 214-219.

Discussion:

Central Control of the Pituitary-Adrenal Axis II

Renate de Jong

Different disciplines such as psychology, physiology, neuroscience, endocrinology, and immunology contribute to the puzzle of defining, categorizing and studying "the conditions that constitute sufficient psychobiological challenge with a potential to result in behavioral and/or physiological impairments and which, given the opportunity, the organism will defend against" (1) - to cite a definition avoiding the term "stress." Most researchers in these different disciplines use a specific language and focus on discrete variables within specific research strategies using their own phenomenological "window" to interpret experimental results.

The four papers which are the subjects of this discussion are written by researchers from different disciplines, but, in contrast, they are oriented towards interdisciplinary research. They conceive of specific biological and psychological variables as being interrelated, and they discuss the implications of their concepts and findings beyond their own field. It is the achievement of the authors to outline how other disciplines can profit from their specific findings, and to set incentives to pursue further in the attempt to complete the puzzle of interactions between internal biological and psychological, as well as external environmental events.

Ursin's approach consisted of formulating a model and the conceptualization and operationalization of biological and psychological events within this model. The results of this effort can be used as valuable "tool" to generate hypotheses and to set up experiments involving critical features of both biological and psychological variables. Murison and Overmier demonstrated very elegantly how the changing of environmental stimuli and learning histories modulates coping behavior as well as different bodily responses in animal models. Learning/conditioning as well as motivational variables are central to Ursin's conceptual framework as well as to Murison's and Overmier's series of experiments.They can be called stimulus-oriented regarding their main alley of manipulating independent variables. Their results, however, are correlational in terms of responses on different levels (psychological, endocrinological, physiological). Thus one can learn about the strength of relationships in given contexts, but the mechanisms by which these interrelationships are produced still remain unclear.

Fehm and Voigt and Long and Holaday, on the other hand, elucidate some mechanisms involved in the regulation of the pituitary-adrenal axis. If one is interested in the responses of organisms to challenging events, the work of both teams sets the incentive to more closely operationalize and control the state of the organism at the time of and during the course of "psychobiological challenge."

Ursin, like many other researchers in the field, is confronted with the existence of many ill-defined concepts being pursued rather independently from each other (e.g., stress, activation, coping, learned helplessness, disease concepts). One of the main targets of interdisciplinatory research surely is to relate these concepts by an empirical network of results. One could do this without a model, but probably would waste time by accumulating experimental knowledge without any heuristic guideline. Ursin offers such a model and, at the same time, presents operational definitions for the concepts involved. He partly bases his formulation on very plausible assumptions derived from other theories. An example is the assumption of "set points" for particular variables at particular times, by which "activation" is self-regulated in a biologically adaptive way. His formulation is partly based on a series of experimental findings. This applies for example to the differential use of the concepts of predictability (relating to stimulus expectancy), and control/controllability (relating to response outcome expectancy). This differentiation may be an important step towards clarifying the discussion of results in the "learned helplessness" paradigm (1). Research regarding psychosomatic diseases in clinical samples will profit from the operationalizations of anxiety- and fear-reducing variables, "coping," and "defense." The conceptualization and prediction of certain types of helplessness, hopelessness and psychosomatic disease as the psychological and/or biochemical correlates of "sustained activation" may lead to innovative experiments. These operationalizations allow predictions regarding defined types of activation and regarding the consequences of short versus prolonged exposure to aversive or challenging stimulus situations.

Ursin concludes that his definitions are not the only possible ones. Perhaps, other researchers (such as the discussant) may object to a concept of coping which narrows this term to "positive outcome expectancy resulting from previously successful responses." They perhaps would not exclude responses without a history of contingencies perceived previously, and they would not exclude behavioral responses from the coping concept. This does not argue, however, against a concept which specifically defines "positive outcome expectancy resulting from previously successful responses." The model encompasses a lot of knowledge which should help to avoid "blind alleys" of research or may help in understanding conflicting findings.

While Ursin's contribution to interdisciplinatory research helps to reflect on and generate assumptions leading to relevant biopsychological experiments, Murison's and Overmier's work is a fine example for what we can learn from experiments performed within such a conceptual framework. Murison's and Overmier's results allow specific predictions regarding either synchronicity (parallel rises or decreases of both corticosterone and ulceration responses) or desynchronicity. A "periodic table" as presented by Overmier (1) can be considered helpful in pursuing this research. Among the four classes of outcome in the experiments presented here, there are two types of synchronicity and desynchronicity respectively: "strengthening of ulceration effects/relative reduction of corticosterone effects" and "weakening of the ulceration effect/relative strengthening of the corticosterone response."

If one tries to classify the independent variables and the situational context of these experiments, particularly those with desynchronicity, several assumptions arise:

1) The ulceration response may be an index of lack of active coping and/or lack of anticipation of active coping by motor responses.
2) The corticosterone response may be more closely related to learning or information processing: Corticosterone levels are low if active coping is predictable *and* if active coping is of no use but waiting is, since the termination of the stimulation is predictable; corticosterone levels are high if there are no signals for either one of these alternatives, and the search by the organism to obtain cues has to go on.
3) As the up *and* down of corticosterone levels can signal processes leading to ulceration, it is probably the time course that is critical: No ulceration if corticosterone is fluctuating; risk of ulceration if there is a critical time period of steady state in the corticosterone response without response feedback.

In addition to the characteristics of independent variables in Overmier's "periodic table," perhaps familiarity/newness, time intervals of aversive events, degree of motor feedback, and cues of the experimental setting as well as handling characteristics (that is, signals perhaps not explicitly varied in a design) are additional sources contributing to differential outcomes.

Murison and Overmier by looking into the literature on stress-induced analgesia (SIA) point to the possible role of opioid-mediated inhibition of gastric secretion, whereby the organism copes with aversive events in series and prepares against forthcoming aversive events. Each month, however, we extend our knowledge on new agents, functional systems, peptides, or interactions of peptides with neurotransmitters, and this demands a continuous displacement, redefinition or refinement of concepts such as the opioid-mediation hypothesis. Thus we are probably far from knowing the exact mechanisms by which the organism manages the fine adjustments necessary to cope with specific events, as will become clear in discussing the approaches of Fehm and Voigt and Long and Holaday which deal more specifically with yet other regulatory systems contributing to and complicating pituitary-adrenal activities.

As a concluding comment on the theoretical and empirical work of Ursin and Murison and Overmier, the potential of learning theory paradigms in human and animal research should be stressed.

Murison and Overmier reasoned that "subjecting animals to explicit conditioning procedures prior to a final stressor session somehow activates a mechanism whereby later stress-induced activation of the pituitary-adrenal axis has an inhibitory effect on gastric ulceration." One suggestion is, to look more closely into mechanisms inherent in classical conditioning. This viewpoint emerges if one considers classical conditioning as a flexible adaptional process with dynamically changing stimuli and responses in multiple response systems. Hollis (2) summarized this functional conceptualization of thc traditional paradigm. She states in her "prefiguring hypothesis": "Pavlovian conditioning appears to involve more than mere 'predictability'... The result of such conditioning is the eventual elicitation of a response, the conditional response or CR, which actually *precedes* the occurrence of the biologically important event and which, if it is a skeletal behavior, is often *directed at the conditional stimulus (CS)*" (2, p. 2) and "...the CR does not involve the same response system as the unconditioned response (UCR) ... may change over the course of conditioning and may vary with both the intensity ... and type of the CS as well as the timing of CS and UCS events ... and can be even in the opposite direction of the UCR."

If this applies to the experiments reported, it would mean that given previous experiences in stress-induced activation of the pituitary-adrenal axis with associated activation of ulceration process as the UCR, a CR might develop which inhibits further ulceration. The paradigm thus would imply responses in different directions or the possibility of adaptional desynchronicity between response systems. There is good evidence from other systems suggesting that CR's are indeed anticipatory and of functional meaning (and not accidental false starts). Siegel (3, 4) could demonstrate this Pavlovian conditioning phenomenon in his analysis of drug tolerance and drug withdrawal processes. The CR's were compensatory ones, that is CR's opposite in direction to the UCR's (drug-induced effects). Solomon (5, 6) has generalized these and other findings and assumes that emotional processes in general are characterized by "opponent processes."

A second point among the same line of reasoning applies to phenomena observed after "backward conditioning" procedures: Backward conditioning has only been reported in experiments employing aversive UCS. Pavlov (1928, see 2) suggests that backward conditioning might produce CRs initially and "with a sufficient number of pairings, a backward CS might become inhibitory, "that it decreases the probability of a particular CR," or "a backward CS signals a period of time, until the next UCS-CS trial, in which the threat of danger is absent."

Translated into the paradigms of experiments using "safety-signals," the CR produced initially might have been the activation of the pituitary-adrenal axis associated with ulceration rise. But with sufficient numbers of pairings the backward CS (pituitary-adrenal activation) might become inhibitory regarding the conditioned ulceration response.

The inhibitory response elicited by a backward CS is seen by Hollis as the "learned" manifestation of a compensatory CR, "the compensatory response, whose function it is to reduce the physiological turmoil ... induced by aversive stimulation ... and this response may move forward in time." This interpretation may help to explain the "safety-signals" results, and may cast some new light on learning mechanisms involved in stress-induced analgesia (SIA).

Fehm's and Voigt's work contributes to our understanding of the mechanisms of corticosteroid feedback regulation of pituitary ACTH secretion in both patients with known deficiencies in endogenous cortisol regulation and healthy subjects. They demonstrated in Addison's patients as previously shown in animal models that one has to discriminate a first rate-sensitive inhibitory response to corticosteroid-induced ACTH-release and a second dose-sensitive mechanism after a latency period. These results not only help us to understand one feature of Cushing's disease (change in the rate-sensitive but not the dose-sensitive mechanism), but may lead to new treatment approaches based on the assumption that the rate-sensitive mechanism is mediated by catecholaminergic neurons, whose action can be modified by neuroactive drugs.

Their second series of findings in normal subjects cast serious doubt on an assumption typically found in "stress" on cortisol, namely that ACTH is the main or even single mediator of the release of this steroid. As the authors demonstrate very elegantly in men, the rhythms of cortisol secretion during the day, and particularly the physiological phenomena of circadian cortisol peaks (morning peak, midday surge), seem to be mediated by extrapituitary mechanisms given at least the permissive effect of a small amount of ACTH. These findings have important implications for researchers looking at cortisol levels and rate changes as indices or correlates of a biopsychological challenge to the organism. If it is true that ACTH-induced cortisol bursts only occur after extreme challenges, such as insulin-induced hypoglycemia or surgical stress, important questions have to be answered before continuing along the old pathways of "stress"-research:

1) What is the relation between ACTH-dependent and -independent cortisol secretion particularly during the "early morning peak," the "midday surge" of plasma cortisol, the methamphetamine-, and the CRF-induced secretion?
2) If ACTH-independent cortisol secretion is inhibited most of the time and disinhibited during critical periods of the day and/or in periods with a critical functional meaning, what does that mean for ACTH-dependent disinhibitory processes? Does an ACTH-independent system pose limits on the experimental manipulation of the ACTH-dependent regulation? Is there perhaps a buffering effect against stress-induced cortisol secretion changes during these critical time periods?
3) What are the specific trigger events for ACTH-independent secretion?

The main implication for researchers focussing on the understanding of mechanisms is to detect the nature of these extrapituitary mechanisms.

Bohus (7) concluded that the neuroendocrine hypothalamic-pituitary-adrenal system affects limbic-midbrain functions through complex hormonal and neural mechanisms. Long's and Holaday's findings may complicate the understanding of these relationships even more. They focus on the blood brain barrier, which has not yet received much attention as a flexible mediatory system. In showing that adrenal corticosteroids can affect the permeability of the blood brain barrier, they point to the functional implications of having such a dynamic interface between central and peripheral physiological events and processes. Thus, there is now evidence that corticosteroids not only act directly via specific receptors and pathways in discrete brain regions but can also exert an indirect effect on central nervous system physiology and behavior by modulating the access of humoral substances.

The thoughts and findings of Long and Holaday, Fehm and Voigt, Murison and Overmier as well as Ursin do not point to solutions in our understanding of the relationships between external stimuli, behavioral and physiological responses and the internal biopsychological state of individual organisms. But they offer fruitful perspectives for future studies of these complex and puzzling relationships. Miller, Galanter, and Pribram (8) have spent a funded year to write "Plans and Structures of Behavior" which had an important influence on research perspectives. It would be attractive to think about these researchers from different fields spending enough time combining their efforts.

References

1. Overmier, J.B.: This volume.
2. Hollis, K.L. (1982). Pavlovian conditioning of signal-centered action patterns and autonomic behavior: A biological analysis of function. Advances in the study of behavior, Vol. 12. Academic Press, N.Y.
3. Siegel, S. (1979). The role of conditioning in drug tolerance and addiction. In J.D. Keehen (Ed.), Psychopathology in animals: Research and implications. Academic Press, N.Y., p. 143-168.
4. Siegel, S. (1979). Pharmacological learning and drug dependence. In D.J. Osborne, M.M. Gruneberg & J.R. Eiser (Eds.), Research in psychology and medicine. Academic Press, N.Y., p. 127-134.
5. Solomon, R.L. (1977). An opponent-process theory of motivation: IV. The affective dynamics of addiction. In J.D. Maser & M.E.P. Seligman (Eds), Psychopathology: Experimental models. Freeman, San Francisco.
6. Solomon, R.L. (1980). The opponent-process theory of acquired motivation. The costs of pleasure and the benefits of pain. Am. Psychol., 35: 691-712.
7. Bohus, B.: This volume.
8. Miller, G.A., Galanter, E.H. & Pribram, K.H. (1960). Plans and the structure of behavior. Holt, Rinehart & Winston, N.Y.

7.
Brief Communications

Interaction of Expectancy and Physiological Stressors in a Laboratory Model of Panic

Anke Ehlers, Jürgen Margraf and Walton T. Roth

In the field of anxiety research much attention has recently been focused on panic attacks. They are considered important for the classification and treatment of anxiety disorders (1, 2). Since natural panic attacks are difficult to study in a laboratory setting, reliable laboratory models of panic are desirable. Sodium lactate infusion and carbon dioxide (CO_2) inhalation have been proposed as specific physiological provocations for panic attacks (3-5). However, several issues remain unresolved. It is controversial whether biological challenges such as lactate or CO_2 specifically affect patients prone to panic attacks. Furthermore, the specificity of these stressors as opposed to so-called nonspecific stress tests has not been tested. Finally, it is possible that response to these physiological challenges is mediated by cognitive variables such as expectancy (6). Our study was designed to shed some light on these questions.

Methods

Subjects

Sixteen patients (15 women, 1 man) and 18 control subjects (17 women, 1 man) were recruited by newspaper advertisements. Patients met DSM-III criteria for Panic Disorder or Agoraphobia with Panic Attacks as determined by the Structural Clinical Interview for DSM-III - Upjohn version (7).

Control subjects described themselves as "non-anxious" and had to be free of any history of psychiatric problems as determined by structured interviews. The groups were matched for age (mean ± standard deviation in years: 34.5 ± 9.4 for patients, 35.1 ± 11.1 for controls). Age ranged from 22 to 59 years in each group.

Procedure

Testing took place in a sound attenuated, electrically shielded chamber. The subjects sat alone and could not see the laboratory personnel during the test periods, but could communicate with them by intercom at any time. Identical, written instructions were used for patients and controls. After a baseline of 15

The study was supported by the Veterans Administration and the Upjohn Company.

min (quiet sitting), the Cold Pressor Test and Mental Arithmetic were presented in balanced order. During the Cold Pressor Test, subjects had to immerse their dominant foot in ice water (4°C) for one minute. The mental Arithmetic task lasted 5 min and consisted of serial subtractions of 13 starting at 7683. Each of these tests was preceded by a 4 min anticipation period and was followed by a 7 min recovery period. After these "non-specific" stress tests, subjects were exposed to the CO_2 challenge using a single-blind protocol similar to that of Gorman et al. (5). After 15 min of room air (placebo), 5.5% CO_2 in room air was given for 20 min. CO_2 and room air were administered through a continuous positive air pressure (C-PAP) gas mask. Gas tanks and other equipment were located in a room adjacent to the recording chamber. Continuous monitoring ensured that a stable CO_2 concentration above 5% was delivered. The CO_2 inhalation was terminated before 20 min if subjects reported severe anxiety and asked to stop. In any case, recording was continued for a recovery period of 15 min after the end of the CO_2 inhalation, while subjects were breathing room air.

Subjects were familiar with the laboratory environment since they had participated in another test session on the previous afternoon (Day 1). On this test day, subjects had to wear the gas mask for 6 min knowing that they would only breathe room air. Expectancy effects were assessed by comparing subjects' responses to wearing the gas mask in anticipation of the CO_2 challenge (Day 2), and on this previous occasion (Day 1) when subjects did not expect a panic challenge test.

Assessment

Heart rate (HR) and blood pressure (BP) were measured automatically at regular intervals (Accutorr 2, Datascope Corporation). HR and BP were measured every 4.5 min during baselines, every 2 min during the Cold Pressor Test and Mental Arithmetic, and every 2.5 min during the CO_2 challenge. Subjective anxiety was assessed by an eleven-point Anxiety Rating (AR) scale. Subjects were instructed to fill out one AR scale each time after the blood pressure cuff was completely deflated. They were given a supply of these rating scales prior to the test runs. Subjects indicated which test was most unpleasant. They also rated the similarity of CO_2-induced effects to a usual panic attack (patients) or to the most extreme anxiety experienced (controls). Results of other physiological and self-report variables will be reported elsewhere.

Data Analysis

Repeated measures analysis of variance (ANOVA) with the Greenhouse-Geisser correction was used for calculating statistical significance. Separate analyses were performed for the baseline, Cold Pressor, Mental Arithmetic, and CO_2 paradigms. Effects of the stressors would appear as significant effects of the factor Time (changes over time points). Different reactions of patients and controls would appear as significant interactions between the factors Group and

Time. Since a few subjects stopped the CO_2 inhalation before 20 min, there were some missing data. The last measurement taken during the CO_2 inhalation was used as an estimate for missing time points.

To assess possible expectancy effects, responses to wearing the mask while breathing room air for the previous test day (Day 1, no anticipation of panic challenge) and for the CO_2 test day (Day 2, just prior to the CO_2 challenge) were compared with the respective baselines. Demand to stop the CO_2 inhalation and ratings of similarity and unpleasantness were tested using Fisher's exact probability and chi^2 tests, respectively. If not mentioned otherwise, the results reported here meet the significance level of 0.05. All significance levels are two-tailed.

Results

Response to Different Stressors

Figures 1 to 4 show the results for subjective anxiety, heart rate, systolic and diastolic blood pressure. Both the Cold Pressor and Mental Arithmetic produced considerable and highly significant increases in subjective anxiety and cardiovascular arousal. During these tests and at baseline, patients were significantly more anxious and had higher heart rates than controls. Response to Cold Pressor and Mental Arithmetic did not differ significantly between patients and controls.

CO_2 inhalation led to highly significant increases in subjective anxiety and cardiovascular arousal in both groups.

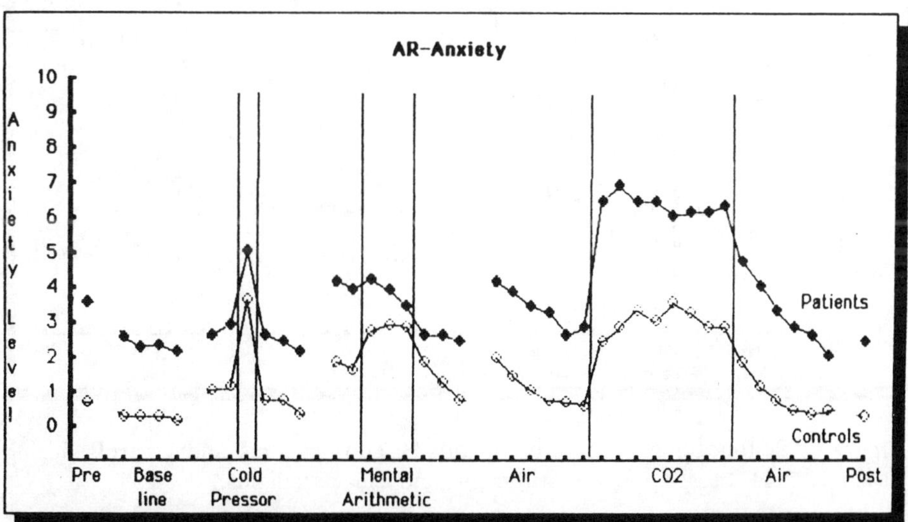

Figure 1. Self-reported anxiety for patients and controls during baseline, Cold Pressor, Mental Arithmetic, and CO_2 paradigms.

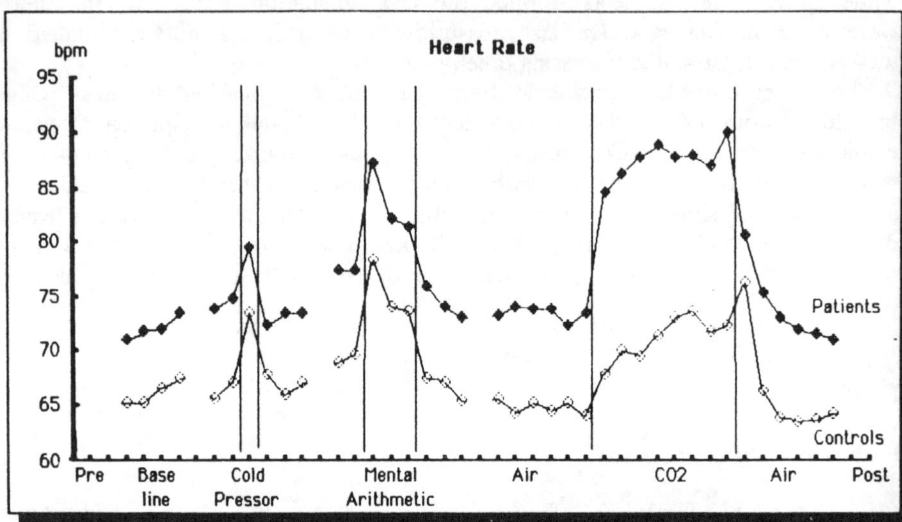

Figure 2. Heart rate in beats per minute (bpm) for patients and controls during baseline, Cold Pressor, Mental Arithmetic, and CO_2 paradigms.

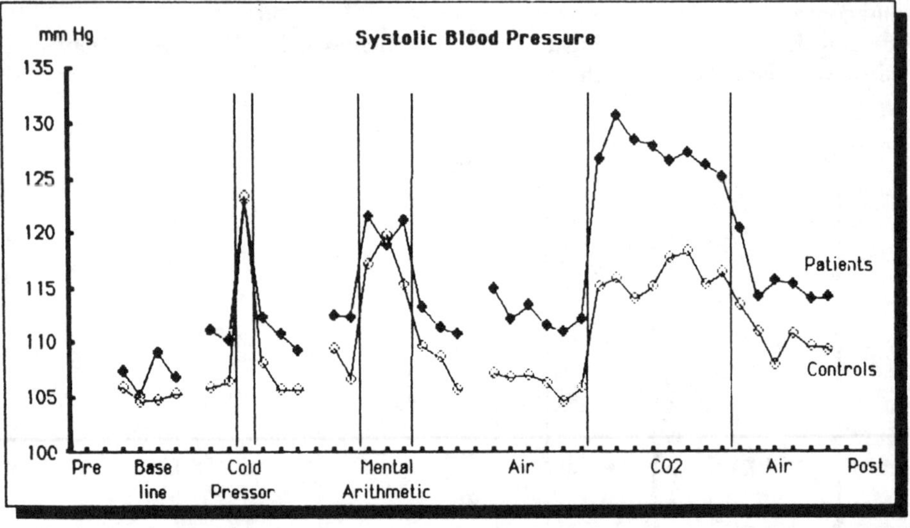

Figure 3. Systolic blood pressure (in mm Hg) for patients and controls during baseline, Cold Pressor, Mental Arithmetic, and CO_2 paradigms.

The reactions of patients and controls were similar. The only exception was that patients showed faster, but not larger increases in heart rate and systolic

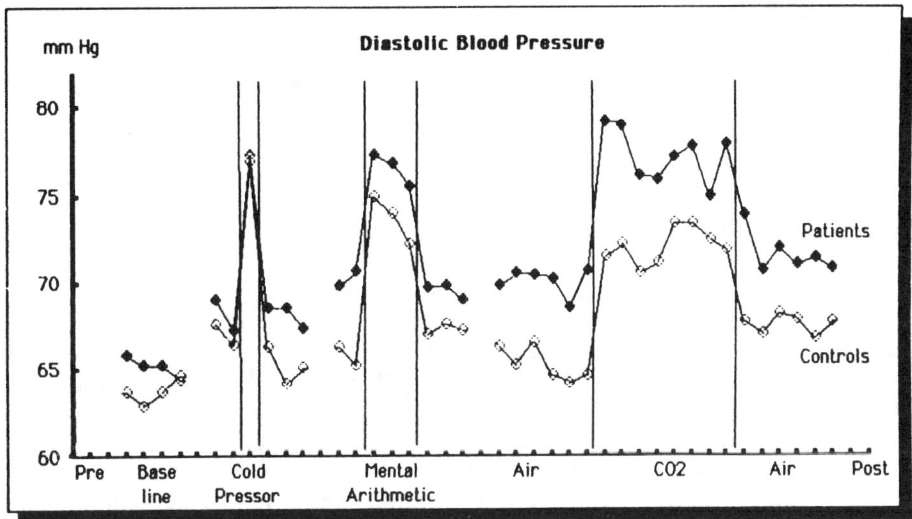

Figure 4. Diastolic blood pressure (in mm Hg) for patients and controls during baseline, Cold Pressor, Mental Arithmetic, and CO_2 paradigms.

blood pressure than controls, leading to significant Group x Time interactions in the ANOVAs.

Three patients and one control asked to stop the inhalation before the full 20 min. This difference is not significant (Fisher's exact probability test). These subjects had higher baseline levels of anxiety than subjects who completed the CO_2 inhalation. The majority of subjects reported that the CO_2 inhalation was the most unpleasant test (75% of the patients, 72% of the controls). Sixty-nine percent of the patients compared to 44% of the controls rated the effects of CO_2 as similar to usual panic attacks/extreme anxiety. This difference is not significant (chi^2 test).

Differential Expectancy Effect While Wearing Gas Mask

During the previous test session when subjects did not expect any panic challenge (Day 1), wearing the gas mask produced increases in anxiety compared to baseline, but no increases in cardiovascular measures. Both groups responded in the same way. In contrast, patients and controls responded differently to wearing the mask just prior to CO_2, that is, in anticipation of a panic challenge (Day 2). On this occasion, significant cardiovascular responses were observed. Patients showed larger increases in systolic and diastolic blood pressure, leading to significant Group x Time interactions. For heart rate, the interaction was only marginally significant ($p<0.08$). Heart rate increased slightly in the patient group and decreased slightly in the control group. Self-reported anxiety increased in both groups.

Discussion

Our results confirm Gorman et al. (5) in that prolonged inhalation of CO_2 raises anxiety levels and cardiovascular arousal in patients prone to panic attacks. Contrary to their findings, however, the rises also occurred in healthy control subjects. Furthermore, very few subjects, three patients and one control, asked to stop the procedure because of panic. The major difference between the groups were baseline or tonic level differences on all measures during the whole experiment. This replicates our earlier findings with lactate infusion (8).

Although the Cold Pressor Test and Mental Arithmetic are not usually considered panic provocations, both produced considerable increases in subjective anxiety and cardiovascular arousal. Some subjects found these stressors even more disturbing than the CO_2 inhalation although the duration of these tests was much shorter. These findings cast doubt on the specificity of CO_2 inhalation as an anxiety provocation method.

Wearing the gas mask and breathing room air produced increases in cardiovascular arousal only when CO_2 was expected. These expectancy effects were stronger in the patient group. These results underline the necessity to consider expectancy as a mediating variable in the interpretation of panic induction studies (6).

In conclusion, response to CO_2 inhalation was shown to be an effective laboratory model of anxiety. However, our results cast doubt on the specificity of CO_2 inhalation as a physiological trigger for panic. Furthermore, response to CO_2 cannot be regarded as a biological marker of a person's proneness to panic attacks. Expectancy effects were shown to be crucial mediating variables in laboratory models of panic attacks.

References

1. American Psychiatric Association. (1980). Diagnostic and statistical manual of mental disorders. Third edition. APA, Washington, D.C.
2. Klein, D.F. (1981). Anxiety reconceptualized. In D.F. Klein & J. Rabkin (Eds.), Anxiety: New research and changing concepts. Raven Press, N.Y.
3. Liebowitz, M.R., Fyer, A.J., Gorman, J.M., Dillon, D., Appleby, I.L., Levy, G., Anderson, S., Levitt, M., Palij, M., Davies, S.O. & Klein, D.F. (1984). Lactate provocation of panic attacks: I. Clinical and behavioral findings. Arch. Gen. Psychiat., 41: 764-770.
4. Liebowitz, M.R., Gorman, J.M., Fyer, A.J., Levitt, M., Dillon, D., Levy, G., Appleby, I.L., Anderson, S., Palij, M., Davies, S.O. & Klein, D.F. (1985). Lactate provocation of panic attacks: II. Biochemical and physiological findings. Arch. Gen. Psychiat., 42: 709-719.
5. Gorman, J.M., Askanazi, J., Liebowitz, M.R., Fyer, A.J., Stein, J., McKinney, J.M. & Klein, D.F. (1984). Response to hyperventilation in a group of patients with panic disorder. Am. J. Psychiat., 141: 857-861.
6. Margraf, J., Ehlers, A. & Roth, W.T. (1986). Sodium lactate infusions and panic attacks: A review and critique. Psychosom. Med., 48: 23-51.
7. Spitzer, R.L. & Williams, J.B. (1983). Structured clinical interview for DSM-III - Upjohn version (unpublished manual). N.Y. State Psychiatric Institute, N.Y. (SCID-UP 10/15/83).
8. Ehlers, A., Margraf, J., Roth, W.T., Taylor, C.B., Maddock, R.J., Sheikh, J., Kopell, M.L., McClenahan, K.L., Gossard, D., Blowers, G.H., Agras, W.S. & Kopell, B.S. (1986). Lactate infusions and panic attacks: Do patients and controls respond differently? Psychiatry Res., 17: 295-308.

Psychological and Electrophysiological Evidence for Vasopressin Effects in Human Memory

Gabriele Fehm-Wolfsdorf, Jan Born, Karl Heinz Voigt and Horst-Lorenz Fehm

Many hormones have been found to possess properties that are distinct from their classical endocrine functions. Among these, the neurohypophyseal hormones, vasopressin (VP) and oxytocin with their well-known chemical, cytological, and cellular physiological actions (1), have been found to alter behavior by acting on central nervous system functions. Evidence that VP may have beneficial effects on memory was accumulated in animal studies using paradigms of conditioned avoidance behavior or retrograde amnesia. In these studies, very low amounts of VP-related peptides administered cerebroventricularly resulted in resistance to extinction (2, 3). Although negative findings were infrequently reported from laboratories other than Utrecht, vehement criticisms were made of de Wied's central vasopressin-memory hypothesis (4). Firstly, the assumption that peripheral administration of VP acted directly on the CNS was questioned. Instead, it was suggested that its influences were mediated by peripheral actions, e.g., by vasopressor actions (5). Secondly, alternatives to the memory hypothesis interpretation have been proposed, e.g., that VP affects reinforcement mechanisms, and modulates arousal level (6).

Human studies have mainly focused on the treatment of patients suffering from memory deficits. Until now, the results have been inconclusive. The rate of success in clinical trials may be no higher than chance as long as there is no agreement as to what particular stage of information processing is improved by the substance. Hence it seems appropriate, at first, to specify the effects of VP on central nervous activity in normal humans.

Methods and Results

To define the exact psychological operations affected by VP and by oxytocin (which is presumed to have opposite effects), we performed a series of studies combining the methods of experimental psychology and psychophysiology. After a baseline session and before the experimental session, subjects received 20 I.U. of lysin-vasopressin as intranasal spray for three days. All treatments were held double-blind. Study I and II (7, 8) included 10 male student volunteers per treatment group, with study II containing an additional oxytocin treatment group. In study III (9) a single person was tested within 12 sessions after

This research was supported by Deutsche Forschungsgemeinschaft.

randomized intake of LVP or placebo. Study IV (10) used a co-twin control design with 17 pairs of monozygotic twins participating in two sessions each. We followed several lines of evidence across these experiments:

Does VP Enhance Memory Functions?

Study I and II employed a classical paradigm for the analysis of long-term versus short-term memory functions. Subjects heard lists of 15 common German nouns at a rate of 1 item/2 sec. The words they still remembered at the end of the list had to be written down either immediately (immediately free recall) or after an interpolating activity (delayed free recall). In the latter condition the enhanced recall of the most recent items from short-term storing ("recency effect" in free recall) breaks down. In this experiment, recall from long-term memory was not affected by the VP treatment. But the peptide was found to influence immediate recall performance. While placebo subjects from baseline to experimental session gained in recall from short-term store, i.e., enhanced recall of the most recent items, peptide subjects, by contrast, improved in long-term store, recalling more items from the beginning of the list (Figure 1).

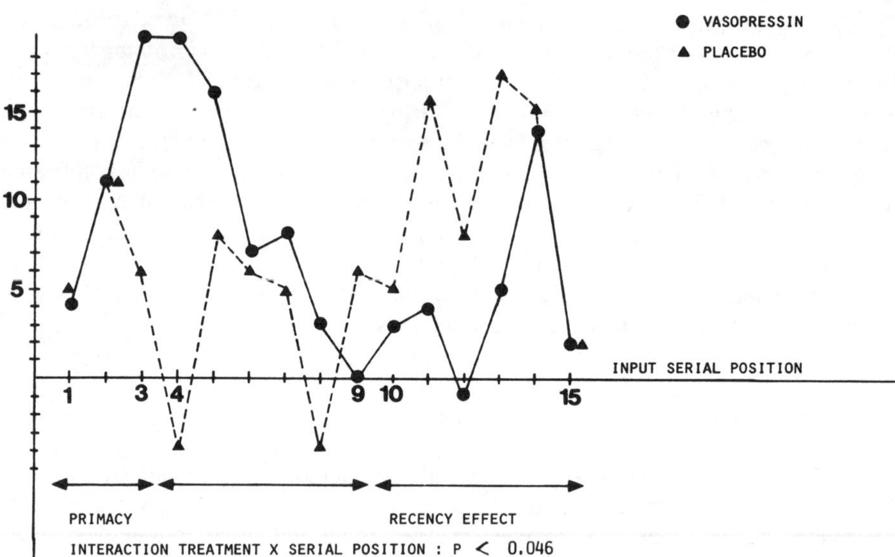

Figure 1. Number of words recalled correctly: Difference from baseline to session 2.

Since there was no treatment effect on delayed recall performance, an interpretation of this interaction as an enhancement of long-term memory but not short-term store seemed not to be justified. Baddeley and Hitch (11) proposed that the recency effect could reflect a retrieval strategy of the subject. In study II, therefore, we controlled for this variable. Subjects first had some training on the memory task, and were required to adopt the strategy of starting recall with the last few items. In fact, homogenizing the subjects' recall strategies by this procedure led to the disappearance of the differential peptide effects obtained in study I. Overall recall of the VP treated group was not significantly higher compared to controls, but significantly better than the performance in the oxytocin group which was worse than baseline values. That VP does not induce any memory enhancement superior to placebo was also confirmed by results from the single case study (III) including the same immediate recall task.

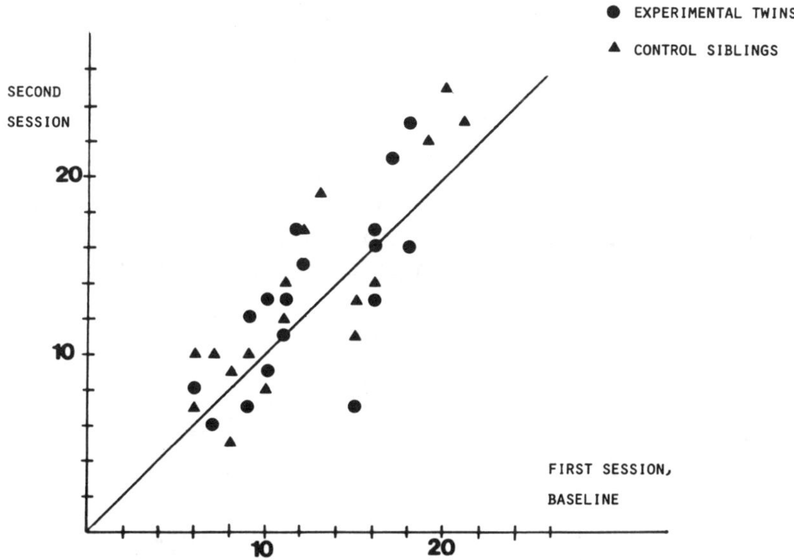

Figure 2. Number of words recalled correctly: Correlation of performance between sessions.

Some authors argued that beneficial effects of the peptide on memory might be visible only in states of deficiency. In study IV we therefore experimentally induced a quasi-amnesic state in normal subjects (12). When subjects concentrate on their lip-movements during speaking the items of the list they can only remember half as many items compared to controls. Treatment with VP, however, did not compensate for this deficiency. With monozygotic twins participating in this study the negative findings appeared to be even more valid: The number of items recalled correctly was highly correlated between twins, $r=0.67$ first session, $r=0.75$ second session. Figure 2 shows that performance of session 2 could be well predicted from the recall in session 1, even after peptide treatment in the second session. This confirmed that there was no apparent effect of the VP treatment.

Are the Behavioral Effects of VP Mediated by Peripheral Changes?

As already mentioned it has been argued that behavioral effects after peripheral administration of VP might be the consequence of peripheral alterations. With regard to vasopressor actions of the peptide, studies have focused on blood pressure as a possible intervening variable. The respective results showing parallel influences on extinction of conditioned behavior and on blood pressure elevation, however, rely on extremely high doses of VP. During the course of study IV we measured blood pressure and heart rate repeatedly and could not detect any change in these variables by VP. This is in line with studies which failed to find any change in endocrine function with doses typically used in behavioral studies on VP (13).

Does VP Exert Arousing Effects, and Is its Administration Aversive?

Support for the view that VP acts as a negative reinforcer comes from studies by Ettenberg et al. (14). They reported that VP injection produced a conditioned taste aversion, and that rats avoided a distinctive place which had previously been paired with VP administration. From this and other results Gash and Thomas concluded that emotional/motivational factors might be influenced by VP which indirectly led to modulations of cognitive functioning.

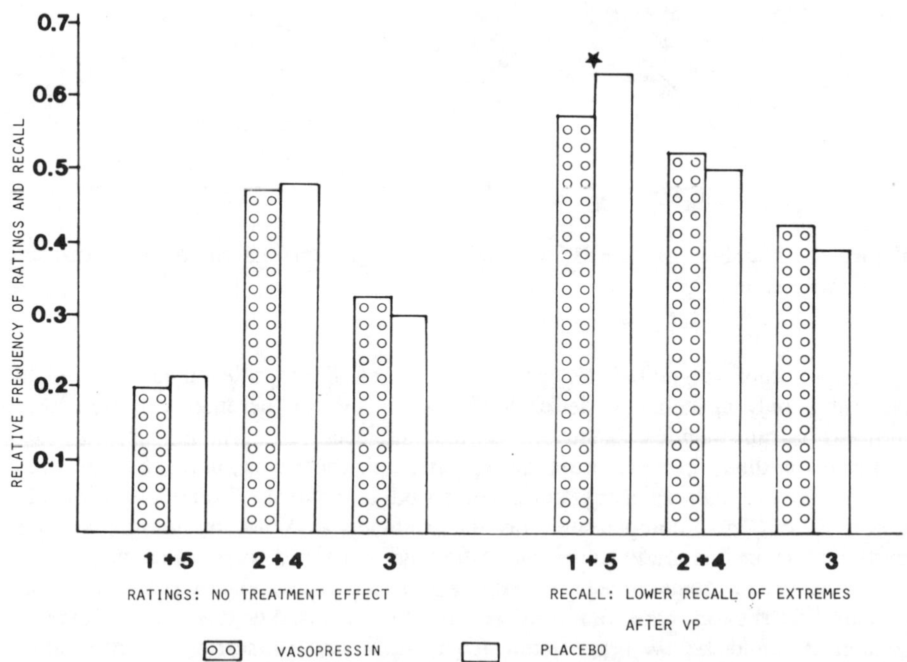

Figure 3. Ratings and recall of items according to their emotional value.

Transferring this to human verbal memory performance we would expect a more negative ("unpleasant") classification of verbal material with subsequent better recall of "negative" items after treatment with VP. In study IV subjects rated every item of a list according to its subjective emotional value on a five-point scale reaching from "very pleasant" to "very unpleasant." These ratings did not differ between the treatment groups. Results concerning recall are summarized in Figure 3. Neutral words had the lowest relative frequency of recall in both groups. The treatment did not affect recall of "pleasant" versus "unpleasant" words, except that VP treated subjects recalled significantly less items previously assigned to extreme ratings (see Figure 3: Ratings 1+5; $chi^2=5.9$; 2; 95%=5.9).

From this results it may be concluded that VP induced some subject arousal which, on top of the arousal induced by extreme items, exceeded an optimal level for recall performance, thus impairing it. In this view performance is assumed to depend on arousal in an inverted-U shaped curve (law of Yerkes-Dodson). However, as no exact relations between the level of arousal and most specific measures of task performance have been demonstrated, the arousal concept often seems to be misused to explain performance enhancements post hoc.

Influences of VP on arousal, in addition, would not explain outcomes of the single case study (IV) where treatment with VP enhanced performance in some tasks (e.g., shortened reaction times in the Stroop task), leaving performance in others unaffected (e.g., Sternberg task and free recall). The pattern of variables affected by the neuropeptide treatment in this study rather pointed to a role of VP in earlier stages of information processing.

How to Localize the Influence of VP During the Course of Information Processing?

Behavioral measures such as reaction time, number of successful trials, etc., only roughly compare CNS input and output of an otherwise black box. In contrast, recording of the EEG during a distinct task performance provides a continuous measure of processing. Special waveforms of the stimulus evoked potentials can be associated with psychological concepts. In study IV, subjects performed a dichotic listening task providing electrophysiological measures of selective attention (15). Subjects heard sequences of tone pips of different pitchs in each ear, 800 or 1200 Hz respectively. Interspersed among these frequent "standard" tones were rare "target" tones of a slightly higher pitch. Subjects were required to covertly count the target tones in one ear, ignoring all tones in the other, the unattended ear. EEG recordings were obtained from electrode locations along the midline from frontal, central and parietal leads. Auditory evoked potentials were averaged for attended and unattended standard and target stimuli, separately. The course of the evoked potential was mainly changed within the range of 180 to 220 msec after stimulus onset. VP induced a negative shift of the amplitudes within this latency range. Figure 4 demonstrates that this negative shift was more apparent after the rare target stimuli, and occurred no matter if these stimuli were attended to or not. Increased negativity at that particular latency range - independently from voluntary selective attention towards stimuli - led us to the assumption that VP primarily affected the autonomic processing of stimulus deviance.

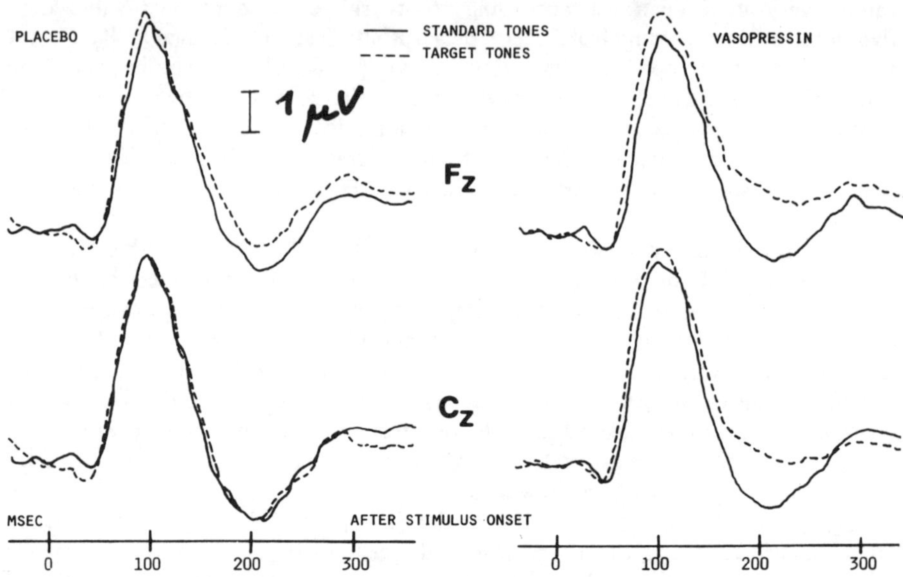

Figure 4. Auditory evoked potentials after different treatments.

Conclusion

To specify the behavioral effects of vasopressin in normal human central nervous functioning, a series of studies including tasks from experimental psychology and psychophysiology measures was performed. Results obtained with subjects of different age, sex, and social status fail to show any memory enhancing properties of VP treatment. Selectively attending to stimuli, too, does not seem to be the process primarily affected by VP. Influences of VP become evident rather early in the course of information processing when incoming stimuli are matched with previous ones. Autonomic responding to deviant stimuli can be described as pre-attentive mechanism (16) enabling fast stimulus-oriented reacting of the organism. Future research should clarify thc role of vasopressin in this mechanism.

References

1. Cross, B.A. & Leng, G. (1983). The neurohypophysis: Structure, function and control. Prog. Brain Res., 60. Elsevier, Amsterdam.
2. De Wied, D. (1983). Central actions of neurohypophysial hormones. In B.A. Cross & G. Leng (Eds.), The neurohypophysis: Structure, function and control. Prog. Brain Res., 60. Elsevier, Amsterdam, p. 155-167.
3. Van Wimersma Greidanus, T.B., Van Ree, J.M. & De Wied, D. (1983). Vasopressin and memory. Pharmacol. Ther., 20: 437-458.

4. Gash, D.M. & Thomas, G.J. (1983). What is the importance of vasopressin in memory processes? Trends Neurosci., 60: 197-198.
5. Le Moal, M., Dantzer, R., Mormede, P., Baduel, A., Lebrun, C., Ettenberg, A., Van der Kooy, D., Wenger, J., Deyo, S., Koob, G.F. & Bloom, F.E. (1984). Behavioral effects of peripheral administration of arginine vasopressin: A review of our search for a mode of action and a hypothesis. Psychoneuroendocrinology, 9, 4: 319-341.
6. Saghal, A. (1984). A critique of the vasopressin-memory hypothesis. Psychopharmacology, 83: 215-228.
7. Fehm-Wolfsdorf, G., Voigt, K.H. & Fehm, H.L. (1983). Human memory and lysin-vasopressin: A psychological study. In E. Endröczi, L. Angelucci, D. De Wied, & U. Scapagnini (Eds.), Neuropeptides and psychosomatic processes. Academiai Kiado, Budapest, p. 81-88.
8. Fehm-Wolfsdorf, G., Born, J., Voigt, K.H. & Fehm, H.L. (1984). Human memory and neurohypophyseal hormones: Opposite effects of vasopressin and oxytocin. Psychoneuroendocrinology, 3: 285-292.
9. Fehm-Wolfsdorf, G., Born, J., Voigt, K.H. & Fehm, H.L. (1984). Behavioral effects of vasopressin. A single case study. Neuropsychobiology, 11: 49-53.
10. Fehm-Wolfsdorf, G., Born, J., Voigt, K.H. & Fehm, H.L. (1985). Vasopressin does not enhance memory processes: A study in human twins. Peptides, 6: 297-300.
11. Baddeley, A.D. & Hitch, G.J. (1977). Recency reexamined. In S. Dornic (Ed.), Attention and performance VI. Erlbaum, Hillsdale, N.J., p. 647-667.
12. Graf, P., Mandler, G. & Haden, P.E. (1982). Simulating amnesic symptoms in normal subjects. Science, 218: 1243-1244.
13. Rousselle, J., Lacranjan, J., Dubey, L., Audibert, A. & Felber, J.P. (1979). Central effects of vasopressin in man, not mediated by ACTH release. Acta Endocrinol., Suppl., 225, 411.
14. Ettenberg, A., Van der Kooy, D., Le Moal, M., Koob, G.F. & Bloom, F.E. (1982). Can aversive properties of (peripherally-injected) vasopressin account for its putative role in memory? Behav. Brain Res., 7: 331-350.
15. Born, J., Fehm-Wolfsdorf, G., Schiebe, M., Birbaumer, N., Fehm, H.L. & Voigt, K.H. (1985). An ACTH 4-9 analog impairs selective attention in man. Life Sci., 36: 2117-2125.
16. Neisser, U. (1974). Kognitive Psychologie. Klett, Stuttgart.

Effects of Restraint on Adjuvant Arthritis in Two Strains of Rats

Wolfgang Klosterhalfen and Sybille Klosterhalfen

The possible influence of psychological factors in the pathogenesis of rheumatoid arthritis has frequently been discussed. Thus, in addition to "arthritic personality," stress also has been considered to play a role in the etiology and course of this immune disease (1). This view, which is based on correlative studies, is supported by experimental results suggesting that various stressors may affect immune responses in animals and humans (2, 3). However, it is not yet possible to predict results of stress treatments on the development of experimentally induced arthritis in animals. The few experiments published to date yielded conflicting results. Thus, in a pioneering paper, Amkraut et al. (4) reported that crowding enhanced adjuvant arthritis (AA) in Fisher rats. However, in Sofia's study (5), crowding had suppressive effects on AA in Sprague-Dawley rats. Rogers et al. showed that type II collagen-induced arthritis was suppressed in Wistar rats by transportation plus social stimulation (6), but was aggravated by noise (7). In our own experiments on the effects of several putative stressors on the course of AA, neither housing conditions, nor social stimulation, nor noise had reliable effects on the degree of hind paw swelling (the major clinical symptom of the disease) in Wistar rats (unpublished data).

It seemed therefore appropriate to choose a presumably more powerful stressor, restraint to test the idea noted above. Restraint procedures comparable to ours (see below) have been shown to result in significant changes in plasma corticosterone, prolactin, and growth hormone (8). Furthermore, because the divergent results of the cited experiments on arthritis may partly be due to the use of different strains across experiments, and because there is evidence that stress may act differentially on resistance to disease in different strains (9), a comparison was made on the effects of restraint on AA in two strains of rats.

General Method

AA was induced by a subplantar injection of 0.1 ml of complete Freund's adjuvant (CFA, Behringwerke, Marburg) under light ether narcosis on day 0. The degree of swelling in both hind paws was determined by two "blind" and independent observers on days 12, 14, 16, 18, and 20. A scale of nine standards

We wish to thank J.B. Overmier and H.-J. Steingrüber for their helpful comments on an earlier version of the manuscript.

(range: 0 to 4, intervals: 0.5) of dental-acrylic-casted alginate impressions was used from other arthritic hind paws (interrater reliability for the injected paws: r = 0.90 to 0.95).

Animals were restrained for 2h/24h in perforated plastic tubes (16 x 5 cm) which could be opened at both ends. Stressed animals had no access to food and water during restraint. Thus, the term "restraint" is used here as a short hand for a more complex stress procedure. In order to leave home cage animals as undisturbed as possible, food and water were not removed while stressed animals were restraint. (A pilot study revealed that food and water deprivation for 2h/24h for 1 week, compared to no deprivation, does not affect body weight gain.)

ANOVA's were calculated for injected hind paws; for the non-injected hind paws Halperin U-tests for censored samples were used. ANOVA's were also calculated to test for a reduction in body weight gain which may be regarded as a crude stress indicator.

Experiment 1

Methods and Results

Twenty-four male Long Evans (LE, inbred, SPF) and 24 male Wistar rats (W, outbred, SPF) were housed 2/cage with food and water *ad lib.* At the end of an adaptation week, mean body weights were 231 g (LE) and 263 g (W), respectively. In both strains, pairs of rats were matched for body weight and then randomly assigned to Groups R (restraint) or HC (home cage).

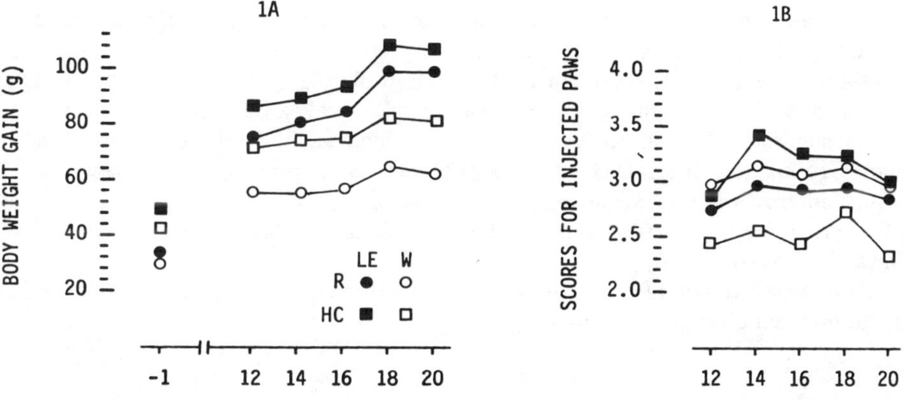

Figure 1. Body weight gain (1A) and scores for the injected hind paws (1B) on different days before and after the induction of AA in groups LE-R, LE-HC, W-R, and W-HC.

Groups LE-R and W-R were restrained for 2h in the mornings of days -7 to -1; groups LE-HC and W-HC were left undisturbed. On day 0, all animals were injected with CFA.

As a consequence of the stress procedure, Groups R gained significantly less weight than Groups HC from Day -8 to Day -1 ($F(1,44)=55.7$, $p<0.001$); weight gain was also reduced in the restraint groups on Days 12 to 20 ($F(1,44)=6.2$, $p<0.05$). There was no significant "restraint x strain" interaction (see Figure 1A).

Figure 1B shows the degree of swelling in the injected hind paws on Days 12 to 20. Restraint had no significant main effect; however, there was a significant "restraint x strain" interaction ($F(1,44)=13.1$, $p<0.001$): while restraint suppressed paw swelling in LE, the opposite was true for W, i.e., the stress procedure resulted in an enhancement of hind paw swelling. Restraint reduced the number of swellings in the uninjected hind paws: 16 of 24 unrestrained but only 8 of 24 restrained rats showed (typically minor) signs of inflammation; a Halperin U-test revealed that the degree of swelling differed significantly between restrained and unrestrained groups ($p<0.05$).

Experiment 2

The aim of this experiment was to test whether the structure of findings seen in Experiment 1 could be replicated under somewhat modified conditions. In an attempt to increase the effects of stress, animals were restrained during their more active (dark) period.

Methods and Results

All procedural details were the same as in Experiment 1 except for the following changes: The animals' light-dark cycle was reversed (from Day -33 until the end of the experiment). Restraint took place on Days -6 to -1. On Day -7 mean body weights were 258 g (LE) and 245 g (W), respectively.

As suggested by Figure 2A, Groups R gained significantly less body weight than Groups HC from Day -7 to -1 ($F(1,44)=26.1$, $p<0.001$); the "restraint x strain" interaction was significant, i.e., stress effects were more pronounced in LE ($F(1,44)=7.9$, $p<0.01$). Restraint had no effects on relative body weight during Days 12 to 20 ($ps<0.10$).

Restraint did not affect swelling either in the injected (s. Figure 2B) or in the uninjected hind paws (all $ps>0.10$).

Discussion

Reduced body weight gain in Groups R on Day -1 is consistent with the idea that restraint was an effective stressor in both strains. Stress effects on body weight seem, however, not to be closely related to the course of AA.

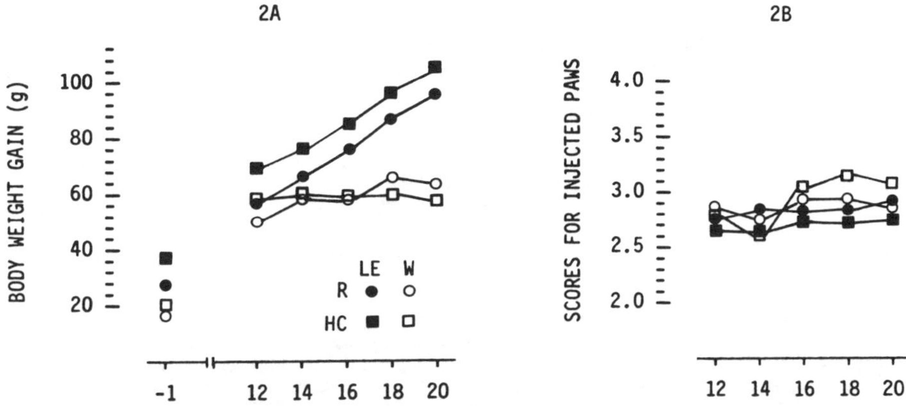

DAYS BEFORE AND AFTER INDUCTION OF ADJUVANT ARTHRITIS

Figure 2. Body weight gain (2A) and scores for the injected hind paw (2B) on different days before and after the induction of AA in groups LE-R, LE-HC, W-R, and W-HC.

In separate experiments, our restraint procedure left rectal temperature essentially unchanged; therefore, it seems unlikely that the effects of restraint on AA were mediated by changes in body temperature.

The differential stress effects seen in the injected hind paws in Experiment 1 suggest that both genetic and environmental factors played a role. For example, the two strains could have produced different hormonal response patterns and/or their immune systems could have responded differently to hormonal changes. It is also conceivable that restraint was more intense in Wistar rats because these animals had higher body weights than Long Evan rats.

Stress effects in the uninjected paws were less dramatic (which might be due to a floor effect) and were not strain-specific. The dissociation of stress effects in the injected versus uninjected hind paws in Wistar rats suggests that the presumed strain specific hormonal and/or immunological responses also have strain specific *courses* (in the uninjected hind paws, AA develops later).

Restraint did not have any effects on the development of AA in Experiment 2 and this may be because the light-dark reversal served itself as a stressor (cf. 10) which may have masked any additional stress effects due to restraint. Alternatively, the light-dark reversal may have modified the effects of restraint. These interpretations are consistent with the results of another experiment with Wistar rats in which enhancing effects of restraint on AA were abolished when mild tail shock was added to restraint (11). So far, the effects of stress on inflammatory joint diseases in animals are poorly understood. The implications of stress related brain-immune system interactions are, however, so important that every effort should be made to elucidate the conditions that produce predictable stress effects in experimental immune diseases (12) such as AA.

References

1. Anderson, K.O., Bradley, L.A., Young, L.D., McDaniel, L.K. & Wise, C.M. (1985). Rheumatoid arthritis: Review of psychological factors related to etiology, effects, and treatment. Psychol. Bull., 98: 358-387.
2. Ader, R. (Ed.) (1981). Psychoneuroimmunology. Academic Press, N.Y.
3. Ballieux, R.E. & Heijnen, C.J.: This volume.
4. Amkraut, A.A., Solomon, G.F. & Kraemer, H.C. (1971). Stress, early experience and adjuvant-induced arthritis in the rat. Psychosom. Med., 33: 203-214.
5. Sofia, R.D. (1980). The effect of overcrowding stress on the development of adjuvant-induced polyarthritis in the rat. J. Pharm. Pharmacol., 32: 874-875.
6. Rogers, M.P., Trentham, D.E., McCune, W.J., Ginsberg, B.I., Rennke, H.G., Reich, P. & David, J.R. (1980). Effect of psychological stress on the induction of arthritis in rats. Arthritis Rheum., 23: 1337-1342.
7. Rogers, M.P., Trentham, D.E., Dynesius-Trentham, R., Daffner, K. & Reich, P. (1983). Exacerbation of collagen arthritis by noise stress. J. Rheumatol., 10: 651-654.
8. Kant, G.J., Bunnell, B.N., Mougey, E.H., Pennington, L.L. & Meyerhoff, J.L. (1983). Effects of repeated stress on pituitary cyclic AMP, and plasma prolactin, corticosterone and growth hormone in male rats. Pharmacol. Biochem. Behav. 18: 967-971.
9. Friedman, S.B. & Glasgow, L.A. (1973). Interaction of mouse strain and differential housing upon resistance to Plasmodium berghei. J. Parasitol., 59: 851-854.
10. Kort, W.J. & Weijam, J.M. (1982). Effect of chronic light-dark shift stress on the immune response of the rat. Physiol. Behav., 29: 1083-1087.
11. Klosterhalfen, W., Klosterhalfen, S. & Hampel, U. (in press). Restriktionsstress und Adjuvans-Arthritis: Ein psychoimmunologisches Experiment. In W. Miltner, W.D. Gerber & K. Mayer (Eds.), Verhaltensmedizin. Ergebnisse und Perspektiven interdiziplinärer Forschung. Springer-Verlag, Heidelberg.
12. Fox, B.H. (1985). Disease is a stepchild in psychoneuroimmunology. Invited commentary on R. Ader & N. Cohen. CNS-immune system interactions: Conditioning phenomena. Behav. Brain. Sci., 8: 400.

The Role of Hypothalamic Norepinephrine in the Control of Corticosterone Secretion in Rat

Hendrik Lehnert, Daniel K. Reinstein and Richard J. Wurtman

In previous experiments we have demonstrated that acute and dietary administration of the essential amino acid l-tyrosine - the circulating precursor for brain norepinephrine (NE) - alleviates sequelae of uncontrollable stress such as behavioral depression and depletion of NE in specific brain areas, e.g., hypothalamus and locus coeruleus (1, 2). Tyrosine was not found to be effective under normal conditions, it only exerted its effects like restoring locomotor activity and repleting NE concentrations via an enhanced supply of substrate in the state of neuronal activation.

An augmented secretion of corticosterone has long been described as another consequence of an acute stress in rats. Since numerous studies suggested roles for NE and epinephrine (E) in the secretion of ACTH and corticosterone (3-5) most likely by inhibiting CRF secretion, we reasoned that a depletion of hypothalamic NE in a stressful event might diminish the tonic inhibition of CRF release and thus participate in the elevation of plasma corticosterone following an acute stress.

The aim of this study was thus to investigate, whether preventing these neurochemical changes by dietary l-tyrosine administration could also prevent the rises in plasma corticosterone.

Methods

L-tyrosine was administered in a high-tyrosine diet, where the casein was supplemented with four times as much free tyrosine and consumed for three consecutive days.

The stress procedure consisted of an electric tail-shock delivered for 5 sec every 30 sec at 20 V intensity (1-2 mA) over a period of 60 minutes. The animals were then allowed to recover for 10 minutes before behavioral testing began. Behavioral activity was then assessed using an open-field/hole-poke apparatus that was unfamiliar to the animal and was rated by an independent observer. Four behavioral categories were measured: Locomotion, hole-poking, standing on the hindlegs and grooming.

Tyrosine and plasma corticosterone were determined fluorometrically, NE by high-performance liquid-chromatography and ACTH by radioimmunoassay.

Results

Stress alone significantly decreased locomotion and exploratory behavior, while the group receiving tyrosine and stress was not different from controls. Grooming as a possibly ACTH dependent behavior was increased in stressed animals receiving a normal diet.

Hypothalamic tyrosine was doubled in both the stressed and unstressed groups receiving tyrosine when compared to both control groups. The stress procedure significantly reduced the concentration of hypothalamic NE in control animals receiving no tyrosine, while the high-tyrosine diet restored NE levels in stressed rats almost to normal (Figures 1 and 2).

Pituitary and plasma levels of ACTH tended to increase, but did not reach statistical significance. Plasma corticosterone levels were significantly elevated in the stressed animals receiving a normal diet; the high-tyrosine diet markedly attenuated the stress-induced increase in corticosterone secretion. In no case had tyrosine alone (i.e., without stress) any effect (Figure 3).

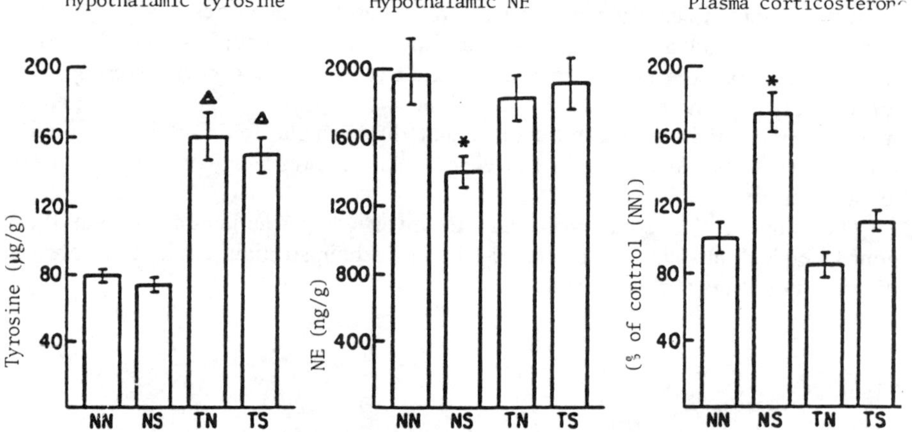

Figures. Effects of tyrosine and stress on hypothalamic tyrosine and norepinephrine and on plasma corticosterone.

Groups: NN (normal diet, no stress), NS (normal diet, stress),
TN (high-tyrosine diet, no stress), TS (high-tyrosine diet, stress)

Symbols: * different from other groups
△ different from NN and NS

Discussion

These data demonstrate that tyrosine supplementation not only prevents the behavioral deficits and regional brain NE depletion caused by an acute stress, but also suppresses the stress-induced rise in plasma corticosterone levels. This effect of tyrosine on stress-induced corticosterone secretion may be exerted by supplementing activated noradrenergic with their circulating precursor and thereby repleting hypothalamic NE concentrations. The mechanisms by which the physiological activity of catecholaminergic neurons is coupled to their ability to respond to supplementary tyrosine probably involves the activation of tyrosine-hydroxylase, which uncouples the relation between the enzyme and its tetrahydrobiopterin cofactor (whose availability may be rate-limiting for catecholamine biosynthesis under basal conditions) and decreases the enzyme's susceptibility to end-product inhibition (6).

Thus, these data provide further evidence that hypothalamic CRF secretion might - at least under stressful conditions - be under inhibitory control of hypothalamic NE.

Since in human depression decreases in brain NE (7, 8), elevations in plasma cortisol and cerebrospinal fluid levels of CRF-like immunoreactivity (9) have been observed, it might be important to further explore tyrosine's role in the treatment of depression.

References

1. Reinstein, D.K., Lehnert, H., Scott, N.A. & Wurtman, R.J. (1984). Tyrosine prevents behavioral and neurochemical correlates of acute stress in rats. Life Sci., 34: 2225-2231.
2. Lehnert, H., Reinstein, D.K., Strowbridge, B.W. & Wurtman, R.J. (1984). Neurochemical and behavioral consequences of acute, uncontrollable stress: Effects of dietary tyrosine. Brain Res., 303: 215-223.
3. Rose, J.C., Goldsmith, P.C., Holland, F.J., Kaplan, S.L. & Ganong, W.F. (1976). Effect of electrical stimulation on the canine brain stem on the secretion of ACTH and growth hormone. Neuroendocrinology, 22: 352-362.
4. Ganong, W.F. (1980). Neurotransmitters and pituitary function: Regulation of ACTH secretion. Fed. Proc., 39: 2923-2930.
5. Mezey, E., Kiss, J.Z., Skirboll, L.R., Goldstein, M. & Axelrod, J. (1984). Increase of corticotropin-releasing factor staining in rat paraventricular nucleus neurons by depletion of hypothalamic adrenaline. Nature, 310: 140-141.
6. Roth, R.H., Morgenroth, V.H. & Salzmann, P.M. (1975). Tyrosine hydroxylase: Allosteric activation induced by stimulation of activated noradrenergic neurons. Naunyny Schmiedeberg's Arch. Pharmacol., 289: 327-334.
7. Maass, J.W. (1975). Biogenic amines and depression. Arch. Gen. Psychiatry, 32: 1357-1361.
8. Leonard, B.E. (1982). Current status of the biogenic amine theory of depression. Neurochem. Int., 4: 339-350.
9. Nemeroff, C.B., Widerlöv, E., Bissette, G., Wallens, H., Karlsson, J., Eklund, K., Kilts, C.D., Loosen, P. & Vale, W. (1984). Elevated concentrations of CSF corticotropin-releasing factor-like immunoreactivity in depressed patients. Science, 226: 1342-1344.

Major Depression:
A Behavioral Analysis of Core Symptoms

John I. Nurnberger, Joseph N. Hingtgen and Morris H. Aprison

Some clinicians, as well as laboratory and clinical investigators continuously question the validity of using animal models in order to gain insights into the affective disorders. A central problem with such models is that the total behavioral complex as repeatedly confirmed not only in extended clinical observations, but also emphasized in the clinical research literature, is not represented. Recently proposed models, (1, 2) are closer approximations but still fall short of the behavioral ideal.

Since the current interests of two of the authors (Hingtgen and Aprison) working in the field of depression concern the use of an animal model to study this illness, a decision was made to join with a psychiatrist (Nurnberger) and systematically analyze the characteristic behavioral repertoires most commonly manifest in human major depression. Investigators attempting to describe once again the depressive state might be discouraged by the historically relevant comment (3) as follows:

> It seems as if the psychiatric profession has taken for granted that all that can be known about depressions has already been discovered and thoroughly described. As a matter of fact, one finds that clinically relatively little new has been added to the description of depressions in general since antiquity. Textbook descriptions of this entity are stereotyped accounts which have been copied from book to book and have been repeated from generation to generation.

This statement could be repeated with equal relevance at the present time, twenty-five years later. Therefore, we feel it is necessary to use a new approach, one that incorporates the total spectrum of representative behavioral symptoms. Such an analysis should provide the basis for an evaluation of current models of depression. In addition, this profile of depression could provide for expanding a current model or developing a new one, either of which generate a more meaningful animal model for use in future studies of depression.

A Functional Analysis of Characteristic Behaviors in Human Major Depression

A review of the clinical testimony (4, 5) suggests two conspicuous factors as determining the behavioral deficits in major depressions in man (see Table 1). Factor I is expressed in the central experience of a depressed individual as

Supported in part by grant from the Association for the Advancement of Mental Health Research and Education, Inc.

being totally uncoupled from or uncontrolled by basic positive unlearned and learned reinforcement contingencies.

Table 1. Central features of a behavioral analysis of human major depression: A two-factor model.[1]

I. Loss of Control by Positive Reinforcers	
A. Primary (unlearned) reinforcers:	Eating, excretory, sleeping and sexualy behaviors.
B. Conditioned (learned) reinforcers:	Persons, places, times, and behaviors associated with pleasure and joy.
II. Overcontrol by Aversive Reinforcers	
A. Primary reinforcers:	Guilt, worthlessness, hopelessness, helplessness, etc.
B. Conditioned reinforcers:	Certain factors associated with occurrence and treatment of depression.

Thus, the patient suffering from a major depression is joyless, pleasure-free, with total loss of savor for: (1) eating functions, (2) excretory functions, (3) sleeping functions, (4) sexual functions, (5) social recreational activities, and (6) work activities. Factor II includes all elements of Factor I, but adds the condition that the patient is also under the tyrannical domination and control of *aversive* contingencies.

We will now consider Factor I in the behavioral model of human depression (major, unipolar) as manifested in six activities no longer controlled by primary or conditioned positive reinforcers (see Table 2).

Eating Behavior

The depressed patient characteristically loses pleasure in eating. In "retarded" depression, representing approximately one-seventh of all clinical major depressions (6) there is a reduction of appetite as well as enjoyment of food, a reduction of all customary eating behaviors, and a loss of body weight. In the much more common (about 85%) "agitated" type of major depression, manifested by anxious, hostile, paranoid components (6) there is often an increase in eating behavior but of an atypical sort. Some of these individuals exhibit bulimic type patterns. In two separate populations of bulimic patients investigated for presence of major depression from 25-75% of the total satisfied diagnostic criteria for major depression (7, 8).

1. The authors have studied DSM-III but the present description given above is an attempt at ordering the observational data in terms of behavioral principles to facilitate comparison to animal models.

Table 2. Factor I: Loss of control by primary (unlearned) or conditioned (learned) positive reinforcers.

	Patient Type	
A. Primary behavior (unlearned positive reinforcing contingencies)	Behavioral retardation type[1] 15%	Behavioral agitation type[1] 85%
1. Eating behavior - loss of savor	Appetite and food consumption decreased; body weight decreased	Some may manifest increased eating, especially "junk foods" at odd times; body weight may be increased
2. Excretory activity loss of pleasurable relief	Constipation; obstipation	May manifest loose to waterly stools; bloody stools (rare)
3. Sleeping functions - absence of refreshment	Early morning arousals with tortuors occupations	Difficulty in falling asleep and staying asleep; ready rousability
4. Sexual behaviors - no erotic arousal or orgasmic fulfillment	Decreased sexual interest and activity; irregular or absent menses in female; loss of erectile potency in males	May exhibit perversly excessive sexual activity without savor or pleasure
B. Conditioned behavior (learned positive reinforcing contingencies)		
1. Recreational and social outlets - withdrawl of interest; absence of pleasurable participation	No recreational or social outlets pursued or desired; e.g., decreased or absent TV viewing	Compulsive, repetitive, superstitious rituals; behavior not goal oriented
2. Work and other conditioned positive reinforcing contingencies	For this items (B2) there is no difference between the retardation type patient and the agitated type: This loss involves all persons, places, time and circumstances and behaviors historically associated with pleasure and joy.	

1. Characteristics of these types refer to the worst case; patients may exhibit mildest to most severe forms, as well as few or many of these behaviors.

Some reveal extreme food idiosyncracies or almost total aversion seen in anorexia nervosa (8, 9). Other patients show additional alterations of customary eating behavior of an atypical type. The pattern of eating changes with rejection of breakfast and lunch and an increase in eating beginning late in the afternoon or early evening, with increased intake of high caloric, so-called "junk" foods. A resultant gain in weight occurs. Here, again, there is a little or no savor for food. Obesity and depression have been associated; significantly in the same patient. Twenty percent (10) to thirty percent (11) of a grossly obese population are reported to exhibit depressive symptoms.

Excretory Behavior

Both types of depressed patient (retarded and agitated) exhibit a total loss of pleasure in bowel excretory activities. In the retarded mode, constipation, fecal retention and occasionally even intestinal obstruction are seen, while in the agitated mode, loose, watery and frequently diarrheal stools are the rule (12).

Sleeping Behavior

In the third customary avenue of positive reinforcement, that is, having a refreshing sleeping experience, there is a critical disturbance (13). Most characteristic is a loss of refreshment and renewal which customarily follows a normal night's sleep of whatever pattern. In the retarded form of depression the patient frequently awakens in the late night or early morning hours and can then not fall back to sleep. While awake the patient is beset by insoluble worries and painful preoccupations, particularly focused on problems recently encountered or anticipated in the unwelcome morning. In the agitated form of depression the sleep disturbance is even more pervasive. In this instance the patient has difficulty falling asleep as well as in staying asleep, with uniformly ready rousability and painful mental preoccupations during all periods of restless wakefulness. It is this distressing sleep experience, sometimes extended over weeks or even months, which makes many patients dread even the prospect of trying to sleep. This behavior occasions not only increasing dependence on sleeping medications, but also precipitates desperate searches for sleep with excessive sleep medication and alcohol occasionally with a fatal outcome. Suicide by this route is one of the common methods in the United States.

Sexual Behavior

A very potent avenue of personal pleasure, social joy, and release is to be found in the exploitation of various sexual outlets. This positive reinforcement contingency is very early and sensitively compromised in depressed patients and provides the symptomatic indicator of the beginning of a major depressive episode, even when other cardinal symptoms may not have fully manifested themselves. In the retarded type of depression there is (a) turning away, frequently with aversion, from all customary sexual stimulation, with (b) loss of erectile capacity and potency in the male, and (c) irregular to absent menses in the female. In the agitated type of major depression there occasionally may be excessive sexual acting out and compulsive sexual behavior inconsistent with the ethical standards of the individual prior to the onset of depression. Further, there is no savor in the sexual activities that are pursued by the patient. There are even examples of excessive Don Juanism activities or acting out of prostitution fantasies in the agitated depressed patient.

Recreational, Social and Work Outlets

Extensive and varied recreational, social and work outlets are certainly characteristic of individuals in our culture who become vulnerable to major depression. Major depression is associated with a total loss of interest and turning away from these customary outlets with not only no free and spontaneous participation, but with an active aversion for such participation (14). In the retarded form of depression, these outlets are not exploited, and sometimes this even extends to television viewing. These individuals actually have an aversion to TV. In the agitated form of depression, characteristically repetitive ritualistic behaviors may be strongly maintained without any clear goal or orientation and with no participating joy, release, and savor. Many of these ritualistic repertoires have the strength and perverse durability of neurotic, obsessive-compulsive magical rituals (15), and may, in some instances, be vested with a pseudoreligious significance because of the underlying sense of intense guilt and sinfulness in such depressed individuals (see Table 2).

A second major behavioral modifier (Factor II) which is operative in human depressions is that individuals appear to be under the tyrannical domination of aversive contingencies (see Table 3).

It will be noted from the resume of Factor I that we are dealing with an individual who is effectively uncoupled from the control of positively reinforcing contingencies. The other side of this behavioral analysis must include the control which aversive contingencies obviously exert on the individual with major depression. In almost all patients with major depression there appears to be a deep and consuming conviction of unspeakable guilt (4). This peculiar conviction of guilt probably serves as the mechanism for the aversive control in this clinical condition just as punishment, or the anticipation of punishment or the prospect of escaping anticipated punishment, serves as a potent contingency in all types of aversive animal behavior control. Guilt, of course, makes punishment mandatory. Hence the many ritualistic, magical and symbolic behaviors which are elaborated and maintained, permit alleviation of intense distress. They permit the avoidance, postponement or escape from the punishment which is all to obviously deserved. Many subjects under such aversive tyranny fail to escape and of course finally ultimately visit an absurd justice on themselves through self-destruction. The fact is that over 25,000 people in the United States die by the suicidal route each year (16). What fraction of this total is represented by patients with major depression is not known.

Because of the prepotency of primary aversive contingencies operating in the depressed state, many important persons in the environment acquire conditioned aversive control over the patient's behavior (Table 3). Thus, the psychotherapist who is seen regularly during an intensely symptomatic period may acquire conditioned aversive properties which tend to prolong symptomatic distress. One of us (Nurnberger) has noted impressive improvement when such a patient was transferred to a second therapist during a prolonged vacation.

Table 3. Factor II: Overcontrol by primary (unlearned) or conditioned (learned) aversive reinforcers.[2]

A. Overcontrol by Aversive Contingencies
1) Awareness of consuming guilt.
2) Conviction of worthlessness.
3) Hopelessness, helplessness, rejection of proffered help.
4) Overpowering need for self-punishment, leading to suicidal activities.
B. Overcontrol by Conditioned Aversive Contingencies
1) The long-term therapist.
2) The somatic forms of therapy used such as drugs, ECT, etc.
3) Persons, places, times and other circumstances associated with experience of depression and agony.

Conditioned aversive properties may also be associated with various somatic therapies such as drugs and electroconvulsive therapy (ECT). Thus, ineffective medication (or sometimes even effective medication) may acquire negative associations with the symptoms of depression. In a similar manner a long series of ECT also has been observed to acquire aversive properties.

There are also instances in which family members, living circumstances, places of work, etc. have been repeatedly paired with the experience of depressive anguish. These acquire the power to sustain or prolong distress. Even the spouse with whom the long agony has been intimately shared can acquire conditioned aversive properties contributing to the chronicity of symptoms.

Discussion

Of most importance is the fact that in all of the published stereotypical animal models of depression which include 30 or more (see most recent reviews, 1, 2) none has been based on a systematic behavioral analysis of the symptoms of depression encountered in the clinical state. This lack is reflected in four of the most interesting and recently cited models involving, for example, olfactory bulbectomy (17, 18), anhedonia (18), learned helplessness (19), and postsynaptic hypersensitive serotonergic receptors (20-23). It is also noteworthy that no

2. The descriptions under Factor II are manifested by both retarded and agitated types.

critical evaluation of the symptoms of depression prior to our current formulation utilizes a comprehensive multimodal analysis of the behaviors of depressed patients which include not only the usual clinical symptomatology (i.e., sleeping, eating, excretory and sexual behaviors), but also the involved unifying behavioral concepts (i.e., uncoupling from positive reinforcement contingencies and control by primary and conditioned aversive contingencies).

The analysis of available data concerning core changes observed clinically in the syndrome of major depression revealed not only critical alterations in important behavioral repertoires, but also overall changes in schedules of reinforcement (24). Changes associated with the loss of control of human behavior by positive reinforcers, including not only the primary effects on eating, excretory, sleeping, and sexual behaviors, but also intimately associated effects on conditioned positive reinforcers as indicated in Table 1, do not elicit substantial question or debate. These alterations reflect clinical changes which have been described repeatedly½not only in the classical literature of depression but also in standard textbook descriptions of depression, and even the more recent behavioral descriptions incorporated in DSM III criteria (25). All are, however, most clearly reflective of the clinical subtype: Retarded depression.

The important fact is that such symptoms do not accurately reflect the changes associated with the more common agitated, hostile, paranoid, or anxious depressions (70-75%, see Table 2). The manifestation of agitated depression will be questioned by some. Thus, the inclusion of bulimic patterns in the agitated depressive category (7) might be debated, though there is independent supportive data for this (26). The presence of ruminative bsessive-compulsive behavioral patterns in unipolar depression has been investigated recently (15). Clinical records on a substantial population of inpatients revealed 110 with a primary discharge diagnosis of obsessive-compulsive illness. Thirty of these met acceptable criteria for primary depression. The authors suggested that obsessions and compulsions in this circumstance appeared to be secondary although the criteria for determining primary or secondary categorization were not provided. Our behavioral agitated type of depressive is perhaps most clearly reflected in the two sub-categories of Matussek (5), referred to by them as mental depression and aggressive-irritated depression. Finally, nowhere in the clinical literature are there substantiated references to the occurrences of paradoxical sexual behaviors as accompaniments of major depression, agitated type. These changes are indicated by direct clinical observation by one of us (Nurnberger).

Based on the analysis presented in this paper the authors feel that any model of depression under investigation should be tested for as many of the factors noted in Tables 2 and 3 as possible. It is interesting that the literature contains investigations where many of the parameters listed in these tables such as sleeping, eating, and sexual behavior have been studied by neurobiologists, but for different reasons than testing a model of depression. It is, therefore, of great interest to us that several of the neurotransmitters have been implicated in many of these normal physiological functions in animals and man as well as in the abnormal depressive state.

It should be apparent that several of the factors listed in Tables 2 and 3 cannot easily be tested. For example, we do not understand how guilt can be induced or measured in animals. It would seem that in man, it is very difficult to disassociate guilt from chronic anticipation of punishment. If this is true, and if one can equate the two in the case of animals, then it might be possible to test this concept.

The clinically orientated researcher may have a problem with the development of animal models of depression. Such an individual often suffers from the bias that the behavioral changes and deficits associated with clinical depression should ideally be the foundations of the behavioral programs and schedules used to generate the model. However, a closer scrutiny of the time course of symptomatic development in most major depressions would argue more strongly for the intervention of a disturbed metabolic process as the major instigator of symptomatic breakdown with the behavioral changes resulting from the chemical changes. It is now imperative for researchers in this field to try to measure more of these behavioral factors in their proposed model to see how close the fit is to the clinical picture. For example, in order to improve the hypersensitive serotonergic postsynaptic receptor model developed in our laboratories (20-23) we are attempting to measure as many as possible of the parameters listed in Tables 2 and 3 in addition to changes in behavioral response rates.

References

1. Jesberger, J.A. & Richardson, J.S. (1985). Animal models of depression: Parallels and correlates to severe depression in humans. Biol. Psychiat., 20: 764-784.
2. Willner, P. (1984). The validity of animal models of depression. Psychopharmacology, 83: 1-16.
3. Grinker, R.R., Miller, J., Sabshin, M., Nunn, R. & Nunnally, J.C. (1961). The phenomena of depressions. Hoeber, N.Y.
4. Leckman, J.F., Weissman, M.M., Prusoff, B.A., Caruso, K.A., Merikangas, K.R., Pauls, D.L. & Kidd, K.K. (1984). Subtypes of depression. Family study perspectives. Arch. Gen. Psychiat., 41: 833-838.
5. Matussek, P., Soldner, M. & Nagel, D. (1981). Identification of the endogenous depressive syndrome based on the symptoms and the characteristics of the course. Brit. J. Psychiat., 138: 361-372.
6. Overall, J.E., Hollister, L.E., Johnson, M. & Pennington, V. (1966). Nosology of depression and differential response to drugs. J. Am. Med. Assoc., 195: 946-948.
7. Brotman, A.W., Herzog, D.B. & Woods, S.W. (1984). Antidepressent treatment of bulimia: The relationship between bulimia and depressive symptomatology. J. Clin. Psychiat., 45: 7-9.
8. Herzog, D.B. (1984). Are anorexic and bulimic patients depressed? Am. J. Psychiat., 141: 1594-1597.
9. Viesselman, J.O. & Roig, M. (1985). Depression and suicidality in eating disorders. J. Clin. Psychiat., 46: 118-124.
10. Halmi, K.A., Long, M., Stunkard, A.J. & Mason, E. (1980). Psychiatric diagnosis of morbidly obese gastric bypass patients. Am. J. Psychiatry, 137: 470.
11. Hopkinson, G. & Bland, R.C. (1982). Depressive syndromes in grossly obese women. Can. J. Psychiat., 17: 213-215.
12. Weiss, K.J., Schwarz, H.J. & Berrettini, W.H. (1982). Phenelzine treatment of depression with chronic diarrhea. J. Clin. Psychiat., 43: 250-251.
13. Cicchetti, D.V. & Prusoff, B.A. (1983). Reliability of depression and associated symptoms. Arch. Gen. Psychiat., 40: 987-990.
14. Clark, D.C., Cavanaugh, S.A. & Gibbons, R.D. (1983). The core symptoms of depression in medical and psychiatric patients. J. Nerv. Ment. Dis., 171: 705-713.

15. Coryell, C. (1981). Obsessive-compulsive disorder and primary unipolar depression. Comparisons of background, family history, course and mortality. J. Nerv. Ment. Dis., 169: 220-224.
16. Statistical Abstracts of U.S., 105th ed., 1985.
17. Cairncross, K.D., Cox, B., Forster, C. & Wren, A.F. (1978). A new model for the detection of antidepressant drugs: Olfactory bulbectomy in the rat compared with existing models. J. Pharmacol. Methadaka, 1: 131-143.
18. Katz, R.J. (1982). Animal models of depression: Parallels and correlates to severe depression: Pharmacological sensitivity of a hedonic deficit. Pharmacol. Biochem. Behav., 16: 965-968.
19. Telner, J.I. & Singhal, R.L. (1984). Psychiatric proress. The learned helplessness model of depression. J. Psychiat. Res., 18: 207-215.
20. Aprison, M.H. & Hingtgen, J.N. (1981). Hypersensitive serotonergic receptors: A new hypothesis for one subgroup of unipolar depression derived from an animal model. In B. Haber, S. Gabay, S. Alivisatos & M. Issidorides (Eds.), Serotonin-current aspects of neurochemistry and function. Plenum Press, N.Y., p. 627-656.
21. Aprison, M.H. & Hingtgen, J.N. (1986). A hypersensitive serotonergic receptor theory of depression: The role of stress. In R.C.A. Frederickson, H.C. Hendrie, J.N. Hingtgen & M.H. Aprison (Eds.), Neuronal control of bodily function - Basic and clinical aspects: I. New concepts of regulation of autonomic, neuroendocrine and immune systems. Martinus-Nijhof, Boston.
22. Aprison, M.H., Hingtgen, J.N. & Nagayama, H. (1982). Testing a new theory of depression with an animal model: Neurochemical-behavioral evidence for postsynaptic serotonergic receptor involvement. In S. Langer, R. Takahashi, T. Seqawa & M. Briley (Eds.), New vistas in depression. Pergamon Press, Oxford, p. 171-178.
23. Aprison, M.H., Takahashi, R. & Tachiki, K. (1978). Hypersensitive serotonergic receptors involved in clinical depression - A theory. In B. Haber & M.H. Aprison (Eds.), Neuropharmacology and behavior. Plenum Press, N.Y., p. 23-53.
24. Ferster, C.B. (1973). A functional analysis of depression. Am. Psychol., 28: 857-870.
25. American Psychiatric Association (1980). Diagnostic and Statistical Manual of Mental Disorders (DSM III) (3rd ed.), American Psychiatric Association, Washington.
26. Hudson, J., Jeffer, P. & Pope, J. (1982). Bulimia related to affective disorder by family history and response to the dexamethasone suppression test. Am. J. Psychiat., 137: 695-698.

Epileptic Neuronal Activity: Involvement of Calcium Ions

Jörg Walden, Erwin-Josef Speckmann and Otto W. Witte

Seizure potentials in the EEG are associated with typical membrane potential changes of cortical neurons directly involved in epileptic activity. These membrane potential changes, labeled as paroxysmal depolarization shifts, consists of a steep depolarization leading to a burst of action potentials, of a plateau-like diminution of the membrane potential and of a final repolarization (1-4). Reports in the literature suggest that calcium ions are involved in the generation of these epileptic neuronal potentials (5). For a further analysis calcium channel blocking agents were applied intracellularly and systemically (6, 7).

Methods and Results

The investigations were performed on the motor and somatosensory cortex of the anesthetized and artificially ventilated rat. Focal epileptic activity induced by local application of penicillin served as the seizure model. Calcium channel blocking agents were applied into the intracellular space of single neurons by ionophoresis or by pressure pulses through the recording microelectrode and to the extracellular space of the epileptic neuronal population by perfusion (push-pull-technique) of the lateral cerebral ventricle. Excitatory postsynaptic potentials were elicited in cortical neurons by stimulation of the thalamus; evoked potentials of the somatosensory cortex were elicited by stimulation of the sciatic nerve.

After topical penicillin application, focal epileptic activity appeared which persisted for several hours. When the focus was fully established, the calcium channel blocker D890, found to be specific in invertebrate preparations (8), was injected into cortical neurons. A typical experiment is displayed in Figure 1.

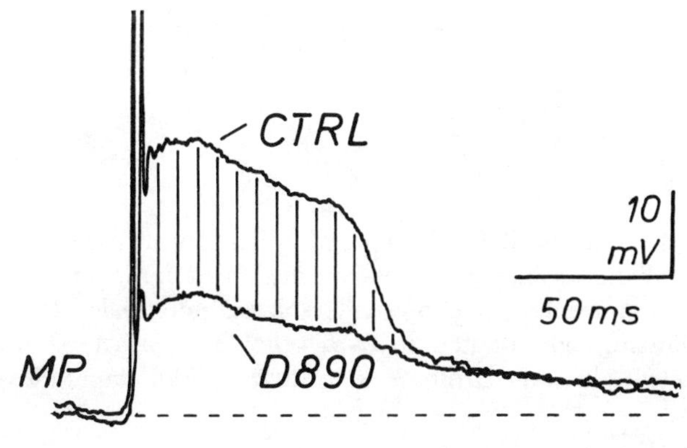

Figure 1. Paroxysmal depolarization shifts before (CTRL) and after the intra-cellular application of the calcium channel blocking agent D890. MP: Membrane potential. Action potentials are truncated.

It shows that the intracellular injection of D890 reduced the amplitude of the paroxysmal depolarizations by up to 55% of the control values. In a few experiments the first injections of D890 led to an increase of the amplitude of the paroxysmal depolarizations whereas further injections decreased the amplitude. Excitatory postsynaptic potentials elicited in non-epileptic animals were found not to be altered by the calcium antagonist (9).

In a further series of experiments it was examined whether a systemic administration of the calcium antagonist verapamil influences the epileptic activity of neuronal populations. After the establishment of the epileptic focus the calcium antagonist verapamil was applied into the lateral ventricle. Such an experiment is demonstrated in Figure 2.

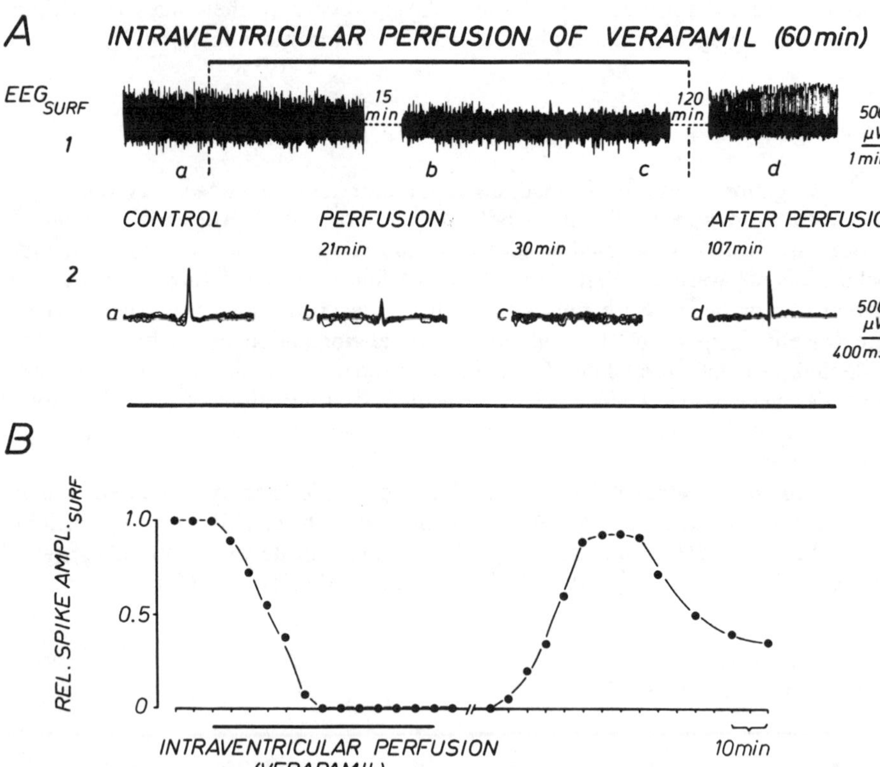

Figure 2. Reduction of the amplitudes of focal interictal epileptiform discharges in the surface EEG (EEG_{surf}) during intraventricular perfusion of verapamil. A: Inkwriter recordings *(1)* and superimposition of single seizure potentials at an expanded time scale *(2)*. Tracings are related to each other by characters. B: Evaluation of the experiment in A. Ordinate: Relative spike amplitudes ($Ampl._{surf}$).

With verapamil perfusion epileptic potentials were reduced in amplitude and were finally abolished. The seizure potentials reappeared 60 to 120 min after the end of the perfusion. Together with the decrease of the amplitude of seizure potentials, the frequency of occurrence was diminished. In a few experiments the decrease in amplitude was preceded by an accentuation. But also in these cases a final depression below control level occurred. Somatosensory evoked potentials elicited in non-epileptic animals were increased rather than decreased by verapamil perfusion (10).

Discussion

The present findings show that epileptic EEG potentials and their cellular correlates are finally decreased after administration of calcium antagonists. The depressive effect is restricted to epileptic potentials since excitatory post-synaptic potentials as well as somatosensory evoked potentials in non-epileptic animals were not decreased by the calcium antagonists.

The transient enhancement of seizure potentials induced by application of calcium antagonists could, in principle, be due to a transient increase in calcium entry during paroxysmal depolarizations. This effect may occur when a high calcium leakage of the neuronal membrane preexists. Since a high concentration of calcium ions is reported to reduce the calcium influx (11, 12), the application of the calcium antagonist may be thought to disinhibit the calcium current in a first step and decrease the calcium entry in a following one. A further explanation is that the calcium activated potassium current is depressed transiently to a greater extent than the calcium current.

The present findings demonstrate that calcium antagonists counteract epileptic neuronal activity. First reports in the literature reveal that the calcium antagonist flunarizine given as an add-on therapy is also effective in human epilepsy (13).

References

1. Jasper, H.H., Ward, A.A. & Pope, A. (1969). Basic mechanisms of the epilepsies. Little, Brown & Co.
2. Klee, M.R., Lux, H.D. & Speckmann, E.-J. (1982). Physiology and pharmacology of epileptogenic phenomena. Raven Press, N.Y.
3. Speckmann, E.-J. & Caspers, H. (1979). Origin of field potentials. Thieme, Stuttgart.
4. Speckmann, E.-J. & Elger, C.E. (1983). Epilepsy and motor system. Urban and Schwarzenberg, München.
5. Lux, H.D. & Heinemann, U. (1983). Consequences of calcium-electrogenesis for the generation of paroxysmal depolarization shift. In E.-J. Speckmann & C.E. Elger (Eds.), Epilepsy and motor system. Urban and Schwarzenberg, München, p. 100-119.
6. Witte, O.W., Speckmann, E.-J. & Walden, J. (1984). Contribution of calcium and calcium-dependent membrane currents to focal epileptic discharges in neocortical ne rons of the rat. Cell Calcium, 5: 311.
7. Walden, J., Speckmann, E.-J. & Witte, O.W. (1985). Suppression of focal interictal epileptiform discharges by intraventricular perfusion of the calcium antagonist. Electroencephalogr. clin. Neurophysiol., 61: 299-309.

8. Walden, J., Witte, O.W., Speckmann, E.-J. & Elger, C.E. (1984). Reduction of calcium currents in indentified neurons of helix pomatia: Intracellular injection of D890. Comp. Biochem. Physiol., 77C: 211-217.
9. Witte, O.W., Speckmann, E.-J. & Walden, J. (1985). Wirkungen eines Calciumkanalblockers und eines Calciumchelators auf epileptische Entladungen einzelner Neurone im motorischen Cortex der Ratte. In R. Kruse (Ed.), Epilepsie 84. Einhorn-Presse-Verlag, p. 451-456.
10. Walden, J., Speckmann, E.-J. & Witte, O.W. (1984). Effect of the calcium antagonist verapamil on spontaneous and evoked bioelectric activity of the cerebral cortex. Pfügers Arch., 402, R36.
11. Eckert, R. & Chad, J.E. (1984). Inactivation of calcium channels. Prog. Biophys. mol. Biol., 44: 215-267.
12. Walden, J., Witte, O.W. & Speckmann, E.-J. (1982). A calcium-dependent potassium current induced by pentylenetetrazol in snail neurons. Pflügers Arch., 394, R49.
13. Overweg, J., Binnie, C.D., Meyer, H., Meinardi, H., Schmalty, S.T.M. & Wauquier, A. (1984). Double-blind placebo-controlled trial of flunarizine as add-on therapy in epilepsy. Epilepsia, 25: 217-222.

Effects of Benzodiazepam on Salivary Cortisol under Experimental Stress

Dirk H. Hellhammer, Ingmar Gutberlet,
Jürgen Konermann, Uta Müller and Ludger Rolf

Cortisol is considered an important mediator of psychological stress on organic functions. Psychological factors, such as unpredictability, uncertainty, novelty, anxiety, and suspense seem to be potent stimuli for a release of this steroid (1). However, under psychological stimulation, only some individuals respond with an increase of cortisol while others do not. Psychological and physiological factors have been discussed to contribute to this phenomenon (2).

In animal experiments, it was shown that diazepam prevented the stress induced increase of cortisol without affecting baseline levels (3). These data suggest a relationship between benzodiazepine receptors, anxiety, and cortisol release. Thus, we were interested to investigate effects of benzodiazepam on cortisol release and anxiety under experimental stress in men.

Methods

Sixty healthy adult men between the ages of 18 and 24 years participated in the experiment. Three groups (N=20) were formed at random, and were then subdivided into four subgroups (N=5). All members of each subgroup underwent the experiment together on two consecutive days. All experimental sessions were conducted between 8:00 and 9:30 p.m. Each session started with the intake of a drug, which was either lorazepam (1 mg), alprazolam (0.5 mg), or placebo. Neither the conductor of the experiment, nor the probands knew which kind of drug was administered. The probands then watched a movie (an animal film and surfing instructions, respectively) for a period of 60 min. The subjects were then asked to fill in a questionnaire (German version of the Spielberger State Anxiety Questionnaire; STAI; 4), and to salivate into a disposable tube over a period of five minutes. For the next ten minutes, a stressful film was presented to the subjects (scenes from "Shining" or "Halloween", respectively), and two other samples of saliva were collected during intervals of 5 min. After the film had ended, probands were asked to fill in the STAI-questionnaire again, and then collected another sample of saliva over the next 5 min. Group I received lorazepam and placebo, group II alprazolam and placebo, and group III lorazepam and alprazolam in random order. Films and drugs were randomly distributed over

This study was supported, in part, by the Deutsche Forschungsgemeinschaft (He 1013/2-2).

all three groups. Saliva samples were stored at -20° C prior to being analyzed by radioimmunoassay with a commercial kit (Mallinckrodt Diagnostica). All samples of each individual were analyzed in one assay to minimize variability of results. The mean intraassay variability was 3.7 %.

With respect to their cortisol response within the first stimulation interval, subjects were classified as either "responders" or "non-responders", according to criteria defined elsewhere (5). Statistical analysis was performed by ANOVA and discriminant analysis.

Results

In group I, 13 responders and 7 non-responders could be discriminated under placebo conditions. Significant differences between the two groups could be shown under placebo ($p = 0.0002$), but not under lorazepam treatment. Thus, lorazepam seems to prevent a response of salivary cortisol to film stimulation in these subjects (see Figure 1). Subgroups were not different with respect to their self-reported state anxiety under these conditions. 5 of the 20 probands still showed a cortisol increase under lorazepam; however, these subjects already showed a simular response under placebo conditions, and no significant difference could be verified for the treatment conditions in these men.

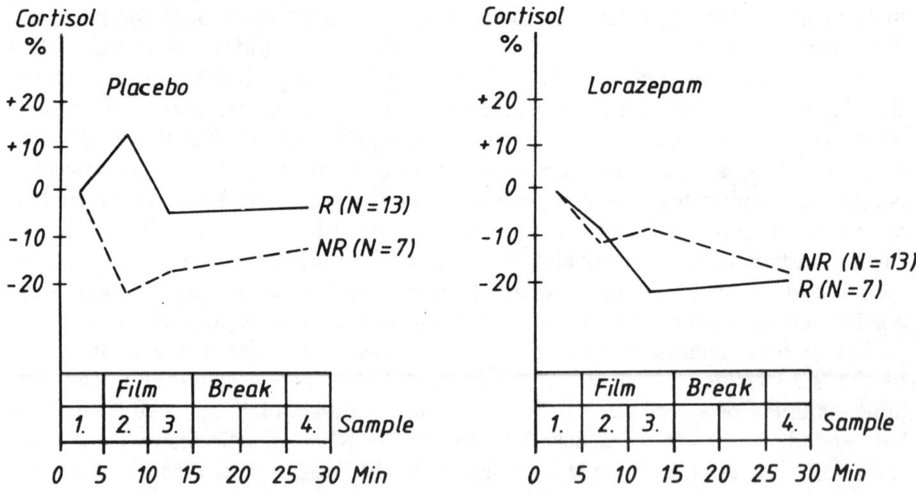

Figure 1. Percentual deviations of salivary cortisol from individual baseline levels over the experimental period of 20 min under placebo and lorazepam treatment, respectively. R = Responders under placebo conditions (N=13); NR = Non-responders under placebo conditions (N=7).

In group II, alprazolam also tends to prevent a cortisol increase in responders, but these changes were not significant. Interestingly, responders reported significantly less state-anxiety under placebo but not under alprazolam treatment before stimulation ($p = 0.024$).

In group III, no significant differences could be observed between treatment effects of alprazolam and lorazepam. Eight subjects of this group showed a cortisol response under both lorazepam and alprazolam pretreatment.

As verified by ANOVA and t-test, we can exclude effects of the sequence of film presentation, the sequence of drug administration, as well as a possible influence of the experimentor on the results reported for the three groups.

Discussion

About half of our 40 subjects, who were treated with placebo emitted a cortisol response under film stimulation. Under these conditions, however, the response occured only within the first but not the second stimulation interval. These data support our previous observations on a rapid and short first cortisol response to psychological stimulation in about half of experimental subjects (5).

In these responders, lorazepam prevented the increase of salivary cortisol. These data suggest a relationship among benzodiazepine receptors, anxiety, and cortisol release. The septo-hippocampal system is a likely candidate modulating these effects, since this part of the limbic system has numerous benzodiazepine receptors (6), and seems to be involved in the release of cortisol under psychological stress (7).

Although treated with benzodiazepines, some subjects still showed a cortisol response under film stimulation. In group III, these effects were persistent under both drug treatments. This may suggest that the dosage given was insufficient to eliminate the cortisol rise in most of the responders in this group. In group I, for example, there were still five subjects which fullfilled response criteria under lorazepam treatment, and all of them have also been responders under placebo conditions. Furthermore, treatment with a relatively small dose of 0.5 mg alprazolam showed a tendency toward suppression of the salivary cortisol response. From these observations, one may conclude that a higher dosage of benzodiazepines would be more effective in eliminating an increase of cortisol under such experimental conditions.

Results of the psychological test used in this study (STAI) were not sufficient to demonstrate a consistent relationship between state-anxiety, cortisol secretion, and drug effects. There is a tendency, however, that responders report higher state anxiety before but not after stimulation. So far, we are unable to detect psychological factors which could explain part of the variance between responders and non-responders in this experimental design.

References

1. Mason, J.W. (1968). A review of psychoendocrine research on the pituitary-adrenal cortical system. Psychosom. Med., 30: 576-607.

2. Rose, R.M. (1984). Overview of endocrinology of stress. In G.M. Brown et al. (Eds.), Neuroendocrinology and psychiatric disorders. Raven Press, N.Y., p. 95-122.
3. Ida, Y. et al. (1984). The effect of diazepam on NA turnover in brain regions of stressed and non-stressed rats. Neurochem. Res., 9: 1167.
4. Laux, L. et al. (1981). Das State-Trait-Inventar. Beltz, Weinheim.
5. Hellhammer, D.H. et al. (1987). Measurement of salivary cortisol under psychological stimulation. In J.N. Hingtgen et al. (Eds.), Advanced methods in psychobiology. Hogrefe, Toronto, p. 281-289.
6. Robertson, H.A. (1980). The benzodiazepine receptor: The pharmacology of emotion. Can. J. Neurol. Sci., 7: 243-245.
7. Bohus, B. (1975). The hippocampus and the pituitary-adrenal system. In R.L. Isaacson & K.H. Pribram (Eds.), The hippocampus. Plenum Press, N.Y., p. 323-374.

8.

Overview and Outlook

Overview of the Symposium

Herbert Weiner

It is a source of wonder that the last two Symposia have been held at all. Those familiar with the history of the topic of the role of social, behavioral and psychological factors in health and disease could not have predicted 30 years ago that we would be talking today about some of the brain mechanisms which mediate their relationships. Although vast gaps in our knowledge still exist, one may discern what current research strategies seem most promising, how to conceptualize the phènomena under study, and pick the variables which may most productively be employed in order to close these gaps.

In summarizing this Symposium, I am forced to be selective; my remarks undoubtedly are biased. If some of the presentations are not cited, I must apologize to their authors; it is not that they are not worthy of citation, but because I could not do full justice to them.

Specifying the "Stressor": Injury and Fear - Abnormal Responses

The first lesson to be learned from this Symposium is the need to specify rigorously the nature of the independent variable (or "stressor") in order to analyze further the brain mechanisms that mediate its effect. The failure to do so has characterized all of "stress" research. Selye (1) believed that any noxious stimulus produces a general response (the "adaptation syndrome"). It has taken 50 years to refute this thesis: Behavioral and physiological responses are discriminated. Smelik (2), for example, has demonstrated that physical damage to an animal releases the corticotrophin releasing (CRH) and adrenocorticotrophic (ACTH) hormones, and corticosterone. That is to say, the *anterior* pituitary secretes under such conditions.

On the other hand, fear-inducing stimuli, mediated either by suppression of dopaminergic or by increased ß-adrenergic activity in the hypothalamus, release ß-endorphin, and the melanocyte stimulating hormone (MSH) from the *intermediate* lobe of the hypophysis. Yet prolactin (PRL) is also secreted.

No intermediate lobe exists in man. Nonetheless, a paper has just appeared that reports on the effects of cardiac arrest on human beings. During this experience, γ_3-MSH, ß-endorphin, ACTH, PRL and cortisol were secreted (3).

The point of Smelik's presentation must not get lost: In the rat highly discriminated hormonal patterns are generated in response to different "stressors." This is all the more remarkable because ACTH, ß-lipotropin (LPH), a family of

Supported in part by the John D. and Catherine T. MacArthur Foundation Grant on "Health-Promoting and Health-Damaging Behaviors."

MSH's, and ß endorphin all derive from the same precursor molecule - proopiomelanocortin (POMC). POMC is under CRH control; yet in the rat the two former (ACTH, LPH) derive from the cells of the anterior pituitary, the two latter from the cells of the intermediate lobe. Each of these are differently regulated.

Fehm (4) raised the regulation of cortisol release by ACTH in man to a new level of complexity. His work is of profound significance in clarifying a number of puzzles. He has shown that normally, cortisol is not only under the control of ACTH. The early morning peak and the lunch-time increase of cortisol are dissociated from any increase in ACTH (granting that its difficult assay is reliable). What other regulators of cortisol secretion could there be? Is there, for example, a neural (dopaminergic?) innervation to the adrenal cortex?

Of equal significance, is that in Cushing's disease cortisol stimulates ACTH secretion. This suggests that a positive feedback sustains the disease process. What is more the usual negative feedback effect of cortisol (in Addison's disease) can be converted into a positive one by desipramine.

What is true for Cushing's disease may also hold true for some forms of severe depression, in which mean cortisol levels are high, or for anorexia nervosa with elevated cortisol production rates.

Specifying the Stressor: Parameters of Electric Shock - Immune Responses

To return to the main thesis that "stress" responses are not global. In Lewis' and his colleagues' work (5) we find that intermittent electrical shock (120 shocks every 10 seconds) applied to a rat produces a naloxone-reversible analgesia. Whereas continuous shock (120 shocks every second) produces an analgesia uninfluenced by naloxone. Presumably, the former releases endorphins while at the same time it suppresses natural killer (NK) cell activity *and* accelerates the death of animals injected with a mammary ascites tumor; continuous shock does not have such effects (6).

The exquisite specificity of the outcomes of these two forms of shock is further indicated by the fact that the analgesia produced by continuous shock mainly depends on spinal mechanisms (mediated by glycine and/or substance P?) whereas intermittent shock is inferred to release endorphins (being naloxone reversible). In turn, it is assumed but not proven, that endorphins suppress NK cell activity.

Ballieux and Heijnen (7) remind us that we must be even more specific: α- and ß-endorphins have different effects on immune function - the former inhibits antibody formation to ovalbumen and the latter enhances it and also modulates T-helper cell function. In Shavit's system it must still be shown that the NK-cell assay is valid *in vivo* not only *in vitro.* Furthermore, intermittent foot shock presumably releases more than the endorphins; in fact, PRL is also released. The mammary ascites tumor cells are PRL-sensitive. Bernton, Meltzer and Holaday (8) presented data to suggest that tumoricidal macrophages are activated by PRL, which stimulates the release of lymphokines from T-cells. T-cells in turn contain PRL receptors.

Were it not for Felten's important work (9), we could only be searching for the hormonal mediation of intermittent shock. He and his co-workers have reminded us that the immune system (including bone marrow, thymus, spleen, gut and lymph nodes) is also under neuronal control. Post-ganglionic noradrenergic fibers run between the lymph nodules in lymphatic gut tissue. They traverse the area which contains plasma, enterochromaffin and T-cells. In addition to noradrenalin, roles for serotonin, acetylcholine and vasopressin in the regulation of these immunocompetent cells in the gut have been found. Such cells are also mobile, and are "sent" to the spleen. Felten's work adds another level of complexity to the process of immunoregulation. Not only do T-cells regulate ("help" or "suppress") B-cells, but lymphokines transform T-effector cells into specific cytotoxic cells, and lymphokines (such as γ-interferon, and interleukin-2) regulate NK-cell function. Local regulation of lymphocytes and plasma cells may occur directly by amine-transmitters and peptides, or indirectly by influencing (enterochromaffin) cells that secrete chemicals that influence immunologically competent cells. The latter in turn are influenced by a variety of peptides and steroid hormones and by neural discharge, both acting at a distance. Conversely, a variety of feedback loops from the immune system and its products (including interleukin-l, CRH-like peptide, "cachectin" and antibody) influence hypothalamic cells.

Integrated Cardiovascular Responses to Various Contingencies: Brain Circuits

Not only are endocrine and immune responses exquisitely discriminated, and specific to the particular stimulus or contingency, but cardiovascular responses are also. Jänig (10) reminded us of Darwin's (11) contribution which was to point out that behavior and physiology consists of an indivisible whole - one did not "cause" the other: That is, fear did not raise the heart rate (HR), or diastolic blood pressure (BP), they were each part of an integrated pattern.

Two major advances have occurred in our understanding of the circulation:

1) Circulatory patterns (not only single measurable variables) are differentiated. The pattern in anticipation of, and during exercise is different than during orthostasis.
2) Different brain circuits subserve and regulate these integrated circulatory patterns.

To be specific: Exercise elicits an increase in HR and systolic and diastolic BP; Stroke volume (SV) and the cardiac output (CO) rise; blood flow through muscle is greater; but the peripheral resistance (PR) falls. During the assumption of the upright position HR, mean BP, and PR are raised, SV falls, CO shows little change, but blood flow in the carotid artery increases while it is diminished in the great vessels in the lower parts of the body. Oral examinations elicit still another pattern. The cat about to fight another one manifests a circulatory pattern different than during the actual fight (12). While preparing to fight, during which the cat may paw the air, BP does not change, HR and CO fluctuate and blood flow in the mesenteric, renal and iliac arteries is reduced. During the actual fight - especially when prolonged and intense- BP, CO and HR increase, vasoconstriction in the renal and mesenteric arteries is intense, but dilatation of the iliac arteries occurs.

Such dilatation (presumably to increase the blood supply to muscle) was first described (13) during the "defense" reaction. This behavior, homologous to Darwin's cat terrified by, and prepared to fight a dog, is associated with increases in BP, CO, HR and SV and a reduced blood flow to viscera but increased muscle blood flow.

The "defense" reaction can be produced by stimulation of the lateral hypothalamus, close to the entry of the fornix. The integrated circulatory response elicited by orthostasis is subserved by a neural circuit that begins in the vestibular apparatus, passes *via* the 8th nerve and vestibulocerebellar pathways to the cerebellum, the paramedian reticular and vasomotor medullary neurons and then down the spinal cord (14). The circulatory response to exercise is believed to pass from the motor cortex, to the subthalamus, posterior hypothalamus and ventral brain stem (15). By lesioning, the fields (H_2) of Forel the circulatory changes in anticipation of exercise are abolished, but those during exercise are unchanged. As Jänig also pointed out, Smith and his colleagues (16) have dissociated the (electric) shock-related motor behaviors (bar-pressing) from the increased HR, BP and CO during a conditioned emotional response. Only the cardiovascular (not the motor) responses after placing the lesion in the posterior hypothalamus, were affected; and the circulatory responses elicited by feeding or exercise were not.

What can be learned from this new information? Although Darwin was correct that behavior and physiology form an indivisible composite, analytic studies of the kind carried out by Smith teach us that separate pathways in the brain, subserve behavior and cardiovascular responses. Even the responses of peripheral sympathetic nerves are highly discriminated. This is the message of Jänig's (10), and Wallin's (17) presentations. Sympathetic discharge to muscle, producing vasoconstriction, is under the control of baroreceptor (and phrenic nerve) activity to regulate BP. Whereas, the sympathetic innervation to the skin, involved in the regulation of blood flow, sweating and body temperature, is influenced by the ambient temperature, vibratory and tactile stimulation, and the emotions.

Organ Systems also Regulate Themselves

As is the case of the immune system, each system or organ also regulates its own activity. The enteric nervous system does so by a series of interneurons, and of peptides. But the motor activity of the gut is also regulated by post-ganglionic autonomic neurons, and by food. Wienbeck (18) pointed out that a carbohydrate meal stimulates gastric propulsive motor activity, which in turn is regulated by negative feedback from the duodenum. Cholecystokinin-8 and secretin also delay gastric emptying. On the other hand, pentagastrin suppresses the migratory motor complex of the small intestine, and stimulates its post-digestive motility pattern.

Malliani (19) also reminded us of this principle - one that holds true for every other organ system. Cardiac and aortic sympathetic, and vagal afferent activity, stimulated either by the stretching of myocardial fibers or the thoracic aorta, or injection of bradykinin into the lumen of the coronary arteries, depresses baroreceptor reflexes, and interacts with efferent, supraspinal input. Thus, narrowing the coronary arteries of the mechanical distension of the aorta (as pressure rises within it) increases the firing rate in delta-sympathetic efferents to raise BP, HR and left ventricular pressure. Inhibitory vagal, efferent reflex activity (similarly stimulated), counteracts these cardiovascular responses.

Effects of Various Contingencies on Self-Regulation

Yet the matter is, again, more complex. Although, local sympathetic cardiac reflexes attenuate baroreceptor reflexes - designed to lower BP and HR - they are in turn modified by behaviors or the behavioral state of the organism. The sensitivity of the baroreceptor reflex is blunted with age, during exercise (20), and mental arithmetic (21). It is greatest during sleep, intermediate during feeding, and least during mild exercise (22). To make the matter even more complicated, it is apparent that investigators need to take into account the context in which they do experiments. Lown and Verrier (23) have shown that ventricular arrhythmias (VA) could be produced in dogs by stimulation of the two main brain stem vasomotor (sympathetic and parasympathetic) centers. The threshold for producing VA was modified by classical aversive stimulation. The thresholds for the induction of VA were much lower when tested in the experimental apparatus than in the home cage.

Wesemann (24) reminded us that circadian rhythms - even to the level of the binding of serotonin to its receptors - of every physiological function exist. He pointed out that disease might be associated with a phase shift of one or other rhythm. Indeed, such phase shifting of BP at night is seen in some hypertensive patients. It also occurs in the polycystic ovary syndrome with regard to luteinizing hormone patterns.

In addition, the manner in which hormones (vasopressin, LH and PRL) are regulated may be different at different body weights (25, 26), which in turn affect circadian rhythms of, at least, some hormones. These insights are important in planning experiments and assessing their results: Investigators must take into consideration the time of day, and the setting of their experiments.

The Setting: Laboratory versus Field Experiments

The problem of the setting in which human "stress" experiments are carried out is a particularly vexing one. The physiological effects of "stressors" - such as those described by Siegrist (27) and Ursin (28) - could not possibly be carried out in the laboratory. How could one mimic the kind of routinized, excessive, paced, boring work carried out year-in, year-out in the modern factory that causes distress in workers, and is a major risk factor for coronary heart disease, in a laboratory? (Other risk factors of less magnitude such as an excess of low density lipoproteins are, of course, also present.)

As Dimsdale (29) has pointed out, "stressors" in the laboratory (e.g., "flooding") produced no secretion of "stress" hormones but they may do so in the "field" (28). In the field, hormone secretion or patterns also depend on additional variables, including the quality of the performance, and the social status of the individual in a group.

Specifying the "Stressors": Social Status, Social Interactions and the Dominance-Submission Dichotomy

One of the important lessons learned in this Symposium is that the study of the social status, etc., of an animal can be related to the "spontaneity" of behavior (30), but also to very specific hormonal and immunological changes. It is another research strategy that is powerful in furthering our insights into brain and other mechanisms.

When the dominant rat in a colony is confronted by an intruder its serum testosterone levels rise; the intruder and the more submissive members of the colony, however, manifest no such rise. They secrete PRL, α-MSH and ß-endorphin - hormones of the intermediate lobe of the hypophysis, put out in response to frightening stimuli (2). And Ballieux and Heijnen (7) reported that a dominant rat's splenic lymphocytes incorporate the greatest amount of thymidine after mitogenic stimulation; the subdominant animal less; and the once-dominant animal cast out of the colony the least of all. The largest number of T-suppressor cells is found in the outcast animal, and the least in the dominant. In fact, a linear (and inverse) relationship exists between the number of these cells and the status of the animal in the social hierarchy. (Because a change in status of an animal produces an alteration of these two immune parameters, the animal's social status cannot be a product of the functioning of its immune system).

We know from other observations, that the dominant (male) rodent patrols its territory, and is the first to eat and mate. Cools (30) so elegantly showed that it initiates and emits much more "spontaneous" motor behavior, independent of external clues. These behaviors are enhanced by the administration of a dopamine (DA) agonist, and diminished by striatal injury. Under these conditions - when DA neurons are destroyed, - and the gabaminergic content of the *substantia nigra* is reduced, such movements are only initiated by visual and proprioreceptive cues. Cools also presented data to show that specific social interactions and their ensuing behaviors are associated with specific changes in the norepinephrine (NE) content of *N. accumbens*. The intruding rat confronted with one, housed in its home cage, freezes - a situation conducive to an increase in NE content of this nucleus. If the two animals fight, and the intruder is defeated no change in NE content occurs.

Specifying the Stressor: Disruption of Social Relationships (Separation and Bereavement)

The fourth and final research strategy, only briefly touched upon in this Symposium, is that of experimentally disrupting the social relationships of animals early in life. It has taught us about the many facets of the interaction of the mother and its infant (31), and about the disease consequences of the disruption of their relationship (32). This line of work has had two additional outcomes. It has:

1) Added substance to the observations that separation or bereavement may impair the health of human beings.
2) Allowed neurobiologists to investigate how one aspect of the mother-infant interaction is subserved by the olfactory apparatus.

To make a long story short, the attachment of the infant rat to the mother's nipple is assured by a pheromone secreted by her areolar glands. Destruction of the infant's olfactory epithelium with zinc sulphate renders the infant incapable of attachment and thus suckling. Teicher et al. (33) has shown that during suckling a small group of neurons in the accessory olfactory bulb is activated. This line of investigation should allow a further analysis of the neuronal pathways that link the smell of the pheromone to suckling behavior.

Destruction of the olfactory epithelium in the 15-day-old rat has the same effects as separating it from the mother. The separated infant rat is at high risk for gastric erosions when restrained or not fed at 30 days (32). The production of gastric erosions is associated with a fall in body temperature.

In fact, one may divide the various animal models of erosion formation into two groups: Those which are associated with an increase in body temperature (e.g., the rat with a lateral hypothalamic lesion) and a second group into which it falls (e.g., the rat restrained in cold and the prematurely separated rat). (34).

We know that hypothermia is a powerful stimulus to the release of the thyrotropin releasing hormone (TRH), whose highest concentration is found in the dorsal motor nucleus of the vagus nerve. It is now clear that TRH injected at this site or into the IVth ventricle, increases gastric secretion and motility and produces gastric erosions (34). Thus, TRH may be one mediating mechanism in producing gastric erosions in hypothermic rats.

But the matter is again more complex. As Glavin (35) pointed out, depletion of brain NE (by RO4-1284) enhances gastric erosions produced by cold-restraint. This result is not as surprising as it might seem, because such a depletion also enhances gastric motility.

The Coordination of Behavior and Physiology

Permit me a digression. It is remarkable that TRH is found where it is in the medulla. But as one ponders on this finding, one concludes that nature is truly wise. A fall in body temperature increases basal metabolism, fueled by a rise in caloric intake (i.e., food). Food intake in turn stimulates gastric secretion. Therefore, TRH coordinates behavior (food intake), digestion and an increased metabolism when body temperature falls.

Other peptides also coordinate behavior and the physiology of the body. Angiotensin II promotes salt and water intake and raises BP. In a hypovolemic animal one would wish for just such a coordinating mechanism. GNRH in the female rat integrates the mating stance ("lordosis behavior") and the release of pituitary gonadotrophins leading to ovulation. Thus some peptides integrate behavior and physiology which are one and indivisible; although they can be decomposed by experimental techniques.

Effects of Bereavement in Man

Bereavement has been cited as a major "stressor," and as the context in which some persons develop disease, visit physicians more, take more medications, or become depressed (36). However, these observations have so far failed to specify with enough precision what the bereaved person is bereft of, to describe with sufficient accuracy the different responses - grief, pathological grief, etc., to bereavement - and to provide us with a physiology of bereavement over the short and long term.

Lieberman (37) has shown that the effects on parents of losing a child continue for, at least, 7 years and manifest themselves over that time as an increased morbidity (27% of their sample), and more family discord and disruption. The effects of such a loss of a child are greater and last longer, than the loss of a spouse or a parent.

The effects of bereavement are also age- and gender-related, and are much more likely to impair health than produce disease (36). One form of ill-health was described by Fielding (38). It is fairly clear that the irritable (functional) bowel disorders (IBS) are a syndrome. Patients with IBS whose initial complaints are lower abdominal pain, constipation and diarrhea also manifest symptoms of upper gastrointestinal tract dysfunction. They also have a high incidence of anxiety and depression, and evidence of low pulse rates, increased forearm blood flow and increased responses to the cold pressor test. They are liable to headaches, or they hyperventilate and have musculoskeletal pains. They are, in short, people in ill-health. Whitehead (39) reported that their behavior may very well be learned: Their illnesses in childhood were rewarded. He also reminded us that some patients with IBS are particularly sensitive to distension of the colon, and the contractile response to distension lasts longer. On the other hand, some patients with IBS have mainly a decreased transit time of a bolus travelling from the mouth to the cecum: "Stresses" have this effect in some persons (8).

The Problem of Disease Induction

Some still maintain that disease is the linear outcome of "stressors" (28). My own reading of the data differs from this point of view. The basis of the disagreement is, that the predisposition to disease is to be found in organ-specific, local regulatory disturbances. This axiomatic statement is supported by the fact that bronchial hyperreactivity is the *sine qua non* for bronchial asthma; it is due to an excessive responsiveness to acetylcholine of the post-ganglionic, muscarinic receptor of the bronchial musculature. A number of regulatory disturbances have also been described in peptic duodenal ulcer (40). These consist of the failure of gastric hydrochloric acid to suppress gastrin production by the antrum, an excessive acid secretory response to histamine and aminoacids, ·or an accelerated transit time, etc. And Fehm (4) presented the example of cortisol having a positive (rather than a negative) feedback effect on ACTH secretion in Cushing's disease. The predisposition to some infections lies at times with an incapacity to produce antibodies in the agammaglobulinemias, or because T-helper cells do not "aid" B-cells to secrete them.

We need to understand the interaction of these organ-specific, regulatory disturbances with the outputs that emanate from the brain and which "stressors" specifically activate to produce disease. My suspicion is that when "stressors" are brought into action, but when *no* predisposing local, regulatory disturbances obtain, illness is produced in some but not in other persons. This hypothesis may be all wrong but might be worth testing.

Therefore, one might conclude that "stressors" with their specific and integrated effects on behavioral and physiological systems, mediated by the brain and its neuronal and hormonal outputs, do not linearly produce disease. They only do so in a non-linear manner in interaction with organ-specific disturbances which are either genetically programmed, or are the product of early experience (31, 32).

References

1. Selye, H. (1946). The general adaptation syndrome and the diseases of adaptation. J. Clin. Endocrinol., 6: 117.
2. Smelik, P.G.: This volume.
3. Wortsman, J., Frank, S., Wehrenberg, W.B., Petra, P.H. & Murphy, J.E. (1985). Gamma$_3$-melanocyte-stimulating hormone immunoreactivity is a component of the neuroendocrine response to maximal stress (cardiac arrrest). J. Clin. Endocrinol. Metab., 61: 355-360.
4. Fehm, H.L., Voigt, K.H. & Born, J.: This volume.
5. Lewis, J.W., Cannon, J.T. & Liebeskind, J.C. (1980). Opioid and non-opioid mechanisms of stress analgesia. Science, 208: 623.
6. Shavit, Y., Lewis, J.W., Terman, G.W., Gale, R.P. & Liebeskind, J.C. (1984). Opioid peptides mediate the suppressive effect of stress on natural killer cell cytoxicity. Science, 223: 188.
7. Ballieux, R.E. & Heijnen, C.J.: This volume.
8. Bernton, E.W., Meltzer, M.S. & Holaday, J.W.: This volume.
9. Aravich, P.F., Davis, B.J., Sladek, C.D., Felten, S.Y. & Felten, D.L.: This volume.
10. Jänig, W.: This volume.
11. Darwin, C. (1872). The expression of the emotions on man and animals. University of Chicago Press, Chicago. (Reprinted 1965).
12. Zanchetti, A., Baccelli, G. & Mancia, G. (1976). Fighting, emotion and exercise: Cardiovascular effects in the rat. In G. Onesti, M. Fernandez & K.E. Kim (Eds.), Regulation of blood pressure by the central nervous system. Grune & Stratton, N.Y.
13. Abrahams, V.C., Hilton, S.M. & Zbrozyna, A. (1964). The role of active muscles vasodilatation in the alerting stage of the defense reaction. J. Physiol. (London), 171: 189.
14. Doba, N. & Reis, D.J. (1974). Role of the cerebellum and the vestibular apparatus in regulation of orthostatic reflexes in the cat. Circulation Res., 34: 9.

15. Cohen, D.H. (1981). Cardiovascular neurobiology: The substrate for biobehavioral approaches to hypertension. In Joint U.S.A.-U.S.S.R. Symposium, Hypertension: Biobehavioral and epidemiological aspects. U.S. Department of H.H.S., Bethesda, MD, p. 93.
16. Smith, A.O., Astley, C.A., DeVito, J.L., Stein, J.M. & Walsh, K.E. (1980). Functional analysis of hypothalamic control of the cardiovascular responses accompanying emotional behavior. Fed. Proc., 39: 2487.
17. Wallin, B.G.: This volume.
18. Wienbeck, M., Enck, P. & Erckenbrecht, J.F.: This volume.
19. Lombardi, F., Ruscone, T.G., Malfatto, G. & Malliani, A.: This volume.
20. Bristow, J.D., Brown, E.B.Jr., Cunningham, D.J.C., Howson, M.G., Petersen, E.S., Pickering, T.G. & Sleight, P. (1971). Effect of bicycling on the baroreflex regulation of pulse interval. Circulation Res., 28: 582.
21. Brooks, D., Fox, P., Lopez, R. & Sleight, P. (1978). The effect of mental arithmetic on blood pressure variability and baroreflex sensitivity in man. J. Physiol. (London), 280: 75.
22. Stephenson, R.B., Smith, O.A. & Scher, A.M. (1981). Baroreceptor regulation of heart rate in baboons during different behavioral states. Am. J. Physiol., 241: R277.
23. Lown, B., Verrier, R. & Corbalan, R. (1973). Psychologic stress and threshold for repetitive ventricular response. Science, 182: 834.
24. Wesemann, W.: This volume.
25. Quigley, H.E., Sheehan, K.L., Casper, R.F. & Yen, S.S.C. (1980). Evidence for increased dopaminergic and opioid activity in patients with hypothalamic hypogonadotrophic amenorrhea. J. Clin. Endocrinol. Metab., 50: 949.
26. Gold, P.W., Kaye, W., Robertson, G.L. & Ebert, M.H. (1983). Abnormalities in plasma and cerebrospinal fluid arginine vasopressin in patients with anorexia nervosa. N. Engl. J. Med., 308: 1117.
27. Siegrist, J., Matschinger, H. & Siegrist, K.: This volume.
28. Ursin, H.: This volume.
29. Dimsdale, J.E. (1984). Generalizing from laboratory studies to field studies of human stress physiology. Psychosom. Med., 46: 463.
30. Cools, A.R.: This volume.
31. Hofer, M. (1984). Relationships as regulators. Psychosom. Med., 46: 183.
32. Weiner, H. (1982). The prospects for psychosomatic medicine: Selected topics. Psychosom. Med., 44: 491.
33. Teicher, M.H., Stewart, W.B., Kauer, J.S. & Shepherd, G.M. (1980). Suckling pheromone stimulation of a modified glomerular region in the developing rat olfactory bulb revealed by the 2-deoxyglucose method. Brain Res., 194: 530.
34. Weiner, H., Novin, D., Grijalva, C.V., Taché, Y., & Garrick, T. (1985). Neurobiologic and psychobiologic mechanisms in gastric function and ulceration. West. J. Med., 143: 207.
35. Glavin, G.: This volume.
36. Weiner, H. (1985). The concept of stress in the light of studies on disasters, unemployment, and loss: A critical analysis. In M. Zales (Ed.), Stress in health and disease. Brunner/Mazel, N.Y.
37. Lieberman, M. Personal communication
38. Fielding, J.F. (1985). Lecture held at the Second International Symposium on Neuronal Control of Bodily Processes. Bielefeld.
39. Whitehead, W.E.: This volume.
40. Grossman, M.I. (1978). Abnormalities of acid secretion in patients with duodenal ulcer. Gastroenterology, 75: 524.

General Discussion:

Research Goals in Behavioral Medicine

Roman Ferstl

In 1977 the Yale Conference defined *Behavioral Medicine* as the field concerned with the development of behavioral-science knowledge and techniques relevant to the understanding of physical health and illness, and the application of this knowledge and these techniques to prevention, diagnosis, treatment, and rehabilitation. Psychosis, neurosis, and substance abuse were included only insofar as they contribute to physical disorders as an end point (1).

Explicitly, as a description of a scientific enterprise and as a demand for further bio-behavioral research, the present conference has shown a certain degree of agreement with this definition. Implicitly, it appears to me that there are at least two problem areas which I want to pinpoint in my comments. First, I want to concentrate on some methodological considerations regarding the definition and use of the concept of models. As a second point I would like to comment on the problem of stress and specificity. Finally, I develop two research goals in behavioral medicine, which I have identified from a behaviorist's point of view during the presentations of the last three days.

Interdisciplinary research in bio-behavioral areas covering physiology, immunology, neuroanatomy, endocrinology, and psychology is often inhibited in its communication by the use of a pseudo-common language. A typical example of this obstacle is - at least in my eyes - the sometimes misleading use of the term "model." Even at this conference the concept of a model was used in a very divergent and confusing way. Sometimes it was defined as:

- a set of hypotheses,
- a certain preparation or technique,
- an experimentally induced behavior, or
- an experimentally induced biological state.

One could enlarge this list by examples from the literature on experimental psychopathology (2), biological psychiatry (3), and other disciplines. In all of these cases the problems in understanding the others' scientific approach rarely arise from the use of different technical terms or from the altering state of theoretical basic knowledge. They stem rather in a certain sense from the undefined use of a single term. According to Webster, a "model" is *A small copy or representation of an existing or planned object, as a ship, building, etc.* Of course, nowadays, micro-models of biological structures are an exception. We refer rather to macro-models as enormously blown-up plans and structures of e.g., transmitter actions at the synaptic cleft. But in both cases a logical principle is at work: The abstract description of common features of a structure. Understanding the degree of representativeness of such a model or - in other words - knowing the degree of similarity between the model's features and the supposed domain of its validity is a necessary condition for a better communication among researchers in related disciplines. In bio-behavioral research this requires at least information about, or better, a rating of the following four criteria (cf. papers presented by Dr. Cools and Dr. Henn):

1) Information about the degree of the model's identity with behavior.
2) A rating of the objectivity of measurement.
3) Information about pharmacological or physiological similarity.
4) Data on internal, external, and ecological validity of the model.

I believe that further conferences on neuronal control of bodily functions, should ask participants to comment on these four points for every single model presented, increasing not only the understanding between, but also the discussions across disciplines.

A second problem, which I came across in several presentations of this conference belongs to the questions of stress and specificity of responses. I think we are still faced with the old contradiction between general activation and stress theory (4, 5) and the well-known response specificity, which was first reported by Malmo and Shagass (6). While general activation and stress theory states that all kinds of stressors initiate a common pattern of physiological arousal and adaptive response, specificity theories try to discriminate at least between stimulus specific responses (SSR) which depend on a causal relation between stressor and response (e.g., thermo-regulation) and an individual response specificity (ISR), which is defined as an individual pattern, which is independent of the different stimuli or stressors used in the experimental situation. Subjects with a tendency to display ISR respond physiologically with a relatively constant hierarchy of diverse autonomic parameters (7). In psychophysiology this type of experimental study is usually designed and analyzed in the form of a multivariate analysis of variance. A group of subjects is repeatedly confronted with a series of different cognitive tasks (e.g., mental arithmetics, recognition, recall, etc.) and physical stressors (e.g., ice-water, loud noise, etc.) while several autonomic and CNS-functions are recorded. Specificity is then explained in terms of variance and the lower the degree of rest-variance, the better one can infer the different types of specificities. In the case of studies that try to identify specific health risks (as demonstrated in Dr. Siegrist's paper) or specific mechanisms, I would expect a high degree of practicability for such research designs. Nevertheless, no causal model can be derived from such experimentation. This would require a different kind of statistical analysis such as is offered now with the type of log-linear models (8).

Turning back to the topic I was asked to comment on by the organizers of this conference, I have to admit that I had expected to hear at least some speculations on the application of new techniques in treatment or prevention. But obviously, this would have gone to far beyond the scope of this conference. I think it also was rather wise to stay with basic research and to skip around the attractive sounds of Scylla and Charybdis' land of therapeutic applications of basic techniques. Nevertheless, there were two significant and, for a behaviorist, promising groups of results that can be considered as the starting point for future research. We have scattered examples from the literature for each of these: The impact of social hierarchy and social stressors on the course of human diseases and the extension of learning paradigms in neuroimmunomodulation.

We have heard from Dr. Cools that changes in the dopaminergic system have an immediate consequence on the social ranks of monkeys in colonies. Dr. Ballieux cited some impressive data from Dr. Bohus' group, which demonstrated the relation of social ranks and the proliferation response to Con A. Even when there is no way to link these results, I think both should increase our sensitivity for research that is directed towards the functional dependence of physiological regulations from social relations (ranks) and stressors (inhibition or disinhibition of behavior by rank orders). It is a well-known fact from psychological studies on the treatment of psychosomatic disorders, that those patients who increase their social competence have a better prognosis for their follow-up status. Can this be explained by mechanisms like the one we heard of? I would definitely suggest that these kinds of studies represent the most promising research goals in behavioral medicine.

The second suggestion for another research goal maybe pure speculation. In the presentations of Dr. Felten, Dr. Ballieux, and Drs. Bernton and Holaday we have learned about the increasing evidence for neuronal and humoral regulation of the immune system. Most recently the results of Besedovsky et al. (9), indicate evidence for a bidirectional regulation of CNS and immune functions. It may be too early, too stupid, or too much science fiction: But there should be a way for a behavioral regulation at least of some immune system reactions. As the Klosterhalfens have demonstrated in their excellent contribution, adjuvans arthritis as an experimental phenomenon can be either enhanced or inhibited by an unreinforced presentation of a saccharine-vanilla solution previously paired with cyclophosphamide (10). If classical conditioning is effective in immunomodulation, why shouldn't there be a way for operant control of the same phenomenon? The technique of biofeedback-experimentation offers the best rationale for testing this hypothesis. I think it would be worthwhile to speculate about it.

References

1. Schwartz, G.E. & Weiss, S.M. (1977). Yale Conference on Behavioral Medicine. DHEW Publications No. (NIH) zu-1424.
2. Kimmel, H.D. (Ed.) (1971). Experimental psychopathology. Academic Press, N.Y.
3. Van Praag, H.M. (Ed) (1981). Handbook of biological psychiatry. Marcel Dekker, N.Y./ Basel.
4. Duffy, E. (1962). Activation and behavior. Wiley, N.Y.
5. Selye, H. (1956). The stress of life. McGraw-Hill, N.Y.
6. Malmo, R.B. & Shagass, C. (1949). Physiologic study of symptom mechanisms in psychiatric patients under stress. Psychosom. Med., 11: 25-29.
7. Lacey, J.I. (1967). Somatic response patterning and stress: Some revisions of activation theory. In M.H. Appley & R. Trumbull (Eds), Psychological stress: Issues in research. Appleton-Century-Crofts, N.Y.

8. Jöreskog, K.G. & Sörbom, D. (1981). LISREL-analysis of linear structural relationships by the method of maximum likelihood. National Educational Resources, Chicago, Ill.
9. Besedovsky, H.O., Del Rey, A.E. & Sorkin, E. (1983). What do the immune system and the brain know about each other? Immunology Today, 4: 342-356.
10. Ader, R. & Cohen, N. (1985). CNS-immune system interactions: Conditioning phenomena. Brain Behav. Sci., 8: 379-426.

Author Index

This index contains the page numbers of the respective reference sections in which the author is mentioned. The numbers in ( ) represent the reference numbers on that page.